Four week loan
Benthyciad pedair wythnos

Please return on or before the due date to avoid overdue charges
*A wnewch chi ddychwelyd ar neu cyn y dyddiad a nodir ar eich llyfr os
gwelwch yn dda, er mwyn osgoi taliadau*

- 5 MAR 2008		
0 4 AUG 2008	2 4 JAN 2011	
1 9 NOV 2008		
	0 7 FEB 2011	
1 6 JAN 2009		
1 1 FEB 2009		
0 8 APR 2009		
1 9 OCT 2009		
0 1 FEB 2010		
1 1 OCT 2010		

http://library.cardiff.ac.uk
http://llyfrgell.caerdydd.ac.uk

Pain in Neonates and Infants

Pain Research and Clinical Management series

Other volumes in this series:

PAIN RESEARCH AND
CLINICAL MANAGEMENT

Pain in Neonates and Infants

THIRD EDITION

Edited by

KJS Anand MBBS DPhil
Professor of Pediatrics, Anesthesiology, Pharmacology and Neurobiology
Morris and Hettie Oakley Endowed Chair of Critical Care Medicine
UAMS College of Medicine
and
Director
Pain Neurobiology Laboratory
Arkansas Children's Hospital Research Institute
Little Rock, Arkansas
USA

BJ Stevens RN PhD
Professor of Nursing and Medicine
University of Toronto
The Hospital for Sick Children
Signy Hildur Eaton Chair in Pediatric Nursing Research
and
Associate Chief of Nursing (Research)
Toronto, Ontario
Canada

PJ McGrath OC PhD FRSC
Professor of Psychology, Pediatrics and Psychiatry
Canada Research Chair
Dalhousie University
and
CIHR Distinguished Scientist
Psychologist
IWK Health Centre
Halifax, Nova Scotia
Canada

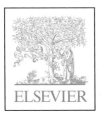

ELSEVIER

EDINBURGH LONDON NEW YORK OXFORD PHILADELPHIA ST LOUIS SYDNEY TORONTO 2007

ELSEVIER

First edition 1993
Second edition 2000
This edition 2007

ISBN–10: 0-444-52061-9
ISBN–13: 978-0-444-52061-6

British Library Cataloguing in Publication Data
A catalogue record for this book is available from the British Library

Library of Congress Cataloging in Publication Data
A catalog record for this book is available from the Library of Congress

Notice

ELSEVIER your source for books, journals and multimedia in the health sciences
www.elsevierhealth.com

Working together to grow libraries in developing countries

www.elsevier.com | www.bookaid.org | www.sabre.org

ELSEVIER BOOK AID International Sabre Foundation

For Elsevier:

Commissioning Editors: Elly Tjoa, Timothy Horne
Development Editor: Hannah Kenner
Project Manager: Joannah Duncan
Design Direction: Stewart Larking

Printed in China

The publisher's policy is to use **paper manufactured from sustainable forests**

Preface

In 1993, the 1st Edition of *Pain in Neonates* began with the optimistic note that 'The clinical management of pain associated with the care of newborns and young infants is at the threshold of dramatic change ...' Although dramatic changes in the assessment and clinical management of neonatal pain occurred in the 1990s, the field was still largely dominated by small, single-center studies or individual investigators focusing on specific areas of their interest, making sequential advances and observations. The expanded research and clinical interests focused on neonatal pain were summarized in the 2nd Edition of *Pain in Neonates*, published in 2000 and containing 15 chapters. That edition added significantly to relevant neonatal pain topics and summarized the recent research evidence and clinical interest in this field.

Although major advances in pain assessment and the provision of analgesia or anesthesia to neonates and older infants have occurred since 1993, it is clearly evident that we lack a deeper understanding of the different types of pain during early life, leading to significant limitations in our ability to assess or effectively treat some of the commonly occurring types of infant pain. Furthermore, what we do know is not always translated into practice in an effective and timely way. Limited changes occur in medical or nursing practices unless clinical findings are supported by changes in health policy, economic considerations and consumer activism. If we expect dramatic improvements in patient outcomes, we must also attend to structural and contextual issues at the individual, institutional and society levels. Therefore, it is imperative that recent advances from neonatal and infant pain research be summarized and presented to students in health sciences programs, practicing clinicians at the bedside, basic scientists at the laboratory bench, and behavioural scientists at the observation window or testing station, taking the above challenges into consideration.

Other developments since the previous edition include: larger teams of investigators that have coalesced around major research areas, increasing realization of the long-term global developmental effects of early pain or stress, and the availability of newer tools such as genomics and proteomics for the study of infant pain. It is also evident that more and more infants, beyond the neonatal period, are being hospitalized in the Neonatal Intensive

Care Unit (NICU), community settings or elsewhere, with minimal information available on the assessment or management of pain in this population. Other textbooks focused on pediatric pain or pain in adults may devote limited space to neonatal pain, but do not adequately address the pain occurring in older infants. This 3rd Edition has therefore been updated and expanded to include new topics related to infant and neonatal pain in a variety of settings and contexts, while retaining many features from previous editions and changing the title to *Pain in Neonates and Infants*.

Until recently, the label of pain was denied neonates and infants, no matter how intense, or how frequent, or how prolonged these experiences were. The current definition of pain states that use of the word pain needs to be learned through experiences in early life. An alternative view is that the perception of pain is an inherent quality of life itself, and thus is applicable to all infants and neonates. Although a subjective interpretation or verbal description of pain may be learned from previous painful experiences, its perception does not require prior experience even in the first instance. It seems intuitive that pain perception cannot be a learned capability if pain is the primary sensation that guards the organism against damage from its external or internal environment. The first experience of tissue injury is painful, in much the same way that touch, smell, vision, or hearing occur without the need for learning and memory. Cognitive interpretation of these sensations, however, will develop via the contextual factors associated with them.

Few areas in health care can boast of the scientific advances that have occurred in the assessment and management of infant pain over the past few years. A natural consequence of rapid progress is that major differences may exist between current scientific knowledge and current clinical practice. Whereas clinical practices may have changed drastically over the past decade, there remain multiple clinical situations where outdated practices are continued. It is still commonplace for premature neonates to be subjected to multiple invasive procedures during routine NICU care or receive postoperative intensive care, without adequate analgesia or behavioural, physical or environmental interventions. The clinical and physiological consequences of such clinical practices are becoming clearer. This book was written for clinicians and clinical and basic science researchers, to provide a single, comprehensive source for recent advances in neonatal and infant pain: its science and application, policy and practice, and assessment and management. The impact of this issue will depend on whether this information is relevant or not, whether it will be used to initiate changes in clinical practice at unit, institutional and policy levels, and whether it will stimulate greater impetus for research in this area.

We present the 3rd Edition as *Pain in Neonates and Infants* with the hope that it will fulfill its promise of enhancing and further advancing the knowledge related to pain in infancy.

K. J. S. Anand
B. J. Stevens
P. J. McGrath

List of contributors

Marilyn Aita RN
PhD student
School of Nursing
McGill University
Montreal, Quebec
Canada

Rene Albertyn PhD
Senior Researcher in Paediatric Pain
Division of Paediatric Surgery
School of Paediatric and Adolescent Health
Red Cross War Memorial Children's Hospital
University of Cape Town
Cape Town
South Africa

Elie D Al-Chaer MS PhD JD
Associate Professor of Pediatrics, Neurobiology and Developmental Sciences
UAMS College of Medicine
Biomedical Research Center
Little Rock, Arkansas
USA

K J S Anand MBBS DPhil
Professor of Pediatrics, Anesthesiology, Pharmacology and Neurobiology
Morris and Hettie Oakley Endowed Chair of Critical Care Medicine
UAMS College of Medicine
Director
Pain Neurobiology Laboratory
Arkansas Children's Hospital Research Institute
Little Rock, Arkansas
USA

Brian J Anderson PhD FANZCA FJFICM
Associate Professor of Anaesthesiology
University of Auckland
Paediatric Anaesthetist/Intensivist
Auckland Children's Hospital
Auckland
New Zealand

Ronald G Barr MA MDCM FRCPC
Professor of Pediatrics
Faculty of Medicine
University of British Columbia
4480 Oak Street, L408
Vancouver, British Columbia
Canada

Simon Beggs PhD
Assistant Professor
Faculty of Dentistry
University of Toronto
Research Associate
The Hospital for Sick Children
Toronto, Ontario
Canada

Adnan T Bhutta MBBS FAAP
Instructor, Pediatric Critical Care Medicine and
Cardiology
University of Arkansas for Medical Sciences
Co-Medical Director
Cardiovascular Intensive Care Unit
Arkansas Children's Hospital
Little Rock, Arkansas
USA

Adrian T Bosenberg MD MBChB DA(SA) FFA(SA)
Professor
Department of Paediatric Anaesthesia
Red Cross War Memorial Children's Hospital
University of Cape Town
Cape Town
South Africa

Marsha Campbell-Yeo RN MN CNNP
Neonatal Nurse Practitioner
IWK Health Centre
Halifax, Nova Scotia
Canada

Christine T Chambers PhD
Assistant Professor and Canada Research Chair
Departments of Pediatrics and Psychology
Dalhousie University and IWK Health Centre
Halifax, Nova Scotia
Canada

Lenora J Duhn RN MSc
Acting Director, Nursing Research
Kingston General Hospital
Kingston, Ontario
Canada

Nicholas M Fisk PhD, MD
Professor
Institute of Reproductive and Developmental Biology
Imperial College London
Hammersmith Campus
Du Cane Road
London
UK

Maria Fitzgerald PhD
Professor of Developmental Neurobiology
Pediatric Pain Research Group
Department of Anatomy and Developmental Biology
University College London
London
UK

Shuvo Ghosh MD FAAP
Assistant Professor, Pediatrics
Child Development Program
McGill University
Montreal Children's Hospital
Montreal, Quebec
Canada

Sharyn Gibbins RN PhD
Director of Interdisciplinary Research
Sunnybrook and Women's Hospital
Toronto, Ontario
Canada

Vivette Glover MA PhD DSc
Professor of Perinatal Psychobiology
Institute of Reproductive and Developmental Biology
Faculty of Medicine
Imperial College London
London
UK

Ruth Eckstein Grunau PhD RPsych
Associate Professor of Pediatrics
University of British Columbia
Senior Scholar
Michael Smith Foundation for Health Research
Vancouver, British Columbia
Canada

Richard Whit Hall MD FAAP
Associate Professor
Department of Pediatrics
University of Arkansas for Medical Sciences
Division of Neonatology
Little Rock, Arkansas
USA

Nicholas H G Holford MB ChB MSc MRCP(UK)
FRACP
Associate Professor
Department of Pharmacology and Clinical
Pharmacology
University of Auckland
Auckland
New Zealand

Paul E Hyman MD
Professor of Pediatrics
Chief
Pediatric Gastroenterology
University of Kansas Hospital
Kansas City, Kansas
USA

C Celeste Johnston RN DEd FCAHS
James McGill Professor
School of Nursing
McGill University
Montreal, Quebec
Canada

Linda Johnston RN PhD
Chair of Neonatal Nursing Research
The Royal Children's Hospital and
Associate Head (Research)
School of Nursing
University of Melbourne
Melbourne, Victoria
Australia

John Lantos MD FAAP
Chief
Division of General Pediatrics
University of Chicago
Chicago, Illinois
USA

Margot A Latimer RN
Ferasi Fellow
McGill University
Montreal, Quebec
Canada
Research Associate
Interdisciplinary Research Department
IWK Health Centre
Halifax, Nova Scotia
Canada

Shoo K Lee MBBS FRCPC PhD
Director
Centre for Healthcare Outcomes Research
Capital Health Authority
Walter C Mackenzie Health Sciences Centre
8440 112 Street
Edmonton, Alberta
Canada

Inge de Liefde MD
Trainee Anaesthetist
Department of Anesthesiology
Erasmus Medical Center
Sophia Children's Hospital
Pain Expertise Center
Rotterdam
The Netherlands

Patrick J McGrath OC PhD FRSC
Professor of Psychology, Pediatrics and Psychiatry
Canada Research Chair
Dalhousie University
CIHR Distinguished Scientist
Psychologist
IWK Health Centre
Halifax, Nova Scotia
Canada

Kathryn J McNaughton
Research Assistant
School of Nursing
McGill University
Montreal, Quebec
Canada

William Meadow MD PhD
Department of Pediatrics
University of Chicago
Chicago, Illinois
USA

Marcia L Meldrum PhD
Co-Director, John C Liebeskind History of Pain Project
Co-Investigator, UCLA Pain Study Group
UCLA
Los Angeles, California
USA

Christine Newman MD
Staff Neonatologist and Palliative Care Physician
The Hospital for Sick Children
Assistant Professor
Department of Paediatrics
University of Toronto
Toronto, Ontario
Canada

Timothy F Oberlander MD(TP) FRCP(c)
Associate Professor
Department of Paediatrics
University of British Columbia
Developmental Paediatrician
Children's & Women's Health Centre of BC
BC Research Institute
Vancouver, British Columbia
Canada

Arne Ohlsson MD MSc FRCPC FAAP
Director, Evidence-Based Neonatal Care and
Outcomes Research
Department of Pediatrics
Mount Sinai Hospital
Toronto, Ontario
Canada

Rebecca R Pillai Riddell PhD
Assistant Professor
Department of Psychology
York University
Toronto, Ontario
Canada

Heinz Rode PhD MD
Professor and Pediatric Surgeon
Head of Department of Pediatric Surgery
Red Cross War Memorial Children's Hospital
University of Cape Town
Cape Town
South Africa

Maria Rugg RN MN AXNP CHPCN(C)
Clinical Nurse Specialist/Nurse Practitioner
Palliative and Bereavement Care Program
Advanced Practice Nurses
The Hospital for Sick Children
Toronto, Ontario
Canada

Navil Sethna MD
Professor of Anesthesiology and Pediatrics
Harvard Medical School
Department of Anesthesia
Children's Hospital
Boston, Massachusetts
USA

Vibhuti Shah MD MRCP FRCPC
Staff Neonatologist
Assistant Professor
Department of Paediatrics
Mount Sinai Hospital
Toronto, Ontario
Canada

Wendy F Sternberg PhD
Associate Professor of Psychology
Department of Psychology
Haverford College
Haverford, Pennsylvania
USA

Bonnie J Stevens RN PhD
Professor
Faculties of Nursing and Medicine
University of Toronto
Signy Hildur Eaton Chair in Pediatric Nursing
Research
Associate Chief of Nursing (Research)
The Hospital for Sick Children
Toronto, Ontario
Canada

Santhanam Suresh MD FAAP
Associate Professor of Anesthesiology and Pediatrics
Feinberg School of Medicine
Northwestern University
Attending Anesthesiologist
Children's Memorial Hospital
Chicago, Illinois
USA

Anna Taddio BScPhm MSc PhD
Scientist
Departments of Pharmacy and Population Health
Sciences
The Hospital for Sick Children
Assistant Professor
Faculty of Pharmaceutical Sciences
University of Toronto
Toronto, Ontario
Canada

Jenny Thomas MD MBChB FFA(SA)
Paediatric Anaesthesiologist
Senior Specialist in Anaesthesia
Department of Paediatric Anaesthesia
Red Cross War Memorial Children's Hospital
University of Cape Town
Cape Town
South Africa

Dick Tibboel MD PhD
Director of Research
Intensive Care in Childhood
Erasmus Medical Center
Sophia Children's Hospital
Department of Pediatric Surgery
Rotterdam
The Netherlands

Jennie CI Tsao PhD
Associate Research Psychologist
Pediatric Pain Research Program
UCLA
Los Angeles, California
USA

Mai Thanh Tu MSc
Visiting Scholar
Centre for Community Child Health Research
Vancouver, British Columbia
Canada

Anita M Unruh BScOT MSW PhD
Professor of Health and Human Performance and
Occupational Therapy
Dalhousie University
IWK Health Centre
Halifax, Nova Scotia
Canada

John N van den Anker MD PhD FCP FAAP
Executive Director
Pediatric Pharmacology Research Unit
Chief
Division of Pediatric Clinical Pharmacology
Children's National Medical Center
Professor of Pediatrics, Pharmacology and Physiology
George Washington University School of Medicine
and Health Sciences
Washington DC
USA

Monique van Dijk PhD RN
Research Psychologist
Department of Pediatric Surgery
Erasmus Medical Center
Sophia Children's Hospital
Pain Expertise Center
Rotterdam
The Netherlands

Ron H N van Schaik PhD
Department of Clinical Chemistry
Erasmus Medical Center
Rotterdam
The Netherlands

Lonnie K Zeltzer MD
Professor of Pediatrics and Anesthesiology
Director, Pediatric Pain Management Program
UCLA
Los Angeles, California
USA

Contents

1

An overview of pain in neonates and infants

Bonnie J Stevens
K J S Anand
Patrick J McGrath

INTRODUCTION

In each of the first two editions of *Pain in Neonates*, we enthusiastically anticipated that we were on the threshold of dramatic improvement in the clinical management of pain in newborns. Now, over a decade later, we have seen significant increases in our knowledge of pain in neonates and important strides have been made towards the desired practice changes. Advances have been made especially in relation to our understanding of pain mechanisms, the immediate and short-term consequences of pain, the proliferation of pain assessment measures and effective pain management strategies; particularly for acute neonatal pain. Specifically, since the 2nd edition of this book in 2000, we have witnessed: (a) important discoveries related to the spinal, central and behavioural mechanisms of pain during early human development (fetus, neonate, infant, toddler); (b) a clearer understanding of the consequences of pain to infants born very prematurely and adaptational processes that transpire over time; (c) acknowledgement that pain in infants exists beyond acute procedural and postoperative pain and includes persistent pain that may be due to inflammatory, visceral or perhaps central sources; (d) the emergence of new, unique indicators for pain assessment in the youngest and most vulnerable infant populations; and (e) significant progression in determining the safety and efficacy of a variety of pharmacological, physical, environmental and behavioural interventions both alone and in combination. Furthermore, international recognition and efforts by professional, national and local organizations have developed pain management guidelines, based on systematic reviews or meta-analyses, that have had a considerable impact on pain assessment and management in neonates and young infants.

Despite these advances, a major reorientation in the clinical management of neonatal pain that was predicted 6 years ago in the 2nd edition of *Pain in Neonates* and predicted to either prevent or ameliorate pain and its consequences in infants has not totally materialized. Neonatal pain is acknowledged as an entity almost universally in the medical, nursing, psychological, neuroscience, social, bioethical, philosophical, political and legal literature and across clinical or home settings and professional or lay care providers. Yet, there are still many neonates or older infants in Neonatal Intensive Care

Units (NICUs), hospital wards, or community and home settings who suffer needlessly from acute, prolonged, persistent and perhaps even chronic pain.

To address this reality, we have expanded the scope of this 3rd edition to encompass the broadest scope of pain from the earliest stages of fetal development and viability in the external uterine environment to those infants who progress beyond the neonatal period and are faced with acute, repetitive or persistent pain in the first year of life (Fig. 1.1). Many conditions related to the neonatal period require ongoing surgical, medical, or other interventions (e.g. physical therapy) for several months after NICU or hospital discharge. These infants may remain technology-dependent at home or in chronic care facilities, with continued exposure to pain (Slonim et al. 2000, Marcin et al. 2001). Large numbers of infants with congenital malformations or genetic/metabolic disorders also require surgical and other interventions during infancy. Expanding the scope of this edition to include older infants, therefore, provides a more comprehensive approach to understanding and addressing pain in infants and should be of use to multiple stakeholders who are involved with infants, their parents and families, institutions and society in relation to pain in this population.

Since the year 2001, when the United States Congress declared the upcoming decade as the Decade of Pain, there has been an exponential growth of pain research across all ages and stages of development including neonates and infants. Massive growth has occurred in biological, clinical, epidemiological, ethical and legal circles such that it is almost impossible to compile a comprehensive list of the discoveries and achievements in this opening overview. *Only highlights from the past six years that are particularly noteworthy will be highlighted here.* These highlights are excerpted from subsequent chapters in this book, to facilitate a logical understanding from developmental biology to applied clinical science, to exploit this knowledge for more effective pharmacological, behavioural and environmental means of pain management, and to

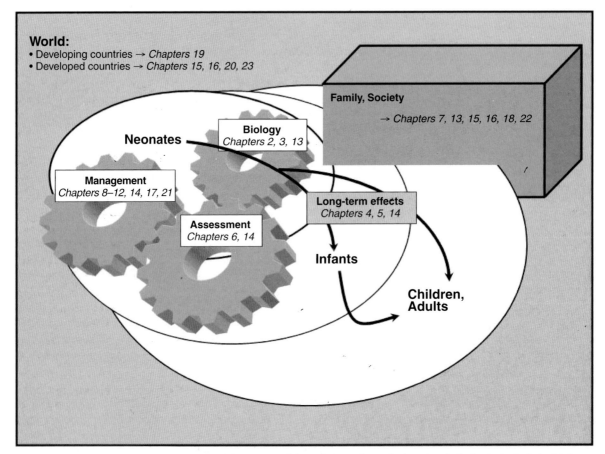

Figure 1.1 Diagrammatic representation of the scope of this edition, where the 'mechanics' of pain include its biology, assessment and management in neonates and infants. Progressively increasing ovals represent the stages of development in neonates, infants and older age groups, with arrows denoting long-term effects across these stages, all of which are supported within the context of family and society, and contained within developing and developed countries of the world.

focus attention on the care provider, ethical, legal and policy issues.

DEVELOPMENT

Developmental neurobiologists have strengthened our realization that infants from a very young age can experience pain and demonstrate specific pain behaviours (Chapters 2 and 3). The development of nociceptive pathways at the peripheral and spinal level, along supraspinal centres to the cortex, the balancing of inhibitory and excitatory synaptic transmission in developing pain pathways, and the short-term and long-term effects of early tissue damage on the developing nervous system have received significant attention in the past few years (Narsinghani and Anand 2000, Fitzgerald 2005). In preterm infants, pain responses were thought to be largely subcortical, with functional maturation of higher brain centres being required to produce a pain experience, but recent and ongoing studies show acute pain activates the sensory cortex even in the smallest preterm infants (Bartocci et al. 2005, Fitzgerald 2005). Cells in the dorsal horn are more excitable than in more mature individuals. The cutaneous receptive fields of dorsal horn cells are larger and overlapping (Torsney and Fitzgerald 2002) and there is prolonged hypersensitivity following skin injury in infancy. These neurophysiological properties result in reduced spatial discrimination, temporal and spatial summation, with increased input to tertiary cells (e.g. motor neurons, thalamic neurons), which contribute to an enhanced sensitivity and lower behavioural thresholds in early infancy (Anand 1998). The most immature infants have the lowest thresholds and widespread reflex responses at the spinal level; thus reflecting the predominance of excitatory over inhibitory synaptic transmission (Fitzgerald 2005). Descending inhibitory and facilitatory mechanisms from the brainstem and thalamus, which regulate the sensitivity of spinal-bulbospinal loops, are also immature in the small infant (Fitzgerald and Koltzenburg 1986, Ren et al. 1997). While these features may increase the sensitivity to acute pain, they may also protect the infant from persistent, neuropathic or central pain (Howard et al. 2005). The most important caveat with premature or older infants is that noxious information is processed within a pain-processing system in constant change during development.

CONSEQUENCES OF PAIN

Abnormal or excessive neural activity related to pain and injury during the postnatal period have long been proposed to cause long-term changes in somatosensory and pain processing (Anand 1997, 2000, Fitzgerald and Walker 2003). The long-term alterations following injury during a critical period of early neonatal life are likely to reflect plasticity in the anatomical, neuro-chemical and physiological characteristics of peripheral and central sensory pathways (Chapter 4).

There have been considerable advances in understanding the effects of early pain, with significant convergence between results in the human and animal studies. Neurobiological development in newborn rats approximates that of a 22-week gestation human fetus, thus providing a good model for prematurity (Clancy et al. 2001). Pain/injury in the neonatal rat has developmentally regulated long-term effects that do not occur following pain exposure at later ages. Effects of early pain exposure are evident at all levels of pain systems (Fitzgerald 2005). The direction and extent of effects related to repetitive pain in the immature organism depend on the type of pain stimulus and timing (Bhutta et al. 2001, Bhutta and Anand 2002, Ren et al. 2004).

Models of repetitive pain, inflammation, skin wounding, visceral stimulation or surgery in early life in rodents and other species have noted multiple alterations in the neonate and in the adult nervous system, correlated with specific behavioural phenotypes depending on the timing and nature of the insult (Chapter 5, Sternberg et al. 2005). Although there are some discrepancies in the long-term consequences of pain, produced by using different animal models of neonatal pain, the consensus is that early periods of development are especially vulnerable to the long-term effects of acute or repetitive pain exposures (Anand 2000, Anand and Scalzo 2000). Nociceptive and antinociceptive neural circuitry undergoes substantial changes during the early neonatal period, and therefore remains vulnerable to the effects of incident noxious stimulation.

Controlled experimental studies of the long-term consequences of early somatic or visceral pain in the rodent or human species are relatively recent additions to the literature, spurred in part by the recognition of frequent pain occurring in the NICU. The research suggests that early pain experience may account for a portion of the variability in pain thresholds and pain behaviours (both at the site of injury, and overall sensitivity), as well as stress-related behaviours and physiological responses, and their underlying neuro-endocrine substrates. Research highlighted in Chapters 4 and 5 describes the responsiveness of the developing nervous system to stimulation during critical periods just before and after birth.

PAIN ASSESSMENT

A systematic review of infant pain assessment measures by Duhn and Medves (2004) indicates that there are dozens of univariate, multivariate and composite measures for assessing pain in infants. This extremely rapid proliferation of measures with varying degrees of psychometric testing, feasibility and clinical utility addresses the need for infant pain measures (previously thought to be a major impediment to optimal pain management) and the dilemma of the lack of an available gold standard for infant pain measurement.

Pain assessment is an essential prerequisite to safe and efficacious management (Chapter 6). Given that there is no biological marker for assessing pain in any age group (Warnock and Lander 2004), physiological, bio-behavioural and behavioural indicators need to be considered as surrogate markers for self-report in infancy. The greatest steps forward were the assessment of acute procedural and postoperative pain and the inclusion of physiologic biomarkers of pain and stress such as heart rate variability (Oberlander and Saul 2002) and cortisol (Yamada et al. 2006). However, we still lack a single biologic measure or a small cadre of universally accepted, valid, reliable, feasible and clinically useful measures that would provide the basis for assessing all types of pain in neonates and infants. Additionally, the focus has been on psychometric testing, with a paucity of work on feasibility, clinical utility (Stevens and Gibbins 2002), clinical meaningfulness (sensitivity/specificity) (Shah et al. 2004) and the clinical attribution of pain by care providers (Pillai Riddell and Craig 2004).

Persistent, acute and chronic pain still pose substantial measurement challenges. This challenge is particularly salient in the most vulnerable populations including extremely low-birth-weight infants, infants at risk for neurological impairment, critically ill infants and those requiring supportive and/or palliative care (Chapter 18). The challenge is equally perplexing for professional care providers and families. In this 3rd edition, parenting of infants in pain is addressed by Pillai Riddell and Chambers in Chapter 22. Parents seem to confront a more emotionally distressing, ambiguous and challenging task than health professionals, given their personal investment and lack of technical knowledge about infant pain. In some cases, however, parents may be more knowledgeable about their infant's pain cues and thus be in a unique position to advocate for appropriate pain management for their infants. In addition to providing a review of the sparse research that has been conducted on this topic to date with both full-term and preterm infants, this chapter provides an overview of theoretical perspectives on parent–infant relationships that can be used to guide future research on this important topic.

PAIN INTERVENTIONS

Many interventions have been proposed to decrease pain and its effects on the developing infant. In this volume, there is a major focus on the advances in pharmacologic (Chapters 8, 9, 10 and 11), physiologic, behavioural and environmental (Chapter 12) interventions for pain relief. A novel feature is the consideration and applicability of complementary and alternative therapies for infant pain management (Chapter 21), which are now frequently used for older age groups (Eisenberg et al. 2002, Cherkin et al. 2003, Madsen et al. 2003).

Safe and effective pain treatment in neonates and young infants requires a thorough understanding of various developmental aspects of drug disposition and metabolism (Chapter 8). In general, the phenotypic variation in drug disposition and metabolism is based on constitutional, genetic and environmental factors. Clearance of most medicines is decreased in neonates as compared to adults and older children. This can be attributed to the immaturity of renal function as well as a decreased capacity of drug-metabolizing enzymes (Hines and McCarver 2002, Kearns et al. 2003). Moreover, the disposition and action of many drugs are polygenically determined events whereby polymorphisms in drug-metabolizing enzymes, transporters and receptors cooperatively determine the spectrum of drug response ranging from no effect (therapeutic failure) to suprapharmacologic effect (drug toxicity) (Evans and McLeod 2003, Weinshilboum 2003).

The genetic and epigenetic regulation of drug-metabolizing enzymes, receptors and regulatory proteins involved in antinociception in neonates and young infants is addressed in Chapter 8. Research into the pharmacogenetics and pharmacogenomics of transporters, receptor systems, and cell signaling will further elucidate the developmental events that affect the treatment of pain in neonates and young infants. Increasing knowledge of the regulation of genes involved in the disposition and action of analgesic drugs in animals and adults is, however, still far from a reality in daily neonatal and paediatric clinical practice. To date, minimal prospective data are available on the distribution of the different polymorphisms in neonates treated for different kinds of pain. Moreover, the impact of disease on the disposition and action of analgesic drugs in this vulnerable patient population has never been evaluated. Finally, the consequences of race and ethnicity as it relates to the appropriate (most effective and safe) choice of analgesic drugs needs to be elucidated. The incorporation of this important and crucial information into dosing regimens of different pain medicines in this young age group will result in more personalized pain management.

A surge of interest in developmental pharmacology, methods for scaling paediatric pharmacokinetic (PK) parameters from individual drug studies in adults and children of all ages is improving current drug management in the first year of life. In Chapter 9, the pharmacokinetic and pharmacodynamic changes after birth are explored along with pharmacological models and reviews of analgesic drugs commonly used in early infancy. Anderson and Holford conclude that growth and developmental changes account for major pharmacokinetic differences between children and adults. Additional differences in neonates and infants are largely attributable to maturational parameters, which can be represented by gestational age or post-conceptional age. Pharmacodynamic factors that may influence the clinical response to analgesics in early life remain poorly defined.

In Chapter 10, Taddio explores the evidence for systemic administration of two commonly used opioids, morphine and fentanyl. Clearly, there is now sufficient evidence to justify the use of systemic opioid analgesics for the management of moderate and severe pain in this population. However, unanswered questions remain regarding optimal utilization of these drugs in the clinical setting. For instance, there are unresolved issues regarding the most appropriate measures of analgesic efficacy and dosing regimens for individual infants. In addition, most recent studies do not support the routine use of opioids in neonates that are ventilated or undergoing skin-breaking procedures. In contrast, there is clear documentation of the adverse effects of opioid analgesia, including hypotension and respiratory depression (Bhandari et al. 2005, Hall et al. 2005). Clearly, more research is needed to determine the clinical factors that determine analgesic effectiveness and methods to maximize the risk:benefit ratio. Hopefully, these initiatives will lead to improved pain management in infants and improved outcomes.

The context in which the neonate experiences pain is multidimensional and complex. How environmental and contextual factors affect pain perception and response in neonates is only in its infancy (Chapter 12). Presence and tactile contact of parents and siblings with the infant (e.g. skin to skin contact during painful procedures) promote physiological stability and quiet state, opening avenues for exploring their effects on pain experienced during infancy (Johnston et al. 2003). Physical aspects of the context such as reduction of light and noise also enhance physiological stability and may consequently decrease the pain response. Finally, the complex work environment of the NICU affects staff performance, which will affect pain management; thus, there is an ever-increasing challenge of decreasing the gap between knowledge and practice necessitating novel strategies

such as one-to-one coaching (Johnston et al. 2006). Direct links between the work environment, interactive knowledge translation strategies and pain experience in the neonate have not been specifically studied (Sharek et al. 2006). We do know that the contextual environment in which pain is experienced does influence pain response in neonates, including critically ill preterm neonates, especially those undergoing multiple painful events.

The strength of existing evidence is also a crucial component that influences the quality of pain management. In Chapter 17, Ohlsson and Shah address the value of systematic reviews and meta-analyses as a means of evaluating the effectiveness of pain-relieving interventions through randomized controlled trials. The question of how this evidence can be utilized in clinical decision making is paramount and is explored using a synopsis approach (evidence based on reviews and individual studies) to the clinical question 'Do local anaesthetics reduce pain associated with venepuncture in neonates/infants?'

The general premise underlying all interventions is that improved prevention and more aggressive treatment of pain will diminish not only the pain and suffering of the infant but also will minimize immediate and future consequences. However, as one example, it is important to note that sucrose, with over three dozen randomized controlled trials, has not led to a well-defined administration and dosage template that is effective and safe for all infant populations (Johnston et al. 2002, Stevens et al. 2004). Whether or not ongoing pharmacologic or non-pharmacological treatments provide clinical benefits or harm to preterm infants in the NICU needs to be further investigated. Conversely, since the central nervous system and endocrine systems are relatively more mature at the time of pain exposure in full-term or older infants, under-treated pain may have different effects. Currently it is unclear to what extent changes are pain-specific or reflect combined pain and stress in human infants.

PAIN IN SPECIAL SITUATIONS AND CIRCUMSTANCES

The applicability of what we have learned concerning capacity for pain in the extrauterine environment and its applicability to the fetal environment where the issues of conscious awareness and the ability to experience pain are currently under scrutiny (Mellor et al. 2005). With the ever-increasing incidence of fetal surgery, it is reasonable to ask whether the fetus is capable of feeling pain (Chapter 13). For the fetus to feel pain there must be functional connections between the peripheral nociceptive receptors and the sites in the brain necessary for conscious pain perception. It is incorrect to assume that fetal pain perception must activate the same structures as those used for pain processing by human adults. The fetus or neonate is not a 'little adult' and many structures or mechanisms used for pain processing during fetal or neonatal life are unique and completely different from those used by adults. The immature pain system may play a signalling role during fetal development and may use neural elements available at that time to fulfil this role. The current evidence, although still limited, makes it very unlikely that the fetus can feel pain before 17 weeks and very likely after 26 weeks. Glover and Fisk (Chapter 13) suggest that it is possible that some sensory experience of pain may start by about 20 weeks. The possibility of fetal pain should be considered in relation to fetal interventions, terminations in the second half of gestation, and possibly also for traumatic births. This enquiry, however, will generate research about the most appropriate drugs to use, what doses to use, and how to deliver them.

Novel additions to this 3rd edition are the inclusion of chapters on infant colic (Chapter 7) and visceral pain (Chapter 14). Ghosh and Barr remind us that, although infant colic is common, there is still no predominant etiology that can explain the large majority of the cases. The symptoms may be a manifestation of several primary disturbances. However, the bulk of the present literature strongly suggests that infants with colic are generally free of organic pathology (Barr and Geertsma 2002, Lobo et al. 2004) and there is little evidence that infants with colic actually experience pain during crying episodes (Barr and Geertsma 2002). The behaviours exhibited in infant colic are present in normally developing infants, merely lesser in intensity or frequency. This means that for most infants, colic is a phenomenon within the spectrum of normative infant behaviour. Nevertheless, it is one of the most common complaints raised by parents and continues to present a difficult challenge in the clinical setting. Until there is a better understanding of the mechanisms involved in excessive crying and associated behaviours, a variety of management strategies will continue to be attempted. The most important issue is appropriate reassurance and the prevention of secondary consequences such as caregiver anxiety and depression and the one truly tragic consequence of inappropriate caregiver responses to crying; shaken baby syndrome. Current theories about factors that may incite colic symptoms and new recommendations for the management and reduction of infant colic are a source of controversy.

Visceral pain (Chapter 14) is caused by disorders of the stomach, kidney, gallbladder, urinary bladder, intestines, pancreas, spleen and liver. Such pain, often poorly described and associated with nausea, is caused in hollow viscera by distension from obstruction by atresia, stenosis, tumour, ischaemia, inflammation and muscle spasm. Causes are age-related, e.g. necrotizing enterocolitis mostly occurs in preterm neonates, intussusception is most common between 4 and 24 months, but rare beyond that except in children with cystic fibrosis or polyps. In Chapter 14, Al-Chaer and Hyman provide a comprehensive basic and clinical overview of the mechanisms and approach to the evaluation and treatment of the neonate and infant with visceral pain. We hope that this chapter will trigger a search for novel methods to evaluate and treat visceral pain in infants.

Pain in vulnerable infants and those requiring palliative care (Chapter 18) is addressed within the context of the Vulnerable Populations Model (Flaskerud and Winslow 1998) with attention to the major relationships between resource availability, relative risk and health status. Although significant advances in infant pain assessment and management research should extend equally to infants at the extreme lower limit of viability, those at risk for varying degrees of neurological impairment, those who are critically ill and those at the end of life, to date, researchers have generally not included this population in their research studies. Therefore, our knowledge of the validity of existing pain measures and the efficacy and safety of pharmacological, physical, behavioural, environmental and supportive therapies, although implemented effec-tively with healthy infants, are relatively unknown in these infants. Effective pain assessment and management of vulnerable infants, including those receiving end of life care, needs to become a major priority of researchers and healthcare providers in settings that accommodate vulnerable infants and their families.

Finally, infant pain in developing countries, using South Africa as an example, is addressed in Chapter 19. This is an especially important addition to the book as little attention has been given to developing countries that often lack the resources and infrastructure for pain research and therapy. As relevant examples, this chapter addresses the challenges associated with the management and assessment of pain in HIV-positive infants as well as in burn-injured infants from predominantly a South African perspective. Although clinicians in other developing countries (e.g. India) show a detailed understanding of pain physiology, assessment and management in infants (Mathew and Mathew 2003), very little research is published on the specific management of pain in neonates and infants in developing countries. Analgesics may be prescribed but they are often not given at all or not given appropriately. Nursing units are plagued with chronic understaffing and the level of nursing training varies enormously. From a societal perspective, we need to employ the lessons learned from research on pain in infants to address the specific clinical questions related to the developing world. There is an urgent need for international collaboration to combine knowledge and resources between developed and developing world partners.

ETHICAL, LEGAL AND POLICY IMPLICATIONS

The treatment of pain in neonates and infants raises passionate concerns that are ethically controversial (Chapter 15). Neonatal intensive care is an idealistic attempt to treat each newborn life as of inestimable value and has been one of the most phenomenally successful medical developments of the last century. Some of the ethical controversies associated with neonatal intensive care focus on the implications of saving babies with debilitating chronic conditions. Other controversies focus on the painful nature of many interventions and the lack of attention to analgesic treatment for those painful procedures. The problem is that most interventions are of uncertain efficacy and associated with both costs and risks. Furthermore, pain relief is a difficult goal to precisely quantify so it is not always clear whether the risks and costs are associated with commensurate benefits.

In Chapter 15, the approaches to this topic from the two previous editions of this book are compared. Lantos and Meadow conclude that the ethical issues associated with the treatment of neonatal pain have gotten harder, rather than easier, as a result of recent scientific studies. Put simply, treatments that work well enough to relieve pain seem to worsen other outcomes. We know from both surgical experience and from experiences in adult ICUs that we can control pain in most instances. However, to do so in the NICU would likely require higher doses of opioids or other drugs than those that most health professionals feel comfortable administering. Such doses pose the risk of leading to more complications and higher mortality rates. The judgement about the ethics of such treatment must turn on the assessment of three factors – pain relief, effect of treatment on mortality, and the effect of treatment on long-term morbidity.

In Chapter 20, issues that deal with health policy and economics related to neonatal pain are addressed. These issues are rooted in the premise that any therapy must be evaluated both by its benefits and its costs, and caregivers must constantly ask themselves whether their treatment is appropriate, how much is too much, under what conditions is it appropriate to provide

sedation and analgesia, and at what cost. Unfortunately, measuring and managing pain in babies is challenging, and applying a valuation to pain is even more so. These are difficult issues that raise dilemmas with respect to policy development, and particularly for babies who cannot speak for themselves.

Several reasons underlie these issues. First, there is a general lack of emphasis and information about the prevalence, treatment and outcomes of pain in infants among both the public and health professional constituencies in order to define any policy issues. Second, it is difficult to reach consensus about how best to evaluate and measure neonatal pain, when to treat, what therapies to use, and how best to manage pain over time. Third, there are limited methods to tailor treatments for individual babies because of differences in comorbidities, drug metabolism and drug interactions (Glasziou 2002), as well as huge differences across the range of infant development. Fourth, the majority of analgesic medications used in children are 'off-label' (i.e. not tested or labeled for safety and efficacy in infants and children, as required by the US Food and Drug Administration (FDA) regulations), because of difficulties associated with ethics and evaluation of drugs in the paediatric population (Anand et al. 2005). Fifth, there are unique organizational, financial and legal barriers to developing and implementing the most appropriate treatments. For instance, the small size of the market for neonatal therapeutic agents is a deterrent to conducting expensive clinical trials and leads to the phenomenon of 'orphan drugs', for which there is a need but not a sufficiently large market to entice development by pharmaceutical industries (Peabody et al. 1995). Sixth, current knowledge translation processes for healthcare professionals to update their procedures and therapies remain largely ineffective and slow. Finally, there are cultural, societal and economic considerations that apply to pain management in specific populations of newborns and older infants.

SUMMARY

The overall aim of this edition is to review what is currently known about the science and practice of *Pain in Neonates and Infants* (see Fig. 1.1). We also strive to stimulate greater interest, explore novel ideas, and generate new directions for research, knowledge translation, and change in clinical practice. Although knowledge of the advantages, limitations, technical problems and relative risks/benefits with various pain-relieving techniques continue to evolve, we encourage all who care for neonates to evaluate and apply the best available evidence in the care of their young patients. This volume provides a starting point for those professionals interested in improving their knowledge, communication, critical analyses and decision making with regard to pain in neonates and infants in hospital, community and home settings. Our ultimate goal is to prevent, minimize or ameliorate pain and its consequences for all infants.

REFERENCES

Anand KJS. (1997). Long-term effects of pain in neonates and infants. In: Jensen TS, Turner JA, Wiesenfeld-Hallin Z (eds). Proceedings of the 8th World Congress on Pain, Vol. 8, pp. 881–892. IASP Press, Seattle, Washington DC.

Anand KJS. (1998). Clinical importance of pain and stress in preterm neonates. Biol Neonate 73: 1–9.

Anand KJS. (2000). Pain, plasticity, and premature birth: a prescription for permanent suffering? Nat Med 6: 971–973.

Anand KJS, Scalzo FM. (2000). Can adverse neonatal experiences alter brain development and subsequent behavior? Biol Neonate 77: 69–82.

Anand KJS, Aranda J, Johnston CC, et al. (2005). Analgesia for neonates: Study design and ethical issues. Clin Ther 27: 813–843.

Barr RG, Geertsma A. (2002). Colic: the pain perplex. In: Schecter NL, Berde CB, Yaster M (eds). Pain in Infants, Children, and Adolescents, pp. 751–764. Lippincott Williams & Wilkins, Baltimore, MD.

Bartocci M, Bergqvist LL, Lagercrantz H, et al. (2005). Pain activates cortical areas in the preterm newborn brain. Pain 122: 109–117.

Bhandari V, Bergqvist LL, Kronsberg SS, et al. (2005). Morphine administration and short-term pulmonary outcomes among ventilated preterm infants. Pediatrics 116: 352–359.

Bhutta AT, Anand KJS. (2002). Vulnerability of the developing brain: Neuronal mechanisms. Clin Perinatol 29: 357–372.

Bhutta AT, Rovnaghi CR, Simpson PM, et al. (2001). Interactions of inflammatory pain and morphine treatment in infant rats: Long-term behavioral effects. Physiol Behav 73: 51–58.

Cherkin DC, Sherman KJ, Deyo RA, et al. (2003). A review of the evidence for the effectiveness, safety, and cost of acupuncture, massage therapy, and spinal manipulation for back pain. Ann Intern Med 138: 898–906.

Clancy B, Darlington RB, Finlay BL. (2001). Translating developmental time across mammalian species. Neuroscience 105: 7–17.

Duhn L, Medves J. (2004). A systematic integrative review of infant pain assessment tools. Adv Neonatal Care 4: 126–140.

Eisenberg DM, Cohen MH, Hrbek A, et al. (2002). Credentialing complementary and alternative medical providers. Ann Intern Med 137: 965–973.

Evans WE, McLeod HL. (2003). Pharmacogenomics – drug disposition, drug targets and side effects. New Engl J Med 348: 538–549.

Fitzgerald M. (2005). The development of nociceptive circuits. Nat Rev Neurosci 6: 507–520.

Fitzgerald M, Koltzenburg M. (1986). The functional development of descending inhibitory pathways in the dorsolateral funiculus of the newborn rat spinal cord. Brain Res 389: 261–270.

Fitzgerald M, Walker S. (2003). The role of activity in developing pain pathways. In: Dostrovsky JO, Carr DB, Koltzenburg M (eds). Proceedings of the 10th World Congress on Pain. Progress in Pain Research and Management, Vol. 24. IASP Press, Seattle, Washington DC.

Flaskerud JH, Winslow BJ. (1998). Conceptualizing vulnerable populations health related research. Nurs Res 47: 69–78.

Glasziou PR. (2002). Analgesia and public health: what are the challenges? Am J Ther 9: 207–213.

Hall RW, Kronsberg SS, Barton BA, et al. (2005). Morphine, hypotension and adverse outcomes in preterm neonates: Who's to blame? Pediatrics 115: 1351–1359.

Hines RN, McCarver DG. (2002). The ontogeny of human drug-metabolizing enzymes: Phase I oxidative enzymes. J Pharmacol Exp Ther 300: 355–360.

Howard RF, Walker SM, Mota PM, et al. (2005). The ontogeny of neuropathic pain: postnatal onset of mechanical allodynia in rat spared nerve injury (SNI) and chronic constriction injury (CCI) models. Pain 115: 382–389.

Johnston CC, Walker CD, Boyer K. (2002). Animal models of long-term consequences of early exposure to repetitive pain. Clin Perinatol 29: 395–414.

Johnston CC, Stevens B, Pinelli J, et al. (2003). Kangaroo care is effective in diminishing pain response in preterm neonates. Arch Pediatr Adolesc Med 157: 1084–1088.

Johnston CC, Gagnon A, Rennick J, et al. (2006). Coaching one-to-one for pain practices of pediatric nurses. J Pediatr Nurs (under review).

Kearns GL, Abdel-Rahman SM, Alander SW, et al. (2003). Developmental pharmacology – drug disposition, action, and therapy in infants and children. New Engl J Med 349: 1157–1167.

Lobo ML, Kotzer AM, Keefe MR, et al. (2004). Current beliefs and management strategies for treating infant colic. J Pediatr Health Care 18: 115–122.

Madsen H, Andersen S, Nielsen RG, et al. (2003). Use of complementary/alternative medicine among paediatric patients. Euro J Pediatr 162: 334–341.

Marcin JP, Slonim AD, Pollack MM, et al. (2001). Long-stay patients in the pediatric intensive care unit. Crit Care Med 29: 652–657.

Mathew PJ, Mathew JL. (2003). Assessment and management of pain in infants. Postgrad Med J 79: 438–443.

Mellor DJ, Diesch TJ, Gunn AJ, et al. (2005). The importance of "awareness" for understanding fetal pain. Brain Res Rev 49: 455–471.

Narsinghani U, Anand KJS. (2000). Developmental neurobiology of pain in neonatal rats. Lab Animal 29: 27–39.

Oberlander TF, Saul JP. (2002). Methodological considerations for the use of heart rate variability as a measure of pain reactivity in vulnerable infants. Clin Perinatol 29: 427–443.

Peabody JW, Ruby A, Cannon P. (1995). The economics of orphan drug policy in the US. Can the legislation be improved? Pharmacoeconomics 8: 374–384.

Pillai Riddell RR, Craig KD. (2004). Understanding caregivers' attributions of infant pain. J Pain 5: 106.

Ren K, Blass EM, Zhou Q, et al. (1997). Suckling and sucrose ingestion suppress persistent hyperalgesia and spinal Fos expression after forepaw inflammation in infant rats. Proc Nat Acad Sci USA 94: 1471–1475.

Ren K, Anseloni V, Zou SP, et al. (2004). Characterization of basal and re-inflammation-associated long-term alteration in pain responsivity following short-lasting neonatal local inflammatory insult. Pain 110: 588–596.

Shah V, Ipp M, Sam J, et al. (2004). Eliciting the minimal clinically important difference in the pain response from parents of newborn infants and nurses. Pediatr Res 55: 519.

Sharek PJ, Powers R, Koehn A, et al. (2006). Evaluation and development of potentially better practices to improve pain management of neonates. Pediatrics (in press).

Slonim AD, Patel KM, Ruttimann UE, et al. (2000). The impact of prematurity: a perspective of pediatric intensive care units. Crit Care Med 28: 848–853.

Sternberg WF, Scorr L, Smith LD, et al. (2005). Long-term effects of neonatal surgery on adulthood pain behavior. Pain 113: 347–353.

Stevens B, Gibbins S. (2002). Clinical utility and clinical significance in the assessment and management of pain in vulnerable infants. Clin Perinatol 29: 459–468.

Stevens B, Yamada J, Ohlsson A. (2004). Sucrose for analgesia in newborn infants undergoing painful procedures. The Cochrane Database of Systematic Reviews. Issue 3. CD001069.PUB2.

Torsney C, Fitzgerald M. (2002). Age-dependent effects of peripheral inflammation on the electro-physiological properties of neonatal rat dorsal term neurons. J Neurophysiol 87: 1311–1317.

Warnock F, Lander J. (2004). Foundations of knowledge about neonatal pain. J Pain Symptom Manage 27: 170–179.

Weinshilboum R. (2003). Inheritance and drug response. New Engl J Med 348: 529–537.

Yamada J, Stevens B, de Silva N, et al. (2006). Hair cortisol as a biologic indicator of chronic stress in hospitalized neonates. Pediatr Res E-PAS 2006: 59: 5578. 509.

2

Development of peripheral and spinal nociceptive systems

Simon Beggs
Maria Fitzgerald

INTRODUCTION

The study of pain in infants, from the underlying neurobiological mechanisms to effective, successful management in the clinic has grown over the last two decades into an extremely active and important field. A key conceptual change has been the realization that infants can experience pain and show strong pain behaviour. In the past the consensus was that the immaturity of the nervous system was such that infants effectively did not feel pain and consequently analgesia for potentially painful interventions was unnecessary. It is now fully accepted that infants are not only capable of experiencing pain, but that there are potential long-term adverse effects on sensation and behaviour (Fitzgerald and Howard 2003).

Further advances in successful pain management in infants are dependent upon increasing our understanding of the key neurobiological mechanisms that govern the development of the somatosensory nervous system and its response to potentially painful stimuli.

PAIN BEHAVIOUR IN THE NEONATE

Functional connectivity of somatosensory circuitry is a prerequisite of any behavioural response to a peripheral sensory stimulus. The study of pain behaviours in fetal and neonatal animals is restricted to examination of reflex responses that can only be elicited once the primary afferent, dorsal horn neuron, motor neuron circuitry synaptic connections are complete. Reflex responses can be elicited to both tactile and noxious stimuli. It is important not to interpret these responses as evidence of pain perception, but as an indication of the degree of maturation of somatosensory circuitry and sensitivity to peripheral stimuli.

At birth cutaneous reflex responses are prevalent, albeit diffuse. In the neonatal rat a pinprick stimulus to the hindpaw elicits movement of the whole body, involving wriggling, rolling and simultaneous responses from fore- and hindlimbs. These responses reduce as the rat matures becoming more restricted to an isolated leg or foot movement. Exaggerated cutaneous responses in newborns compared to adults has been shown in rat, cat and human studies (Ekholm 1967, Fitzgerald et al. 1988). Thresholds are lower, such that the elicitation of a flexor reflex response does not always require a noxious stimulus as in the adult, and the reflex muscle contractions are more synchronized and long-lasting. Repeated skin stimulation results in considerable hyperexcitability or sensitization with generalized movement of all limbs. Comparative studies of the flexor reflex in premature and full-term human infants and newborn rat pups showed that reflex thresholds are very low in preterm infants but increase with post-conceptional age (PCA) (Fitzgerald et al. 1988). Repeated stimulation sensitizes this but the phenomenon declines after 29–35 weeks PCA in the human and postnatal day 8 (P8) in the rat (Andrews and Fitzgerald 1994).

Thresholds for withdrawal from heat stimuli are also lower in younger animals (Lewin et al. 1993, Falcon et al. 1996, Marsh et al. 1999). The response to formalin has a tenfold higher sensitivity in neonatal rats compared to weanlings (Teng and Abbott 1998), although up until P10 the responses are predominantly 'non-specific' whole body movements, rather than more 'specific' flexion reflexes with shaking and licking the affected area, which predominate from then on. The classic biphasic response to formalin (Dubuisson and Dennis 1977) is not apparent in the rat pup until P15, coinciding with the overall depression in the response (Guy and Abbott 1992).

Receptive fields of hindlimb flexor muscles are large and disorganized in younger animals resulting in inappropriate limb withdrawal responses to noxious stimuli (Fitzgerald and Jennings 1999, Schouenborg 2003). Directional tail flick responses to precise laser stimulation of the tail show high error rates for the first 10 postnatal days, gradually improving to adult levels within 3 weeks (Waldenstrom et al. 2003), indicative of the fine-tuning of excitatory and inhibitory synaptic connectivity in the spinal cord over the postnatal period. Preterm human infant limb and abdominal withdrawal reflexes show a similar lack of tuning (Andrews and Fitzgerald 1994, 2000, Andrews et al. 2002). Unilateral abdominal skin stimulation evokes bilateral limb flexion in very young babies. With increasing PCA this is reduced to unilateral flexion and finally no limb movement, the response restricted to abdominal muscle contraction (Andrews et al. 2002).

Despite their importance in early behaviour, reflex responses cannot be equated with true pain experience, which must involve the cortex and cognitive brain function. It follows that stronger reflexes do not necessarily mean more pain and are likely to reflect the absence of the normal inhibitory control that higher brain structures exert at more mature stages to 'dampen' spinal excitability. The role of exaggerated reflex responsivity to noxious stimuli may well be protective and beneficial to an animal that is as yet not equipped to perceive and organize a more directed response to the stimulus. This is supported by the observation that although infants of 26–31 weeks gestational age show co-ordinated facial responses to noxious stimuli (Craig et al. 1993), younger gestational age is associated with less reactivity in facial expression, suggesting that the youngest infants are less able to display more complex affective reactions to noxious stimuli (Stevens et al. 1994). To better understand the maturation of pain pathways it is necessary to investigate further the ontogeny of the underlying neuronal connections.

DEVELOPMENT OF PRIMARY SENSORY AFFERENTS

The specification of primary sensory neurons is the first stage in the development of the somatosensory pathways that will transmit sensory stimuli from the periphery to the higher areas of the central nervous system (CNS). Nociceptive neurons are specified extremely early in development; as neural crest cells still migrating into positions and before even being committed to a neuronal or glial lineage. As such they develop as nociceptive neurons without influence from either central or peripheral targets (Zirlinger et al. 2002). Primary sensory neurons that make up the dorsal root ganglia (DRG) are born segmentally in a rostrocaudal progression starting at around embryonic day 12 (E12). The two broad subdivisions of DRG neurons are born separately: the large-diameter cells that give rise to A-fibres and express the neurotrophin receptors trkB and trkC appear first, followed by the smaller-diameter, C-fibre-producing cells that express trkA (Altman and Bayer 1984, Kitao et al. 1996). The development of these two populations is under the control of separate transcription factors of the neurogenin family from the outset. Neurogenin (ngn)1 is required for small, C-fibre neurons and ngn2 for the larger, A-fibre cells (Ma et al. 1999). Within the C-fibre population there are two distinct subpopulations, distinguished by their expression of peptides. Peptidergic cells appear before non-peptidergic cells; the transcriptional control of this process remains unclear, however (Kitao et al. 1996). Many more DRG neurons are born than will survive into adulthood. The number of neurons increases up until the time of birth and is followed by a 15–20% loss over the first postnatal week (Coggeshall et al. 1994) coinciding with the final innervation of the skin by the peripheral afferents of the DRG neurons. The survival of the neurons is dependent upon their access to neurotrophic factors produced by both peripheral (e.g. skin) and central targets (Kirstein and Farinas 2002).

CUTANEOUS INNERVATION

Outgrowth of axons from DRG sensory neurons occurs before birth and reflects the two waves of neurogenesis of the parent neurons. Large-diameter A-fibres form an initial nerve plexus and are followed by the smaller-diameter C-fibres (Jackman and Fitzgerald 2000). This growth is extremely accurate, with each DRG innervating somatotopically appropriate dermatomes from the outset, under the control of a number of signalling molecules (Dickson 2002). Although precise, there is an initial hyperinnervation of the skin, extending beyond the dermis into the epidermal surface. These exuberant projections subsequently withdraw to leave the adult situation (Jackman and Fitzgerald 2000).

PERIPHERAL CUTANEOUS RECEPTORS

All the functional afferent types seen in the adult are therefore present in the rat hindlimb at birth, although their maturity depends on the receptor type they innervate (Fitzgerald 1987, Fitzgerald and Fulton 1992) and the individual stimulus modality (Koltzenburg 1999). Sensory end organs that transduce low-threshold mechanosensation, such as Merkel cells and Meissner's corpuscles, mature over a prolonged period postnatally, despite the A-fibres that innervate them being the first to be present in the skin (English et al. 1980). Hair follicle innervation by A-fibres does not begin until P7 in rats and 28 weeks PCA in humans (Payne et al. 1991). The low-threshold mechano-receptors are the most immature of all cutaneous receptors at birth, exhibiting low firing frequency and amplitude of response (Fitzgerald 1985a). High-threshold mechanoreceptors, innervated by A-delta fibres and which in the adult respond maximally to noxious mechanical stimulation are also distinguishable in the neonate, but have reduced peak firing frequencies. Polymodal nociceptors, which have C-fibre axons and respond to mechanical, thermal and chemical noxious stimuli, appear to be fully mature in terms of threshold, pattern and frequency of firing at birth (Fitzgerald 1987) suggesting that the mechanisms of transduction are already in place and functional. The receptor TRPV1, which is essential for the detection of noxious thermal and chemical stimuli is as abundant at P2 as in the adult rat. Similarly the ATP receptor $P2X_3$, also implicated in noxious sensory processing, is present in the neonatal DRG (Guo et al. 2001). The tetrodotoxin-resistant sodium channel Nav1.8 is expressed in developing C-fibres as early as E17 and reaches adult levels by P7 (Benn et al. 2001). Adult nociceptors respond to a large array of endogenous molecules, such as bradykinin, serotonin, substance P, etc., and further research will elucidate whether these molecules are active at neonatal stages of development.

CENTRAL INNERVATION

In the rat lumbar spinal cord, the first sensory neuron-derived afferents to penetrate the cord are the large-diameter fibres that will eventually transduce proprioceptive and low-threshold mechanical stimuli. These fibres enter the dorsal horn grey matter at E13, considerably earlier than C-fibre projections, which only appear at E19 (Fitzgerald 1987). From the outset, C-fibres terminate in a somatotopically precise manner in lamina I and II of the superficial dorsal horn (Fitzgerald and Swett 1983, Ozaki and Snider 1997). As with the staggered specification of the sub-populations of C-fibre afferent neurons, the non-peptidergic small C-fibres appear to form synaptic connections in the dorsal horn later than the peptidergic sub-population, with synaptic terminals only detectable at the electron microscopy (EM) level at P5 (Pignatelli et al. 1989). This relatively late formation of functional synapses suggests that despite the early maturation of nociceptive functionality in the periphery, central nociceptive processing remains immature in the neonate and immediate postnatal period. It is clear that despite the presence of C-fibres in the dorsal horn during the late embryonic period, the maturation of synaptic connectivity occurs later. In vivo experiments have shown that electrical stimulation of A-fibres can evoke action potentials in superficial dorsal horn cells as early as P3, but that C-fibre-evoked activity is not seen until P10 (Fitzgerald 1988, Jennings and Fitzgerald 1998). This failure to elicit action potentials is not due to an absence of functional C-fibre synapses during the first postnatal week as capsaicin application can evoke glutamate release in the dorsal horn, suggesting that TRPV1-expressing nociceptive afferents have formed functional synapses. However, the robustness of this effect increases between P5 and P10, which is consistent with a proliferation of C-fibre synaptic inputs during this time (Baccei et al. 2003).

As with C-fibres, A-fibre innervation of the dorsal horn is somatotopically precise from the outset. However the laminar organization is not, with A-fibre terminals growing beyond the final adult pattern into superficial laminae (Fitzgerald et al. 1994, Beggs et al. 2002, Pattinson and Fitzgerald 2004). The adult pattern, where lamina II is exclusively occupied by C-fibre terminals, occurs with a gradual withdrawal of the dorsally projecting A-fibres during the first 3 postnatal weeks (Fitzgerald et al. 1994, Beggs et al. 2002). Synaptic connectivity of these transient A-fibres in lamina II has been confirmed at the EM level

(Coggeshall et al. 1996) and correlates with the high incidence of A-fibre-evoked monosynaptic responses seen in lamina II neurons in young rats (Park et al. 1999, Nakatsuka et al. 2000) and activation of c-fos expression by low-intensity stimulation at P3 but not P21 (Jennings and Fitzgerald 1996). Furthermore, repeated low-intensity mechanical or A-fibre stimulation can lead to sensitization of dorsal horn cell responses beyond the period of stimulation, a phenomenon that is never seen in the adult (Jennings and Fitzgerald 1998).

The postnatal 'fine-tuning' of A-fibres is an activity-dependent process requiring activation of NMDA receptors. Adult rats that had received chronic blockade of lumbar dorsal horn NMDA receptors by the local application of the antagonist MK801 from birth showed increased A-fibre-evoked responses in lamina II neurons with reduced mechanical thresholds to an innocuous stimulus, while C-fibre input and noxious heat responses were unaffected (Beggs et al. 2002). Competition for synaptic space between A- and C-fibres may underlie the withdrawal. If the majority of C-fibre inputs are destroyed by neonatal capsaicin treatment, the exuberant superficial A-fibre projections persist into adulthood (Park et al. 1999, Torsney et al. 2000). The inference here is that the A-fibres lose the competition for the synaptic space within lamina II and withdraw, leaving only C-fibres. The underlying mechanism may involve the postnatal increase in A-fibre frequency leading to a mismatch of pre- and postsynaptic activity at A-fibre/lamina II neuron synapses, leaving them to be increasingly driven by low-frequency C-fibre input.

DEVELOPMENTAL CHANGES IN SENSORY PROCESSING IN THE DORSAL HORN

Understanding the development of all the key components of spinal cord circuitry is necessary to elucidate the mechanisms underlying the developmental changes observed in nociceptive processing. In the adult central nervous system somatosensory processing comprises a fine balance of sensory afferent input, local inhibitory and excitatory control on dorsal horn projection neurons as well as descending inhibitory and facilitatory modulation (Fig. 2.1). The development and maturation of each of these components will affect the nociceptive responsivity of the animal.

Within the dorsal horn itself, development occurs in a ventrodorsal gradient such that motoneurons are born first, followed by deep dorsal horn neurons and substantia gelatinosa (SG) and finally lamina I neurons (Altman and Bayer 1984). Interneurons and supraspinal projection neurons develop at approximately the same time, appearing first at E13. However,

projection neurons are fully developed in advance of the interneurons, at E14 compared to E16 (Bicknell and Beal 1984).

In the newborn, the synaptic linkage between afferents and dorsal horn cells is still weak and electrical stimulation often evokes only a few spikes at long and variable latencies (Fitzgerald 1985a, Jennings and Fitzgerald 1998). However, in many respects neonatal rat dorsal horn cells are more excitable than in the adult. At birth dorsal horn cells possess large peripheral cutaneous receptive fields, which decrease in size over the first 2 postnatal weeks (Fitzgerald 1985a, Torsney and Fitzgerald 2002). Natural stimulation of these receptive fields at early postnatal ages can evoke long-lasting excitation and prolonged after-discharge, which can lower the threshold to subsequent stimuli, but is absent by P21 (Jennings and Fitzgerald 1998). The result of these properties is that otherwise weak cutaneous inputs are made more effective centrally, suggesting an imbalance of excitation and inhibition compared to the mature spinal cord. This clearly offers a substrate for the exaggerated low-threshold cutaneous reflexes observed in the neonatal rat and human described earlier, and also illustrates the importance of understanding the development of excitation and inhibition within the spinal cord at the synaptic level.

DEVELOPMENT OF EXCITATORY SYNAPTIC TRANSMISSION IN THE DORSAL HORN

Many neurotransmitters and signalling molecules involved in nociceptive processing are expressed early in the developing nervous system but do not reach adult levels for a considerable period. More importantly, receptors are frequently transiently overexpressed or expressed in areas during development where they are not seen in the adult. While low levels of neurotransmitters will clearly result in reduced function, widespread, high-density receptor expression and distribution will result in non-specific or quite different function in the neonate compared to the adult. This will clearly impact on both pain behaviour in the neonate and the effects of analgesics in controlling pain.

It is well established that glutamate is the major excitatory neurotransmitter in the central nervous system, both in terms of normal function and nociception (Dickenson 1997). The development of the various glutamate receptor mechanisms is therefore of prime importance in neonatal pain.

NMDA receptors

The neonatal spinal cord has a higher concentration of NMDA receptors in the grey matter than is observed

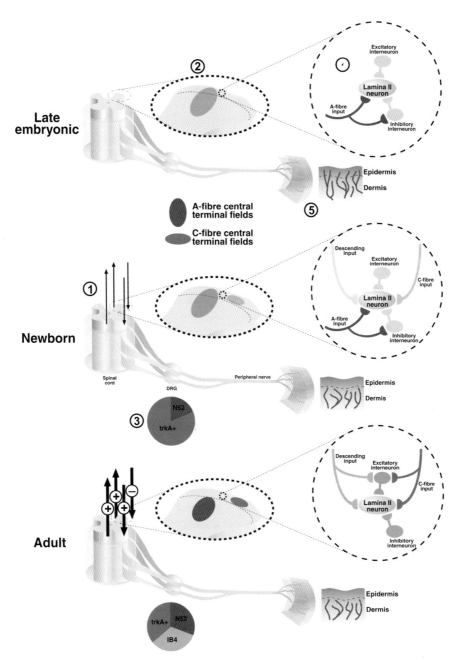

Figure 2.1 (1) In early postnatal life, descending fibres are present but inhibitory and excitatory influences are weak or absent. The connections gradually strengthen, becoming fully functional at the end of the third postnatal week. (2) A-fibres are the first primary afferents to enter the dorsal horn grey matter and are present during the last few embryonic days. Their distribution is diffuse, with exuberant, more superficial projections gradually retracting over the first 3 postnatal weeks. C-fibres are present in the dorsal horn during late embryonic stages, but only enter the grey matter 2–3 days before birth. Unlike A-fibres, they project to topographically appropriate regions in lamina II of the spinal cord as soon as they enter. C-fibre synaptic connectivity is present, although very weak, at the time of birth, with connections strengthening over the first 2 postnatal weeks. (3) At birth the majority (~80%) of DRG neurons express the NGF receptor trkA. Over the first postnatal week this population reduces, with approximately half of these neurons losing their trkA expression and beginning to express receptors for GDNF (identifiable as the IB4-binding population). (4) The balance of excitation and inhibition in the superficial dorsal horn develops postnatally, through changes in both local interneuron circuitry and descending fibres. A-fibre input is stronger in the neonate and weakens as the influence of C-fibre input increases. (5) Primary afferent innervation of the skin occurs earlier than central projections. By late embryonic stages primary afferents of all classes have reached the skin and innervate through the dermis into the epidermis. These projections die back during the immediate perinatal period to leave the full adult situation of dermal innervation present soon after birth.

in older animals. All laminae in the dorsal horn are uniformly labelled with NMDA-sensitive [^{3}H] glutamate until P10–12, when higher densities gradually appear in substantia gelatinosa (SG) so that by P30 the binding is confined to the SG as seen in the adult. A similar situation has been reported in the human spinal cord (Kalb and Fox 1997).

NMDA receptors are comprised of different subunits; NR1 and NR2A–D. Changes in expression of these subunits occur during embryonic and postnatal development (Audinat et al. 1994). Activity-dependent postnatal shifts from NR2B to NR2A expression have been shown to occur in many areas of the central nervous system, resulting in accelerated decay rates of NMDA excitatory postsynaptic currents (EPSCs) (Philpot et al. 2001). These rapid decay rates are seen in SG throughout the postnatal period, suggesting a high prevalence of NR2A expressing NMDA receptors from birth (Bardoni et al. 1998). However, receptor affinity for NMDA decreases with postnatal age as does NMDA-evoked calcium efflux in rat SG neurons. This reduction is delayed following neonatal capsaicin treatment suggesting that C-fibre afferent activity regulates the postnatal maturation of NMDA receptors (Hori and Kanda 1994).

Pure NMDA synapses ('silent synapses') have been identified in the neonatal superficial dorsal horn but are absent in the adult (Bardoni et al. 1998, Li and Zhuo 1998, Baba et al. 2000). It has been suggested that they may play an important role in excitability in postnatal SG neurons (Bardoni et al. 2000).

AMPA receptors

As with NMDA, AMPA receptors are highly expressed in the neonatal dorsal horn before being subsequently down-regulated to adult levels (Jakowec et al. 1995). Again, subunit changes occur postnatally although little is known of the functional role of immature AMPA receptors in neonatal pain.

DEVELOPMENT OF INHIBITORY SYNAPTIC TRANSMISSION IN THE DORSAL HORN

The development of the inhibitory circuitry and its connections is as fundamentally important to nociception as excitatory input. The main inhibitory neurotransmitters in the dorsal horn of the adult are GABA and glycine, both of which are predominantly released from intrinsic interneurons (Todd and Spike 1993). GABA is synthesized from glutamate by the glutamic acid decarboxylases (GAD65 and GAD67). Both of these enzymes can be detected in early development, first appearing at E11 and increasing up to birth (Somogyi et al. 1995). However, GABA itself is not expressed in the superficial dorsal horn until E17–18

(Ma et al. 1992). From this stage the number of GABA-expressing cells increases over the first postnatal weeks before declining to adult levels by P21 (Schaffner et al. 1993).

Glycine is also detected at early stages of development in the spinal cord, with the mature pattern of expression evident by E12, and remaining constant through to adulthood (Berki et al. 1995).

Both glycine and GABA are packaged into synaptic vesicles by the same transporter (Gasnier 2000) and they have been shown to be released together in the spinal cord resulting in mixed GABA/glycine-receptor-mediated inhibitory postsynaptic currents (IPSCs) (Jonas et al. 1998). These mixed IPSCs are only seen in immature dorsal horn neurons between P8 and P23, after which they are down-regulated such that mature IPSCs are mediated by either GABA or glycine receptors, but not both (Chery and DeKoninck 1999, Keller et al. 2001). However, during the immediate postnatal period in the first postnatal week, lamina II neurons exhibit only GABA IPSCs, despite possessing functional glycine receptors (Baccei and Fitzgerald 2004).

An extremely important feature of GABA receptor activation in the developing CNS is that it can be excitatory rather than inhibitory. Chloride levels within neurons are controlled, to an extent, by the action of the potassium chloride co-transporter (KCC2). Expression of this co-transporter increases postnatally and as a consequence chloride ions are pumped out of neurons, maintaining a low concentration of chloride intracellularly. This maintains the chloride ion reversal potential more negative than resting membrane potential, such that GABA$_A$R activation results in chloride efflux and hyperpolarization of the neuron. This is the fundamental ionic basis of GABAergic inhibition. In immature neurons intracellular chloride levels are higher due to the low expression of KCC2. As a result, the reversal potential for chloride is shifted more positive than the resting potential, rendering GABA less inhibitory (Ben-Ari 2002). A sub-population of neonatal dorsal horn neurons depolarize in response to GABA, the response only becoming exclusively hyperpolarizing by P6–7 (Baccei and Fitzgerald 2004). In the hippocampus GABA$_A$R activation provides a major excitatory drive during development (Ben-Ari et al. 1989). The situation in the spinal cord is not as extreme, with the chloride reversal potential never reaching action potential threshold (Baccei and Fitzgerald 2004), such that GABA remains inhibitory, albeit less effectively than in the adult. It remains possible that spinal GABAergic stimulation has an important role in neurotransmission at embryonic stages (Serafini et al.

1995). At birth the reduced inhibitory drive of GABA may have an effect through sub-threshold depolarization leading to activation of voltage-gated calcium channels (Reichling et al. 1994) and release of the NMDA receptor magnesium block (Khazipov et al. 1997). It has been suggested that the increases in intracellular calcium concentrations that these mechanisms would produce may well be vital for a number of important developmental processes, e.g. synapse formation/elimination/remodelling and neuronal differentiation (Wang et al. 1994).

THE DEVELOPMENT OF DESCENDING PAIN PATHWAYS

Brainstem descending pathways form a major mechanism in the control of pain transmission (Ren and Dubner 2002, Gebhart 2004). Axons from brainstem nuclei appear to grow down the spinal cord well before birth (Cabana and Martin 1984). Injections of horseradish peroxidase into lumbosacral spinal cord of the neonatal rat label brainstem nuclei with similar density to that seen in the adult (Leong 1983, Fitzgerald and Koltzenburg 1986, Fitzgerald et al. 1987) but it is unclear at what stage these axons begin producing collaterals that innervate the dorsal horn and make synapses with their target cells. Mapping degenerating axons and synaptic endings following thoracic hemisections of the spinal cord at various postnatal stages suggests that descending axon collaterals innervate the intermediate and central grey from birth but that they are not found in the dorsal horn until P15 (Gilbert and Stelzner 1979).

Descending inhibitory pathways travelling from the brainstem via the dorsolateral funiculus (DLF) of the spinal cord to the dorsal horn grow down the spinal cord early in fetal life, but they do not extend collateral branches into the dorsal horn for some time. Stimulation of the DLF fails to produce descending inhibition of C-fibre-evoked activity in neonatal rats before P9, but high-intensity stimulation produces descending inhibition at P18. By P22–24 more typical adult responses were observed (Fitzgerald and Koltzenburg 1986). Similarly the inhibition of C- and A-delta activity in the dorsal horn by periaqueductal grey (PAG) stimulation via the DLF that is clearly observed in adults (Basbaum and Fields 1978) cannot be produced in rat pups before P21 (van Praag and Frenk 1991). Diffuse noxious inhibitory control (DNIC), measured as a reduction in noxious evoked dorsal horn c-fos expression in the presence of an inflammatory stimulus elsewhere on the body, also develops between P12 and P21 (Boucher et al. 1998).

The delayed postnatal onset of functional descending inhibition, despite the presence of DLF terminals in the dorsal horn may be due to immaturity of neurotransmitter–receptor interactions or delayed maturation of critical interneurons. It has been suggested that the maturation of descending inhibition is dependent upon afferent C-fibre activity, because rats treated with capsaicin at birth have reduced inhibitory controls compared with adults (Cervero and Plenderleith 1985). The lack of descending inhibition in the neonatal dorsal horn means that there is no endogenous analgesic system to 'dampen' noxious inputs as they enter the CNS and their effects may therefore be more profound than in the adult. It also explains why stimulus-produced analgesia from the PAG is not effective until P21 in rats (van Praag and Frenk 1991).

OPIOID ACTIONS IN THE DEVELOPING CNS

Of particular importance to the management of paediatric pain is the developmental pharmacology of opioid analgesia, in particular the development of opioid receptor interactions in the developing nervous system.

The analgesic potency of morphine in mechanical sensory tests is significantly greater in neonatal animals compared with adults (Nandi et al. 2004). The opposite situation persists for thermal nociceptive thresholds, with increasing analgesic potency occurring between P3 and P21 (Marsh et al. 1999). Codeine analgesia is also developmentally regulated, having low efficacy in the early postnatal period (Williams et al. 2004).

Opioids interact with three opioid receptors; μ, δ and κ. The endogenous opioid peptides, comprised of the enkephalin, dynorphin and endorphin families are ligands for the three receptors but show no specificity for individual receptors (Dickenson 1994). Autoradiographic studies have shown that μ receptor binding in the adult is restricted to the superficial laminae, whereas in the first 2 postnatal weeks there is widespread binding throughout the dorsal horn (Kar and Quirion 1995, Rahman et al. 1998). κ receptor binding follows a similar pattern to μ receptor; widespread embryonically and then down-regulated after the first postnatal week. Conversely, δ receptor binding does not occur until the postnatal period (Rahman et al. 1998).

Opioid receptors are also expressed by primary sensory neurons, and as with dorsal horn neurons, considerable postnatal reorganization occurs with their expression. μ receptor protein is expressed by a far greater proportion of DRG neurons in the first postnatal week compared to P21 (Beland and Fitzgerald 2001b). Their expression profile reveals that they are expressed in both small C neurons and large Aβ cells in the first postnatal week, gradually becoming more restricted to smaller cells by P21 (Beland and Fitzgerald 2001b). However, the proportion of small C cells that are sensitive to μ-agonists remains the same throughout postnatal development (Nandi et al. 2004). This result offers an explanation for the disparity in selectivity and sensitivity of morphine with postnatal age on mechanical and thermal tests. Furthermore, if the μ-receptor distribution in human neonates is as in the rat, it may be a key factor in the increased responsiveness of human neonates to opioids.

DEVELOPMENT OF CONNECTIONS IN HIGHER CENTRES

Behavioural measurements of flexor reflexes provide important information on the reactions of human and animal neonates to noxious stimulation and analgesic efficacy. However, these flexor reflexes can never be equated to representing a true 'pain experience'. To do so requires functional maturation and involvement of higher brain centres. Human infants display particular facial expressions associated with tissue insult (Grunau and Craig 1987, Johnston et al. 1993), crying characteristics (Grunau et al. 1990) and body movements and posture (Johnston et al. 1993). Behavioural state and severity of illness influence these responses (Stevens et al. 1994). In contrast to spinal cord reflex responses, younger gestational age is associated with less reactivity in facial expression to heel lance (Johnston et al. 1995) and it has been suggested that below 32 weeks they appear to be largely subcortical in origin (Oberlander et al. 2002). Stronger reflexes, in other words, do not necessarily signify more pain; they may be a consequence of the absence of normal inhibitory control of higher brain structures over spinal systems.

The development and maturation of peripheral and spinal components of nociceptive processing outlined thus far are far better understood than for the ascending projections to the supraspinal regions essential for pain perception. In the rat, dorsal horn projection cells begin to grow axons prenatally (Bicknell and Beal 1984, Fitzgerald et al. 1991) and afferents reach the thalamus at E19. Thalamocortical projections exit the thalamus by E16 and form functional connections in the cortical plate by E18–19 (Higashi et al. 2002). By birth, thalamic axons have extended into the cortex in a topographically precise manner (Agmon et al. 1995, Rebsam et al. 2002). The spatial distribution of thalamic synapses onto cortical neurons is established by P11 in the somatosensory cortex of the mouse (Lev et al. 2002). In the human fetus, the major afferent fibre projections to the cortex

accumulate below the cortical plate between 22 and 26 weeks, gradually penetrating after 26 weeks. Somatosensory potentials evoked by electrical stimulation can be observed by 29 weeks (Klimach and Cooke 1988), although very little is known of the cortical response to pain in human infants.

THE DEVELOPMENT OF PAIN ASSOCIATED WITH INFLAMMATION AND TISSUE INJURY

Plasticity of the nervous system in response to tissue injury has been well documented and includes changes in gene expression and in the structural and functional organization of somatosensory networks. These changes in turn lead to the increased neuronal excitability that underlie persistent pain, hyperalgesia and allodynia. The chronic effects of tissue injury in infancy are less well understood.

Repeated heel lances in newborn infants cause peripheral tissue injury and elicit hyperalgesia as shown by a reduction in the threshold of cutaneous reflexes. This hyperalgesia may last for days or even weeks in the presence of the injury (Fitzgerald et al. 1988, 1989). The mechanical threshold required to elicit reflex responses decreases significantly following surgery (Andrews and Fitzgerald 2002). These phenomena can also be exhibited in rat pups; treatment with mustard oil and carrageenan produces a mechanical hyperalgesia at P3 that increases with postnatal age (Jiang and Gebhart 1998, Howard et al. 2001).

In the adult rat, inflammation-induced hyperalgesia is accompanied by changes in both peripheral and central components of nociceptive processing. Much evidence suggests the same situation occurs in neonates. Injection of carrageenan into the hindpaw of newborn rat pups increases calcitonin gene-related peptide (CGRP) expression in small and large sensory neurons (Beland and Fitzgerald 2001a), while complete Freund's adjuvant (CFA) injections in the newborn led to increased CGRP afferents in the superficial dorsal horn 2 weeks later (Ling et al. 2003). This treatment also induces an acute expansion of the terminal field of sciatic nerve central projections in lamina II (Walker et al. 2003). Electrophysiological evidence from postnatal rats supports this evidence, with dorsal horn neurons following peripheral carrageenan-induced inflammation exhibiting increases in A-fibre-evoked sensitization, spontaneous activity and response magnitude at all ages up to P21 (Torsney and Fitzgerald 2002).

Full-thickness skin wounds on the hindpaw of neonatal rats result in a dense hyperinnervation of the wound site by both A- and C-fibres that persist into adulthood (Reynolds and Fitzgerald 1995). This hyperinnervation has a functional consequence as mechanical thresholds are reduced 6–12 weeks later, long after the original injury has healed. A similar injury performed in the adult has only a small and transient response in comparison to that which occurs if the injury occurs in the first postnatal week. The hyperinnervation and subsequent hypersensitivity appear to occur independently of ongoing activity, with application of a local anaesthetic to the nerve at the time of injury having no preventative effect (De Lima et al. 1999). Evidence suggests a permissive role of neurotrophic factors in initiating the hyperinnervation (Constantinou et al. 1994, Beggs et al. unpublished observations). Clearly these findings have profound clinical implications for the consequences of tissue injury in neonates.

THE DEVELOPMENT OF PAIN ASSOCIATED WITH NERVE INJURY

The developing nervous system is much more vulnerable to peripheral injury than in the adult. Sciatic nerve transection in the neonatal rat causes the rapid death of ~75% of axotomized neurons, compared to a 30% cell loss in the adult over a much extended time course. There appears to be at least an apoptotic component to this cell death, with cells labelling positively for the apoptotic marker TUNEL within 1 day of transection (Oliveira et al. 1997, Whiteside et al. 1998). There is no direct evidence for central cell death following peripheral nerve injury, although reduced somatodendritic growth of spinal projection neurons after sciatic nerve injury occurs (Fitzgerald and Shortland 1988).

As a result of the death of dorsal root ganglion cells the central dorsal root terminals of adjacent intact nerves sprout in the spinal cord to occupy areas normally exclusively devoted to the sectioned nerve (Fitzgerald 1985b, Fitzgerald et al. 1990, Reynolds and Fitzgerland 1992, Shortland and Fitzgerald 1994). These new sprouts form inappropriate functional connections with dorsal horn cells in areas far outside their normal termination area, permanently distorting the somatosensory system with a greater proportion than normal devoted to inputs surrounding the denervated skin. In the short term this may be a useful compensatory device to restore sensory input from an area of the body surface in which it has been lost, but the long-term effects of a permanent alteration in the sensory mapping of the body may be detrimental. The effects of nerve injury in the developing rat nervous system have been shown not to be confined to primary afferent nerve, but to spread to postsynaptic dorsal horn cells and from there up to higher levels of the central nervous system including the cortex and corticospinal tract.

The epidemiology of neuropathic pain in infants and children is not well understood. Brachial plexus injuries occurring in infants during delivery do not appear to result in chronic neuropathic pain (Anand and Birch 2002). However, recent reports show that phantom pain occurs in the majority of paediatric amputees and is significantly underreported in medical records (Krane and Heller 1995).

Peripheral nerve injuries do not seem to evoke neuropathic pain behaviour in neonatal rats in contrast to the pronounced behavioural changes seen in adults. Tight ligation of the L5–L6 spinal nerves during the first 2 postnatal weeks produced only transient mechanical allodynia, while nerve injury at P21 evoked the prolonged neuropathic pain behaviours that characterize the adult (Lee and Chung 1996). In addition, sciatic nerve damage before P21 is not associated with autotomy (self-mutilation) as in adults (Anand 1992). A study of pain behaviour in the spared nerve injury (SNI) model suggests that the onset of mechanical allodynia occurs after P21 (Howard et al. 2005). The above results suggest that the mechanisms underlying neuropathic pain develop during the postnatal period. Further investigations into how nerve injury-induced plasticity differs between the immature and mature nervous system may aid the development of improved therapeutic strategies to treat chronic pain.

LONG-TERM CONSEQUENCES OF NEONATAL INJURY AND PAIN

The immediate postnatal period is critical to the development of spinal sensory systems. Key molecular components; receptors, channels and signal transduction pathways associated with sensory transmission are highly developmentally regulated postnatally. Accompanying these changes are profound structural and functional alterations of sensory connections. It has become clear in recent years that the nervous system undergoes extensive development postnatally and it is dependent upon neural activity. Furthermore, normal postsynaptic reorganization requires defined patterns of afferent input. As a consequence abnormal or excessive activity related to pain and injury during the immediate postnatal period have the potential to cause long-term changes in somatosensory and pain processing (Fitzgerald and Walker 2003).

Preterm infants in intensive care can receive hundreds of invasive procedures and although much care is taken to achieve adequate levels of analgesia, this is frequently a problem (Anand and Porter 1998). One report estimated that infants aged 28–32 weeks PCA experience 2–10 invasive procedures per day (Johnston et al. 1997), while a previous study of 54 neonates recorded more than 3000 invasive procedures during the hospital stay (Barker and Rutter 1995). There is considerable concern that such early pain experiences may alter subsequent pain responses (Porter et al. 1999, Anand 2000) although clinical studies supporting this can be hard to interpret due to confounding factors such as gestational age at birth, length of intensive care stay, intensity of the stimulus and parenting style.

Neonatal circumcision is associated with increased pain responses during inoculation in 4–6-month-old infants and is partially reversed by the use of local anaesthetic (Taddio et al. 1997). In addition, extremely low-birth-weight infants (ELBW) are more likely to exhibit somatization (unexplained stomach aches, headaches or other complaints) than full-term infants at 4.5 years old although this has resolved at 8–10 years (Grunau et al. 1994). In a blinded study of referred abdominal hypersensitivity in infants with visceral pain, increased sensitivity was still present 3 months after corrective surgery (Andrews et al. 2002). However, other studies have reported unaltered or even decreased pain sensitivity in children previously exposed to repeated painful procedures (Oberlander et al. 2000) and further studies in this area are required.

While many of the nervous system responses to local tissue damage resolve after the injury is healed, tissue damage during a critical period in newborn rodents can cause prolonged alterations in somatosensory function into adult life.

The consequences of neonatal injury in rodents depend on the type of injury and the modality of sensation under investigation. Repetitive paw needle prick in the first postnatal week produces heat hyperalgesia several weeks later (Anand et al. 1999, Johnston and Walker 2003). Neonatal hindpaw inflammation has a pronounced effect on the behavioural and dorsal horn cellular response to a second inflammatory challenge well into adulthood (Ruda et al. 2000, Tachibana et al. 2001, Ren et al. 2004), but does not produce heat or mechanical hyperalgesia beyond the first week (Alvares et al. 2000, Walker et al. 2003). Chemical or mechanical irritation of the colon in P8–P21 rats, on the other hand produces a persistent visceral hypersensitivity in the adult (Al-Chaer et al. 2000). Skin wounds in the newborn also have prolonged effects: the skin remains hypersensitive long after the wound has healed (Reynolds and Fitzgerald 1995) and the size of the dorsal horn receptive field increases for at least six weeks (Torsney and Fitzgerald 2002).

Neonatal injury can also have the opposite effect. Both repetitive foot shock (Shimada et al. 1990) and repeated formalin injections into neonatal paws (Bhutta et al. 2001) lead to a generalized heat hypoalgesia in adulthood. Furthermore, hindpaw inflammation causes a generalized and slow-developing reduction in baseline sensitivity all over the body in response to mechanical and thermal stimuli that provides a background to the enhanced inflammatory responses described above (Ren et al. 2004). The early onset inflammatory hyperalgesia and the later onset baseline hypoalgesia only occur if the original inflammatory stimulus is applied within the first 10 days of life and both responses last into adulthood.

Although it is not known how these long-term changes in pain behaviours develop, candidate mechanisms might include alterations in synaptic connectivity and signalling in postnatal nociceptive pathways, and changes in the balance of inhibition versus excitation as described earlier.

Long-term hypoalgesia over the whole body is likely to arise from an alteration or resetting of the stress response (Ren et al. 2004), as exposure to stress during the perinatal period is known to influence adult nociceptive behaviour (d'Amore et al. 1995, Sternberg and Ridgway 2003). This could be viewed as a useful adaptive behaviour in response to early trauma. Any long-term sensitization that occurs at segmental level could be masked and require a strong stimulus such as reinflammation to uncover it.

Animal models offer an invaluable route to understanding and unravelling the role that early pain experience has in the long term. These studies have also highlighted the complexities of designing appropriate studies and their interpretation. The consequences of neonatal injury have been shown to be critically dependent upon the nature of the stimulus (Fitzgerald and Walker 2003).

The long-term alterations in pain behaviours following injury during a critical period of early neonatal life likely reflect plasticity in the anatomical, neurochemical and physiological characteristics of peripheral and central sensory pathways. Infant pain has traditionally been poorly understood and undertreated and much remains to be understood. Further study of the developmental neurobiology of the multiple mechanisms underlying pain processing can only lead to improvements in our understanding and future treatments specific to young infants.

REFERENCES

Agmon A, Yang LT, Jones EG, et al. (1995). Topological precision in the thalamic projection to neonatal mouse barrel cortex. J Neurosci 15: 549–561.

Al-Chaer ED, Kawasaki M, Pasricha PJ. (2000). A new model of chronic visceral hypersensitivity in adult rats induced by colon irritation during postnatal development Gastroenterology 119: 1276–1285.

Altman J, Bayer SA. (1984). The development of the rat spinal cord. Adv Anat Embryol Cell Biol 85: 1–164.

Alvares D, Torsney C, Beland B, et al. (2000). Modelling the prolonged effects of neonatal pain. Prog Brain Res 129: 365–373.

Anand KJS. (2000). Pain, plasticity and premature birth: a prescription for permanent suffering? Nat Med 6: 971–973.

Anand KJS, Porter FL. (1998). Epidemiology of pain in neonates. Res Clin Forums 20: 9–18.

Anand KJS, Coskun V, Thrivikraman KV, et al. (1999). Long-term behavioral effects of repetitive pain in neonatal rat pups. Physiol Behav 66: 627–637.

Anand P. (1992). Lack of chronic pain and autotomy in young children and rats after peripheral nerve injury: the basis of a new plasticity theory of chronic pain. J Neurol 239 Suppl 2: S12.

Anand P, Birch R. (2002). Restoration of sensory function and lack of long-term chronic pain syndromes after brachial plexus injury in human neonates. Brain 125: 113–122.

Andrews K, Fitzgerald M. (1994). The cutaneous withdrawal reflex in human neonates: sensitization, receptive fields and the effects of contralateral stimulation. Pain 56: 95–101.

Andrews K, Fitzgerald M. (2000). Flexion reflex responses in biceps femoris and tibialis anterior in human neonates. Early Hum Dev 57(2): 105–110.

Andrews K, Fitzgerald M. (2002). Wound sensitivity as a measure of analgesic effects following surgery in human neonates and infants. Pain 99: 185–195.

Andrews KA, Desai D, Dhillon HK, et al. (2002) Abdominal sensitivity in the first year of life: comparison of infants with and without prenatally-diagnosed unilateral hydronephrosis. Pain 100: 35–46.

Audinat E, Lambolez B, Rossier J, et al. (1994). Activity-dependent regulation of N-methyl-D-aspartate receptor subunit expression in rat cerebellar granule cells. Eur J Neurosci 6: 1792–1800.

Baba H, Doubell TP, Moore KA, et al. (2000). Silent NMDA receptor-mediated synapses are developmentally regulated in the dorsal horn of the rat spinal cord. J Neurophysiol 83: 955–962.

Baccei ML, Fitzgerald M. (2004). Development of GABAergic and glycinergic transmission in the neonatal rat dorsal horn. J Neurosci 24: 4749–4757.

Baccei ML, Bardoni R, Fitzgerald M. (2003). Development of nociceptive synaptic inputs to the neonatal rat dorsal horn: glutamate release by capsaicin and menthol. J Physiol 549: 231–242.

Bardoni R, Magherini PC, MacDermott AB. (1998). NMDA EPSCs at glutamanergic synapses in the spinal cord dorsal horn of the postnatal rat. J Neurosci 18: 6558–6567.

Bardoni R, Magherini PC, MacDermott AB. (2000). Activation of NMDA receptors drives action potentials in superficial dorsal horn from neonatal rats. Neuroreport 11: 1721–1727.

Barker DP, Rutter N. (1995). Exposure to invasive procedures in neonatal intensive care unit admissions. Arch Dis Child Fetal Neonatal Ed 72: F47–48.

Basbaum AI, Fields HL. (1978). Endogenous pain control mechanisms: review and hypothesis. Ann Neurol 4: 451–462.

Beggs S, Torsney C, Drew LJ, et al. (2002). The postnatal reorganization of primary afferent input and dorsal horn cell receptive fields in the rat spinal cord is an activity-dependent process. Eur J Neurosci 16: 1249–1258.

Beland B, Fitzgerald M. (2001a). Influence of peripheral inflammation on the postnatal maturation of primary sensory neuron phenotype in rats. J Pain 2: 36–45.

Beland B, Fitzgerald M. (2001b). Mu- and delta-opioid receptors are downregulated in the largest diameter primary sensory neurons during postnatal development in rats. Pain 90: 143–150.

Ben Ari Y. (2002). Excitatory actions of gaba during development: the nature of the nurture. Nat Rev Neurosci 3: 728–739.

Ben Ari Y, Cherubini E, Corradetti R, et al. (1989). Giant synaptic potentials in immature rat CA3 hippocampal neurones. J Physiol 416: 303–325.

Benn SC, Costigan M, Tate S, et al. (2001). Developmental expression of the TTX-resistant voltage-gated sodium channels Nav1.8 (SNS) and Nav1.9 (SNS2) in primary sensory neurons. J Neurosci 21: 6077–6085.

Berki AC, O'Donovan MJ, Antal M. (1995). Developmental expression of glycine immunoreactivity and its colocalization with GABA in the embryonic chick lumbosacral spinal cord. J Comp Neurol 362: 583–596.

Bhutta AT, Rovnaghi C, Simpson PM, et al. (2001). Interactions of inflammatory pain and morphine in infant rats: long-term behavioral effects. Physiol Behav 73: 51–58.

Bicknell HR, Beal JA. (1984). Axonal and dendritic development of substantia gelatinosa neurons in the lumbosacral spinal cord of the rat. J Comp Neurol 226: 508–522.

Boucher T, Jennings E, Fitzgerald M. (1998). The onset of diffuse noxious inhibitory controls in postnatal rat pups: a C-Fos study. Neurosci Lett 257: 9–12.

Cabana T, Martin GF. (1984). Developmental sequence in the origin of descending spinal pathways. Studies using retrograde transport techniques in the North American opossum (Didelphis virginiana). Brain Res 317: 247–263.

Cervero F, Plenderleith MB. (1985). C-fibre excitation and tonic descending inhibition of dorsal horn neurones in adult rats treated at birth with capsaicin. J Physiol 365: 223–237.

Chery N, de Koninck Y. (1999). Junctional versus extrajunctional glycine and GABA(A) receptor-mediated IPSCs in identified lamina I neurons of the adult rat spinal cord. J Neurosci 19: 7342–7355.

Coggeshall RE, Pover CM, Fitzgerald M. (1994). Dorsal root ganglion cell death and surviving cell numbers in relation to the development of sensory innervation in the rat hindlimb. Brain Res Dev Brain Res 82: 193–212.

Coggeshall RE, Jennings EA, Fitzgerald M. (1996) Evidence that large myelinated primary afferent fibers make synaptic contacts in lamina II of neonatal rats. Brain Res Dev Brain Res 92: 81–90.

Constantinou J, Reynolds ML, Woolf CJ, et al. (1994). Nerve growth factor levels in developing rat skin:

upregulation following skin wounding. Neuroreport 5: 2281–2284.

Craig KD, Whitfield MF, Grunau RV, et al. (1993). Pain in the preterm neonate: behavioural and physiological indices. Pain 52: 287–299. Erratum in: Pain 54: 111.

d'Amore A, Mazzucchelli A, Loizzo A. (1995). Long-term changes induced by neonatal handling in the nociceptive threshold and body weight in mice. Physiol Behav 57: 1195–1197.

De Lima J, Alvares D, Hatch DJ, et al. (1999). Sensory hyperinnervation after neonatal skin wounding: effect of bupivacaine sciatic nerve block. Br J Anaesth 83: 662–664.

Dickenson AH. (1994). The localization and mechanisms of action of opioids. Eksp Klin Farmakol 57: 3–12.

Dickenson AH. (1997). Excitatory amino acids and pain. In: Besson J-M, Dickenson AH (eds). Handbook of Experimental Pharmacology, Vol.130, pp. 173–176. The Pharmacology of Pain. Springer Verlag, Berlin.

Dickson BJ. (2002). Molecular mechanisms of axon guidance. Science 298: 1959–1964. Erratum in: Science (2003) 299: 515.

Dubuisson D, Dennis SG. (1977). The formalin test: a quantitative study of the analgesic effects of morphine, meperidine, and brain stem stimulation in rats and cats. Pain 4: 161–174.

Ekholm J. (1967). Postnatal changes in cutaneous reflexes and in the discharge pattern of cutaneous and articular sense organs: a morphological and physiological study in the cat. Acta Physiol Scand 297 [Suppl]: 1–130.

English KB, Burgess PR, Kavka-Van Norman D. (1980). Development of rat Merkel cells. J Comp Neurol 194: 475–496.

Falcon M, Guendellman D, Stolberg A, et al. (1996). Development of thermal nociception in rats. Pain 67: 203–208.

Fitzgerald M. (1985a). The post-natal development of cutaneous afferent fibre input and receptive field organization in the rat dorsal horn. J Physiol 364: 1–18.

Fitzgerald M. (1985b). The sprouting of saphenous nerve terminals in the spinal cord following early postnatal sciatic nerve section in the rat. J Comp Neurol 240: 407–413.

Fitzgerald M. (1987). Prenatal growth of fine-diameter primary afferents into the rat spinal cord: a transganglionic tracer study. J Comp Neurol 261: 98–104.

Fitzgerald M. (1988). The development of activity evoked by fine diameter cutaneous fibres in the spinal cord of the newborn rat. Neurosci Lett 86: 161–166.

Fitzgerald M, Fulton B. (1992). The physiological properties of developing sensory neurons. In: Scott SA, (ed). Sensory Neurons. pp. 287–306. Oxford UP, New York.

Fitzgerald M, Howard R. (2003). The neurobiological basis of pediatric pain. In: Schechter N, Berde C, Yaster M (eds). Pain in Children and Adolescents, 2nd Edn. pp. 19–42. Lippincott, Williams & Wilkins, Philadelphia.

Fitzgerald M, Jennings E. (1999). The postnatal development of spinal sensory processing. Proc Natl Acad Sci USA 96: 7719–7722.

Fitzgerald M, Koltzenburg M. (1986). The functional development of descending inhibitory pathways in the dorsolateral funiculus of the newborn rat spinal cord. Brain Res 389: 261–270.

Fitzgerald M, Shortland P. (1988). The effect of neonatal peripheral nerve section on the somadendritic growth of sensory projection cells in the rat spinal cord. Brain Res 470: 129–136.

Fitzgerald M, Swett J. (1983). The termination pattern of sciatic nerve afferents in the substantia gelatinosa of neonatal rats. Neurosci Lett 43: 149–154.

Fitzgerald M, Walker S. (2003). The role of activity in developing pain pathways. In: Dostrovsky JO, Carr DB, Koltzenburg M (eds).Vol. 24. Proceedings of the 10th World Congress on Pain. Progress in Pain Research and Management. IASP Press, Seattle, Washington DC.

Fitzgerald M, King AE, Thompson SW, et al. (1987). The postnatal development of the ventral root reflex in the rat; a comparative in vivo and in vitro study. Neurosci Lett 78: 41–45.

Fitzgerald M, Shaw A, MacIntosh N. (1988). Postnatal development of the cutaneous flexor reflex: comparative study of preterm infants and newborn rat pups. Dev Med Child Neurol 30: 520–526.

Fitzgerald M, Millard C, McIntosh N. (1989). Cutaneous hypersensitivity following peripheral tissue damage in newborn infants and its reversal with topical anaesthesia. Pain 39: 31–36.

Fitzgerald M, Woolf CJ, Shortland P. (1990). Collateral sprouting of the central terminals of cutaneous primary afferent neurons in the rat spinal cord: pattern, morphology, and influence of targets. J Comp Neurol 300: 370–385.

Fitzgerald M, Reynolds ML, Benowitz LL. (1991). GAP-43 expression in the developing rat lumbar spinal cord. Neuroscience 41: 187–199.

Fitzgerald M, Butcher T, Shortland P. (1994). Developmental changes in the laminar termination of A fibre cutaneous sensory afferents in the rat spinal cord dorsal horn. J Comp Neurol 348: 225–233.

Gasnier B. (2000). The loading of neurotransmitters into synaptic vesicles. Biochimie 82: 327–337.

Gebhart GF. (2004). Descending modulation of pain. Neurosci Biobehav Rev 27: 729–737.

Gilbert M, Stelzner DJ. (1979). The development of descending and dorsal root connections in the lumbosacral spinal cord of the postnatal rat. J Comp Neurol 184: 821–838.

Grunau RV, Craig KD. (1987). Pain expression in neonates: facial action and cry. Pain 28: 395–410.

Grunau RV, Johnston CC, Craig KD. (1990). Neonatal facial and cry responses to invasive and non-invasive procedures. Pain 42: 295–305.

Grunau RV, Whitfield MF, Petrie JH, et al. (1994). Early pain experience, child and family factors, as precursors of somatization: a prospective study of extremely premature and full term children. Pain 56: 353–359.

Guo A, Simone DA, Stone LS, et al. (2001). Developmental shift of vanilloid receptor 1 (VR1) terminals into deeper regions of the superficial dorsal horn: correlation with a shift from TrkA to Ret expression by dorsal root ganglion neurons. Eur J Neurosci 14: 293–304.

Guy ER, Abbott FV. (1992). The behavioral response to formalin in preweanling rats. Pain 51: 81–90.

Higashi S, Molnar Z, Kurotani T, et al. (2002). Prenatal development of neural excitation in rat thalamocortical projections studied by optical recording. Neuroscience 115: 1231–1246.

Hori Y, Kanda K. (1994). Developmental alterations in NMDA receptor-mediated [Ca2+]i elevation in substantia gelatinosa neurons of neonatal rat spinal cord. Brain Res Dev Brain Res 80: 141–148.

Howard R, Walker S, Mota P, et al. (2005). The ontogeny of neuropathic pain: postnatal onset of mechanical allodynia in rat spared nerve injury (SNI) and chronic constriction injury (CCI) models. Pain 115: 382–389.

Howard RF, Hatch DJ, Cole TJ, et al. (2001). Inflammatory pain and hypersensitivity are selectively reversed by epidural bupivacaine and are developmentally regulated. Anesthesiology 95: 421–427.

Jackman, A, Fitzgerald, M. (2000). The development of peripheral hindlimb and central spinal cord innervation by subpopulations of dorsal root ganglion cells in the embryonic rat. J Comp Neurol 418: 281–298.

Jakowec MW, Yen L, Kalb RG. (1995). In situ hybridization analysis of AMPA receptor subunit gene expression in the developing rat spinal cord. Neuroscience 67: 909–920.

Jennings E, Fitzgerald M. (1996). C-fos can be induced in the neonatal rat spinal cord by both noxious and innocuous peripheral stimulation. Pain 68: 301–306.

Jennings E, Fitzgerald M. (1998). Postnatal changes in responses of rat dorsal horn cells to afferent stimulation: a fibre-induced sensitization. J Physiol 509: 859–868.

Jiang MC, Gebhart GF. (1998). Development of mustard oil-induced hyperalgesia in rats. Pain 77: 305–313.

Johnston CC, Walker CD. (2003). The effects of exposure to repeated minor pain during the neonatal period on formalin pain behaviour and thermal withdrawal latencies. Pain Res Manag 8: 213–217.

Johnston CC, Stevens B, Craig KD, et al. (1993). Developmental changes in pain expression in premature, full-term, two- and four-month-old infants. Pain 52: 201–208.

Johnston CC, Stevens BJ, Yang F, et al. (1995). Differential response to pain by very premature neonates. Pain 61: 471–479.

Johnston CC, Collinge JM, Henderson SJ, et al. (1997). A cross-sectional survey of pain and pharmacological analgesia in Canadian neonatal intensive care units. Clin J Pain 13: 308–312.

Jonas P, Bischofberger J, Sandkuhler J. (1998). Corelease of two fast neurotransmitters at a central synapse. Science 281: 419–424.

Kalb RG, Fox AJ. (1997). Synchronized overproduction of AMPA, kainate, and NMDA glutamate receptors during human spinal cord development. J Comp Neurol 384: 200–210.

Kar S, Quirion R. (1995). Neuropeptide receptors in developing and adult rat spinal cord: an in vitro quantitative autoradiography study of calcitonin gene-related peptide, neurokinins, mu-opioid, galanin, somatostatin, neurotensin and vasoactive intestinal polypeptide receptors. J Comp Neurol 354: 253–281.

Keller AF, Coull JA, Chery N, et al. (2001). Region-specific developmental specialization of GABA-glycine cosynapses in laminas I-II of the rat spinal dorsal horn. J Neurosci 21: 7871–7880.

Khazipov R, Leinekugel X, Khalilov I, et al. (1997). Synchronization of GABAergic interneuronal network in CA3 subfield of neonatal rat hippocampal slices. J Physiol 498: 763–772.

Kirstein M, Farinas I. (2002). Sensing life: regulation of sensory neuron survival by neurotrophins. Cell Mol Life Sci 59: 1787–1802.

Kitao Y, Robertson B, Kudo M, et al. (1996). Neurogenesis of subpopulations of rat lumbar dorsal root ganglion neurons including neurons projecting to the dorsal column nuclei. J Comp Neurol 371: 249–257.

Klimach VJ, Cooke RW. (1988). Maturation of the neonatal somatosensory evoked response in preterm infants. Dev Med Child Neurol 30: 208–214.

Koltzenburg M. (1999). The changing sensitivity in the life of the nociceptor. Pain Suppl 6: S93–102.

Krane EJ, Heller LB. (1995). The prevalence of phantom sensation and pain in pediatric amputees. J Pain Symptom Manage 10: 21–29.

Lee DH, Chung JM. (1996). Neuropathic pain in neonatal rats. Neurosci Lett 209: 140–142.

Leong SK. (1983). Localizing the corticospinal neurons in neonatal, developing and mature albino rat. Brain Res 265: 1–9.

Lev DL, Weinfeld E, White EL. (2002). Synaptic patterns of thalamocortical afferents in mouse barrels at postnatal day 11. J Comp Neurol 442: 63–77.

Lewin GR, Ritter AM, Mendell LM. (1993). Nerve growth factor-induced hyperalgesia in the neonatal and adult rat. J Neurosci 13: 2136–2148.

Li P, Zhuo M. (1998). Silent glutamatergic synapses and nociception in mammalian spinal cord. Nature 393: 695–698.

Ling QD, Chien CC, Wen YR, et al. (2003). The pattern and distribution of calcitonin gene-related peptide (CGRP) terminals in the rat dorsal following neonatal peripheral inflammation. Neuroreport 14: 1919–1921.

Ma W, Behar T, Barker JL. (1992). Transient expression of GABA immunoreactivity in the developing rat spinal cord. J Comp Neurol 325: 271–290.

Ma Q, Fode C, Guillemot F, et al. (1999). Neurogenin1 and neurogenin2 control two distinct waves of neurogenesis in developing dorsal root ganglia. Genes Dev 13: 1717–1728.

Marsh D, Dickenson A, Hatch D, et al. (1999). Epidural opioid analgesia in infant rats I: mechanical and heat responses. Pain 82: 23–32.

Nakatsuka T, Ataka T, Kumamoto E, et al. (2000). Alteration in synaptic inputs through C-afferent fibers to substantia gelatinosa neurons of the rat spinal dorsal horn during postnatal development. Neuroscience 99: 549–556.

Nandi R, Beacham D, Middleton J, et al. (2004). The functional expression of mu opioid receptors on sensory neurons is developmentally regulated; morphine analgesia is less selective in the neonate. Pain 111: 38–50.

Oberlander TF, Grunau RE, Whitfield MF, et al. (2000). Biobehavioral pain responses in former extremely low birth weight infants at four months' corrected age. Pediatrics 105: e6.

Oberlander TF, Grunau RE, Fitzgerald C, et al. (2002). Does parenchymal brain injury affect biobehavioral pain responses in very low birth weight infants at 32 weeks' postconceptional age? Pediatrics 110: 570–576.

Oliveira AL, Risling M, Deckner M, et al. (1997). Neonatal sciatic nerve transection induces TUNEL labeling of neurons in the rat spinal cord and DRG. Neuroreport 8: 2837–2840.

Ozaki S, Snider WD. (1997). Initial trajectories of sensory axons toward laminar targets in the developing mouse spinal cord. J Comp Neurol 380: 215–229.

Park JS, Nakatsuka T, Nagata K, et al. (1999). Reorganization of the primary afferent termination in the rat spinal dorsal horn during post-natal development. Brain Res Dev Brain Res 113: 29–36.

Pattinson D, Fitzgerald M. (2004). The neurobiology of infant pain: development of excitatory and inhibitory neurotransmission in the spinal dorsal horn. Reg Anesth Pain Med 29: 36–44.

Payne J, Middleton J, Fitzgerald M. (1991). The pattern and timing of cutaneous hair follicle innervation in the rat pup and human fetus. Brain Res Dev Brain Res 61: 173–182.

Philpot BD, Sekhar AK, Shouval HZ, et al. (2001). Visual experience and deprivation bidirectionally modify the composition and function of NMDA receptors in visual cortex. Neuron 29: 157–169.

Pignatelli D, Ribeiro-da-Silva A, Coimbra A. (1989). Postnatal maturation of primary afferent terminations in the substantia gelatinosa of the rat spinal cord. An electron microscopic study. Brain Res 491: 33–44.

Porter FL, Grunau RE, Anand KJ. (1999). Long-term effects of pain in infants. J Dev Behav Pediatr 20: 253–261.

Rahman W, Dashwood MR, Fitzgerald M, et al. (1998). Postnatal development of multiple opioid receptors in the spinal cord and development of spinal morphine analgesia. Brain Res Dev Brain Res 108: 239–254.

Rebsam A, Seif I, Gaspar P. (2002). Refinement of thalamocortical arbors and emergence of barrel domains in the primary somatosensory cortex: a study of normal and monoamine oxidase a knock-out mice. J Neurosci 22: 8541–8552.

Reichling DB, Kyrozis A, Wang J, et al. (1994). Mechanisms of GABA and glycine depolarization-induced calcium transients in rat dorsal horn neurons. J Physiol 476: 411–421.

Ren K, Dubner R. (2002). Descending modulation in persistent pain: an update. Pain 100: 1–6.

Ren K, Anseloni V, Zou SP, et al. (2004). Characterization of basal and re-inflammation-associated long-term alteration in pain responsivity following short-lasting neonatal local inflammatory insult. Pain 110: 588–596.

Reynolds ML, Fitzgerald M. (1992). Neonatal sciatic nerve section results in thiamine monophosphate but not substance P or calcitonin gene-related peptide depletion from the terminal field in the dorsal horn of the rat: the role of collateral sprouting. Neuroscience 51: 191–202.

Reynolds ML, Fitzgerald M. (1995). Long-term sensory hyperinnervation following neonatal skin wounds. J Comp Neurol 358: 487–498.

Ruda MA, Ling QD, Hohmann AG, et al. (2000). Altered nociceptive neuronal circuits after neonatal peripheral inflammation. Science 289: 628–631.

Schaffner AE, Behar T, Nadi S, et al. (1993). Quantitative analysis of transient GABA expression in embryonic and early postnatal rat spinal cord neurons. Brain Res Dev Brain Res 72: 265–276. Erratum in: Brain Res Dev Brain Res 1993: 295.

Schouenborg J. (2003). Somatosensory imprinting in spinal reflex modules. J Rehabil Med 41 Suppl: 73–80.

Serafini R, Valeyev AY, Barker JL, et al. (1995). Depolarizing GABA-activated Cl- channels in embryonic rat spinal and olfactory bulb cells. J Physiol 488: 371–386.

Shimada C, Kurumiya S, Noguchi Y, et al. (1990). The effect of neonatal exposure to chronic footshock on pain-responsiveness and sensitivity to morphine after maturation in the rat. Behav Brain Res 36: 105–111.

Shortland P, Fitzgerald M. (1994). Neonatal sciatic nerve section results in a rearrangement of the central terminals of saphenous and axotomized sciatic nerve afferents in the dorsal horn of the spinal cord of the adult rat. Eur J Neurosci 6: 75–86.

Somogyi R, Wen X, Ma W, et al. (1995). Developmental kinetics of GAD family mRNAs parallel neurogenesis in the rat spinal cord. J Neurosci 15: 2575–2591.

Sternberg WF, Ridgway CG. (2003). Effects of gestational stress and neonatal handling on pain, analgesia, and stress behavior of adult mice. Physiol Behav 78: 375–383.

Stevens BJ, Johnston CC, Horton L. (1994). Factors that influence the behavioral pain response of premature infants. Pain 59: 101–109.

Tachibana T, Ling QD, Ruda MA. (2001). Increased Fos induction in adult rats that experienced neonatal peripheral inflammation. Neuroreport 12: 925–927.

Taddio A, Katz J, Ilersich AL, et al. (1997). Effect of neonatal circumcision on pain response during subsequent routine vaccination. Lancet 349: 599–603.

Teng CJ, Abbott FV. (1998). The formalin test: a dose-response analysis at three developmental stages. Pain 76: 337–347.

Todd AJ, Spike RC. (1993). The localization of classical transmitters and neuropeptides within neurons in laminae I-III of the mammalian spinal dorsal horn. Prog Neurobiol 41: 609–645.

Torsney C, Fitzgerald M. (2002). Age-dependent effects of peripheral inflammation on the electro-physiological properties of neonatal rat dorsal horn neurons. J Neurophysiol 87: 1311–1317.

Torsney C, Meredith-Middleton J, Fitzgerald M. (2000). Neonatal capsaicin treatment prevents the normal postnatal withdrawal of A fibres from lamina II without affecting fos responses to innocuous peripheral stimulation. Brain Res Dev Brain Res 121: 55–65.

van Praag H, Frenk H. (1991). The development of stimulation-produced analgesia (SPA) in the rat. Brain Res Dev Brain Res 64: 71–76.

Waldenstrom A, Thelin J, Thimansson E, et al. (2003). Developmental learning in a pain-related system: evidence for a cross-modality mechanism. J Neurosci 23: 7719–7725.

Walker SM, Meredith-Middleton J, Cooke-Yarborough C, et al. (2003). Neonatal inflammation and primary afferent terminal plasticity in the rat dorsal horn. Pain 105: 185–195.

Wang J, Reichling DB, Kyrozis A, et al. (1994). Developmental loss of GABA- and glycine-induced depolarization and Ca2+ transients in embryonic rat dorsal horn neurons in culture. Eur J Neurosci 6: 1275–1280.

Whiteside G, Doyle CA, Hunt SP, et al. (1998). Differential time course of neuronal and glial apoptosis in neonatal rat dorsal root ganglia after sciatic nerve axotomy. Eur J Neurosci 10: 3400–3408.

Williams DG, Dickenson A, Fitzgerald M, et al. (2004). Developmental regulation of codeine analgesia in the rat. Anesthesiology 100: 92–97.

Zirlinger M, Lo L, McMahon J, et al. (2002). Transient expression of the bHLH factor neurogenin-2 marks a subpopulation of neural crest cells biased for a sensory but not a neuronal fate. Proc Natl Acad Sci USA 99: 8084–8089.

3 Development of supraspinal pain processing

K J S Anand
Elie D Al-Chaer
Adnan T Bhutta
Richard Whit Hall

OVERVIEW OF SUPRASPINAL PAIN PROCESSING

Accumulating evidence over the past 40 years has discarded the Cartesian view of pain as a 'hard-wired' system, which transmits pain impulses along peripheral sensory nerves, spinothalamic and thalamocortical pathways, to the somatosensory cortex (Lee et al. 2005). Beginning from the Gate Control Theory of pain (Melzack and Wall 1965) and substantiated by multiple lines of clinical and neurophysiological data (Nathan and Rudge 1974, Dickenson 2002, Defrin et al. 2005), the pain system is now viewed as a dynamic, inter-active system creating an interoceptive view of body integrity. Pain perception involves multilayered networks of nociceptors, nerve fibres, neurons and glia, distributed in multiple spinal and supraspinal areas, forming diverse feed-back and feed-forward loops, whereby the participation, function and neuro-chemical profiles of these cellular elements are constantly modified by external and internal cues (Price 2000, Woolf and Salter 2000). Signalling of pain at any stage of development depends not only on the context and characteristics of the painful stimulus, but also on the behavioural state and cognitive demands at that time (Price 2000).

Current pain research shows that the neonate or infant is not a 'little adult', that the structures and mechanisms used for pain processing during early development are unique and different from those used for adult pain processing, and that many of these structures or mechanisms are not maintained beyond specific periods of early development (Narsinghani and Anand 2000, Fitzgerald 2005). The immature pain system thus plays a signalling role during each stage of development and uses neural elements available at that time to fulfil this role (Glover and Fisk 1996). The lack of pain-specific thalamocortical connections in the fetus or preterm neonate was used to argue against pain perception in early development (Lee et al. 2005). This is a simplistic line of reasoning, which ignores clinical data showing that ablation or stimulation of the somatosensory cortex does not alter pain perception in adults, whereas that of the thalamus does (Nandi et al. 2002, 2003, Craig 2003a, Brooks et al. 2005). Supraspinal pain processing and regulation of the spinal–brainstem–spinal loops that mediate descend-ing facilitation or inhibition very likely depend on distributed activity in cortical and subcortical areas (Craig 2003b, 2003c).

PAIN PROCESSING IN THE BRAINSTEM

Areas of the brainstem provide the first supraspinal integration of visceral and somatic nociceptive signals from the spinal cord, receive input directly from the trigeminal, vagal and glossopharyngeal sensory systems, mediate homeostatic changes in bodily functions associated with pain, while receiving active regulatory inputs in real time from cortical, subcortical and thalamic areas. Pain processing may be described in the medullary, pontine and midbrain centres, with minimal or no information during the different stages of fetal, neonatal and infant development. Although some of these areas are beginning to be studied during development, most of the information below has been collated from studies in adult humans and rats. Ascending and descending pathways from brainstem loci to the spinal dorsal horn are summarized in Figure 3.1.

Medulla

Development of the medullary nuclei
By the fifth week of gestation, fusion of the dorsal lips of the neural plate results in the formation of three primary cerebral vesicles, the most caudal of which

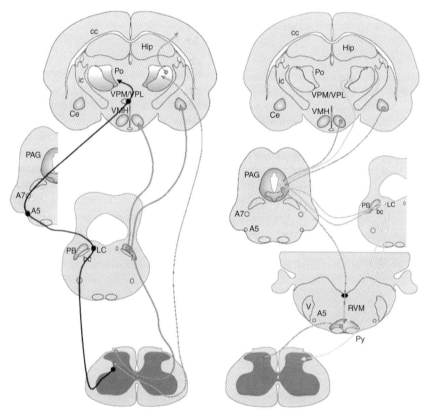

Figure 3.1 Supraspinal pathways ascending from (left panel) and descending to (right panel) the spinal dorsal horn: *Ascending pain pathways* include the spinothalamic pathway (light), spinoparabrachial pathway (darker), and spinoreticular pathway (black). Spinothalamic pathways distribute nociceptive information to the ventral thalamus and cortical areas mediating attention, discrimination and affect. Spinoparabrachial pathways mainly originate from the superficial dorsal horn and connect with various nuclei in the parabrachial complex, which are mainly associated with emotional affect, emotional behaviour and autonomic controls. Other ascending pathways and nerve tracts are not shown to maintain clarity. *Descending pain pathways* originate from the limbic system (amygdala), medial and posterior thalamus, and periventricular hypothalamus and mostly converge in the midbrain periaqueductal grey (PAG). Neurons from the ventrolateral PAG project to the parabrachial complex, locus coeruleus and the rostral ventromedial medulla (RVM) to mediate the modulatory, antinociceptive and autonomic responses following painful stimulation. Most projections from the brainstem to the spinal dorsal horn are bilateral, although only unilateral connections are shown for the sake of clarity. (A, adrenergic nucleus; bc, brachium conjunctivum; cc, corpus callosum; Ce, central nucleus of the amygdala; Hip, hippocampus; ic, internal capsule; LC, locus coeruleus; PB, parabrachial area; Po, posterior group of thalamic nuclei; Py, pyramidal tract; RVM, rostral ventromedial medulla; V, ventricle; VMH, ventral medial nucleus of the hypothalamus; VPL, ventral posteriolateral nucleus of the thalamus; VPM, ventral posteriomedial nucleus of the thalamus.)

is the rhombencephalon or hindbrain. This is marked by two ventral folds, the midbrain flexure rostrally and the cervical flexure caudally. The rhombencephalon then develops a dorsal fold called the pontine flexure, which divides it into the lower myelencephalon developing into the medulla oblongata and the upper metencephalon, from which both the cerebellum and the pons will develop. Like the spinal cord, limiting sulci also divide the lateral walls of the hindbrain and midbrain into the dorsolateral and ventrolateral laminae, the cell columns which correspond to the dorsal and ventral horns of the spinal cord and primarily give rise to the sensory and motor nuclei respectively. By the tenth week of gestation, cell columns of the dorsolateral lamina are interrupted and displaced by differential growth patterns, by the appearance and growth of fibre tracts and by active neuronal migration, to form the general visceral afferent nuclei (e.g., dorsal vagal nucleus), special visceral afferent nuclei (e.g., nucleus of the tractus soltarius), and general somatic afferent nuclei (e.g., the trigeminal nuclei), all of which are involved in pain processing. With this neuronal migration, the thin ventral lamina is invaded by decussating fibre tracts and neuroblasts and thickens to form the median and dorsal raphe. The lower half of the myelencephalon takes no part in forming the fourth ventricle, therefore its development closely resembles the spinal cord, where the dorsolateral lamina forms the nuclei gracilis et cuneatus, the medullary reticular nuclei and the raphe magnus nucleus. For detailed analyses of these early developmental events, anatomical studies have been correlated with ultrafast magnetic resonance imaging (MRI) and cranial ultrasonography during fetal and neonatal life (Pigadas et al. 1981, Muller and O'Rahilly 1997, Stazzone et al. 2000).

Rostral ventromedial medulla (RVM)

The RVM is a major component of the pain modulatory circuitry, exerting inhibitory and facilitatory effects on pain neurotransmission, in addition to relaying the modulatory effects from higher brainstem sites, such as the periaqueductal grey (PAG) and locus coeruleus (LC). This region of the medulla includes the midline nucleus raphe magnus (NRM), the medullary reticular formation, dorsal raphe nucleus, lateral reticular nucleus (LRN), nucleus reticularis gigantocellularis pars alpha (GiA) and the nucleus paragigantocellularis lateralis (LPGi). Bilateral nociception-specific neurons exhibit graded responses to increasing bladder or colorectal distension, suggesting a convergence of visceral sensory information in the lateral reticular nucleus (LRN) (Robbins et al. 2005). Efferent projections from the RVM extend bilaterally to all levels of the spinal dorsal horn, with collateralized and lamina-specific projections to laminae I, II and V. The RVM mediates key inhibitory effects following acute pain and facilitates spinal pain transmission in models of chronic pain. Among RVM neurons recorded in vivo, ON cells show action potentials just prior to a tail flick (pronociceptive activity), whereas OFF cells pause just prior to the tail flick (antinociceptive or analgesic) (Fields 2004). These functions are not specific for pain, but, for example, may also mediate the control of micturition (Baez et al. 2005).

Persistent nociception simultaneously triggers descending facilitation and inhibition from the RVM. In models of inflammation, sensory input from inflamed tissue promotes descending inhibition to attenuate primary hyperalgesia, while inputs from neighbouring tissues promote descending facilitation, thus accentuating secondary hyperalgesia (Vanegas and Schaible 2004). Mechanisms for hyperalgesia include the supraspinal effects of prostaglandins on the midbrain PAG, which expresses prostanoid receptors and synthetic enzymes. Thus, PGE(2) microinjection into the ventrolateral PAG or medial preoptic region (MPO) activated the ON cells and suppressed the firing of OFF cells in the RVM, to mediate descending facilitation (Heinricher et al. 2004a, 2004b). The (primary) hyperalgesia and allodynia of neuropathic pain are also mediated from the RVM, with the inhibition of secondary neuronal pools connected to the PAG, direct or indirect inhibition of RVM OFF cells by κ-opioid agonists (Meng et al. 2005) and the activation of N-type and P/Q-type calcium channels (Urban et al. 2005) in the RVM.

In contrast, μ-opioid agonists activate the OFF cells to mediate descending inhibitory inputs to the spinal dorsal horn (Fields 2000, 2004). There is anatomical and behavioural evidence also that neurotensin activates NTR1-expressing RVM neurons to produce antinociception through release of serotonin in the spinal dorsal horn (Buhler et al. 2005). RVM neurons are relatively resistant to the development of μ-opioid tolerance compared to PAG neurons. For example, repeated microinjections of morphine into the PAG produce a 64% decrease in hot plate latency, but only a 36% drop in latency following RVM microinjections (Morgan et al. 2005). Microinfusion of a cannabinoid (CB1) agonist into the RVM reduced the tail flick-related ON-cell burst, decreased the duration of the OFF-cell pause and increased OFF-cell ongoing activity, to mediate the analgesic effects of cannabinoids (Meng and Johansen 2004).

Dorsal raphe nucleus (DRN)/nucleus raphe magnus (NRM)

Neurons in the DRN and NRM are critically involved in opioid-induced analgesia (Fields 2004) and respond to visceral stimuli (Brink and Mason 2004). The electrophysiological properties of raphe neurons classify them into two general types, primary cells lacking the μ-opioid receptor and secondary cells expressing the μ receptor (Pan et al. 1990). Exposure to opioids, however, inhibits GABAergic synaptic transmission in the primary cells, with opioid analgesia produced by activating primary cells that send descending inhibitory projections to the spinal dorsal horn (Pan et al. 1997). Secondary (opioidergic) NRM neurons also have facilitatory actions on spinal pain transmission through their descending projections (Pan et al. 2000, Porreca et al. 2002, Fields 2004). Thus, both activation of pain-inhibiting primary cells and inhibition of pain-facilitating secondary cells in the NRM may be involved in opioid-induced analgesia. Accumulating evidence shows that the μ receptor-containing cells in the DRN/NRM are also activated in chronic pain conditions associated with hyperalgesia and allodynia (McNally 1999, Porreca et al. 2002, Gebhart 2004). Nociceptin/orphanin FQ (N/OFQ), the endogenous ligand of opioid-like receptor 1 (ORL1), also plays an important role in neuropathic pain. In the chronic constriction injury (CCI) model of neuropathic pain, significant increases in ORL1 mRNA expression occurred in the NRM and DRN, and in the ventrolateral PAG, from 7 to 21 days after injury, the peak period of neuropathic pain (Ma et al. 2005).

Neurochemical lesions of the LC or DRN induce decreases in postictal analgesia, suggesting the involvement of these nuclei in stress-induced analgesia (Freitas et al. 2005). Intraoral sucrose activates neurons in the PAG, the NRM and the DRN, brainstem sites critically involved in descending pain modulation (Anseloni et al. 2005, Miyase et al. 2005). Blockade of postsynaptic serotonergic receptors in the DRN decreased the sucrose-induced analgesia, whereas presynaptic receptor blockade had no effects, indicating that analgesic effects are mediated via descending serotonergic pathways to the dorsal horn (Miyase et al. 2005). The activity of serotonergic neurons in the DRN also increase following peripheral inflammation, which was reversed by blockade of peripheral (but not DRN) mGlu(5) receptors (Palazzo et al. 2004). Thus, peripheral glutamatergic inputs from inflamed tissues may activate these descending serotonergic pathways.

Nucleus tractus solitarius (NTS)

Most of the visceral afferent input seems to converge on the NTS and dorsal vagal nucleus in the medullary centres. These loci are critically involved in descending inhibitory and facilitatory loops to the spinal dorsal horn, autonomic responses to visceral stimulation,

and the phenomena of referred pain and viscerosomatic hyperalgesia. Some evidence for viscerotopic specificity within the NTS exists, although there is considerable overlap. Thus, noxious stimuli indicating myocardial ischaemia project to the caudal NTS (Hua et al. 2004), whereas noxious gastric distension or irritation activates the medial NTS neurons (Liu et al. 2004a). It is interesting that somatic inputs from acupuncture points on the face, which are effective against gastric pain, also project to the medial NTS (Liu et al. 2004a). Moreover, a subpopulation of NTS projection neurons that respond to visceral stimuli may receive somatostatinergic inputs of peripheral, local or supraspinal origins (Gamboa-Esteves et al. 2004). Exposure to previous stress increased neuronal activation in the NTS (with weaker effects in the central nucleus of the amygdala) in response to visceral distension, indicating altered visceral afferent processing in previously stressed rats (de Lange et al. 2005). These long-term effects on NTS signaling may provide an alternative explanation for the long-term effects of gastric suctioning at birth on the prevalence of irritable bowel syndrome during later life (Anand et al. 2004).

Trigeminal nuclear complex

The trigeminal nuclei extend from the spinal sensory nucleus in the medulla and cervical spinal cord, to the principal sensory nucleus in the pons and the mesencephalic nucleus in the midbrain, and have been the focus of intense investigation for orofacial/dental pain. Central sensitization occurs in trigeminal nociceptive pathways, with more robust neuronal hyperexcitability following deep tissue stimulation than cutaneous stimulation. Two distinct regions are activated in the trigeminal sensory nuclei, the subnuclei interpolaris/caudalis transition zone (Vi/Vc) and subnucleus caudalis (Vc). The ventral pole of the Vi/Vc is involved in nociceptive sensory processing from deep tissues, but also in somatovisceral and somatoautonomic processing, activation of the HPA axis, and descending modulation of pain, whereas the Vc is very similar to the spinal dorsal horn, mediating the sensory discriminative aspects of pain (Dubner and Ren 2004). Lamina I neurons in the trigeminal complex project to the thalamic and parabrachial nuclei and express μ-opioid receptors, being the sites of action for opiates that modulate the sensory and/or autonomic aspects of orofacial pain (Mitchell et al. 2004). Many neurons from the ventral Vi/Vc transition zone project to the nucleus submedius of the thalamus (40%), whereas neurons from the caudal Vc and dorsal Vi/Vc project to the pontine parabrachial complex (PBC) (Ikeda et al. 2003).

Early development of pain signalling in trigeminal nuclei is critical, because many painful stimuli experienced by preterm neonates in the orofacial area (Simons et al. 2003) are transmitted to the Vc through the release of glutamate and/or substance P (SP). Newborn mice, corresponding to 23–28-week preterm neonates, showed high densities of SP-positive structures in the marginal (superficial) and magnocellular (deep) layers of Vc. SP staining in the superficial Vc remained unchanged, but decreased with age in the deep layers, with complete absence by 4 weeks of age. Neurokinin 1 receptors (NK1R) exhibited similar distribution patterns to that of SP and remained unchanged during the postnatal period (Aita et al. 2005). Using both extracellular field potential and whole-cell patch-clamp recordings in the superficial layers of Vc in juvenile rats, recent experiments found evidence for long-term potentiation (LTP) via activation of mGluR5. Activation of these receptors triggered a PLC/PKC-dependent signalling cascade, leading to the induction of LTP in primary afferent neurons in the trigeminal (Liang et al. 2005). These LTP mechanisms may contribute to the 'oral aversion syndrome' noted in ex-preterm infants who were exposed to frequent noxious orofacial stimuli during their NICU care.

Pons

The pons develops in the metencephalon, from rhombomeres in the region of the pontine flexure. Ventricular, intermediate and marginal zones are formed at this flexure and the nuclei of the trigeminal, abducens and facial nerves develop in the mantle layer. The grey matter of the formatio reticularis is derived from the ventrolateral lamina, whereas that of the nuclei pontis and locus coeruleus is derived from the dorsolateral lamina by the active migration of neurons from the rhombic lip. The latter origin of these nuclei endows them with mainly sensory functions, with inputs from visceral, autonomic and somatic afferents (Pigadas et al. 1981, Muller and O'Rahilly 1997, Stazzone et al. 2000).

The importance of pontine processing in sensory perception has been under appreciated in the past, but is becoming more evident from clinical examples such as the impairment of spinothalamic pain sensations following a paramedian pontine infarction (Cerrato et al. 2005), abnormal activations of the dorsal pons in patients with visceral pain due to irritable bowel syndrome or those associated with the laterality of migraine headaches (Afridi et al. 2005, Mayer et al. 2005). Differences between ascending projections, originating from the superficial versus deep laminae of the spinal dorsal horn, suggest different types of pain processing in the pons.

Parabrachial complex (PBC)

Spinal projections from lamina I of the dorsal horn make connections with the lateral parabrachial area, from where neurons in the PBC project to the amygdala, hypothalamus, PAG and ventrolateral medulla (VLM) (Gauriau and Bernard 2002). Neurons in the Kolliker-Fuse, lateral crescent, and superior lateral subnuclei of the PBC are connected with medullary respiratory centres and mediate the respiratory activation by acute noxious stimuli (Jiang et al. 2004). Pain-responsive neurons in the external lateral PBC also project to the amygdala, providing inputs for the emotional aspects of pain. Visceral and humoral stimuli cause widespread activation of these parabrachio-amygdaloid neurons, suggesting their involvement in the emotional and homeostatic aspects of pain (Richard et al. 2005). Thus, the lamina I–parabrachial projections mediate the emotional, autonomic and neuroendocrine features of painful stimulation, connecting with key areas of the brain that control the emotional affect (amygdala), emotional behaviour (PAG), and the autonomic adaptation (hypothalamus and VLM) to pain.

Pontine reticular formation

In contrast to lamina I projections, deep laminae of the spinal dorsal horn project to the reticular formation in the caudal pons (including lateral reticular nucleus (LRN), subnucleus reticularis dorsalis (SRD), gigantocellular/lateral paragigantocellular reticular nuclei (NGc), and parabrachial internal lateral subnucleus (PBil)) (Gauriau and Bernard 2002). From their projections, pontine reticular neurons appear to be involved in somatic motor responses, feedback regulation of nociceptive transmission (through a reticulo–spinal loop), arousal and emotional features of pain via medial thalamic and prefrontal cortical connections.

Locus coeruleus/sub-coeruleus (LC/SC)

Noradrenergic neurons in the LC/SC also participate in the descending inhibition of pain via a coeruleo-spinal pathway located in the ventrolateral funiculus (VLF); these axons cross the midline at spinal segmental levels to connect with dorsal horn laminae (I, II, V) inhibiting nociceptive transmission at or remote from the site of injury (Tsuruoka et al. 2004a, 2004b). LC neurons are activated by acute or inflammatory pain, or acute stress-producing analgesia, whereas chronic stress suppresses LC activity to produce hyperalgesia (Imbe et al. 2004, Freitas et al. 2005, Sajedianfard et al. 2005). Corticotropin-releasing factor (CRF) from the paraventricular nucleus of the hypothalamus activates the noradrenergic LC neurons via α,β-methylene-ATP-mediated activation of P2X receptors and up-regulation of ERK kinase in the LC (Sawamura et al. 2003, Fukui et al. 2004, Imbe et al. 2004). Descending modulation of pain is achieved either directly through coeruleospinal pathways or indirectly via LC connections with the pedunculo-pontine nucleus (PPTg), dorsal raphe nucleus, ventro-lateral PAG, or rostral ventromedial medulla (RVM) (Imbe et al. 2004, Freitas et al. 2005).

Midbrain

The midbrain is derived from the mesencephalon, the intermediate primary cerebral vesicle, separated from the prosencephalon and rhombencephalon by slight constrictions in the neural tube. The ventrolateral laminae of the midbrain increase in thickness after the fourth month of gestation to form the cerebral peduncles and also give rise to the oculomotor and tegmental nuclei, whereas neurons of the trochlear and mesencephalic trigeminal nuclei migrate rostrally into the midbrain. Cells of the dorsolateral laminae proliferate to form the corpora bigemina, which are later subdivided into the superior and inferior colliculi. Neurons accumulate in the red nucleus, sub-stantia nigra and reticular tegmental nuclei by the end of the third month, probably originating from both the dorsolateral and ventrolateral laminae – with mixed motor and sensory functions (Muller and O'Rahilly 1997, O'Rahilly and Muller 1999).

Periaqueductal grey
The periaqueductal grey (PAG) is a midline structure surrounding the sylvian aqueduct throughout the midbrain, composed of densely packed heterogeneous neurons distributed into ventrolateral and dorsal groups. Pathways from the midbrain PAG, via the pontine (LC, PBC) and medullary centres (RVM) to the dorsal horn constitute a modulatory system, with important modulatory roles in pain/injury or other homeostatic functions such as sleep/wake or continence/micturition (Craig 2003a, Mason 2005). Both opioid and non-opioid mechanisms of endo-genous analgesia are located in the PAG, mediating different forms of stress-induced analgesia, sucrose-mediated analgesia, or the visceral reactions to pain (Cavun et al. 2004, Anseloni et al. 2005, Hohmann et al. 2005, Ma et al. 2005). Given that few PAG efferents project directly to the spinal dorsal horn, other pathways that mediate the inhibitory effects of PAG stimulation include efferent connections to the RVM, the parabrachial complex, the locus coeruleus and other noradrenergic cell groups (A5, A7) in the brainstem.

Inhibitory effects are mediated via presynaptic opioid (μ-, δ-subtypes), calcitonin gene-related peptide (CGRP1) and cannabinoid (CB1) receptors in the PAG, which inhibit neurotransmission at postsynaptic GABAergic and serotonergic sites (Bartsch et al. 2004, Hahm et al. 2004); whereas descending facilitatory effects are mediated via prostanoid and dopaminergic receptors (D1, but not D2) (Flores et al. 2004, Heinricher et al. 2004a). Differential effects of opioids during development may be dependent on the matu-ration of opioid receptors and descending inhibition from the brainstem, although few studies have included PAG mechanisms in these developmental models (Kinney et al. 1990, Rahman et al. 1998). The clinical importance of PAG neurotransmission, however, was highlighted by the case of a 4-month-old infant with terminal malignancy who had a localized metastasis in the dorsal PAG and required extraordinary doses of intravenous opioids (equivalent to 2680 mg/hour of morphine) in order to achieve adequate analgesia (Collins et al. 1995). Long-term effects of inflammatory pain in infant rats were thought to be mediated via increased expression of serotonergic receptors in the PAG, although their effects on pain modulation remain unclear (Anseloni et al. 2005).

Ventral tegmental area
Neurons in the ventral tegmental area (including those in the anterior pretectal (APtN), pedunculopontine tegmental (PPTg), cuneiform and other midbrain nuclei) play important roles in the dopaminergic re-ward circuitry, but also respond to aversive or noxious stimuli (Kayalioglu and Balkan 2004, Ungless et al. 2004). Efferent projections from these nuclei con-tribute to the pain modulatory system, since stimul-ation of this area produces analgesia and ablation/blockade increases the intensity of acute pain. Within the cholinergic boundaries of the PPTg nucleus, tail pinch excited 33% of neurons, inhibited 20% of neurons, and other neurons were non-responsive, but equal proportions of excited, inhibited, and non-responsive neurons were found in the non-cholinergic cuneiform nucleus (Carlson et al. 2004). Incisional pain activates the descending inhibitory pathways involving the contralateral APtN and PPTg, and the ipsilateral gigantocellularis nucleus (GiA), most likely via descending noradrenergic fibres (Villarreal et al. 2004). Other midbrain mechanisms involved in pain transmission or modulation are not well established and changes during early development have not been studied.

ROLE OF THE THALAMUS

The thalamus functions as a relay station conveying sensory, motor and autonomic information from the spinal cord and brainstem to specific cortical and subcortical regions and vice versa. It arises from cells from the third ventricle neuroepithelium (Altman and Bayer 1979) which then gives rise to diencephalon and is visible in the 6-week human fetus as a swelling (O'Rahilly and Muller 1999). The adult human thalamus arises from three distinct embryonic regions, i.e. epithalamus, ventral thalamus and dorsal thalamus (Gilbert 1935, Jin et al. 2002). The epithalamus gives rise to the stria medullaris, paraventricular nuclei and habenular nuclei. The ventral thalamus gives rise to the reticular nucleus, ventral lateral geniculate nucleus

and zona incerta. The dorsal thalamus gives rise to the complex nuclei which comprise the adult thalamus and are shown in Figure 3.2. The reticular nucleus surrounds the anterior, lateral and ventral parts of the oval-shaped thalamus like a shell. The internal medullary lamina divides the bulk of the thalamus into five major groups which include:

1. The general sensory projection nuclei (ventral posterolateral (VPL)-somatosensory; ventral posteromedial (VPM), the posterior nuclear group

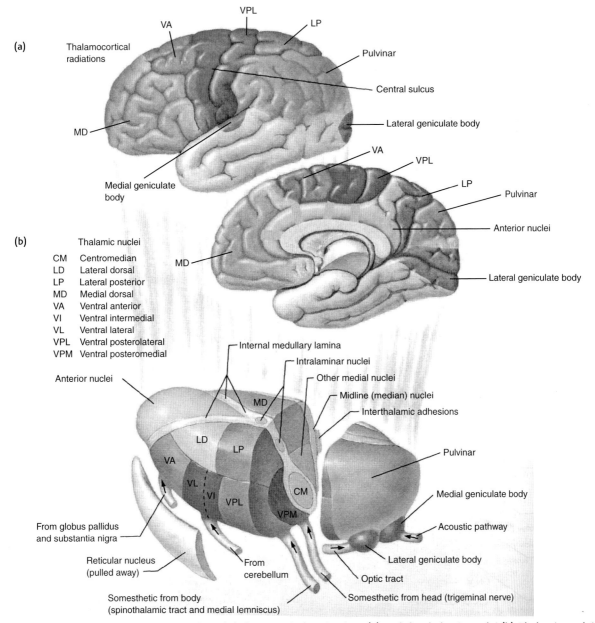

Figure 3.2 Diagrammatic representation of thalamocortical projections (a) and the thalamic nuclei (b). Thalamic nuclei are reciprocally connected with the colour-coded cortical regions. (Reproduced from Netterimages.com with permission from Elsevier.)

(Po) and triangular posterior nucleus (PoT) of the thalamus), which are most clearly involved in pain processing (Gauriau and Bernard 2002);

2. The special sensory projection nuclei (lateral geniculate body – visual; medial geniculate body – auditory);
3. Motor-related nuclei (ventral lateral (VL) and ventral intermedial (VI) – cerebellum; ventral anterior (VA) and VL – basal ganglia);
4. Nuclei related to the autonomic and limbic systems (anterior and lateral dorsal (LD) – cingulate cortex; medial dorsal (MD) – frontal and cingulate cortices); and
5. Nuclei related to the cognitive and association areas (pulvinar and part of MD).

Non-specific thalamic nuclei like the centromedian (CM) and median VA send diffuse connections to widespread regions of the cerebral cortex and other thalamic nuclei. The reticular nucleus of the thalamus helps to regulate the excitability of the thalamic projection nuclei (Felten and Jozefowicz 2003). Most of the thalamic output ends in distributed areas within layer IV of the neocortex.

The thalamus receives most of its nociceptive input from the spinothalamic tract (pain and temperature sensations) and the trigeminothalamic tract. The spinothalamic fibres terminate in distinctive regions of the thalamus including the VPL and the VPM nuclei while the trigeminal fibres terminate in the VL, central lateral nucleus, parafascicular nucleus and the ventral caudal portion of the MD nucleus (MDvc). The ventral posterior nuclei project to the primary and secondary somatosensory cortex while the medial nuclei project to the insular cortex, limbic area and the anterior cingulate cortex (Dostrovsky 2000, Craig 2003a). The role of thalamic nuclei in the supraspinal processing of pain during the fetal and neonatal periods is not clearly established at this time.

The development of the thalamus in fetal animal models and humans has been an area of active investigation in the last 2–3 decades. Thalamocortical development follows a similar sequence in all mammals (Molnar 2000, Clancy et al. 2001). In rats, the thalamus and cortex develop simultaneously and most of the thalamic neurons are formed between embryonic (E) days E13 and E19 which coincides with the period of cortical neuron generation (Lopez-Bendito and Molnar 2003). Substance P (SP)-containing neurons first appear at E14 in the primordium of the epithalamus and extend around the posterior commissure (Inagaki et al. 1982). Soon thereafter, SP-immunoreactivity develops rapidly in the parafascicular and interpeduncular nuclei, bed nucleus of

the stria terminalis, the amygdaloid complex and frontal cortex. Maximum SP expression occurs from P5–P15, with dense representations in the frontal and piriform cortex, the limbic system, thalamic and hypothalamic nuclei (Inagaki et al. 1982, McGregor et al. 1982). The early and abundant expression of opioid (Rahman et al. 1998), nociceptin/orphanin FQ (Ikeda et al. 1998), as well as GABA receptors (Serafini et al. 1998) in the thalamic and brainstem nuclei demonstrates their inhibitory role during development, with direct and indirect effects on modulation of subcortical circuits.

Axons from the dorsal thalamus migrate down through the ventral thalamus and cross the boundary between the diencephalon and telencephalon. They travel in the internal capsule and reach the intermediate zone and subplate of the cortex where they wait until the target layer of the neocortex starts forming (Bolz et al. 1995, Lopez-Bendito and Molnar 2003). The early establishment of thalamocortical connections precedes the connection of peripheral sensory afferents with the dorsal thalamus but parallels the formation of corticothalamic tracts, which connect layers VI and V to the thalamus. There is compelling evidence to suggest that thalamocortical axon growth is guided by expression of various molecules like netrin-1, limbic system-associated membrane protein (LAMP), ephrins (ephrin A-5, A-4 and B-3) and semaphorins whose expression is under control of various regulatory genes and transcription factors and who in turn may be regulated by molecules like fibroblast growth factor 8 (Fgf8) and sonic hedgehog (Shh). Thalamic input is critical for regional specificity within the developing cortex (Bolz et al. 1995). Early ablation of thalamic nuclei leads to alteration in the size and cell number of the neocortex. It is reasonable to suggest that damage to the thalamus during this critical development will lead to altered CNS function including altered pain processing.

DEVELOPMENT AND ROLE OF OTHER SUBCORTICAL AREAS

Hypothalamus

The hypothalamus is important for the integration of descending influences from the cerebral cortex and ascending information from somatic and visceral sources as well as the reticular activating system. Thus, the hypothalamus coordinates behaviours necessary for survival, including the emotional homeostasis and responses to pain. The hypothalamus develops from the ventral portion of the secondary prosencephalon early in gestation. Subsequently the nuclei of the hypothalamus develop from precursor cells through induction of mesoderm, the absence of which can lead to holoprosencephaly (Michaud 2001).

The hypothalamus regulates the autonomic and humoral responses to pain, stress and emotional expression. It forms the ventral wall of the third ventricle and interconnects with the spinal cord and midbrain, the pituitary gland, and with the cerebral cortex through the amygdala and hippocampal formation. In humans, several fibres connect the brainstem and spinal cord with the hypothalamus. The largest of these, the medial forebrain bundle, connects sensory neurons in the spinal cord, laminae VII and VIII, and the trigeminal nucleus to the hypothalamus (Sewards and Sewards 2003). These tracts respond to noxious stimuli in rodents (Hallbeck and Blomqvist 1999, Gauriau and Bernard 2002) and non-human primates (Zhang et al. 1999b) to elicit endocrine responses associated with pain. From the hypothalamus, tracts project to the PAG (Jiang and Behbehani 2001), thalamus, amygdala, and anterior cingulate cortex (Parent 1996, Sewards and Sewards 2003), all of which are important in the modulation of pain (Price 2002). The hypothalamus issues inhibitory and excitatory impulses and is highly organized in the response to pain (Lumb 2002). For example, the hypothalamic tracts differentially connect with the midbrain PAG when stimulated by somatic (escapable) vs. visceral (inescapable) pain. Acute somatic pain increases blood pressure and connects to the dorsolateral/lateral PAG, while visceral pain decreases blood pressure and connects to the ventrolateral PAG. Both excitatory and inhibitory responses to pain are modulated through the hypothalamus to the raphe magnus and PAG (Workman and Lumb 1997, Jiang and Behbehani 2001). Other important connections include the hippocampus, amygdala, anterior cingulate gyrus and the cortex (Lenz et al. 1998, Paulson et al. 2000, Zaichenko et al. 2001, Gauriau and Bernard 2002, Sewards and Sewards 2003).

The hypothalamus secretes numerous hormones responsible for the autonomic response to pain. The effects of stress can be seen as early as 16–20 weeks (see Chapter 13), implying functionality of the hypothalamic–pituitary–adrenal (HPA) axis. The stress response is mediated through the HPA axis and results in increased corticotrophin-releasing hormone which has widespread effects affecting growth and development, immunity and emotional well-being (Charmandari et al. 2003). Other hormones secreted in response to pain include vasopressin, melanocyte-stimulating hormone, catecholamines and beta-endorphin, released in the arcuate nucleus into the cerebrospinal fluid (Bach 1997, Blackburn-Munro and Blackburn-Munro 2003, Charmandari et al. 2003).

The orexins, which are synthesized in the hypothalamus, lead to the descending inhibition of pain (Watanabe et al. 2005). Further, functional MRI studies show that acupuncture specifically activates the hypothalamus and other deep cortical structures, implying a significant role for hypothalamic structures in the modulation of pain in human subjects (Hui et al. 2000, Wu et al. 2002).

Anterior cingulate gyrus

The cingulate cortex contains among the earliest generated cortical neurons, pioneering the corpus callosum (Koester and O'Leary 1994). Sonographic evidence for this structure is present as early as 24 weeks' gestation (Slagle et al. 1989). The anterior cingulate gyrus plays a pivotal role in pain affect and modulation, with inputs from large bilateral receptive fields made up of nociceptive neurons (Sewards and Sewards 2002) via the ventrolateral and medial thalamic nuclei (Bushnell and Duncan 1989, Price 2002). Robust connections with middle and posterior cingular cortex, somatosensory areas, supplementary motor areas and the prefrontal cortex (Price 2002, Vogt 2005) allow probably short- and long-term modulatory roles for this structure as stimulation induces inhibition of the dorsal horn nuclei (Senapati et al. 2005).

In 1962, Folz and White demonstrated a decreased response to pain after cingulotomy. Multiple lines of evidence from neuroimaging techniques reveal anterior cingulate activity with anticipation (Petrovic et al. 2004b, Maihofner et al. 2005, Yaguez et al. 2005), with at least three areas involved in processing a specific pain function including intensity, sensory-integrative and cognitive modulation (Mohr et al. 2005). Further, activation of this area has been utilized to objectively evaluate pain treatments such as acupuncture, opioid and placebo effects (Casey et al. 2000, Petrovic et al. 2002). Indirect evidence for activity in the preterm newborn is shown by anatomic and physiological studies (Slagle et al. 1989, Porter et al. 1998). Experimental evidence suggests that opioid receptors in this area suppress spinothalamic transmission of pain to the forebrain, with tonic inhibitory effects (Liu et al. 2004b). Thus, this area plays a pivotal role in the affective and modulatory responses to infant pain.

Amygdala

Migration of neuroblasts from germinal epithelium forms the amygdala, with differentiation into separate nuclei starting at 12 weeks' gestation (Humphrey 1968). The central, lateral and basolateral nuclei are important in the emotional responses to pain (Bingel et al. 2002, Nakagawa et al. 2003), with visceral pain mediated through the central nucleus and somatic pain mediated through the other nuclei. Even prenatally stressed human infants and experimental animals have effects on this important structure (Weinstock 1997). The central nucleus plays an important role in morphine antinociception (Oliveira and Prado 2001) and also triggers corticotropin-releasing hormone (CRH) release in opiate withdrawal (McNally and Akil 2002) and surgical stress (Bhatia and Tandon 2005), delineating a critical role for the amygdala in the neuroendocrine responses to pain. Through descending pathways that inhibit or enhance painful stimuli, the amygdala alters dorsal horn pain transmission in rats (Fields 2000) and humans, becoming less active with pain conditioning and demonstrating a cognitive response to unavoidable pain (Bornhovd et al. 2002, Petrovic et al. 2004a).

Hippocampus

The hippocampus is important in learning, declarative memory, and chronic pain (McEwen 2001). Hippocampal neurons form synapses as early as 15–16 weeks' gestation in humans with extensive dendritic formation into the marginal and subplate zones (Kostovic et al. 1989). In monkeys, the enterorhinal cortex, which connects the hippocampus with the rest of the cortex, develops in the first half of gestation and generally precedes the development of the neighbouring cortical areas (Berger et al. 1993). It has long been known that hippocampal lesions can alter the perception of pain (Gol and Faibish 1967), but the specific mechanisms are just being revealed. Painful stimuli increase hippocampal activation in a time- and sex-dependent manner in experimental animals (Khanna et al. 2004). Functional neuroimaging has shown that anxiety produced hyperalgesia while appropriate preparation can produce pain modulation in the entorhinal cortex of the hippocampus (Ploghaus et al. 2001). For example, acupuncture prominently decreases hippocampus signal in response to pain (Hui et al. 2000).

Neuropeptides involved in pain transmission, including cortistatin, which induces sleep and interferes with memory, inhibit acetylcholine excitatory actions in the hippocampus (Mendez-Diaz et al. 2004) while orphanin FQ, when injected into the hippocampus inhibits memory at higher levels but facilitates it at lower levels (Sandin et al. 2004). The hippocampus is important in chronic or repetitive pain and stress. The hippocampus has abundant glucocorticoid receptors with biphasic effects on the response to painful and non-painful stress. Stress can inhibit memory through adrenal secretion or endogenous opiate secretion

(Diamond et al. 1994). Steroids, along with other excitatory amino acids, lead to remodelling of neurons in the hippocampus (McEwen 2001). The adverse neurological sequelae triggered by repetitive pain and stress in human preterm neonates may result from changes in this important structure, mediated by glucocorticoids, glutamate and neuropeptides.

Nucleus accumbens

The nucleus accumbens develops in conjunction with the olfactory tubercle in rats early in gestation, with expression of dopamine and cAMP-regulated phosphoprotein between E12 and E14 (Foster et al. 1988, Gustafson et al. 1992). Its role in pain modulation, especially in the suppression of chronic pain, plays an important part in the brain's reward pathway (Barrot et al. 2002), mediated through the amygdala, PAG and RVM (Buchwald et al. 1991). The nucleus accumbens regulates dopamine pathways from the ventral tegmental area, endogenous opioid pathways from the PAG (Van Bockstaele et al. 1995, Altier and Stewart 1999, Lapeyre et al. 2001, Huang et al. 2004) and other neuropeptides including neurotensin and substance P (Benmoussa et al. 1996) in the modulation of pain. This system is so efficient that pain may in some instances be rewarding (Gear et al. 1999, Schmidt et al. 2002a). Opioid receptors (μ-, δ-, but not κ-receptors), dopamine D2 receptors, and calcitonin gene-related peptide (CGRP) receptors play dominant roles in antinociception (Schmidt et al. 2002b, Taylor et al. 2003). There is concern that depletion of dopamine stores or decreased expression of D2 receptors in preterm neonates (Zhang et al. 1999a) may lead to a decreased ability to modulate pain.

ROLE OF CORTICAL AREAS

Painful experiences can only be described in terms of human consciousness. Yet, conscious sensation in general, and pain in particular, is a highly subjective experience with multifaceted processes that involve complex interactions between sensory-discriminative, affective, cognitive and motor dimensions taking place in different areas of the brain. Afferents (see Chapter 2) encode a range of sensory experiences and transmit the information from the periphery to the brain via brainstem nuclei and midbrain structures to the cerebral cortex for higher 'conscious' processing. Sensory discriminative areas are believed to detect the intensity of sensation and its site of origin in the body. Limbic structures allow the sensation to be judged in light of current physical and psychological status and memories of similar past experiences. An emotional response is generated and cognitive judgements are made about coping with the sensation. This section summarizes how basic and clinical studies have advanced our understanding of cortical pain mechanisms.

The cerebral cortex covers almost the entire human brain, owing to its enormous growth and increase in surface area during mammalian evolution. It arises from the most rostral region of the neural tube, the prosencephalon, that later divides into the telencephalon and diencephalon. The dorsal telencephalon gives rise to the cerebral cortex, which comprises the neocortex, paleocortex (piriform cortex) and archicortex (hippocampus), while the ventral telencephalon differentiates into the basal ganglia (Moore and Persaud 1998). The matching of projection and interneuron numbers has apparently been maintained during the expansion of the cerebral cortex in phylogeny even across cortical areas (Winfield et al. 1980), despite prominent differences in the total number of neurons residing in specific layers of distinct cortical areas. In mammals, including mice and humans, cortical areas take the form of radial domains within the cortex that specialize in specific aspects of information processing. However, functional cortical maps are dynamic constructs that are remodelled in detail by behaviourally important experiences throughout life. In fact, the cortex reorganizes its effective local connections and responses with age, following peripheral or central alterations of inputs and in response to behaviour.

Converging evidence from experimental, clinical and neuroimaging data, obtained from adult brains, suggests that a number of cortical areas are involved in human pain processing (Sweet 1982, Willis and Kenshalo 1991). Among those are the primary (S1) and secondary (S2) somatosensory cortex; both receive sensory input from the thalamus. The S1 cortex is located on the postcentral gyrus and extends from the longitudinal cerebral fissure to the lateral sulcus. The S2 cortex is located on the superior bank of the lateral sulcus. Two other areas of the parietal lobe implicated in nociceptive processing are the retroinsular cortex and Brodmann area 7b (Chudler and Bonica 2001).

Somatosensory cortex

The ability to localize both touch and pain in the adult is attributed to the primary somatosensory cortex (S1), based on its fine somatotopic mapping of tactile inputs (Penfield and Rasmussen 1955). Although the role of S1 in the conscious experience of pain still remains a topic of ongoing debate, neurophysiological findings in animals, as well as positron emission tomography (PET), functional magnetic resonance imaging (fMRI) and magneto-encephalography (MEG) studies in humans, implicate S1 in pain localization (Bushnell et al. 1999) and in the differentiation of pain arising from viscera and skin (Strigo et al. 2003).

Results from experimental animal studies clearly indicate participation of S1 in pain processing. Physiological studies in non-human primates revealed nociceptive projections from lateral thalamic nuclei, particularly from the VPL nucleus to S1 (Kenshalo et al. 1980). Single cell recordings in rats (Lamour et al. 1983, Guilbaud et al. 1992, Vin-Christian et al. 1992, Follet and Dirks 1994), and anaesthesized or awake monkeys (Kenshalo and Isensee 1983, Kenshalo et al. 1988, Chudler et al. 1990) demonstrated S1 neurons that responded to somatic and visceral noxious stimuli (Follet and Dirks 1994), localized at the borders between the cytoarchitectonic areas 3b and 1, and 1 and 2 respectively. Most nociceptive S1 neurons had restricted receptive fields arranged somatotopically and their activity correlated with the duration and intensity of stimuli (Kenshalo and Isensee 1983, Lamour et al. 1983, Kenshalo et al. 1988, Chudler et al. 1990), with the intensity of stimulus perception (Kenshalo et al. 1988), as well as with the type of pain – inflammatory (Vin-Christian et al. 1992) or neuropathic (Guilbaud et al. 1992). Studies looking at regional cerebral blood flow have detected changes in the S1 hindlimb area in rats injected with noxious formalin (Morrow et al. 1998) or in response to chronic constriction injury of the sciatic nerve (Paulson et al. 2000). On the other hand, a number of immunocytochemical studies showed a significant increase in Fos expression in S1 (Meaney et al. 1988, Kaminska et al. 1995) following exposure to nociceptive stimuli (however, contrast those with Anand et al. 1999).

Contrary to most S1 cells, nociceptive neurons in the secondary somatosensory area (S2) including the neighbouring area 7b and the retroinsular cortex have mostly large, bilateral receptive fields and poorly encode stimulus intensity. However, only very few neurons have been found in these areas, mainly in the caudal part of S2, that responded to noxious stimuli (Whitsel et al. 1969, Robinson and Burton 1980, Dong et al. 1989, 1994). Anatomic studies indicate that S2 receives projections from lateral thalamic nuclei, mostly from the ventral posterior inferior (VPI) nucleus (Friedman et al. 1986, Stevens et al. 1993).

In contrast to these animal studies, clinical observations of human cortical lesions have shown that patients with cerebral infarcts sparing S1, but affecting the parietal operculum (S2) or the posterior insula and retroinsula, show deficits for mechanical and heat pain (Greenspan et al. 1999, Bowsher et al. 2004), lending weight to a role of S2 in pain processing. In fact, both S1 and S2 have been implicated in a number of PET and fMRI studies on experimental pain (Talbot et al. 1991, Casey et al. 1994, Coghill et al. 1994, 1999, Craig et al. 1996, Derbyshire et al. 1997, Rainville et al. 1997, Davis et al. 1998, Iadarola et al. 1998, Gelnar et al. 1999) in partial contrast to early brain-imaging studies (Jones et al. 1991, Apkarian et al. 1992). Their role has been further emphasized in neuromagnetic recordings of cortical activity (Hari et al. 1997, Ploner et al. 1999, 2000) or scalp-evoked potentials (Bromm and Chen 1995, Spiegel et al. 1996) using different painful stimuli such as thermal heat or laser-radiant heat. Whereas activation of S1 is almost exclusively contralaterally detected following noxious stimulation – in line with a pain-localizing and discriminative-sensory function of this area – the affective-cognitive aspects of pain have been attributed to S2, the cingulate, inferior parietal, prefrontal and insular cortex (Riedel and Neeck 2001).

Using near infrared spectroscopy (NIRS) to monitor brain activity in preterm neonates (28–35 weeks' gestation), tactile and painful stimuli activated the somatosensory cortex (but not the occipital cortex) implying conscious pain perception in preterm neonates (Bartocci et al. 2006). These responses were more pronounced in male vs. female neonates, preterm neonates at lower gestational ages and at older postnatal ages (25–42 hours). A gradual loss of fetal inhibition or increased excitability from exposure to invasive procedures may explain why the older newborns responded with more pronounced increases in cortical activity (Taddio et al. 2002, Liu et al. 2004b). Bilateral activation of somatosensory areas occurred in all infants, regardless of the side of venipuncture. It is likely that the NIRS beam was not exclusively confined to the S1 area, but also sampled other regions such as the S2, insula, ventral premotor area and anterior cingulate cortex, areas that are implicated in bilateral pain processing (Coghill et al. 1999, Ibinson et al. 2004, Ohara et al. 2004). Another study using NIRS found that cortical responses were larger in awake neonates than in sleeping neonates (Cantarella et al. 2005). The lateralization of pain processing, the latency and duration of these responses, their gradations across gestational age, postnatal age and behavioural state (awake vs. asleep), and the neuro-anatomical location of these responses (parietal versus occipital), suggest that cortical processing of acute pain occurs in preterm neonates (Bartocci et al. 2006, Slater et al. 2006).

Other cortical areas

In addition to the somatosensory cortex, several regions of the inferior and anterior parietal cortex, the insular cortex, the anterior cingulate cortex and the medial prefrontal cortex are consistently activated by cutaneous, visceral and intramuscular noxious stimulation (Davis et al. 1997, May et al. 1998, Casey 1999, Willis et al. 1999). In a study on monkeys using fMRI, colorectal distension caused an increase in blood volume in the cingulate, temporal and postcentral gyri, in addition to the cerebellum (Willis et al. 1999). Apart from direct thalamocortical projections to some of these cortical areas, a complex pattern of connections among themselves and indirect inputs from various limbic structures, may explain these results.

Lesion studies have shown that damage restricted to the insula reduces pain affect and appropriate reactions to painful and threatening visual and auditory stimuli but does not influence pain threshold (Berthier et al. 1988, Greenspan et al. 1999). In addition, pain-related activations of the anterior insula from functional imaging studies motivated complementary investigations in experimental animals. Indeed, single-cell recordings and local field potentials in monkeys (Robinson and Burton 1980, Zhang et al. 1999c) revealed nociceptive responses in the insula. These nociceptive neurons had large receptive fields and responded partially to multimodal stimulation, in particular to visceral stimuli (Zhang et al. 1999c). Together, these results clearly indicate that pain processing in the insula does not involve sensory-discriminative functions.

However, chronic pain patients may acquire different or additional mechanisms that require special consideration. For example, in patients with chronic sympathetically mediated pain, abnormal brain responses to pain engage prefrontal/limbic networks more extensively than in acute pain states (Apkarian et al. 2001). In patients with neuropathic pain, brush-induced allodynia activates the contralateral S1 cortex, parietal association (PA) cortex, inferior frontal cortex, bilateral S2 and insula (Maihofner et al. 2004). Plastic changes in the patterns of pain and sensory processing were also observed in patients with complex regional pain syndrome, indicating possible cortical reorganization (Maihofner et al. 2003). In patients with irritable bowel syndrome, both rectal distension and cutaneous heat stimuli evoked greater neural activity in the somatosensory cortex as well as insular, anterior cingulate, posterior cingulate and prefrontal cortical areas, in comparison to age/sex-matched control subjects (Verne et al. 2003).

EMERGING ROLE OF THE CEREBELLUM

Cerebellar neurons develop at two different times from two different matrices: (1) the ventricular epithelium of the cerebellar anlage begins as bilateral elevations on the dorsal aspect of the rostral metencephalon that grow toward the midline and ultimately fuse (Liu and Joyner 2001); it gives rise to all cerebellar neurons except granule cells, by a process of outwardly directed migration, and (2) the cells of the rhombic lip, which give rise to the external granular layer precursors, from which granule cells originate by inward migration. Neurons of the cerebellar nuclei are the first to form, followed by the Purkinje cells, which migrate to their location in the cerebellar cortex. After the Purkinje cells have reached the cortical plate, climbing fibres enter the cerebellum from the inferior olive and begin innervating the Purkinje cells (Crepel et al. 1976).

The cerebellum mainly influences motor behaviour, eye movement and conditioning (Squire et al. 2003). Cerebellar projections are also thought to influence respiration (Xu and Frazier 2000), cognition (Fiez 1996), detection of sensory discrepancy (Blakemore et al. 2001), and prediction of sensory events (Nixon and Passingham 2001). There are no reports of direct cerebellar involvement in neonatal or infant pain; however, cerebellar tumours can sometimes press on sensory pathways in the brainstem causing pain. In the adult cat, stimulation of nociceptive afferent fibres evokes activity in the climbing fibres and neurons of the cerebellum (Ekerot et al. 1987). This stimulation activates somatotopically organized inputs to small cerebellar cortical regions (Gilman et al. 1981) albeit this somatotopy is not continuous. This type of 'fractured somatotopy' suggests that precise topographical relations between adjacent receptive fields do not appear to be preserved (Voogd and Glickstein 1998).

Cerebellar lesions and chemical or electrical stimulation may lead to modulation of nociceptive phenomena. For example, microinjection of morphine into the anterior part of the cerebellum in rats produces profound analgesia (Dey and Ray 1982). These effects can be reversed with intraperitoneal administration of naloxone as well as by focal electrical stimulation of the anterior part of the cerebellum. In monkeys, stimulation of cerebellar areas 'associated with the brachium conjunctivum' causes elevation of nociceptive thresholds (Siegel and Wepsic 1974). In rats, stimulation of the cerebellar cortex (caudal vermis, lobules VI–VII), using electrical or chemical stimulation, increases the firing rate of spinal nociceptive neurons (Saab et al. 2001). However, a role of Purkinje cells in these studies was not confirmed. The intensity of a visceromotor reflex to noxious stimulation increased following cerebellar cortical stimulation, but decreased following stimulation in the fastigial nucleus (Saab and Willis 2002). In contrast, stimulation of the cerebellar cortex in the vermis accentuated the inhibition in the underlying neurons of the fastigial nucleus, resulting in opposite effects. The descending pathways mediating these effects are speculated to be in the brain stem.

Imaging studies have also confirmed an increased cerebellar activity in adult humans following peripheral nociceptive stimulation. fMRI studies have shown increases in blood volume in the cerebellar vermis and lateral regions during the perception of acute heat pain (Casey et al. 1994), the warm-discrimination task (Casey et al. 1996), muscle pain (Svensson et al. 1997) capsaicin-evoked pain and allodynia (Iadarola et al. 1998) (for a review see Saab and Willis (2003)). It remains to be seen whether imaging studies in neonates and infants in pain would show similar or even more pronounced activation of cerebellar structures, given that the cerebellum is involved in learning and coordination of many sensory–motor activities. The immature cerebellum grows rapidly during 24–36 weeks' gestation and this accelerated growth seems to be impeded by premature birth and NICU care. Long-term changes in pain processing and neurodevelopmental outcomes in the survivors of premature birth (see Chapters 4 and 5) may be partly attributable to impaired cerebellar development (Limperopoulos et al. 2005, Messerschmidt et al. 2005).

CONCLUSIONS

There appears to be widespread uncertainty about the ability for supraspinal pain processing in newborn infants, particularly if they are premature. Clinicians and scientists have often characterized infants essentially as unconscious automata (Zelazo 2004), being only capable of reflex responses to pain (Derbyshire and Furedi 1996, Lloyd-Thomas and Fitzgerald 1996). The lack of data on pain-specific thalamocortical connections in the fetus or preterm neonate has been used to argue against the possibility of pain perception in early development (Lee et al. 2005). Although currently limited details are available, the accumulating data suggest that various levels of the brainstem, thalamus, subcortical and cortical areas develop sufficiently early during human gestation to enable supraspinal pain processing in the preterm and term neonate. It is likely that the supraspinal pain mechanisms and structures active during development are unique and different from those used in the mature nervous system. Some of these nociceptive pathways or mechanisms may not be maintained beyond specific periods of early development (Narsinghani and Anand 2000, Fitzgerald 2005). Thus, the immature pain system maintains a signalling role during each stage of development and may use the neural elements available at that time to monitor bodily integrity. Supraspinal pain processing and regulation of the spinal–brainstem–spinal loops that mediate descending facilitation or inhibition very likely depend on distributed activity in cortical and sub-cortical areas. The data reviewed in this chapter may help clinicians and researchers to design clinical studies or experiments to examine the mechanisms underlying supraspinal pain processing, similar to the data available for mechanisms in the peripheral and spinal nervous systems (Chapter 2). Advances in functional neuroimaging, electrophysiology, tract tracing and molecular neuroscience should provide the tools necessary for these future studies. Greater research on supraspinal pain processing will enable the development of improved, specific/sensitive methods for pain assessment and more effective, safer strategies for pain management in preterm and term neonates.

REFERENCES

Afridi SK, Matharu MS, Lee L, et al. (2005). A PET study exploring the laterality of brainstem activation in migraine using glyceryl trinitrate. Brain 128: 932–939.

Aita M, Seo K, Fujiwara N, et al. (2005). Postnatal changes in the spatial distributions of substance P and neurokinin-1 receptor in the trigeminal subnucleus caudalis of mice. Brain Res Dev Brain Res 155: 33–41.

Altier N, Stewart J. (1999). The role of dopamine in the nucleus accumbens in analgesia. Life Sci 65: 2269–2287.

Altman J, Bayer SA. (1979). Development of the diencephalon in the rat. VI. Re-evaluation of the embryonic development of the thalamus on the basis of thymidine-radiographic datings. J Comp Neurol 188: 501–524.

Anand KJS, Coskun V, Thrivikraman KV, et al. (1999). Long-term behavioral effects of repetitive pain in neonatal rat pups. Physiol Behav 66: 627–637.

Anand KJS, Runeson B, Jacobson B. (2004). Gastric suction at birth associated with long-term risk for functional intestinal disorders in later life. J Pediatr 144: 449–454.

Anseloni VC, Ren K, Dubner R, et al. (2005). A brainstem substrate for analgesia elicited by intraoral sucrose. Neuroscience 133: 231–243.

Apkarian AV, Stea RA, Manglos SH, et al. (1992). Persistent pain inhibits contralateral somatosensory cortical activity in humans. Neurosci Lett 140: 141–147.

Apkarian AV, Thomas PS, Krauss BR, et al. (2001). Prefrontal cortical hyperactivity in patients with sympathetically mediated chronic pain. Neurosci Lett 311: 193–197.

Bach FW. (1997). Beta-endorphin in the brain. A role in nociception. Acta Anaesthesiol Scand 41: 133–140.

Baez MA, Brink TS, Mason P. (2005). Roles for pain modulatory cells during micturition and continence. J Neurosci 25: 384–394.

Barrot M, Olivier JD, Perrotti LI, et al. (2002). CREB activity in the nucleus accumbens shell controls gating of behavioral responses to emotional stimuli. Proc Nat Acad Sci USA 99: 11435–11440.

Bartocci M, Bergqvist LL, Lagercrantz H, et al. (2006). Pain activates cortical areas in the preterm newborn brain. Pain 122: 109–117.

Bartsch T, Knight YE, Goadsby PJ. (2004). Activation of 5-HT(1B/1D) receptor in the periaqueductal gray inhibits nociception. Ann Neurol 56: 371–381.

Benmoussa M, Chait A, Loric G, et al. (1996). Low doses of neurotensin in the preoptic area produce hyperthermia. Comparison with other brain sites and with neurotensin-induced analgesia. Brain Res Bull 39: 275–279.

Berger B, Alvarez C, Goldman-Rakic PS. (1993). Neurochemical development of the hippocampal region in the fetal rhesus monkey. I. Early appearance of peptides, calcium-binding proteins, DARPP-32, and monoamine innervation in the entorhinal cortex during the first half of gestation (E47 to E90). Hippocampus 3: 279–305.

Berthier M, Starkstein S, Leiguarda R. (1988). Asymbolia for pain: a sensory – limbic disconnection syndrome. Ann Neurol 24: 41–49.

Bhatia V, Tandon RK. (2005). Stress and the gastrointestinal tract. J Gastroenterol Hepatol 20: 332–339.

Bingel U, Quante M, Knab R, et al. (2002). Subcortical structures involved in pain processing: evidence from single-trial fMRI. Pain 99: 313–321.

Blackburn-Munro G, Blackburn-Munro R. (2003). Pain in the brain: are hormones to blame? Trends Endocrinol Metab 14: 20–27.

Blakemore SJ, Frith CD, Wolpert DM. (2001). The cerebellum is involved in predicting the sensory consequences of action. Neuroreport 12: 1879–1884.

Bolz J, Kossel A, Bagnard D. (1995). The specificity of interactions between the cortex and the thalamus. Ciba Foundation Symposium 193:173–191; discussion 192–199.

Bornhovd K, Quante M, Glauche V, et al. (2002). Painful stimuli evoke different stimulus-response functions in the amygdala, prefrontal, insula and somatosensory cortex: a single-trial fMRI study. Brain 125: 1326–1336.

Bowsher D, Brooks J, Enevoldson P. (2004). Central representation of somatic sensations in the parietal operculum (SII) and insula. Eur Neurol 52: 211–225.

Brink TS, Mason P. (2004). Role of raphe magnus neuronal responses in the behavioral reactions to colorectal distension. J Neurophysiol 92: 2302–2311 Epub 2004.

Bromm B, Chen AC. (1995). Brain electrical source analysis of laser evoked potentials in response to painful trigeminal nerve stimulation. Electroencephalogr Clin Neurophysiol 95: 14–26.

Brooks JC, Zambreanu L, Godinez A, et al. (2005). Somatotopic organisation of the human insula to painful heat studied with high resolution functional imaging. Neuroimage 27: 201–209.

Buchwald JS, Rubinstein EH, Schwafel J, et al. (1991). Midlatency auditory evoked responses: differential effects of a cholinergic agonist and antagonist. Electroencephalogr Clin Neurophysiol 80: 303–309.

Buhler AV, Choi J, Proudfit HK, et al. (2005). Neurotensin activation of the NTR1 on spinally projecting serotonergic neurons in the rostral ventromedial medulla is antinociceptive. Pain 114: 285–294.

Bushnell MC, Duncan GH. (1989). Sensory and affective aspects of pain perception: is medial thalamus restricted to emotional issues? Exp Brain Res 78: 415–418.

Bushnell MC, Duncan GH, Hofbauer RK et al. (1999). Pain perception: is there a role for primary somatosensory cortex? Proc Natl Acad Sci USA 96: 7705–7709.

Carlson JD, Iacono RP, Maeda G. (2004). Nociceptive excited and inhibited neurons within the pedunculopontine tegmental nucleus and cuneiform nucleus. Brain Res 1013(2): 182–187.

Casey KL. (1999). Forebrain mechanisms of nociception and pain: analysis through imaging. Proc Natl Acad Sci USA 96: 7668–7674.

Casey KL, Minoshima S, Berger KL, et al. (1994). Positron emission tomography analysis of cerebral structures activated specifically by repetitive noxious heat stimuli. J Neurophysiol 71: 802–807.

Casey KL, Minoshima S, Morrow TJ, et al. (1996). Comparison of human cerebral activation patterns during cutaneous warmth, heat pain, and deep cold pain. J Neurophysiol 76: 571–581.

Casey KL, Svensson P, Morrow TJ, et al. (2000). Selective opiate modulation of nociceptive processing in the human brain. J Neurophysiol 84: 525–533.

Cavun S, Goktalay G, Millington WR. (2004). The hypotension evoked by visceral nociception is mediated by delta opioid receptors in the periaqueductal gray. Brain Res 1019: 237–245.

Cerrato P, Baima C, Bergui M, et al. (2005). Restricted pain and thermal sensory loss in a patient with pontine lacunar infarction: a clinical MRI study. Eur J Neurol 12: 564–565.

Charmandari E, Kino T, Souvatzoglou E, et al. (2003). Pediatric stress: hormonal mediators and human development. Hormone Res 59: 161–179.

Chudler EH, Bonica JJ. (2001). Supraspinal mechanisms of pain and nociception. In: Loeser JD (ed). Bonica's Management of Pain, 3rd Edn., Chapter 5, pp 153–179. Lippincott, Williams & Wilkins, Philadelphia, PA.

Chudler EH, Anton F, Dubner R, et al. (1990). Responses of nociceptive SI neurons in monkeys and pain sensation in humans elicited by noxious thermal stimulation: effect of interstimulus interval. J Neurophysiol 63: 559–569.

Clancy B, Darlington RB, Finlay BL. (2001). Translating developmental time across mammalian species. Neuroscience 105: 7–17.

Coghill RC, Talbot JD, Evans AC, et al. (1994). Distributed processing of pain and vibration by the human brain. J Neurosci 14: 4095–4108.

Coghill RC, Sang CN, Maisog JM, et al. (1999). Pain intensity processing within the human brain: a bilateral, distributed mechanism. J Neurophysiol 82: 1934–1943.

Collins JJ, Berde CB, Grier HE, et al. (1995). Massive opioid resistance in an infant with a localized metastasis to the midbrain periaqueductal gray. Pain 63: 271–275.

Craig AD. (2003a). Interoception: the sense of the physiological condition of the body. Curr Opin Neurobiol 13: 500–505.

Craig AD. (2003b). A new view of pain as a homeostatic emotion. Trends Neurosci 26: 303–307.

Craig AD. (2003c). Pain mechanisms: labeled lines versus convergence in central processing. Ann Rev Neurosci 26: 1–30.

Craig AD, Reiman EM, Evans A, et al. (1996). Functional imaging of an illusion of pain. Nature 384: 258–260.

Crepel F, Mariani J, Delhaye-Bouchaud N. (1976). Evidence for a multiple innervation of Purkinje cells by climbing fibers in the immature rat cerebellum. J Neurobiol 7: 567–578.

Davis KD, Taylor SJ, Crawley AP, et al. (1997). Functional MRI of pain and attention related activations in the human cingulate cortex. J Neurophysiol 77: 3370–3380.

Davis KD, Kwan CL, Crawley AP, et al. (1998). Functional MRI study of thalamic and cortical activations evoked by cutaneous heat, cold, and tactile stimuli. J Neurophysiol 80: 1533–1546.

Defrin R, Ariel E, Peretz C. (2005). Segmental noxious versus innocuous electrical stimulation for chronic pain relief and the effect of fading sensation during treatment. Pain 115: 152–160.

de Lange RP, Geerse GJ, Dahlhaus M. (2005). Altered brain stem responsivity to duodenal pain after a single stressful experience. Neurosci Lett 381: 144–148.

Derbyshire SW, Furedi A. (1996). Do fetuses feel pain? "Fetal pain" is a misnomer. BMJ 313: 795.

Derbyshire SW, Jones AK, Gyulai F, et al. (1997). Pain processing during three levels of noxious stimulation produces differential patterns of central activity. Pain 73: 431–445.

Dey PK, Ray AK. (1982). Anterior cerebellum as site for morphine analgesia and post-stimulation analgesia. Indian J Phys Pharm 26: 3–12.

Diamond DM, Fleshner M, Rose GM. (1994). Psychological stress repeatedly

blocks hippocampal primed burst potentiation in behaving rats. Behav Brain Res 62: 1–9.

Dickenson AH. (2002). Gate control theory of pain stands the test of time. Br J Anaesthes 88: 755–757.

Dong WK, Salonen LD, Kawakami Y, et al. (1989). Nociceptive responses of trigeminal neurons in SII-7b cortex of awake monkeys. Brain Res 484: 314–324.

Dong WK, Chudler EH, Sugiyama K, et al. (1994). Somatosensory, multisensory, and task-related neurons in cortical area 7b (PF) of unanesthetized monkeys. J Neurophysiol 72: 542–564.

Dostrovsky JO. (2000). Role of thalamus in pain. Prog Brain Res 129: 245–257.

Dubner R, Ren K. (2004). Brainstem mechanisms of persistent pain following injury. J Orofac Pain 18: 299–305.

Ekerot CF, Oscarsson O, Schouenborg J. (1987). Stimulation of cat cutaneous nociceptive fibers causing tonic and synchronous activity in climbing fibers. J Physiol 386: 539–546.

Felten D, Jozefowicz R. (2003). Netter's Atlas of Human Neuroscience. 1st edn. Icon Learning Systems, Teterboro, NJ.

Fields H. (2004). State-dependent opioid control of pain. Nat Rev Neurosci 5: 565–575.

Fields HL. (2000). Pain modulation: expectation, opioid analgesia and virtual pain. Prog Brain Res 122: 245–253.

Fiez JA. (1996). Cerebellar contributions to cognition. Neuron 16: 13–15.

Fitzgerald M. (2005). The development of nociceptive circuits. Nat Rev Neurosci 6: 507–520.

Flores JA, El Banoua F, Galan-Rodriguez B, et al. (2004). Opiate anti-nociception is attenuated following lesion of large dopamine neurons of the periaqueductal grey: critical role for D1 (not D2) dopamine receptors. Pain 110: 205–214.

Follett KA, Dirks B. (1994). Characterization of responses of primary somatosensory cerebral cortex neurons to noxious visceral stimulation in the rat. Brain Res 656: 27–32.

Folz E, White L. (1962). Pain "relief" by frontal cingulotomy. J Neurosurg 19: 89–100.

Foster GA, Schultzberg M, Kokfelt T, et al. (1988). Ontogeny of the dopamine and cyclic adenosine-3′: 5′-monophosphate-regulated phosphoprotein (DARPP-32) in the pre- and postnatal mouse central nervous system. Int J Dev Neurosci 6: 367–386.

Freitas RL, Ferreira CM, Ribeiro SJ, et al. (2005). Intrinsic neural circuits between dorsal midbrain neurons that control fear-induced responses and seizure activity and nuclei of the pain inhibitory system elaborating postictal antinociceptive processes: a functional neuroanatomical and neuro-pharmacological study. Exp Neurol 191: 225–242.

Friedman DP, Murray EA, O'Neill JB, et al. (1986). Cortical connections of the somatosensory fields of the lateral sulcus of macaques: Evidence for a corticolimbic pathway for touch. J Comp Neurol 252: 323–347.

Fukui M, Takishita A, Zhang N, et al. (2004). Involvement of locus coeruleus noradrenergic neurons in supraspinal antinociception by alpha, beta-methylene-ATP in rats. J Pharmacol Sci 94: 153–160.

Gamboa-Esteves FO, McWilliam PN, Batten TF. (2004). Substance P (NK1) and somatostatin (sst2A) receptor immunoreactivity in NTS-projecting rat dorsal horn neurons activated by nociceptive afferent input. J Chem Neuroanat 27: 251–266.

Gauriau C, Bernard JF. (2002). Pain pathways and parabrachial circuits in the rat. Exp Physiol 87: 251–258.

Gear RW, Aley KO, Levine JD. (1999). Pain-induced analgesia mediated by mesolimbic reward circuits. J Neurosci 19: 7175–7181.

Gebhart GF. (2004). Descending modulation of pain. Neurosci Biobehav 27: 729–737.

Gelnar PA, Krauss BR, Sheehe PR, et al. (1999). A comparative fMRI study of cortical representations for thermal painful, vibrotactile, and motor performance tasks. Neuroimage 10: 460–482.

Gilbert M. (1935). The early development of the human diencephalon. J Comp Neurol 62: 81–115.

Gilman S, Bloedel J, Lechtenberg R. (1981). Disorders of the Cerebellum. Davis Company, Philadelphia, PA.

Glover V, Fisk N. (1996). We don't know: better to err on the safe side from mid-gestation. BMJ 313: 796.

Gol A, Faibish GM. (1967). Effects of human hippocampal ablation. J Neurosurg 26: 390–398.

Greenspan JD, Lee RR, Lenz FA. (1999). Pain sensitivity alterations as a function of lesion location in the parasylvian cortex. Pain 81: 273–282.

Guilbaud G, Benoist JM, Levante A, et al. (1992). Primary somatosensory cortex in rats with pain-related behaviours due to a peripheral mononeuropathy after moderate ligation of one sciatic nerve: neuronal responsivity to somatic stimulation. Exp Brain Res 92: 227–245.

Gustafson EL, Ehrlich ME, Trivedi P, et al. (1992). Developmental regulation of phosphoprotein gene expression in the caudate-putamen of rat: an in situ hybridization study. Neuroscience 112: 65–75.

Hahm ET, Lee JJ, Min BI, et al. (2004). Opioid inhibition of GABAergic neurotransmission in mechanically isolated rat periaqueductal gray neurons. Neurosci Res 50: 343–354.

Hallbeck M, Blomqvist A. (1999). Spinal cord-projecting vasopressinergic neurons in the rat paraventricular hypothalamus. J Comp Neurol 411: 201–211.

Hari R, Portin K, Kettenmann B, et al. (1997). Right hemisphere preponderance of responses to painful CO_2 stimulation of the human nasal mucosa. Pain 72:145–151.

Heinricher MM, Martenson ME, Neubert MJ. (2004a). Prostaglandin E2 in the midbrain periaqueductal gray produces hyperalgesia and activates pain-modulating circuitry in the rostral ventromedial medulla. Pain 110: 419–426.

Heinricher MM, Neubert MJ, Martenson ME, et al. (2004b). Prostaglandin E2 in the medial preoptic area produces hyperalgesia and activates pain-modulating circuitry in the rostral ventromedial medulla. Neuroscience 128: 389–398.

Hohmann AG, Suplita RL, Bolton NM, et al. (2005). An endocannabinoid mechanism for stress-induced analgesia. Nature 435: 1108–1112.

Hua F, Harrison T, Qin C, et al (2004). c-Fos expression in rat brain stem and spinal cord in response to activation of cardiac ischemia-sensitive afferent neurons and electrostimulatory modulation. Am J Physiol Heart Circ Physiol 287: H2728–2738, Epub 2004.

Huang EY, Chen CM, Tao PL. (2004). Supraspinal anti-allodynic and rewarding effects of endomorphins in rats. Peptides 25: 577–583.

Hui KK, Liu J, Makris N, et al. (2000). Acupuncture modulates the limbic system and subcortical gray structures of the human brain: evidence from fMRI studies in normal subjects. Hum Brain Map 9: 13–25.

Humphrey T. (1968). The development of the human amygdala during early embryonic life. J Comp Neurol 132: 135–165.

Iadarola MJ, Berman KF, Zeffiro TA, et al. (1998). Neuronal activation during acute capsaicin-evoked pain and allodynia assessed with PET. Brain 121: 931–947.

Ibinson JW, Small RH, Algaze A, et al. (2004). Functional magnetic resonance imaging studies of pain: an investigation of signal decay during and across sessions. Anesthesiology 101: 960–969.

Ikeda K, Watanabe M, Ichikawa T, et al. (1998). Distribution of prepro-nociceptin/orphanin FQ mRNA and its receptor mRNA in developing and adult mouse central nervous systems. J Comp Neurol 399: 139–151.

Ikeda T, Terayama R, Jue SS, et al. (2003). Differential rostral projections of caudal brainstem neurons receiving trigeminal input after masseter inflammation. J Comp Neurol 465: 220–233.

Imbe H, Murakami S, Okamoto K, et al. (2004). The effects of acute and chronic restraint stress on activation of ERK in the rostral ventromedial medulla and locus coeruleus. Pain 112: 361–371.

Inagaki S, Sakanaka M, Shiosaka S, et al. (1982). Ontogeny of substance P-containing neuron system of the rat: immunohistochemical analysis—I. Forebrain and upper brain stem. Neuroscience 7: 251–277.

Jiang M, Behbehani MM. (2001). Physiological characteristics of the projection pathway from the medial preoptic to the nucleus raphe magnus of the rat and its modulation by the periaqueductal gray. Pain 94: 139–147.

Jiang M, Alheid GF, Calandriello T, et al. (2004). Parabrachial-lateral pontine neurons link nociception and breathing. Respir Physiol Neurobiol 143: 215–233.

Jin CY, Kalimo H, Panula P. (2002). The histaminergic system in human thalamus: correlation of innervation to receptor expression. Euro J Neurosci 15: 1125–1138.

Jones AK, Brown WD, Friston KJ, et al. (1991). Cortical and subcortical localization of response to pain in man using positron emission tomography. Proc R Soc Lond B Biol Sci 244: 39–44.

Kaminska B, Mosieniak G, Gierdalski M, et al. (1995). Elevated AP-1 transcription factor DNA binding activity at the onset of functional plasticity during development of rat sensory cortical areas. Brain Res Mol Brain Res 33: 295–304.

Kayalioglu G, Balkan B. (2004). Expression of c-Fos and NADPH-d after peripheral noxious stimulation in the pedunculopontine tegmental nucleus. Neuroreport 15: 421–423.

Kenshalo DR Jr, Isensee O. (1983). Responses of primate SI cortical neurons to noxious stimuli. J Neurophysiol 50: 1479–1496.

Kenshalo DR Jr, Giesler GJ Jr, Leonard RB, et al. (1980). Responses of neurons in primate ventral posterior lateral nucleus to noxious stimuli. J Neurophysiol 43: 1594–1614.

Kenshalo DR Jr, Chudler EH, Anton F, et al. (1988). SI nociceptive neurons participate in the encoding process by which monkeys perceive the intensity of noxious thermal stimulation. Brain Res 454: 378–382.

Khanna S, Chang LS, Jiang F, et al. (2004). Nociception-driven decreased induction of Fos protein in ventral hippocampus field CA1 of the rat. Brain Res 1004: 167–176.

Kinney HC, Ottoson CK, White WF. (1990). Three-dimensional distribution of 3H-naloxone binding to opiate receptors in the human fetal and infant brainstem. J Comp Neurol 291: 55–78.

Koester SE, O'Leary DD. (1994). Axons of early generated neurons in cingulate cortex pioneer the corpus callosum. J Neurosci 14: 6608–6620.

Kostovic I, Seress L, Mrzljak L, et al. (1989). Early onset of synapse formation in the human hippocampus: a correlation with Nissl-Golgi architectonics in 15- and 16.5-week-old fetuses. Neuroscience 30: 105–116.

Lamour Y, Willer JC, Guilbaud G. (1983). Rat somatosensory (SmI) cortex: I. Characteristics of neuronal responses to noxious stimulation and comparison with responses to non-noxious stimulation. Exp Brain Res 49: 35–45.

Lapeyre S, Mauborgne A, Becker C, et al. (2001). Subcutaneous formalin enhances outflow of met-enkephalin- and cholecystokinin-like materials in the rat nucleus accumbens. Naunyn-Schmiedebergs Arch Pharmacol 363: 399–406.

Lee SJ, Ralston HJP, Drey EA, et al. (2005). Fetal pain: A systematic multidisciplinary review of the evidence. JAMA 294: 947–954.

Lenz FA, Rios M, Zirh A, et al. (1998). Painful stimuli evoke potentials recorded over the human anterior cingulate gyrus. J Neurophysiol 79: 2231–2234.

Liang YC, Huang CC, Hsu KS. (2005). Characterization of long-term potentiation of primary afferent transmission at trigeminal synapses of juvenile rats: essential role of subtype 5 metabotropic glutamate receptors. Pain 114: 417–428.

Limperopoulos C, Soul JS, Gauvreau K, et al. (2005). Late gestation cerebellar growth is rapid and impeded by premature birth. Pediatrics 115: 688–695.

Liu A, Joyner AL. (2001). Early anterior posterior patterning of the midbrain and cerebellum. Annu Rev Neurosci 24: 869–896.

Liu JH, Li J, Yan J, et al. (2004a). Expression of c-Fos in the nuceus of the solitary tract following electroacupuncture at facial acupoints and gastric distension in rats. Neurosci Lett 366: 215–219.

Liu J-G, Rovnaghi CR, Garg S, et al. (2004b). Hyperalgesia in young rats associated with opioid receptor desensitization in the forebrain. Euro J Pharmacol 491: 127–136.

Lloyd-Thomas AR, Fitzgerald M. (1996). Do fetuses feel pain? Reflex responses do not necessarily signify pain. BMJ 313: 797–798.

Lopez-Bendito G, Molnar Z. (2003). Thalamocortical development: how are we going to get there? Nat Rev Neurosci 4: 276–289.

Lumb BM. (2002). Inescapable and escapable pain is represented in distinct hypothalamic-midbrain circuits: specific roles for Adelta- and C-nociceptors. (Review) (41 refs) Exp Physiol 87: 281–286.

Ma F, Zie H, Dong ZQ, et al. (2005). Expressions of ORL1 mRNA in some brain nuclei in neuropathic pain rats. Brain Res 1043: 214–217.

Maihofner C, Handwerker HO, Neundorfer B, et al. (2003). Patterns of cortical reorganization in complex regional pain syndrome. Neurology 61: 1707–1715.

Maihofner C, Schmelz M, Forster C, et al. (2004). Neural activation during experimental allodynia: a functional magnetic resonance imaging study. Eur J Neurosci 19: 3211–3218.

Maihofner C, Forster C, Birklein F, et al. (2005). Brain processing during mechanical hyperalgesia in complex regional pain syndrome: a functional MRI study. Pain 114: 93–103.

Mason P. (2005). Deconstructing endogenous pain modulations. J Neurophysiol 93: 1659–1663.

May A, Kaube H, Büchel C, et al. (1998). Experimental cranial pain elicited by capsaicin: a PET study. Pain 74: 61–66.

Mayer EA, Berman S, Suyenobu B, et al. (2005). Differences in brain responses to visceral pain between patients with irritable bowel syndrome and ulcerative colitis. Pain 115: 398–409.

McEwen BS. (2001). Plasticity of the hippocampus: adaptation to chronic stress and allostatic load. Ann NY Acad Sci 933: 265–277.

McGregor GP, Woodhams PL, O'Shaughnessy DJ, et al. (1982). Developmental changes in bombesin, substance P, somatostatin and vasoactive intestinal polypeptide in the rat brain. Neurosci Lett 28: 21–27.

McNally GP. (1999). Pain facilitatory circuits in the mammalian central nervous system: their behavioral significance and role in morphine analgesic tolerance. Neurosci Biobehav Rev 23: 1059–1078.

McNally GP, Akil H. (2002). Role of corticotropin-releasing hormone in the amygdala and bed nucleus of the stria terminalis in the behavioral, pain modulatory, and endocrine consequences of opiate withdrawal. Neurosci 112: 605–617.

Meaney MJ, Sharma S, Sarrieau S, et al. (1988). Postnatal development and environmental regulation of hippocampal glucocorticoid and mineralocorticoid receptors in the rat. Dev Brain Res 43: 158–162.

Melzack R, Wall PD. (1965). Pain mechanisms: a new theory. Science 150: 971–979.

Mendez-Diaz M, Guevara-Martinez M, Alquicira CR, et al. (2004). Cortistatin, a modulatory peptide of sleep and memory, induces analgesia in rats. Neurosci Lett 354: 242–244.

Meng ID, Johansen JP. (2004). Antinociception and modulation of rostral ventromedial medulla neuronal activity by local microinfusion of a cannabinoid receptor agonist. Neuroscience 124: 685–693.

Meng ID, Johansen JP, Harasawa I, et al. (2005). Kappa opioids inhibit physiologically identified medullary pain modulating neurons and reduce morphine antinociception. J Neurophysiol 93: 1138–1144, Epub 2004.

Messerschmidt A, Brugger PC, Boltshauser E, et al. (2005). Disruption of cerebellar development: potential complication of extreme prematurity. Am J Neuroradiol 26: 1659–1667.

Michaud JL. (2001). The developmental program of the hypothalamus and its disorders. Clin Genet 60: 255–263.

Mitchell JL, Silverman MB, Aicher SA. (2004). Rat trigeminal lamina I neurons that project to thalamic or parabrachial nuclei contain the mu-opioid receptor. Neuroscience 128: 571–582.

Miyase CI, Kishi R, de Freitas RL, et al. (2005). Involvement of pre- and post-synaptic serotonergic receptors of dorsal raphe nucleus neural network in the control of the sweet-substance-induced analgesia in adult Rattus norvegicus (Rodentia, Muridae). Neurosci Lett 379: 159–173, Epub 2005.

Mohr C, Binkofski F, Erdmann C, et al. (2005). The anterior cingulate cortex contains distinct areas dissociating external from self-administered painful stimulation: a parametric fMRI study. Pain 114: 347–357.

Molnar Z. (2000). Conserved developmental algorithms during thalamocortical circuit formation in mammals and reptiles. Novartis Foundation Symposium 228: 148–166; discussion 166–172.

Moore KL, Persaud TVN. (1998). The developing human: clinically oriented embryology. 6th edition, WB Saunders Company, Philadelphia, PA.

Morgan MM, Clayton CC, Boyer-Quick JS. (2005). Differential susceptibility of the PAG and RVM to tolerance to the antinociceptive effect of morphine in the rat. Pain 113: 91–98.

Morrow TJ, Paulson PE, Danneman PJ, et al. (1998). Regional changes in forebrain activation during the early and late phase of formalin nociception: analysis using cerebral blood flow in the rat. Pain 75: 355–365.

Muller F, O'Rahilly R. (1997). The timing and sequence of appearance of neuronmeres and their derivatives in staged human embryos. Acta Anatomica 158: 83–99.

Nakagawa T, Katsuya A, Tanimoto S, et al. (2003). Differential patterns of c-fos mRNA expression in the amygdaloid nuclei induced by chemical somatic and visceral noxious stimuli in rats. Neurosci Lett 344: 197–200.

Nandi D, Liu X, Joint C, et al. (2002). Thalamic field potentials during deep brain stimulation of periventricular gray in chronic pain. Pain 97: 47–51.

Nandi D, Aziz T, Carter H, et al. (2003). Thalamic field potentials in chronic central pain treated by periventricular gray stimulation – a series of eight cases. Pain 101: 97–107.

Narsinghani U, Anand KJS. (2000). Developmental neurobiology of pain in neonatal rats. Lab Animal 29: 27–39.

Nathan PW, Rudge P. (1974). Testing the gate-control theory of pain in man. J Neurol Neurosurg Psychiatr 37: 1366–1372.

Nixon PD, Passingham RE. (2001). Predicting sensory events. The role of the cerebellum in motor learning. Exp Brain Res 138: 251–257.

Ohara S, Crone NE, Weiss N, et al. (2004). Attention to pain is processed at multiple cortical sites in man. Exp Brain Res 156: 513–517.

Oliveira MA, Prado WA. (2001). Role of PAG in the antinociception evoked from the medial or central amygdala in rats. Brain Res Bull 54: 55–63.

O'Rahilly R, Muller F. (1999). Minireview: summary of the initial development of the human nervous system. Teratology 60: 39–41.

Palazzo E, Genovese R, Mariani L, et al. (2004). Metabotropic glutamate receptor 5 and dorsal raphe serotonin release in inflammatory pain in rat. Eur J Pharmacol 492: 169–176.

Pan ZZ, Williams JT, Osborne PB. (1990). Opioid actions on single nucleus raphe magnus neurons from rat and guinea-pig in vitro. J Physiol 427: 519–532.

Pan ZZ, Tershner SA, Fields HL. (1997). Cellular mechanism for antianalgesic action of agonists of the kappa-opioid receptor. Nature 389: 382–385.

Pan ZZ, Hirakawa N, Fields HL. (2000). A cellular mechanism for the bidirectional pain-modulating actions of orphanin FQ/nociceptin. Neuron 26: 515–522.

Parent A. (1996). Carpenter's Human Neuroanatomy. 9th edition. Williams & Wilkins, Baltimore, MD.

Paulson PE, Morrow TJ, Casey KL. (2000). Bilateral behavioral and regional cerebral blood flow changes during painful peripheral mononeuropathy in the rat. Pain 84: 233–245.

Penfield W, Rasmussen T. (1955). The Cerebral Cortex of Man. Macmillan Co, New York.

Petrovic P, Kalso E, Petersson KM, et al. (2002). Placebo and opioid analgesia–imaging a shared neuronal network. Science 295: 1737–1740.

Petrovic P, Carlsson K, Petersson KM, et al. (2004a). Context-dependent deactivation of the amygdala during pain. J Cognitive Neurosci 16: 1289–1301.

Petrovic P, Petersson KM, Hansson P, et al. (2004b). Brainstem involvement in the initial response to pain. Neuroimage 22: 995–1005.

Pigadas A, Thompson JR, Grube GL. (1981). Normal infant brain anatomy: correlated real-time sonograms and brain specimens. Am J Roentgenol 137: 815–820.

Ploghaus A, Narain C, Beckmann CF, et al. (2001). Exacerbation of pain by anxiety is associated with activity in a hippocampal network. J Neurosci 21: 9896–9903.

Ploner M, Schmitz F, Freund HJ, et al. (1999). Parallel activation of primary and secondary somatosensory cortices in human pain processing. J Neurophysiol 81: 3100–3104.

Ploner M, Schmitz F, Freund HJ, et al. (2000). Differential organization of touch and pain in human primary somatosensory cortex. J Neurophysiol 83: 1770–1776.

Porreca F, Ossipov MH, Gebhart GF. (2002). Chronic pain and medullary descending facilitation. Trends Neurosci 25: 319–325.

Porter FL, Wolf CM, Miller JP. (1998). The effect of handling and immobilization on the response to acute pain in newborn infants. Pediatrics 102: 1383–1389.

Price DD. (2000). Psychological and neural mechanisms of the affective dimension of pain. Science 288: 1769–1772.

Price DD. (2002). Central neural mechanisms that interrelate sensory and affective dimensions of pain. Mol Interventions 2: 392–403.

Rahman W, Dashwood MR, Fitzgerald M, et al. (1998). Postnatal development of multiple opioid receptors in the spinal cord and development of spinal morphine analgesia. Brain Res Dev Brain Res 108: 239–254.

Rainville P, Duncan GH, Price DD, et al. (1997). Pain affect encoded in human anterior cingulate but not somatosensory cortex. Science 277: 968–971.

Richard S, Engblom D, Paues J, et al. (2005). Activation of the parabrachio-amygdaloid pathway by immune challenge or spinal nociceptive input: a quantitative study in the rat using Fos immunohistochemistry and retrograde tract tracing. J Comp Neurol 481: 210–219.

Riedel W, Neeck G. (2001). Nociception, pain, and antinociception: current concepts. Z Rheumatol 60: 404–415.

Robbins MT, Uzzell TW, Aly S, et al. (2005). Visceral nociceptive input to the area of the medullary lateral reticular nucleus ascends in the lateral spinal cord. Neurosci Lett 381: 329–333.

Robinson CJ, Burton H. (1980). Somatic submodality distribution within the second somatosensory (SII), 7b, retroinsular, postauditory, and granular insular cortical areas of M. fascicularis. J Comp Neurol 192: 93–108.

Saab CY, Willis WD. (2002). Cerebellar stimulation modulates the intensity of a visceral nociceptive reflex in the rat. Exp Brain Res 146: 117–121.

Saab CY, Willis WD. (2003). The cerebellum: organization, functions and its role in nociception. Brain Res Rev 42: 85–95.

Saab CY, Kawasaki M, Al-Chaer ED, et al. (2001). Cerebellar cortical stimulation increases spinal nociceptive responses. J. Neurophysiol 85: 2359–2363.

Sajedianfard J, Khatami S, Semnanian S, et al. (2005). In vivo measurement of noradrenaline in the locus coeruleus of rats during the formalin test: a microdialysis study. Eur J Pharmacol 512: 153–156.

Sandin J, Ogren SO, Terenius L. (2004). Nociceptin/orphanin FQ modulates spatial learning via ORL-1 receptors in the dorsal hippocampus of the rat. Brain Res 997: 222–233.

Sawamura S, Obara M, Takeda K, et al. (2003). Corticotropin-releasing factor mediates the antinociceptive action of nitrous oxide in rats. Anesthesiology 99: 708–715.

Schmidt BL, Tambeli CH, Barletta J, et al. (2002a). Altered nucleus accumbens circuitry mediates pain-induced antinociception in morphine-tolerant rats. J Neurosci 14(11 Pt 1) 22: 6773–6780.

Schmidt BL, Tambeli CH, Levine JD, et al. (2002b). mu/delta cooperativity and opposing kappa-opioid effects in nucleus accumbens-mediated antinociception in the rat. Euro J Neurosci 15: 861–868.

Senapati AK, Lagraize SC, Huntington PJ, et al. (2005). Electrical stimulation of the anterior cingulate cortex reduces responses of rat dorsal horn neurons to mechanical stimuli. J Neurophysiol 94: 845–851.

Serafini R, Maric D, Maric I, et al. (1998). Dominant GABA (A) receptor/Cl-channel kinetics correlate with the relative expressions of alpha2, alpha3, alpha5 and beta3 subunits in embryonic rat neurons. Euro J Neurosci 10: 334–349.

Sewards TV, Sewards MA. (2002). The medial pain system: neural representations of the motivational aspect of pain. (Review) (259 refs) Brain Res Bull 59: 163–180.

Sewards TV, Sewards MA. (2003). Representations of motivational drives in mesial cortex, medial thalamus, hypothalamus and midbrain. (Review) (330 refs). Brain Res Bull 61: 25–49.

Siegel P, Wepsic JG. (1974). Alteration of nociception by stimulation of cerebellar structures in the monkey. Physiol Behav 13: 189–194.

Simons SHP, van Dijk M, Anand KJS, et al. (2003). Do we still hurt newborn babies? A prospective study of procedural pain and analgesia in neonates. Arch Pediatr Adolesc Med 157: 1058–1064.

Slagle TA, Oliphant M, Gross SJ. (1989). Cingulate sulcus development in preterm infants. Pediatr Res 26: 598–602.

Slater R, Cantarella A, Gallella S, et al. (2006). Cortical pain responses in human infants. J Neurosci 26: 3662–3666.

Spiegel J, Hansen C, Treede RD. (1996). Laser-evoked potentials after painful hand and foot stimulation in humans: evidence for generation of the middle-latency component in the secondary somatosensory cortex. Neurosci Lett 216: 179–182.

Squire LR, Bloom FE, McConnell SK, et al. (eds.) (2003). Cerebellum. In: Fundamental Neuroscience, 2nd edn, chapter 32, pp. 841–872. Academic Press, San Diego, CA.

Stazzone MM, Hubbard AM, Bilaniuk LT, et al. (2000). Ultrafast MR imaging of the normal posterior fossa in fetuses. Am J Roentgenol 175: 835–839.

Stevens RT, London SM, Apkarian AV. (1993). Spinothalamocortical projections to the secondary somatosensory cortex (SII) in squirrel monkey. Brain Res 631: 241–246.

Strigo IA, Duncan GH, Boivin M, et al. (2003). Differentiation of visceral and cutaneous pain in the human brain. J Neurophysiol 89: 3294–3303.

Svensson P, Minoshima S, Beydoun A, et al. (1997). Cerebral processing of acute skin and muscle pain in humans. J Neurophysiol 78: 450–460.

Sweet WH. (1982). Cerebral localization of pain. In: Thompson RA, Green JR, (eds). New Perspectives in Cerebral Localization, pp. 205–242. Raven Press, New York.

Taddio A, Shah V, Gilbert-MacLeod C, et al. (2002). Conditioning and hyperalgesia in newborns exposed to repeated heel lances. JAMA 288: 857–861.

Talbot JD, Marrett S, Evans AC, et al. (1991). Multiple representations of pain in human cerebral cortex. Science 251: 1355–1358.

Taylor BK, Joshi C, Uppal H. (2003). Stimulation of dopamine D2 receptors in the nucleus accumbens inhibits inflammatory pain. Brain Res 987: 135–143.

Tsuruoka M, Maeda M, Inoue T. (2004a). Persistent hindpaw inflammation produces coeruleospinal anti-nociception in the non-inflamed forepaw of rats. Neurosci Lett 367: 66–70.

Tsuruoka M, Maeda M, Nagasawa I, et al. (2004b). Spinal pathways mediating coeruleospinal antinociception in the rat. Neurosci Lett 362: 236–239.

Ungless MA, Magill PJ, Bolam JP. (2004). Uniform inhibition of dopamine neurons in the ventral tegmental area by aversive stimuli. Science 303: 2040–2042.

Urban MO, Ren K, Sablad M, et al. (2005). Medullary N-type and P/Q-type calcium channels contribute to neuropathy-induced allodynia. Neuroreport 16: 563–566.

Van Bockstaele EJ, Gracy KN, Pickel VM. (1995). Dynorphin-immunoreactive neurons in the rat nucleus accumbens: ultrastructure and synaptic input from terminals containing substance P and/or dynorphin. J Comp Neurol 351: 117–133.

Vanegas H, Schaible HG. (2004). Descending control of persistent pain: inhibitory or facilitatory? Brain Res Brain Res Rev 43:295–309.

Verne GN, Himes NC, Robinson ME, et al. (2003). Central representation of visceral and cutaneous hypersensitivity in the irritable bowel syndrome. Pain 103: 99–110.

Villarreal CF, Kina VA, Prado WA. (2004). Participation of brainstem nuclei in the pronociceptive effect of lesion or neural block of the anterior pretectal nucleus in a rat model of incisional pain. Neuropharmacol 47: 117–127.

Vin-Christian K, Benoist JM, Gautron M, et al. (1992). Further evidence for the involvement of SmI cortical neurons in nociception: modifications of their responsiveness over the early stage of a carrageenin-induced inflammation in the rat. Somatosens Mot Res 9: 245–261.

Vogt BA. (2005). Pain and emotion interactions in subregions of the cingulate gyrus. Nat Rev Neurosci 6: 533–544.

Voogd J, Glickstein M. (1998). The anatomy of the cerebellum. TINS 21: 370–375.

Watanabe S, Kuwaki T, Yanagisawa M, et al. (2005). Persistent pain and stress activate pain-inhibitory orexin pathways. Neuroreport 16: 5–8.

Weinstock M. (1997). Does prenatal stress impair coping and regulation of hypothalamic-pituitary-adrenal axis? Neurosci Biobehav Rev 21: 1–10.

Whitsel BL, Petrucelli LM, Werner G. (1969). Symmetry and connectivity in the map of the body surface in somatosensory area II of primates. J Neurophysiol 32: 170–183.

Willis WD, Kenshalo DR. (1991). The role of the cerebral cortex in pain sensation. In: Jones EG, Peters A (eds). Cerebral Cortex, Normal and Altered States of Function, vol. 9: 153–212. Plenum, New York.

Willis WD, Al-Chaer ED, Quast MJ, et al. (1999). A visceral pain pathway in the dorsal column of the spinal cord. Proc Natl Acad Sci USA 96(14): 7675–7679.

Winfield DA, Gatter KC, Powell TP. (1980). An electron microscopic study of the types and proportions of neurons in the cortex of the motor and visual areas of the cat and rat. Brain 103: 245–258.

Woolf CJ, Salter MW. (2000). Neuronal plasticity: increasing the gain in pain. Science 288: 1765–1768.

Workman BJ, Lumb BM. (1997). Inhibitory effects evoked from the anterior hypothalamus are selective for the nociceptive responses of dorsal horn neurons with high- and low-threshold inputs. J Neurophysiol 77: 2831–2835.

Wu MT, Sheen JM, Chuang KH, et al. (2002). Neuronal specificity of acupuncture response: a fMRI study with electroacupuncture. Neuroimage 16: 1028–1037.

Xu F, Frazier DT. (2000). Modulation of respiratory motor output by cerebellar deep nuclei in the rat. J Appl Physiol 89: 996–1004.

Yaguez L, Coen S, Gregory LJ, et al. (2005). Brain response to visceral aversive conditioning: a functional magnetic resonance imaging study. Gastroenterology 128: 1819–1829.

Zaichenko MI, Mikhailova NG, Raigorodskii-Yu V. (2001). Neuron activity in the prefrontal cortex of the brain in rats with different typological characteristics in conditions of emotional stimulation. Neurosci Behav Physiol 31: 299–304.

Zelazo PD. (2004). The development of conscious control in childhood. Trends Cogn Sci 8: 12–17.

Zhang J, Penny DJ, Kim NS, et al. (1999a). Mechanisms of blood pressure increase induced by dopamine in hypotensive preterm neonates. Arch Dis Childhood Fetal Neonat Ed 81: F99–F104.

Zhang X, Wenk HN, Gokin AP, et al, Giesler GJ Jr. (1999b). Physiological studies of spinohypothalamic tract neurons in the lumbar enlargement of monkeys. J Neurophysiol 82: 1054–1058.

Zhang ZH, Dougherty PM, Oppenheimer SM. (1999c). Monkey insular cortex neurons respond to baroreceptive and somatosensory convergent inputs. Neuroscience 94: 351–360.

4

Long-term consequences of pain in human neonates

Ruth Eckstein Grunau
Mai T Tu

OVERVIEW

Until recently, nociceptive experiences were rare for neonates. In evolutionary terms, this may be the reason why pain-modulating systems are immature at birth (Winberg 1998). Tremendous advances in medical care in recent decades have led to survival of medically fragile preterm and full-term infants, who are hospitalized sometimes for lengthy periods. The plasticity of the developing nervous system may allow for the greatest impact of pain to occur in the least maturely born infants (Fitzgerald 2005).

Conceptually, pain is on a continuum of stressors from handling to skin-breaking procedures. In preterm infants in the neonatal intensive care unit (NICU), repeated stressful and nociceptive stimulation lead to sensitization whereby pain due to skin-breaking procedures cannot be isolated from stress of tactile stimulation and handling. Therefore in neurophysiologically immature human neonates, it is very difficult to separate specific sensory changes due to neonatal pain exposure from more generalized effects of cumulative stress/pain, on multiple aspects of biobehavioural reactivity. Sensitization to repeated pain is found in full-term healthy infants as well, however in infants who have not experienced surgery or hospitalization, effects may not last as long.

Distinctions between different types of long-term effects of neonatal pain are important. For example, there may be changes in sensory perception specific to certain types of pain, but not mechanical stimulation, and pain may be altered long term with or without changes to other aspects of functioning. The type and extent of effects probably depends on the developmental maturity of the infant at the time the pain occurred, other concomitant clinical factors, the length and extent of exposure to pain, and multiple environmental and contextual factors both concurrently at the time of pain exposure and ongoing during development.

In this chapter we will review evidence for altered pain processing in full-term and preterm infants following neonatal pain exposure, and more broadly altered stress systems and developmental processes in preterm infants. Caregiving profoundly influences mammalian development, therefore the potential for maternal–infant regulators to ameliorate effects of neonatal pain will be addressed.

NOCICEPTION, PAIN PERCEPTION AND LONG-TERM EFFECTS

At the outset, it is important to clarify relationships between infant pain perception and long-term effects of infant pain exposure. Distinctions between re-activity to nociceptive input and pain perception (e.g. Lee et al. 2005) are irrelevant to the issue of long-term effects of pain exposure. Even the most premature neonates show sensitization to stimulation, which is a basic physiological phenomenon of the immature organism's hypersensivity to tactile inputs, together with limited capacity to regulate excitatory and inhibitory systems (Andrews and Fitzgerald 1994, Fitzgerald 2005). Changes in reactivity can be mediated by alterations at the spinal cord level, without involvement of higher centres. Similarly, altered stress hormone expression, and other effects associated with neonatal pain may not involve adult-like higher-order consciousness. These altered systems are signs of implicit biological memory, and the processes engaged may alter the central nervous system and stress physiology without conscious perception of pain.

PAIN AND STRESS IN PRETERM INFANTS IN THE NICU ENVIRONMENT

Procedural pain induces behavioural, physiological and hormonal changes which potentially may influence nociceptive and tactile thresholds, stress physiology and behaviour, and neurodevelopment of the immature organism (Anand 2000, Grunau 2002, 2003). Preterm infants in the NICU are exposed to frequent invasive procedures averaging 2–10 per day for infants from 28–32 weeks post-conceptional age (PCA) (Johnston et al. 1997). The neurophysiological substrates for nociception are functional by mid-gestation, and the lack of inhibitory controls (which develop later), lower pain threshold in extremely pre-term neonates, and sensitization following exposure to further tactile or painful stimuli contribute to hypersensitivity in the least mature preterm infants, leading to ongoing stress and pain (Fitzgerald 2005). Altered excitability may cause seemingly non-noxious tactile stimuli (e.g. routine handling, napkin (diaper) changes, bathing) to be perceived as noxious (Stevens and Gibbins 2002, Stevens et al. 2003, Holsti et al. 2005). For example, reactivity of preterm infants to endotracheal suctioning was greater when more pain exposure occurred on the previous day (Grunau et al. 2000). Further, when clustered nursing care followed blood collection within an hour, the stress of clustered nursing care induced as much biobehavioral reaction as did pain of skin-breaking procedures (Holsti et al. 2005). Therefore, neonatal stress and pain in preterm infants encompasses cumulative effects of repeated procedural pain and spin-off effects of handling, which induces chronic stress in physiologically immature infants.

SENSORY CHANGES: LONG-TERM EFFECTS ON LATER PAIN SENSITIVITY

Preterm infants

Sensitization induces hyper-reactivity in the NICU, however, cumulative exposure to neonatal stress/pain is often associated with decreased behavioural (Johnston and Stevens 1996, Grunau et al. 2001a) and cortisol (Grunau et al. 2005) responses to pain after infants have spent considerable time in the NICU.

Only a few studies have directly compared pain reactivity of former preterm and full-term infants after NICU discharge, in infancy (Oberlander et al. 2000, Grunau et al. 2001b), later in childhood at 9–12 years (Schmelzle-Lubiecki et al. 2005), and in adolescents (Buskila et al. 2003). In these two infant studies, a 'pain naïve' site of blood collection by finger lance was used, and unexpectedly revealed few differences at 4 months corrected chronologic age (CCA) in behavioural or cardiac responses in extremely preterm compared to full-term infants, except for a subgroup of those who were the smallest and sickest in the neonatal period (Oberlander et al. 2000). In contrast, later, at 8 months CCA, there were significant overall differences with the preterm group as a whole showing faster recovery of both facial and cardiac responses (Grunau et al. 2001b), giving an overall impression of less behavioural response in the preterm group. However, unexpectedly, on detailed examination of the pattern over time (see Fig. 4.1), in fact the preterm infants displayed significantly more facial reactivity to the initial finger lance than the full-term infants, and then the groups crossed over to the preterm showing faster recovery. Fast dampening of response (recovery) may be the cues parents used when reporting less pain reactivity in global observations of their preterm toddlers (Grunau et al. 1994a).

In a combined sample of preterm and full-term children, those who had thoracic surgery in infancy displayed decreased pain processing to quantitative sensory testing at age 9–12 years (Schmelzle-Lubiecki et al. 2005). In that study, the injury site in the surgical group showed significantly less mechanical sensitivity, cold and warmth perception than any other area tested. Effects of early infant surgery were not only local, but also evident in other areas, although not to the same extent as in the surgical site. It is not known whether effects would be equally great in the children born full-term compared to preterm, since the sample

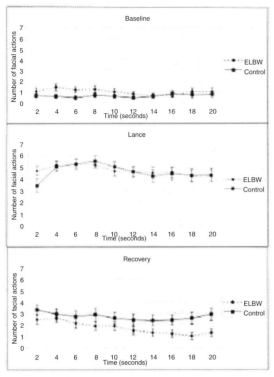

Figure 4.1 Facial response during baseline, finger lance, and recovery at 8 months corrected age (mean facial actions ± SEM). (Reproduced from Grunau et al., 2001b with permission from Elsevier.) (ELBW, extremely low birth weight.)

size was too small in this preliminary sample to examine this question. The methodologies in this initial report were precise and comprehensive; this is landmark work from Maria Fitzgerald's group. In a different study, preterm adolescents had a higher number of tender 'pressure points' and increased sensitivity (Buskila et al. 2003). Importantly, despite altered sensitivity to stimulation, children and adolescents exposed to early pain did not report more pain symptoms in daily life (Buskila et al. 2003, Schmelzle-Lubiecki et al. 2005). In contrast, in a study of health status, preterm-born adolescents reported more functional limitations, including pain, than full-term controls (Saigal et al. 1996). The different findings on self-report of pain between these studies may depend on whether the samples included adolescents with ongoing neurologically based physical problems, such as cerebral palsy. The most compelling evidence for long-term effects is provided by direct sensory testing, however, earlier work using parent report and child responses to pictures of pain are consistent in confirming associations with long-term effects. Parents reported their preterm toddlers born <1000 g were significantly less reactive to everyday bumps and

scrapes, compared to heavier preterm (1500–2499 g) and full-term toddlers (Grunau et al. 1994a). Together these studies suggest central neuroplasticity in the pathophysiology of pain in human infants exposed at an early age. The greater initial facial response in preterm infants evident many months after NICU discharge (Grunau et al. 2001b), in a pain naïve site (finger), implied central sensitization. Furthermore, findings of varying hyper- and/or hyporeactivity to later pain are consistent with animal models varying in nociceptive exposure, timing and type of outcome (Ren et al. 2004). In addition, a pattern of increasing effects across age has also been reported under specific circumstances in animal models, with some effects appearing even post-puberty (Ren et al. 2004). Cumulatively a small body of evidence is emerging demonstrating both local and global long-term consequences of neonatal pain in the NICU on later cortical and thalamic processing in preterm children, however far more studies using direct testing are needed.

Importantly, there is considerable convergence between results in the human findings and the experimental animal literature. Neurobiological development in newborn rats approximates that of the 24-week gestation human fetus, thus providing a good model for prematurity. Pain applied to the neonatal rat has effects not found when pain exposure occurs at later ages. Nociceptive stimulation in rat pups, e.g. repeated pin pricks (Anand et al. 1999), injections of inflammatory agents (Bhutta et al. 2001), surgical cuts (Alvares et al. 2000) induce altered pain thresholds in adulthood. Effects of early pain exposure are evident at all levels of pain systems (Fitzgerald 2005). The direction and extent of effects related to repetitive pain in the immature organism depend on the type of pain stimulus and timing (Ren et al. 2004). Given the multiplicity of influences in the human clinical situation, and lack of controlled circumstances, the animal literature is essential for identifying causal relationships and mechanisms.

Surgery

Studies of long-term effects of surgery in infancy have been informative for understanding long-term effects of infant pain. In healthy full-term male infants, routine neonatal circumcision without pain management was associated with increased sensitivity to vaccination 4 months later, whereas the effect was reduced when circumcision was partially managed with analgesic cream (Taddio et al. 1997). Similarly, surgery in infancy undertaken with appropriate pharmacologic management did not lead to increased pain sensitivity during vaccination subsequently (Peters et al. 2003). Conversely, full-term infants who received multiple skin breaks for blood tests following birth to mothers with gestational diabetes learned to anticipate pain and responded more to venipuncture than controls (Taddio et al. 2002). Furthermore, in a retrospective study, gastric suction at birth was associated with increased incidence of functional intestinal disorders later in life (Anand et al. 2004b). Long-term effects of surgery (hypersensitivity) are greatest when subsequent pain sensitivity is tested in the same region in which the original surgery was performed (Andrews and Fitzgerald 2002, Andrews et al. 2002, Peters et al. 2005, Schmelzle-Lubiecki et al. 2005). These data converge with the results of animal studies which demonstrated that long-term effects differ depending on whether prior tissue damage is re-inflamed or 'pain naïve', and the extent and timing of early insult (Ren et al. 2004, Fitzgerald 2005). In human infants and young children it is challenging to differentiate effects of heightened behavioural, hormonal and metabolic stress responses post surgery due to effects of emotional reactions to a strange environment and separation anxiety, rather than pain per se (Bouwmeester et al. 2001). Taken together these studies suggest alterations in spinal cord connectivity, central sensitization, as well as more generalized changes in stress reactivity.

Somatization

In preschoolers, a higher incidence of unexplained stomachaches, headaches, leg pains, and other somatic concerns ('somatization') was reported in preterm compared to full-term children (Grunau et al. 1994b, Sommerfelt et al. 1996). Surprisingly, however, later at age 9 years (Grunau et al. 1998) and 17 years (Grunau et al. 2004a) the prevalence of somatization did not differ between extremely preterm compared to the full-term children. These later findings are consistent with studies that found no increased report of self-report of pain syndromes in middle childhood (Schmelzle-Lubiecki et al. 2005) or adolescence (Buskila et al. 2003), despite increased sensitivity to induced pain, and no difference in parent report of pain in adolescence (Saigal et al. 2000b). This dissociation between pain sensitivity and pain syndromes such as somatization warrants further investigation of underlying developmental mechanisms, as well as contextual factors such as social modelling.

Stress systems

The hypothalamic–pituitary–adrenal (HPA) axis is highly susceptible to programming during early development (Meaney 2001, Welberg and Seckl 2001, Matthews 2002). In preterm infants, stress exposure related to developmentally 'unexpected' stimulation outside the protective uterine environment, particularly repeated invasive procedures, is ongoing over a prolonged period in the NICU. Activation of the HPA axis is involved with the capacity of the organism to respond to and cope with demands of the environment. Responses of the HPA axis are programmed by experiences early in life, including maternal separation, handling (for a review, see Meaney 2001), and associated with pain exposure (Grunau et al. 2004b, 2005, under review). There are conflicting data on cortisol (the primary human stress hormone) secretion in preterm infants while they are in the NICU. Some studies show higher levels in sick compared to healthy preterm neonates (Economou et al. 1993), whereas others found the highest cortisol levels in the youngest preterm (24–27 weeks gestation) but the lowest levels in the sickest of these infants (Scott and Watterberg 1995). Inappropriately low cortisol levels in preterm infants may be due to multiple factors, including cumulative stress and procedural pain in infants who were in the NICU for many weeks (Grunau et al. 2005).

In general, in full-term neonates, cortisol levels increase in a graded fashion to increasing stress and arousal (Gunnar et al. 1985). Invasive procedures stimulate cortisol release, while aversive but non-invasive events that may be stressful but not painful, such as physical exam, produce a smaller and more variable cortisol response (Gunnar 1989). In the NICU, cortisol responses to stress of routine clustered nursing procedures were examined, showing down-regulation while exposed to ongoing stressors, in infants with the greatest prior procedural pain exposure since birth (Grunau et al. 2005). Later in infancy, cortisol responses have been studied in full-term infants (e.g. Gunnar et al. 1992, 1995, Lewis and Ramsay 1995), but rarely in preterm infants past NICU discharge. There is initial evidence of long-term re-programming in infants born ≤28 weeks gestational age (GA), in that they had significantly high cortisol levels at 8 and 18 months CCA (Grunau et al. 2004b, under review), which is consistent with findings that low birth weight predicted increased cortisol concentrations in adults (Phillips et al. 2000). High salivary cortisol levels across repeated sampling (basal, after introduction of visual novelty, and after developmental assessment) were evident at 8 months CCA (Grunau et al. 2004b). An example of infant-focused attention to visual novelty is provided in Figure 4.2. Among the combined preterm groups at 8 months CCA, a higher number of skin-breaking procedures from birth to term predicted both basal cortisol and cortisol levels during visual novelty, after controlling for early illness severity, duration of supplemental

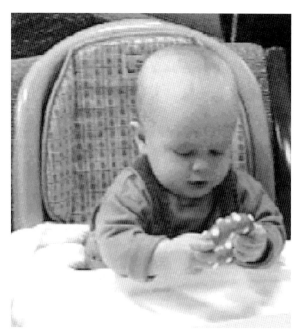

Figure 4.2 Infant attention assessed during toy exploration at age 8 months (corrected for prematurity).

respiratory support and morphine exposure (Grunau et al. 2004b). Importantly, gestational age was not driving these associations, however the effects of a higher number of skin-breaking procedures since birth could not be distinguished from the effects of length of time on mechanical ventilation. Thus the combination of physiological immaturity at birth, stress/pain of repetitive procedures during prolonged mechanical ventilation may contribute to 'resetting' arousal systems in preterm infants. Increased intravenous morphine administration during neonatal hospitalization did not prevent these changes. Findings of higher basal cortisol levels (Grunau et al. 2004b, under review) and higher basal heart rate (Grunau et al. 2001b) in extremely preterm infants suggest resetting of stress physiology. Neonatal reprogramming of stress systems may be one potential mechanism related to altered behaviour, learning and cognition associated with extreme prematurity. Moreover, because the early environment affects vulnerability to diseases later in life (Phillips et al. 2000, Barker 2002), effects of neonatal pain over a prolonged period may have spin-offs for long-term health. Given that prolonged exposure to endogenous corticosteroids is associated with reduced hippocampal volume and cognitive decline, our findings of extended high cortisol levels in extremely low gestational age preterm infants suggests a further possible mechanism, in addition to altered cell death and immature regula-tion of cerebral blood volume

in the NICU proposed previously (Anand 2000), which may contribute to altered neurodevelopment, learning, attention and behaviour in this vulnerable population. Consistent with the results of a major multicentre trial that showed no beneficial effect of intravenous morphine on major outcome at NICU discharge (Anand et al. 2004a), we have found that higher amounts of intravenous morphine do not ameliorate associations between cumulative pain in the NICU and later outcomes in infancy.

Developmental outcomes of prematurity

There is emerging evidence of multiple mechanisms that potentially link neonatal pain in preterm infants to later developmental and behavioural compromise in preterm children, especially in those born prior to the 3rd trimester of fetal life (23–28 weeks gestation).

Survival rates of extremely preterm infants rose substantially in the 1990s, however the rate of developmental problems remains unchanged, and increased survival rates impact the total number of these vulnerable children. Academic achievement of up to 50% of children born <1500 g grams is affected, and attention deficits and anxiety disorders are common (Perlman 2001). While the majority of preterm infants escape major impairment (e.g. blindness, non-ambulatory cerebral palsy, IQ <70), they develop alterations to the brain which are manifested functionally as poorer attention, memory, learning, cognition, motor function, behaviour and academic achievement (e.g. Vohr et al. 1992, Marlow et al. 1993, Hack et al. 1994, Whitfield et al. 1997), and problems persist to late adolescence and beyond (Saigal et al. 2000a, Hack et al. 2002, Grunau et al. 2004a, Rogers et al. 2005).

Neuropsychological studies report impairments across a wide range of cognitive skills in preterm children, notably executive function which includes anticipation, goal selection, planning and organization, self-regulation, attention and utilization of feedback (Anderson et al. 2004). Extremely preterm children with normal IQ are uneasy with novel cognitive challenge as preschoolers (Grunau 2003), and at school age (Whitfield et al. 1997) compared to full-term controls. This likely reflects attention and executive function difficulties related to appraisal and execution of novel and/or challenging tasks. Problems in cognitive and behavioural executive function in preterm children correlated only weakly with birthweight and gestational age 'indicating that other factors must also mediate outcome' (Anderson et al. 2004). We propose that the extent of stress/pain in the NICU is another salient factor.

Prolonged neonatal pain is likely to have a direct impact on the development of systems related to regulation of attention, arousal and emotion. Chronically stressful situations, including neonatal pain, likely inhibit development of integrative self-regulatory processes (Wilson and Gottman 1996, Ryan et al. 1997, Grunau 2003), which may be precursors of dysfunctional attention and higher-order executive processes later in childhood. Preterm infants display delays and deficits in selective visual attention (e.g. Ruff 1988). They show biobehavioural dysregulation (behaviour, cardiac, autonomic, cortisol) during novel learning (Haley et al. 2006, under review), and differences in their range and threshold for optimal states of arousal which facilitate selective and sustained attention and information encoding (Gardner and Karmel 1983), compared to full-term infants. Studies of arousal and attention regulation in preterm infants suggest altered neuropsychological functioning reflecting abnormal patterns of brain organization (Mayes and Bornstein 1997, Davidson et al. 2000). Dysregulation of stress systems may be one contributing factor to underlying deficits in learning, memory and cognition that are typically observed in preterm infants.

Cortisol plays an important role in learning and memory in adult humans and rodents. An inverted U-shaped function has been proposed to account for the positive and negative effects of cortisol on cognitive performance and memory, such that too little or too much impairs, but moderate amounts facilitate performance. Moderate cortisol levels during learning facilitate memory 24 hours later in preterm and full-term infants (Haley et al. 2006). In 4–5-year-old full-term children, chronically high or low levels of cortisol and problems with the up- or down-regulation of cortisol in response to stress are associated with difficulties in executive function (Blair et al. 2005). Altered processing and response to novelty persist across childhood in extremely preterm infants (Whitfield et al. 1997, Grunau 2003). Chronic stress over a prolonged period in neonates implicating reprogramming of stress-sensitive systems and thereby function in the hippocampus, a limbic structure involved in the HPA regulation, may contribute to differences in capacity to self-regulate.

There is an urgent need to move beyond description of problems in this population to address potential mechanisms of brain–behaviour relationships which underlie specific complex processing. Neonatal repetitive pain may contribute to changes in neurodevelopment in infants born very preterm, however this can only be evaluated indirectly in human preterm infants. Anand (2000) described mechanisms which could potentially link repeated pain to neuroanatomic changes, namely the enhanced vulnerability of immature neurons to excitotoxic stress, and that

altered apoptosis, which would change the normally developing cytoarchitecture of the brain. In addition to these structural changes, pain and stress in the NICU appears to induce high endogenous cortisol levels later in infancy (Grunau et al. 2004b, under review), which may be another mechanism whereby neonatal pain potentially may contribute to altered development. However, it must be noted that direct effects of pain on neurodevelopment remain speculative at this time.

Stress and anxiety

Heightened behavioural stress responses to cognitive challenge are evident in extremely preterm children compared to full-term children. Preterm children with normal IQ showed significantly more stress behaviours (e.g. anxious, reacts to failure unrealistically, distrusts own ability, needs constant praise and encouragement to continue) during cognitive assessment (Grunau 2003). These stress behaviours persisted at 9 years (Grunau et al. 1998), independent of IQ. Importantly preterm adolescents appear to be more prone to anxiety and depressive disorders compared to full-term peers (Levy-Shiff et al. 1994, Grunau et al. 2004a). Increased anxiety behaviours are commonly related to early stress in animal models (Meerlo et al. 1996, Vallee et al. 1997). Experimentally induced neonatal stress in rodents (maternal separation) effects changes in prelimbic prefrontal cortex, which is a vulnerable link in neonatal stress exposure and emotion regulation, causing increased excitation and hyper-reactivity (Weller and Feldman 2003). More experimental studies of brain changes following neonatal pain in rodent models are needed.

Sex

Animal studies show sex differences to nociception (Mogil et al. 2000), analgesia (Gear et al. 2003), effects of prenatal stress on later pain (Sternberg and Ridgway 2003), vulnerability to early stress and effects on long-term pain reactivity (Stephan et al. 2002) . In human adults, there are sex differences in effects of opioids (Craft 2003), response to pain (Unruh 1996), and direction of cortisol response (Zimmer et al. 2003). We have found sex differences in relationships between maternal style and parent report of pain sensitivity to everyday bumps and scrapes, in toddlers born extremely preterm (Grunau 2003). Higher pain sensitivity was associated with lower maternal responsivity in boys, but not girls. In general, in animal studies, postnatal stress appears to have greater effects on females (Sternberg and Ridgway 2003), consistent with the higher pain sensitivity in females reported in studies of human adults (Unruh 1996). In rodents, male gonadal hormones may play a protective role in pain perception; moreover female hormones may be related to deficits in pain inhibitory mechanisms (Gaumond et al. 2005). However, importantly, studies of neurodevelopmental outcomes of prematurity have consistently shown more adverse sequelae in boys (e.g. Whitfield et al. 1997). Therefore, it is important to recognize that the mechanisms of long-term outcomes are complex in this population, and that sex effects in the domain of pain sensitivity may differ from those on other aspects of neurodevelopment.

Maternal factors

The primary caregiver is the most important modulator of stimulation (Hofer 1994). There is extensive literature on the influence of maternal behaviours on later stress responses, the development of neural structures and plasticity of functional pathways. The transactional nature of caregiver and infant is fundamental to mammalian development and acquisition of self-regulation (see Walker et al. 2004). Variations in maternal care are key in development of HPA axis and behavioural regulation in rodents (Meaney 2001) and humans (Gunnar 1998), including modulating expression of pain reactivity in infants (Bustos et al. 2005) and young children (Sweet et al. 1999, Chambers et al. 2002).

The untimely birth of a preterm infant impacts parental stress, especially while their infant is in the NICU (Seideman et al. 1997, Levy-Shiff et al. 1998, Klebanov et al. 2001, Franck et al. 2004). Positive adjustment in terms of maternal distress, behaviour toward the infant, and parenting efficacy are associated with positive mother–infant relations and infant development (e.g. Levy-Shiff et al. 1994). Relationships among stress, outcomes and coping are complex (Compas and Thomsen 1999, Klebanov et al. 2001) and probably even more so in preterm infants, who are more sensitive to environmental context at all stages of development. In full-term infants, cortisol activity is sensitive to variations in quality of caregiving (Gunnar and Donzella 2002), and furthermore, stressful maternal life events moderated effects of an intervention programme on child cognitive scores (Klebanov et al. 2001). Following hospital discharge, the quality of mother–infant relations with preterm infants can differ from healthy full-term infants (Beckwith and Rodning 1996, Chapiesky and Evankovich 1997). Preterm infants are described as less alert and less responsive, while their mothers are often more active and directive than full-term mother–infant dyads, presumably to compensate (Macey et al. 1987).

Multiple interacting intrinsic and extrinsic factors potentially ameliorate or exacerbate effects of neo-

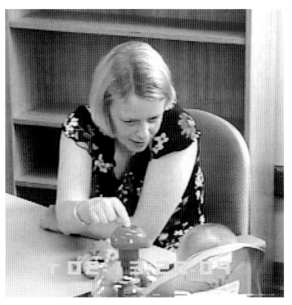

Figure 4.3 Mother–infant interaction assessed during a play session at age 8 months (corrected for prematurity).

natal experience on development. Importantly, in preterm infants born ≤32 weeks gestational age, maternal stress played an important role in mediating relationships of neonatal pain with infant attention (Tu et al. 2005). In that study, positive mother interaction ameliorated negative effects of neonatal pain on attention, but only for mothers who reported lower stress. Figure 4.3 shows a play session during which the mother interacts with her 8-month-old infant, to illustrate methods used in our work. Socioeconomic status (SES) can mediate maternal stress, in turn, affecting quality of maternal behaviours. Low SES and maternal depressive symptoms have been associated with poorer cognitive performance and higher morning cortisol concentrations in children (Lupien et al. 2000, 2001). Studies are needed of various sources of parental stress, and the extent to which caregiver stress may mediate specific effects of neonatal pain.

Caregiver behaviours can partially modify effects of early pain exposure on HPA changes in rodents, as rat pups exposed to neonatal experimental pain elicited increased licking and grooming from their dams, thereby preventing HPA changes, but not other adverse effects (Walker et al. 2003). The influence of parenting is central in developmental psychobiology, and advances have been made in identifying mechanisms of permanent changes in stress systems (Meaney 2001, Sapolsky 2004). Moreover, environmental enrichment in juvenile rats partially reversed effects of neonatal stress (Francis et al. 2002, Bredy et al.

2003). While we recognize the major differences in the human compared to the rat, together these animal studies suggest, in principle, the potential that there may be sufficient plasticity after NICU discharge to ameliorate some of the long-term effects of neonatal pain. Alterations to sensory pain thresholds will probably be less amenable to amelioration from maternal and SES sources than changes to more generalized stress responses.

CONCLUSIONS

Nociceptive systems are functional early, and there is a small body of direct evidence demonstrating that neonatal activation of nociceptive systems is associated with long-term changes in sensory perception of pain. However, the relative vulnerability of biologically immature preterm infants may render them prone to developmentally more pervasive or different long-term effects, in addition to those experienced by full-term infants. Neonatal pain exposure in extremely preterm neonates may re-program fundamental stress systems and may potentially contribute to some aspects of altered brain development. However, current evidence in humans does not address causal links between early pain and neurodevelopment, only tentative associations.

It is important to note that currently there is no evidence to support the use of continuous intravenous morphine in the NICU to prevent major negative sequelae in mechanically ventilated preterm infants. However, a great deal of work remains to be done as to whether or not ongoing pharmacologic treatment is beneficial or harmful to the neurodevelopment of preterm infants in the long run. Conversely, since the central nervous system and endocrine systems are relatively more mature at the time of pain exposure in full-term or older infants, hospitalization with under-treated pain may have different effects. Currently it

is unclear to what extent changes are pain-specific, or reflect combined pain and stress in human infants.

Different aspects of pain systems may or may not be altered, therefore directly evaluating reactivity to a wide range of tactile and nociceptive stimulation is needed. Due to ethical considerations, which constrain inducing pain in young children, testing children exposed to various medical situations including neonatal surgery, is very informative. Differences between groups of children (for example children who did versus did not receive surgery, or preterm versus full-term) reflect multiple factors other than pain. Recent studies of effects of surgery at a young age have contributed substantively to knowledge of long-term effects of pain in both preterm and full-term children on later pain threshold.

In the past few years there have been considerable advances in understanding effects of early pain. Application of precise methods of quantitative sensory testing provides well-controlled, ethically acceptable methods to evaluate thresholds and sensitivity to multiple specific aspects of nociceptive and tactile stimulation, and offers promise with older children. Within a developmental framework, unraveling specific effects of early pain, stress in the interaction with multiple factors continues to be a challenge in clinical populations.

ACKNOWLEDGEMENTS

Ruth Grunau's research is supported by operating grants from the National Institute for Child Health and Human Development (HD39783), the Canadian Institutes for Health Research (MOP42469; MOP68898), and the Human Early Learning Partnership. She is supported by a Senior Scholar Award from the Michael Smith Foundation for Health Research. Mai Tu is supported by the Pain in Child Health CIHR Training grant MOP91869.

REFERENCES

Alvares D, Torsney C, Beland B, et al. (2000). Modelling the prolonged effects of neonatal pain. Prog Brain Res 129: 365–373.

Anand KJS. (2000). Effects of perinatal pain and stress. Prog Brain Res 122: 117–129.

Anand KJS, Coskun V, Thrivikraman KV, et al. (1999). Long-term behavioral effects of repetitive pain in neonatal rat pups. Physiol Behav 66: 627–637.

Anand KJS, Hall RW, Desai NS, et al. (2004a). Effects of pre-emptive morphine analgesia in ventilated preterm neonates: Primary outcomes

from the NEOPAIN trial. Lancet 363: 1673–1682.

Anand KJS, Runeson B, Jacobson B. (2004b). Gastric suction at birth associated with long-term risk for functional intestinal disorders in later life. J Pediatr 144: 449–454.

Anderson PJ, Doyle LW, Victorian Infant Collaborative Study Group. (2004). Executive functioning in school-aged children who were born very preterm or with extremely low birth weight in the 1990s. Pediatrics 114: 50–57.

Andrews K, Fitzgerald M. (1994). The cutaneous withdrawal reflex in human

neonates: sensitization, receptive fields, and the effects of contraleteral stimulation. Pain 56: 95–101.

Andrews K, Fitzgerald M. (2002). Wound sensitivity as a measure of analgesic effects following surgery in human neonates and infants. Pain 99: 185–195.

Andrews KA, Desai D, Dhillon HK, et al. (2002). Abdominal sensitivity in the first year of life: comparison of infants with and without prenatally diagnosed unilateral hydronephrosis. Pain 100: 35–46.

Barker DJ. (2002). Fetal programming of coronary heart disease. Trends Endocrinol Metab 13: 364–368.

Beckwith L, Rodning C. (1996). Duadic processes between mothers and preterm infants. Development at ages 2 to 5 years. Infant Ment Health J 12: 322–333.

Bhutta AT, Rovnaghi C, Simpson PM, et al. (2001). Interactions of inflammatory pain and morphine in infant rats: long-term behavioral effects. Physiol Behav 73: 51–58.

Blair C, Granger D, Razza RP. (2005). Cortisol reactivity is positively related to executive function in preschool children attending head start. Child Dev 76: 554–567.

Bouwmeester NJ, Anand KJ, van Dijk M, et al. (2001). Hormonal and metabolic stress responses after major surgery in children aged 0-3 years: a double-blind, randomized trial comparing the effects of continuous versus intermittent morphine. Br J Anaesth 87: 390–399.

Bredy TW, Humpartzoomian RA, Cain DP, et al. (2003). Partial reversal of the effect of maternal care on cognitive function through environmental enrichment. Neuroscience 118: 571–576.

Buskila D, Neumann L, Zmora E, et al. (2003). Pain sensitivity in prematurely born adolescents. Arch Pediatr Adolesc Med 157: 1079–1082.

Bustos TR, Piira T, Salmon K. (2005). Parent verbal behavior and infant pain during the 6 month immunization injection: Evaluation of a parent based intervention. Abstract presented at the International Association for the Study of Pain, 11th World Congress on Pain, August 21-26th, 2005, Sydney, Australia.

Chambers CT, Craig KD, Bennett SM. (2002). The impact of maternal behavior on children's pain experiences: an experimental analysis. J Pediatr Psychol 27: 293–301.

Chapiesky ML, Evankovich KD. (1997). Behavioral effects of prematurity. Semin Perinatol 21: 221–239.

Compas BE, Thomsen AH. (1999). Coping and responses to stress among children with recurrent abdominal pain. J Dev Behav Pediatr 20: 323–324.

Craft RM. (2003). Sex differences in opioid analgesia: "from mouse to man". Clin J Pain 19: 175–186.

Davidson RJ, Jackson DC, Kalin NH. (2000). Emotion, plasticity, context and regulation: perspectives from affective neuroscience. Psychol Bull 126: 890–909.

Economou G, Andronikou S, Challa A, et al. (1993). Cortisol secretion in stressed babies during the neonatal period. Horm Res 40: 217–221.

Fitzgerald M. (2005). The development of nociceptive circuits. Nat Rev Neurosci 6: 507–520.

Francis DD, Diorio J, Plotsky PM, et al. (2002). Environmental enrichment reverses the effects of maternal separation on stress reactivity. J Neurosci 22: 7840–7843.

Franck LS, Cox S, Allen A, et al. (2004). Parental concern and distress about infant pain. Arch Dis Child Fetal Neonatal Ed 89: F71–F75.

Gardner JM, Karmel BZ. (1983). Attention and arousal in preterm and full-term neonates. In: Field T, Sostek A, (eds). Infants Born at Risk: Physiological, Perceptual and Cognitive Processes pp. 69–98. Grune and Stratton, New York.

Gaumond I, Arsenault P, Marchand S. (2005). Specifity of female and male sex hormones on excitatory and inhibitory phases of formalin-induced nociceptive responses. Brain Res 1052: 105–111.

Gear RW, Gordon NC, Miaskowski C, et al. (2003). Sexual dimorphism in very low dose nalbuphine postoperative analgesia. Neurosci Lett 339: 1–4.

Grunau RE. (2002). Early pain in preterm infants: A model of long term effects. Clin Perinatol 29: 373–394.

Grunau RE. (2003). Self-regulation and behavior in preterm children: Effects of early pain. In: McGrath PJ, Finley A (eds). Pediatric Pain: Biological and Social Context, Progress in Pain Research and Management. Volume 26: pp. 23–55. IASP Press, Seattle, Washington DC.

Grunau RE, Haley DW, Whitfield MF, Weinberg J, Yu W. Altered basal cortisol levels at 3, 6, 8 and 18 months in preterm infants born extremely low gestational age. Under review.

Grunau RVE, Whitfield MF, Petrie JH. (1994a). Pain sensitivity and temperament in extremely low-birth-weight premature toddlers and preterm and full-term controls. Pain 58: 341–346.

Grunau RVE, Whitfield MF, Petrie JH, et al. (1994b). Early pain experience, child and family factors, as precursors of somatization: a prospective study of extremely premature and fulltern children. Pain 56: 353–359.

Grunau RE, Whitfield MF, Petrie J. (1998). Children's judgements about

pain at age 8–10 years: do extremely low birthweight (< or = 1000 g) children differ from full birthweight peers? J Child Psychol Psychiatry 39: 587–594.

Grunau RE, Holsti L, Whitfield MF, et al. (2000). Are twitches, startles, and body movements pain indicators in extremely low birth weight infants? Clin J Pain 16: 37–45.

Grunau RE, Oberlander TF, Whitfield MF, et al. (2001a). Demographic and therapeutic determinants of pain reactivity in very low birth weight neonates at 32 weeks' postconceptional age. Pediatrics 107: 105–112.

Grunau RE, Oberlander TF, Whitfield MF, et al. (2001b). Pain reactivity in former extremely low birth weight infants at corrected age 8 months compared with term born controls. Infant Behav Dev 24: 41–55.

Grunau RE, Whitfield MF, Davis C. (2002). Pattern of learning disabilities in children with extremely low birth weight and broadly average intelligence. Arch Pediatr Adolesc Med 156: 615–620.

Grunau RE, Whitfield MF, Fay TB. (2004a). Psychosocial and academic characteristics of extremely low birth weight (800 g) adolescents who are free of major impairment compared with term-born control subjects. Pediatrics 114: e725–e732.

Grunau RE, Whitfield MF, Weinberg J. (2004b). Neonatal procedural pain exposure and preterm infant cortisol response to novelty at 8 months. Pediatrics 114: e77–e84.

Grunau RE, Holsti L, Haley DW, et al. (2005). Neonatal procedural pain exposure predicts lower cortisol and behavioral reactivity in preterm infants in the NICU. Pain 113: 293–300.

Gunnar M. (1989). Studies of the human infant's adrenocortical response to potentially stressful events. New Dir Child Dev 45: 3–18.

Gunnar M. (1998). Quality of early care and buffering of neuroendocrine stress reactions: potential effects on the developing human brain. Prev Med 27: 208–211.

Gunnar MR, Donzella B. (2002). Social regulation of the cortisol levels in early human development. Psychoneuro-endocrinology 27: 199–220.

Gunnar M, Malone S, Vance G, et al. (1985). Coping with aversive stimulation in the neonatal period: Quiet sleep and plasma cortisol during recovery from circumcision. Child Dev 58: 1448–1458.

Gunnar MR, Herstguard L, Larson M, et al. (1992). Cortisol and behavioral responses to repeated stressors in the human newborn. Dev Psychobiol 24: 487–505.

Gunnar MR, Porter FL, Wolf CM, et al. (1995). Neonatal stress reactivity: Predictions to later emotional temperament. Child Dev 66: 1–13.

Hack M, Taylor HG, Klein N, et al. (1994). School age outcomes in children with birth weights under 750 g. New Engl J Med 331: 753–759.

Hack M, Flannery DJ, Schluchter M, et al. (2002). Outcomes in young adulthood for very-low-birth-weight infants. New Engl J Med 346: 149–157.

Haley DW, Weinberg J, Grunau RE. (2006). Cortisol, contingency learning, and memory in preterm and full-term infants. Psychoneuroendocrinology 31: 108–117.

Haley DW, Weinberg J, Oberlander TF, Grunau RE. Physiological regulation and imitation in six month preterm and full-term infants. Under review.

Hofer MA. (1994). Early relationships as regulators of infant physiology and behavior. Acta Paediatr 397: 9–18.

Holsti L, Grunau RE, Oberlander TF, et al. (2005). Prior pain induces heightened motor responses during clustered care in preterm infants in the NICU. Early Hum Dev 81: 293–302.

Johnston CC, Stevens BJ. (1996). Experience in a neonatal intensive care unit affects pain response. Pediatrics 98: 925–930.

Johnston CC, Collinge JM, Henderson SJ, et al. (1997). A cross-sectional survey of pain and pharmacological analgesia in Canadian neonatal intensive care units. Clin J Pain 13: 308–312.

Klebanov PK, Brooks-Gunn J, McCormick MC. (2001). Maternal coping strategies and emotional distress: results of an early intervention program for low birth weight young children. Dev Psychol 37: 654–667.

Lee SJ, Ralston HJ, Drey EA, et al. (2005). Fetal pain: a systematic multidisciplinary review of the evidence. JAMA 294: 947–954.

Levy-Shiff R, Einat G, Mogilner MB, et al. (1994). Biological and environmental correlates of developmental outcome of prematurely born infants in early adolescence. J Pediatr Psychol 19: 63–78.

Levy-Shiff R, Dimitrovsky L, Shulman S, et al. (1998). Cognitive appraisals, coping strategies, and support resources as correlates of parenting and infant development. Dev Psychol 34: 1417–1427.

Lewis M, Ramsay DS. (1995). Stability and change in cortisol and behavioral responses to stress during the first 18 months of life. Dev Psychobiol 28: 419–428.

Lupien SJ, King S, Meaney MJ, et al. (2000). Child's stress hormone levels correlate with mother's socioeconomic status and depressive state. Biol Psychiatry, 48: 976–980.

Lupien SJ, King S, Meaney MJ, et al. (2001). Can poverty get under your skin? Basal cortisol levels and cognitive function in children from low and high socioeconomic status. Dev Psychopathol 13: 653–676.

Macey TJ, Harmon RJ, Easterbrooks MA. (1987). Impact of premature birth on the development of the infant in the family. J Consult Clin Psychol 55: 846–852.

Marlow N, Roberts L, Cooke R. (1993). Outcome at eight years for children with birth weights of 1250g or less. Arch Dis Child 68: 286–290.

Matthews SG. (2002). Early programming of the hypothalamo-pituitary-adrenal axis. Trends Endocrinol Metab 13: 373–380.

Mayes LC, Bornstein MH. (1997). Attention regulation in infants born at risk. In: Burack JA, Enns JT (eds). Attention, Development and Psychopathology, pp. 97–122. Guildford Press, New York.

Meaney MJ. (2001). Maternal care, gene expression, and the transmission of individual differences in stress reactivity across generations. Ann Rev Neurosci 24: 1161–1192.

Meerlo P, Overkamp GJ, Benning MA, et al. (1996). Long-term changes in open field behavior following a single social defeat in rats can be reversed by sleep deprivation. Physiol Behav 60: 115–119.

Mogil JS, Chesler EJ, Wilson SG, et al. (2000). Sex differences in thermal nociception and morphine antinociception in rodents depend on genotype. Neurosci Biobehav Rev 24: 375–389.

Oberlander TF, Grunau RE, Whitfield MF, et al. (2000). Biobehavioral pain responses in former extremely low birth weight infants at four months corrected age. Pediatrics 105: e6.

Perlman JM. (2001). Neurobehavioral deficits in premature graduates of intensive care - potential medical and neonatal environmental risk factors. Pediatrics 108: 1339–1348.

Peters JWB, Koot HM, de Boer JB, et al. (2003). Major surgery within the first 3 months of life and subsequent biobehavioral pain responses to immunization at later age: A case comparison study. Pediatrics 111: 129–135.

Peters JWB, Schow R, Anand KJS, et al. (2005). Does neonatal surgery lead to increased pain sensitivity in later childhood? Pain 114: 444–454.

Phillips DI, Walker BR, Reynolds RM, et al. (2000). Low birth weight predicts elevated plasma cortisol concentrations in adults from 3 populations. Hypertension 35: 1301–1306.

Ren K, Anseloni V, Zou SP, et al. (2004). Characterization of basal and re-inflammation-associated long-term alteration in pain responsivity following short-lasting neonatal local inflammatory insult. Pain 110: 588–596.

Rogers M, Whitfield MF, Fay TB, et al. (2005). Aerobic capacity, strength, flexibility and activity level in unimpaired ELBW (<800gms) survivors compared to term born controls at 17 years of age. Pediatrics 116: e58–e65.

Ruff HA. (1988). The measurement of attention in high risk infants. In: Vietze PM, Vaughan HG, (eds). Early Identification of Infants with Developmental Disabilities, pp. 282–296. Grune and Stratton, New York.

Ryan RM, Kuhl J, Deci EL. (1997). Nature and autonomy: An organizational view of social and neurobiological aspects of self-regulation in behavior and development. Dev Psychopathol 9: 701–728.

Saigal S, Feeny D, Rosenbaum P, et al. (1996). Self-perceived health status and health-related quality of life of extremely low-birth-weight infants at adolescence. JAMA 276: 453–459.

Saigal S, Hoult LA, Streiner DL, et al. (2000a). School difficulties at adolescence in a regional cohort of children who were extremely low birth weight. Pediatrics 105: 325–331.

Saigal S, Rosenbaum PL, Feeny D, et al. (2000b). Parental perspectives of the health status and health-related quality of life of teen-aged children who were extremely low birth weight and term controls. Pediatrics 105: 569–574.

Sapolsky RM. (2004). Mothering style and methylation. Nat Neurosci 7: 791–792.

Schmelzle-Lubiecki B, Campbell K, Howard R, et al. (2005). The long term consequences of early infant injury and trauma upon somatization processing. Abstract presented at the International Association for the Study of Pain, 11th World Congress on Pain, August 21-26th, 2005, Sydney, Australia.

Scott SM, Watterberg KL. (1995). Effect of gestational age, postnatal age, and illness on plasma cortisol concentrations in premature infants. Pediatric Res 37: 112–116.

Seideman RY, Watson MA, Corff KE, et al. (1997). Parent stress and coping in NICU and PICU. J Pediatr Nurs 12: 169–177.

Sommerfelt K, Troland K, Ellertsen B, et al. (1996). Behavioral problems in low-birthweight preschoolers. Dev Med Child Neurol 38: 927–940.

Stephan M, Helfritz F, Pabst R, et al. (2002). Postnatally induced differences in adult pain sensitivity depend on genetics, gender and specific experiences: reversal of maternal deprivation effects by additional postnatal tactile stimulation or chronic imipramine treatment. Behav Brain Res 133: 149–158.

Sternberg WF, Ridgway CG. (2003). Effects of gestational stress and neonatal handling on pain, analgesia, and stress behavior of adult mice. Physiol Behav 78: 375–383.

Stevens B, Gibbins S. (2002). Clinical utility and clinical significance in the assessment and management of pain in vulnerable infants. Clin Perinatol 29: 459–468.

Stevens B, McGrath P, Gibbins S, et al. (2003). Procedural pain in newborns at risk for neurologic impairment. Pain 105: 27–35.

Sweet SD, McGrath PJ, Symons D. (1999). The roles of child reactivity and parenting context in infant pain response. Pain 80: 655–661.

Taddio A, Katz J, Ilersich AL, et al. (1997). Effect of neonatal circumcision on pain response during subsequent routine vaccination. Lancet 349: 599–603.

Taddio A, Shah V, Gilbert-MacLeod C, et al. (2002). Conditioning and hyperalgesia in newborns exposed to repeated heel lances. JAMA 288: 857–861.

Tu MT, Petrie-Thomas J, Weinberg J, et al. (2005). Maternal stress compounds adverse effects of neonatal pain on the development of HPA axis and cognition in preterm infants. Poster presented at the International Society for Developmental Psychobiology Conference, Washington DC.

Unruh AM. (1996). Gender variations in clinical pain experience. Pain 65: 123–167.

Vallee M, Mayo W, Dellu F, et al. (1997). Prenatal stress induces high anxiety and postnatal handling induces low anxiety in adult offspring: correlation with stress-induced corticosterone secretion. J Neurosci 17: 2626–2636.

Vohr B, Garcia-Coll C, Flanagan P, et al. (1992). Effects of intraventricular hemorrhage and socio-economic status on perceptual, cognitive, and neurologic status of low birth weight infants at 5 years of age. J Pediat 131: 280–285.

Walker CD, Kudreikis K, Sherrard A, et al. (2003). Repeated neonatal pain influences maternal behavior, but not stress responsiveness in rat offspring. Brain Res Dev Brain Res 140: 253–261.

Walker CD, Deschamps S, Proulx K, et al. (2004). Mother to infant or infant to mother? Reciprocal regulation of responsiveness to stress in rodents and the implications for humans. J Psychiatry Neurosci 29: 364–382.

Welberg LAM, Seckl JR. (2001). Prenatal stress, glucocorticoids and the programming of the brain. J Neuroendocrinol 13: 113–128.

Weller A, Feldman R. (2003). Emotion regulation and touch in infants: the role of cholecystokinin and opioids. Peptides 24: 779–788.

Whitfield MF, Grunau RE, Holsti L. (1997). Extreme prematurity (< 800 g) at school age: Multiple areas of hidden disability. Arch Dis Childhood 77: F85–F90.

Wilson BJ, Gottman JM. (1996). Attention - The shuttle between emotion and cognition: Risk, resiliency, and physiological bases. In: Hetherington EM, Blechman EA (eds). Stress, Coping and Resiliency in Children and Families. Erlbaum, Mahwah, NJ.

Winberg J. (1998). Do neonatal pain and stress program the brain's response to future stimuli? Acta Paediatrica 87: 723–725.

Zimmer C, Basler HD, Vedder H, et al. (2003). Sex differences in cortisol response to noxious stress. Clin J Pain 19: 233–239.

5

Long-term consequences of neonatal and infant pain from animal models

Wendy F Sternberg
Elie D Al-Chaer

INTRODUCTION

Clinicians and researchers have long appreciated the marked interindividual variability that exists in pain sensitivity, the efficacy of analgesics, and susceptibility to developing chronic pain conditions. Among the myriad sources of such variability are organismic variables (i.e., those intrinsic to the individual, such as gender, age, hormonal status, genetic variability, and interactions among these factors), the effects of which have been elucidated by carefully controlled laboratory studies (see Bodnar et al. 1988, Mogil et al. 1996, 2000 for reviews). Indeed, genetically based investigations of variability in pain behaviour (and analgesia) have indicated a high degree of heritability of such traits; a substantial portion of variability in these traits can be accounted for by differences in genes. There is much unexplained variance, however, even in the pain-related traits with substantial heritability.

Other investigations have focused instead on environmental factors (those extrinsic to the individual) that contribute to variability in pain-related traits. Of course, these factors operate on a background of genetic variability, but certain identifiable environmental factors (such as the social environment, stressful conditions, light cycle) can affect the observation of pain behaviour in experimental subjects.

What is often overlooked as a potential source of variability in adult pain experience is the individual's life history with noxious stimuli. Pain experience early in life, theoretically, can shape the developing nervous system during the period of heightened plasticity that characterizes early postnatal development. Overproduction of neurons and synapses is the rule during gestational development; postnatal experience refines and prunes those connections, such that only those that are used are retained. What is less clear, in somatosensory systems, is how the principle of use-dependence influences the integrity and competence of peripheral afferents and central modulatory circuitry.

This chapter considers the long-term effects of early noxious stimulation on pain responses and related behaviours using animal models (research involving human neonates is covered in Chapter 4 of this volume). The neonatal rodent represents a useful model for investigation of the long-term consequences of early pain in humans for a number of reasons. Newborn pups are born in a comparatively immature state, with neurological equivalents of cortical areas estimated at the second trimester stage of human brain development (Clancy et al. 2001). Human neonates born at such an early stage of development require extensive medical intervention, much of which is likely to be noxious in nature. Therefore, the study of newborn rodents allows researchers to model the effects of painful manipulations in the neonatal intensive care unit on severely premature infants. Rodents are also useful for ease of study. Laboratory rodents yield large litters of pups after a brief (approximately 3-week) gestation, and they have a rapid rate of postnatal maturation – they are weaned from the dam at around 20 days of age and reach sexual maturity by 6–7 weeks of age. Adult testing typically begins at 10–12 weeks of age in most investigations. Thus, an experiment on long-term consequences of early pain in the laboratory rodent can be accomplished in a few months, rather than the decades required to investigate similar phenomena in human subjects.

PAIN-SENSING CIRCUITS IN THE NEONATAL RODENT

The most important requirement for a successful model of early pain experience is that the functional capacity of pain-sensing circuitry is sufficiently well-developed in the subjects under study. There is ample behavioural and neurological evidence that nociceptive pathways are formed and are functional at birth in humans and in laboratory animals (McLaughlin et al. 1990, Anand 2000a, 2001). Indeed, there is even evidence that preterm humans and newborn rodents exhibit exaggerated nociceptive responses compared to either young (not neonatal) or adult animals (Fitzgerald and Gibson 1984).

Compared to adults (or older juveniles) newborn rodents exhibit enhanced behavioural responses to Von Frey hair stimulation (Fitzgerald et al. 1988), noxious chemical stimuli (Teng and Abbott 1998), and noxious thermal stimuli (Fitzgerald and Gibson 1984, Falcon et al. 1996, Hu et al. 1997, Sternberg et al. 2004), and they demonstrate reduced specificity of peripheral afferents. For example, large-diameter Aβ fibers make synaptic contacts in the superficial spinal cord laminae involved in nociceptive processing in the neonate (Coggeshall et al. 1996), whereas in the adult, these large-diameter afferents are not believed to be involved in direct nociceptive processing. Although direct evidence is lacking, it has been suggested that the enhanced pain behaviour observed in neonatal rodents results from the immaturity of descending pain inhibitory pathways (Fitzgerald and Koltzenburg 1986, Ren et al. 1997, Dubner and Ren 1999). The

sensation of pain is not simply the perceptual outcome of activity in peripheral afferents but also of modulatory mechanisms throughout the central nervous system that can serve to alter the signal, which is ultimately interpreted as pain by the brain. Among these modulatory mechanisms are plastic synapses in the spinal cord that are strengthened by use (providing a plausible mechanism for enhanced responses resulting from exposure to early pain), as well as inhibitory controls that attenuate the signal arising from peripheral afferents. These descending inhibitory controls originate in brainstem loci such as the central grey matter (periaqueductal grey; PAG) with synapses in the rostroventral medulla, and they project down the spinal cord in the dorsolateral funiculus (DLF) to synapse on dorsal horn neurons. This circuitry serves to diminish the ascending signal that will reach the brain. Electrical stimulation of the DLF produces analgesia in adult rodents and in prepubertal juveniles, but not in neonates (Fitzgerald and Koltzenburg 1986). Therefore, one possible mechanism for enhanced pain experience in the neonate is the relative timing of the development of ascending nociceptive vs. descending inhibitory pathways.

Despite the apparent incompetence of descending inhibitory circuitry in the neonate, analgesic responses can be observed following administration of various opiate receptor agonists as early as P0 (day of birth), with increases in analgesia occurring throughout the first week of life (Blass et al. 1993). Morphine, the prototypical μ-opiate agonist, produces near maximal analgesia in tests of nociceptive reflexes (tail-withdrawal test; mechanical withdrawal) on P0, although the analgesic response to supraspinally organized thermal pain responses (Hargreaves et al. 1988) is modest on P0 and increases significantly during the first weeks of life (Sternberg et al. 2004, Nandi and Fitzgerald 2005). As early as P2, substantial analgesia is observed following administration of δ- and κ-opiate agonists (Marsh et al. 1999a, 1999b). Since descending analgesic circuitry is not fully developed in the early neonatal period, these analgesic effects are likely due to the presence of spinal opiate receptors, which appear to be in place at birth. Neonates are also capable of mounting an analgesic response to other opiate ligands and non-opiate analgesics, such as mepiridine, buprenorphine (McLaughlin and Dewey 1994) and isoflurane (Sanders et al. 2005). In some experimental models, the long-term effects of neonatal exposure to painful stimuli (described in detail in the next section) are attenuated by concurrent administration of analgesic agents, highlighting the importance of effective analgesic treatment in the neonate (Bhutta et al. 2001, Sternberg et al. 2005).

One conclusion that may be drawn from the above observations is that nociceptive and antinociceptive neural circuitry undergoes substantial changes during the early neonatal period, and therefore, remains vulnerable to the effects of incident noxious stimulation. It is during the time of cellular differentiation, synapse formation, rearrangement, and retention that neural pathways are the most malleable, as illustrated in numerous studies of the long-term effects of early visual deprivation on adult visual capacity. Most studies investigating basic principles of experience-dependent sensory development involve sensory deprivation, rather than over-stimulation. However, various experimental models in the somatosensory modality have recently been developed to investigate the consequences of early noxious stimulation. The next section describes the experimental models that have been used in laboratory rodents.

NEONATAL PAIN MODELS

Models of early-life incidents, such as repetitive pain, inflammation, skin wounding, visceral stimulation or surgery in rodents and other species have noted multiple alterations in the neonate and in the adult nervous system, correlated with specific behavioural phenotypes depending on the timing and nature of the insult. The general rule in sensation is that sensitivity declines with chronic stimulation (i.e., habituation). However, pain sensation is different from other sensory modalities on many levels, including the way in which nociceptors respond to repeated stimulation (wind-up and sensitization). In response to high levels of activation in nociceptive afferents, central nervous system mechanisms serve to strengthen spinal synapses, leading to enhanced responsiveness to future afferent input. The nociceptive neuronal circuits are generally formed during embryonic and postnatal times when painful stimuli are normally limited and the neural circuitry involved in pain modulation is not yet fully developed. Therefore, the occurrence of persistent inflammation and repetitive pain in the neonate is developmentally unexpected and is likely to have a strong impact on neural development across several critical time points. Although there are some discrepancies in the long-term consequences of pain, produced by using different animal models of neonatal pain, the consensus is that early periods of development are especially vulnerable to the long-term effects of brief or repetitive pain exposures (Anand 1998, 2000b, Anand and Scalzo 2000).

Repeated noxious stimulation

Rat pups that received daily footshock from birth to 21 days of age and reared with no manipulation afterwards showed, after maturation (90–100 days of age), a significant increase in paw-lick latency and in antinociceptive effects of morphine (1.25, 2.5, and 5.0 mg/kg), in comparison with two control groups. These results indicate that exposure to painful foot-shock in the preweanling period has a long-term effect on the sensitivity of rats to painful events (Shimada et al. 1990). In another study, neonatal rat pups were stimulated four times each day from P0 to P7 with either needle pricks or tactile stimuli. Decreased pain latencies were noted at P16 and P22 in the rats exposed to acute pain in the neonatal period, indicating effects of repetitive neonatal pain on subsequent development of the pain system, although no significant differences were observed in the adult rats (Anand et al. 1999). Despite discrepancies in the results of these two studies, which may be due to spinal versus supraspinal measures of pain sensitivity, both studies indicate that brief or repetitive pain exposures during early periods of development can have a long-term effect on the behaviour of the adult.

Inflammatory noxious stimuli

In adult rats exposed to a brief period of inflammation just after birth, the receptive field (areas of skin) supplied by individual dorsal horn neurons was decreased by more than 30% (Rahman et al. 1997), implying permanent alterations in the spinal pain processing for these areas. In a similar model of short-lasting local inflammation (produced by injection of 0.25% carageenan), a long-term hypoalgesia at baseline occurred equally in the previously injured and un-injured paws (Lidow et al. 2001), suggesting centrally mediated mechanisms (Rahman et al. 1997, Liu et al. 2004). After re-inflammation, however, a long-term hyperalgesia occurred in the neonatally injured paw, indicating significant segmental changes in the spinal processing of pain (Ren et al. 2004). The critical window for the generation of both these long-term effects (global hypoalgesia and segmental hyperalgesia) occurred within the first postnatal week in newborn rats and they were also detectable in 120–125 day-old rats (Ren et al. 2004). Subsequent experiments tested the effects of neonatal hindpaw inflammation at P3 or P14 on the visceral and somatic pain sensitivity in adult rats. In P3-treated rats, greater degrees of inhibitory processing of somatic and visceral stimuli were noted during adulthood, but no long-term consequences occurred in the P14-treated rats (Wang et al. 2004a). Inflammation in the adult rat in previously uninjured tissue, however, reversed the relative hypoalgesia resulting from neonatal inflammation and evoked the normal hyperexcitability associated with tissue injury (Wang et al. 2004a).

In an animal model of persistent inflammatory pain, neonatal rat pups were exposed to repeated formalin injections from postnatal days 1–7. The rats exhibited decreased alcohol preference and reduced locomotor activity in adulthood, suggesting that plasticity of the neonatal brain may be causing permanent changes in spinal cord or brain development leading to these behavioural changes (Bhutta et al. 2001). By comparison, neonatal rats treated with complete Freund's adjuvant (CFA), used to produce intense inflammation that lasts for a relatively prolonged period, exhibited as adults increased input onto spinal neuronal circuits, segmental changes in nociceptive primary afferent axons and altered responses to sensory stimulation (Ruda et al. 2000). These rats also showed increased dorsal horn neuronal activity in response to both innocuous and noxious stimuli; the receptive fields were significantly larger in the treated group as compared to the controls (Peng et al. 2003).

Skin wounding

Surgical injury with removal of a small piece of skin was followed by robust sprouting of the local sensory nerve terminals, which resulted in cutaneous hyperinnervation lasting into adulthood. This response was more pronounced when injury occurred at birth in newborn rats (300% increase) as compared to adult rats (50%) and continued to mediate a heightened sensitivity to pain even into adulthood (Reynolds and Fitzgerald 1995). Both hyperinnervation and hypersensitivity were not significantly altered by the application of a regional nerve block at the time of injury, suggesting that regional analgesia, used commonly in clinical practice, is unlikely to prevent the local hyperinnervation that follows surgical skin wounds in newborns (De Lima et al. 1999).

Visceral stimuli

Newborn rat pups exposed to nociceptive or inflammatory treatments of their colons exhibit altered sensory pathways circuitry and a stronger response to pain in adulthood (Al-Chaer et al. 2000). Adult rats exposed to persistent neonatal colon inflammation (produced with mustard oil 2%, injected into the colon lumen at P8–P21) exhibited visceral hypersensitivity in response to colorectal distension and signs of central neural sensitization in the dorsal horn neurons. Similarly adult rats that received neonatal colorectal distension (using an angioplasty balloon inflated inside the descending colon) – a painful stimulus but arguably a reproducible experimental form of physical abuse – showed visceral hypersensitivity associated with central sensitization (Al-Chaer et al. 2000). The visceral hypersensitivity was also associated with

sensitization of primary afferents (Lin and Al-Chaer 2003) and other functional changes in sensory pathways including changes in thalamo-spinal modulation of dorsal horn sensory processes. In adult rats that received neonatal colon pain (P8–P12), a shift in the role of the thalamus was observed. Thalamic stimulation in the region of the ventrobasal complex (VBC) is known to cause inhibition of nociceptive neuronal responses in the dorsal horn under normal conditions (Sorkin et al. 1992); however, in adult rats exposed to neonatal colon pain, thalamic stimulation had largely a facilitatory effect (Saab et al. 2004). In addition to viscerosomatic hypersensitivity and neurophysiological plasticity, adult rats exposed to neonatal colon pain showed changes in metabolic outcomes characterized mainly by disturbances in colon motility and changes in fecal output (Al-Chaer et al. in preparation). These symptoms were observed in the absence of colon inflammation. When combined, these observations mimic to a large extent the symptoms commonly seen in patients with irritable bowel syndrome (IBS) (Al-Chaer and Traub 2002). In fact, a recent study concluded that noxious stimulation caused by gastric suction at birth may promote the development of long-term visceral hypersensitivity and cognitive hypervigilance, leading to an increased prevalence of functional intestinal disorders in later life (Anand et al. 2004). On the other hand, a decrease in exploratory activity was also seen in adult rats treated with neonatal colon pain, who confined themselves to a limited area of an open field. The decrease in exploratory activity was aggravated by stress (Hinze et al. 2002). In general, voluntary exploratory behaviour of animals in a new environment may be used as a measure of discomfort associated with ongoing pain (Palecek et al. 2002), distress and anxiety, sociosexual behaviour (Griebel et al. 1998), or adaptation to or fear of leaving a familiar place, clinically known as agoraphobia, often a co-morbid symptom in patients with IBS. Differential outcomes were studied in male and female rats at different stages of the estrus cycle and early results indicate that female rats have greater sensitivity to nociceptive stimuli, particularly when their circulating estrogen levels are elevated (Wang et al. 2004b).

Such investigations substantiate a long-lasting impact of early postnatal events on the neural processing of sensory information. This includes alterations in the afferent pathways, hyperexcitability or sensitization of the receptive neurons, and possibly a shift in the dynamics of sensory channels and descending controls, which in turn determines the visceral sensitivity of the adult organism and predisposes it to chronic visceral pain.

Surgery

A clinically relevant model of surgical injury in neonates employed a laparotomy under cold anaesthesia on the day of birth, followed by morphine analgesia postoperatively (or a saline control) in mouse pups. Laparotomy produced increased ultrasonic distress vocalizations, but did not change maternal care for these pups. In adulthood, various tests for nociceptive sensitivity showed that neonatal surgery decreased pain behaviour relative to the control groups, and this effect was reversed by postoperative morphine treatment in the neonatal period (Sternberg et al. 2005).

Summary: Long-term effects of neonatal pain on adult pain behaviour

Tissue injury or inflammation in the early neonatal period causes profound and longlasting changes in the pain thresholds and subsequent patterns of pain processing (Anand 2000b). A growing body of literature indicates that repetitive neonatal pain is a cause of change in adult behaviour in animal models. This change ranges from hypoalgesic to hyperalgesic states depending on the nature, time and duration of the neonatal injury and is often associated with plastic changes in sensory circuitry. Change in some of these behaviours may be attributable to long-term changes in the supraspinal processing of pain or altered stress responses (Anand et al. 1999), evidence for which is considered in the next section. However, changes are also seen in the peripheral nervous system and the spinal cord. These widespread changes in behavioural and neuromotor functions imply that the long-term effects of repetitive or prolonged neonatal pain may be pervasive to many parts of the developing brain.

THE STRESS RESPONSE AS A POTENTIAL MEDIATOR OF LONG-TERM EFFECTS OF PAIN

Although adulthood enhancements in pain sensitivity observed at the site of neonatal injury are well understood to result from plastic changes in the relevant spinal cord segments, global changes (most often reductions) in nociceptive sensitivity in body loci distant from the site of neonatal injury are unlikely to be explained by similar mechanisms. Instead, these long-term changes may be a result of activation of the neonatal hypothalamic–pituitary–adrenal (HPA) axis that accompanies noxious stimulation in the newborn. Early life exposure to mild stress exerts protective effects on the brain by decreasing cumulative exposure to the potentially damaging effects of glucocorticoids throughout the lifespan (Meaney et al. 1985). This phenomenon of 'stress-inoculation',

whereby mild neonatal stress exposure reduces stress-related behaviours in adulthood, has been observed prospectively in several animal species, including non-human primates, and retrospectively in studies of resilience to stressors in humans (Parker et al. 2004). On the other hand, severe neonatal stress often results in an adulthood phenotype characterized by a hyperactive stress response (Teicher et al. 2003). Much research has been directed at understanding the mechanisms of early life stress effects on adult behavioural and neuroendocrine endpoints (see Pryce and Feldon 2003 for review).

Certainly, pain experience is capable of producing an acute stress response in newborn humans (Porter et al. 1988) and laboratory animals (Shimada et al. 1990, Sternberg et al. 2005). Neonatal surgery produces ultrasonic distress vocalizations in P0 mice, an effect that is dose-dependently reversed by morphine immediately following surgery (Sternberg et al. 2005). Indeed, the model of footshock as a neonatal noxious stimulus described above was developed as a model of neonatal stress (Shimada et al. 1990); like other noxious stimuli, it too produces a longlasting decrease in basal thermal nociceptive sensitivity. It is plausible, therefore, that neonatal noxious stimuli produce long-term effects via vigorous activation of the HPA axis during an early critical period. Early stress activation, in turn, can affect several systems that are involved in pain behaviour – for example, endogenous opiate systems, emotional reactivity or the HPA axis itself. Lastly, the role of the dam in mediating long-term effects of early stress must be considered (Johnston et al. 2002, Walker et al. 2003).

Long-term effects of non-noxious stressors on pain behaviour

The first part of this hypothesis (that long-term effects of neonatal pain are due to activation of the rat pup's stress response) is supported by the similarity in long-term effects on basal nociception of exposure to both noxious stimuli and innocuous stressors during the neonatal period in rats and mice. Daily handling stress (separation from the dam for 15 minutes) for the first 2 weeks of life elevates thermal withdrawal latencies (indicating a decrease in sensitivity) in adult rats and mice (Smythe et al. 1994, Sternberg and Ridgway 2003), similar to the effects of neonatal surgery, footshock and inflammatory chemicals (Shimada et al. 1990, Lidow et al. 2001, Ren et al. 2004, Sternberg et al. 2005). Chronic stressors applied in adulthood can also induce long-term changes in nociceptive sensitivity. Recently, Bradesi et al. (2005) showed that repeated water-avoidance stress in male Wistar rats resulted in a sustained increase of the nociceptive response to colorectal distension (CRD), consistent with chronic stress-induced visceral hyperalgesia (Bradesi et al. 2005). This long-lasting up-regulation of the nociceptive response was selective for visceral sensitivity, because only a transient effect of the stressor on somatic nociception was observed. Thus, global changes in nociceptive sensitivity may be a manifestation of the long-term effects of neonatal stress. This hypothesis can be tested by the administration of anxiolytics concurrently with noxious stimulation.

Long-term effects of neonatal pain/stress on opiate activity

Indeed, if neonatal stress is the key mediator of the long-term effects of neonatal noxious stimulation, the question of which adult systems are affected in adulthood remains. Previous studies have demonstrated neonatal stressors (noxious or innocuous) to have long-term effects on adult opiate activity in laboratory rodents. If adult levels of circulating endogenous opiate peptides (or expression of opiate receptors) are altered by neonatal stress, one would expect to also observe alterations in basal nociception. Kalinichev and colleagues, using a model of prolonged maternal separation as a neonatal stressor (often characterized as a severe manipulation resulting in enhanced stress responsiveness in adulthood), observed a decrease in morphine analgesia in adult rats exposed to this neonatal manipulation (Kalinichev et al. 2001). Similarly, daily injections of saline for the first 19 days of life resulted in a reduction of morphine anti-nociception in adulthood (Fernandez et al. 1999). In contrast, Shimada et al. (1990) observed an increase in morphine antinociception (attributable to pre-synaptic, rather than receptor-related effects) in adult rats exposed to chronic footshock stress as neonates (arguably, a severe stressor similar to prolonged maternal separation). Likewise, postnatal handling stress (brief separations from the dam and littermates over the first 2 weeks of life) has been reported to elevate the analgesic response to morphine (Sternberg and Ridgway 2003). No investigations have so far reported a reversal of adult alterations in basal nociceptive sensitivity by pretesting treatment with opiate antagonists. Thus, although the hypothesis that adult alterations in basal nociception are due to heightened opiate activity is plausible, it remains a hypothesis.

Long-term effects of neonatal pain/stress on adult stress responses and their relation to pain

Adulthood stress-related behaviours (unrelated to nociception) have also been assessed following neonatal noxious or innocuous stressors. Anseloni et al.

(2005) demonstrated behaviours consistent with low levels of trait anxiety (e.g. open-arm time, number of open-arm entries in the elevated plus maze) in rats that had been treated with an inflammatory stimulus on P3 (but not on P12, indicating that a critical period exists for such changes) (Anseloni et al. 2005). These behaviours were similar to those noted in several other studies of neonatal innocuous stress – adult mice or rats exposed to brief neonatal maternal separation during the first 2 weeks of life displayed markedly reduced stress behaviour following stressor challenge compared to subjects reared under normal animal husbandry conditions (Meaney et al. 1989, Hilakivi-Clarke et al. 1991, Sternberg and Ridgway 2003). Long-lasting changes in stress behaviours may also result from chronic stressors applied in adulthood. The visceral hyperalgesia following chronic repeated adulthood stress described above was associated with increased anxiety-like behaviour and evidence for low-level immune activation of the colon that lasted at least 1 month (Bradesi et al. 2005). Taken together, these results suggest that early adverse experience is capable of altering emotional reactivity to stress in adulthood. Others have shown that noxious manipulations produce no long-term changes in emotionality but the general consensus is that the most severely stressful neonatal manipulations produce alterations in emotional reactivity (see Pryce and Feldon 2003 for review).

The relationship between anxiety levels or emotional reactivity in adulthood and nociceptive responses is not entirely clear. A plausible mechanism which might underlie the long-term visceral hyperalgesia, and elevations in anxiety-like behaviour following stress, as seen by Bradesi and colleagues, is stress sensitization; a phenomenon observed following various types of acute and chronic stressors (Stam et al. 2002). The modulation of the corticotrophin-releasing factor (CRF) and its receptor (CRFR1) might be involved in the phenomenon of stress sensitization (Schwetz et al. 2004), with significant changes in the amygdala and interconnected brainstem nuclei involved in descending pain modulation (e.g. the locus coeruleus, raphe complex). Alternatively, the emotional state of the organism might regulate pain behaviour, such that low anxiety may be responsible for long-term global hypoalgesia in subjects exposed to these neonatal manipulations (Anseloni et al. 2005). Here it is useful to distinguish between trait anxiety (the emotional state characterized by its chronicity) and the acute stress response to environmental perturbation. If, indeed, neonatal noxious experience heightens emotional reactivity to stressor challenge (as opposed to overall trait anxiety) one might expect to observe basal

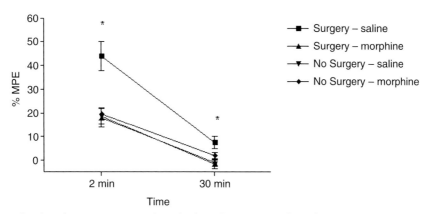

Figure 5.1 Magnitude of analgesia as measured on the hot-plate test, resulting from a 3-min swim in cold water in adult CD-1 mice of both sexes. Groups refer to neonatal treatment condition. Subjects undergoing surgery with no post-operative analgesic treatment exhibit a greater analgesic response to stress than subjects who received post-operative analgesics (morphine 10mg/kg) or subjects who did not receive the surgery (but did experience cold anesthesia and maternal separation). (* indicates significantly larger analgesic response; %MPE, percentage of maximal possible effect.)

hypoalgesia since the testing conditions themselves could trigger endogenous analgesia mechanisms.

This hypothesis has been recently tested by observing the magnitude of stress-induced analgesia (SIA) in subjects that had been exposed to the neonatal surgical procedure described above. As illustrated in Figure 5.1, untreated surgical pain on P0 produced an enhanced analgesic response to stress in mice compared to animals that had undergone the same manipulation with postoperative analgesic treatment (which were no different from untreated controls; Sternberg et al. in preparation). Interestingly, neonatal inflammatory insult results in an up-regulation of serotonin receptor genes in the PAG (a brainstem locus involved in descending pain inhibition), as well as several other genes involved in peptide neurotransmission in this brain region (Anseloni et al. 2005). This up-regulation is consistent with a heightened analgesic response to stress. However, the HPA component of the SIA pathway appears to be down-regulated, as evidenced by reductions in circulating CRF, vasopressin (VAS) and adrenocorticotropic hormone (ACTH) (Plotsky and Meaney 1993, Liu et al. 2000, Anseloni et al. 2005) as well as reductions in the stress behaviours described above.

Mediating effects of maternal behaviour

Finally, although early stressful or noxious experience appears to be capable of producing long-term alterations in physiology that manifest as altered nociceptive sensitivity, the possibility remains that the dam is the key mediator of these long-term changes. Early life manipulations occur during discrete epochs or critical windows, however, the dam interacts with

the pups throughout the entire preweanling period. It is plausible that the experimental manipulations produce changes in maternal behaviour toward the pups that are in fact responsible for the long-term changes in adult behaviour. This hypothesis was explicitly tested in a model of neonatal handling, which showed that enhanced bouts of maternal care following return of handled pups to the nest is the crucial mediating factor for the stress-reducing effects of the manipulation (Lehmann and Feldon 2000).

However, it is not clear whether the models of neonatal pain experience that have been developed produce similar increases in maternal care. Walker et al. (2003) illustrated an increase in maternal care following a neonatal repeated heel stick procedure (designed to mimic the experience of infants under medical care), but did not observe any long-term effects of the procedure (Walker et al. 2003). Neonatal hindpaw inflammation produces an increase in maternal care during the period of active inflammation; however, this increase is followed (and perhaps offset) by a subsequent reduction in care following recovery (Anseloni et al. 2005). Neonatal abdominal surgery produces no obvious alterations in maternal care during the first 90 minutes following reunion (Sternberg et al. 2005). In a more thorough observation of maternal behaviour following neonatal formalin injection into the hindpaw of P0 mice, dams were observed for a period of at least 360 minutes, spanning light and dark cycles following return to the nest of a mixed litter of pups – half of which received an injection of formalin, the other half received an injection of saline to one hindpaw. Maternal care did not vary among the pups in the litter receiving either saline or formalin injections, although the amount of care given (to all pups) was much increased during the light cycle compared to the dark cycle (due largely to an increase in time spent nursing the entire litter of pups during the light cycle) (Sternberg et al. in preparation). Thus, although maternal care may be responsive to pup distress, it is not clear whether dams are capable of directing attention to individual pups within the litter that have undergone particular treatments. More research is clearly necessary (on both dams and adult offspring) to determine the role of maternal care (and the state of littermates) in producing the long-term consequences of early pain.

CONCLUSIONS

Controlled experimental studies of the long-term consequences of early pain in the rodent are relatively recent additions to the literature, spurred in part by long overdue clinical attention to the problem of pain in the NICU. The research reviewed above suggests that early pain experience may indeed account for a portion of the variability in adulthood pain behaviour (both at the site of injury, and overall sensitivity), as well as stress behaviour, and its underlying neuroendocrine substrates. Research such as is described in this review highlights the responsiveness of the developing nervous system to stimulation during an early critical period following birth. As profound as some of these consequences are, the guiding principle for clinical care of the neonate should not be the long-term effects of pain experience, but rather the recognition of the potential for suffering in the individual experiencing pain at the time of the procedure.

REFERENCES

Al-Chaer ED, Traub RJ. (2002) Biological basis of visceral pain: recent developments. Pain 96: 221–225.

Al-Chaer ED, Kawasaki M, Pasricha PJ, et al. (2000) A new model of chronic visceral hypersensitivity in adult rats induced by colon irritation during postnatal development. Gastroenterology 119: 1276–1285.

Anand KJS. (1998) Clinical importance of pain and stress in preterm neonates. Biol Neonate 73: 1–9.

Anand KJS. (2000a) Effects of perinatal pain and stress. Prog Brain Res 122: 117–129.

Anand KJS (2000b) Pain, plasticity, and premature birth: a prescription for permanent suffering? Nat Med 6: 971–973.

Anand KJS (2001) Consensus statement for the prevention and management of pain in the newborn. Arch Pediatr Adolesc Med 155: 173–180.

Anand KJS, Scalzo FM. (2000) Can adverse neonatal experiences alter brain development and subsequent behavior? Biol Neonate 77: 69–82.

Anand KJS, Coskun V, Thrivikraman KV, et al. (1999) Long-term behavioral effects of repetitive pain in neonatal rat pups. Physiol Behav 66: 627–637.

Anand KJS, Runeson B, Jacobson B, et al. (2004) Gastric suction at birth associated with long-term risk for functional intestinal disorders in later life. J Pediatr 144: 449–454.

Anseloni VC, He F, Novikova SI, et al. (2005) Alterations in stress-associated behaviors and neurochemical markers in adult rats after neonatal short-lasting local inflammatory insult. Neuroscience 131: 635–645.

Bhutta AT, Rovnaghi C, Simpson PM, et al. (2001) Interactions of inflammatory pain and morphine in infant rats: long-term behavioral effects. Physiol Behav 73: 51–58.

Blass EMC, Catherine P, Fanselow MS. (1993) The development of morphine-induced antinociception in neonatal rats: A comparison of forepaw, hindpaw, and tail retraction from a thermal stimulus. Pharmacol Biochem Behav 44: 643–649.

Bodnar GJ, Romero MT, Kramer E. (1988) Organismic variables and pain inhibition: roles of gender and aging. Brain Res Bull 21: 947–953.

Bradesi S, Schwetz I, Ennes HS, et al. (2005) Repeated exposure to water avoidance stress in rats: a new model for sustained visceral hyperalgesia. Am J Physiol Gastrointest Liver Physiol 289: G42–53.

Clancy B, Darlington RB, Finlay BL. (2001) Translating developmental time across mammalian species. Neuroscience 105: 7–17.

Coggeshall RE, Jennings EA, Fitzgerald M. (1996) Evidence that large myelinated primary afferent fibers make synaptic contacts in lamina II of neonatal rats. Brain Res Dev Brain Res 92: 81–90.

De Lima J, Alvares D, Hatch DJ, et al. (1999) Sensory hyperinnervation after neonatal skin wounding: effect of bupivacaine sciatic nerve block. Br J Anaesth 83: 662–624.

Dubner R, Ren K. (1999) Endogenous mechanisms of sensory modulation. Pain Suppl 6: S45–53.

Falcon M, Guendellman D, Stolserg A, et al. (1996) Development of thermal nociception in rats. Pain 67: 203–208.

Fernandez B, Alberti I, Kitchen I, et al. (1999) Neonatal naltrindole and handling differently affect morphine antinociception in male and female rats. Pharmacol Biochem Behav 64: 851–855.

Fitzgerald M, Gibson S. (1984) The postnatal physiological and neurochemical development of peripheral sensory C fibres. Neuroscience 13: 933–944.

Fitzgerald M, Koltzenburg M. (1986) The functional development of descending inhibitory pathways in the dorsolateral funiculus of the newborn rat spinal cord. Brain Res 389: 261–270.

Fitzgerald M, Shaw A, MacIntosh N. (1988) Postnatal development of the cutaneous flexor reflex: comparative study of preterm infants and newborn rat pups. Dev Med Child Neurol 30: 520–526.

Griebel G, Perrault G, Sanger DJ. (1998) Limited anxiolytic-like effects of non-benzodiazepine hypnotics in rodents. J Psychopharmacol 12: 356–365.

Hargreaves K, Dubner R, Brown F, et al. (1988) A new and sensitive method for measuring thermal nociception in cutaneous hyperalgesia. Pain 32: 77–88.

Hilakivi-Clarke LA, Turkka J, Lister RG, et al. (1991) Effects of early postnatal handling on brain beta-adrenoceptors and behavior in tests related to stress. Brain Res 542: 286–292.

Hinze CL, Lin C, Al-Chaer ED. (2002) Estrous cycle and stress related variations of open field activity in adult female rats with neonatal colon irritation (CI). Society for Neuroscience Annual Meeting, Washington, DC.

Hu D, Hu R, Berde CB. (1997) Neurologic evaluation of infant and adult rats before and after sciatic nerve blockade. Anesthesiology 86: 957–965.

Johnston CC, Walker CD, Boyer K. (2002) Animal models of long-term consequences of early exposure to repetitive pain. Clin Perinatol 29: 395–414.

Kalinichev M, Easterling KW, Holtzman SG. (2001) Repeated neonatal maternal separation alters morphine-induced antinociception in male rats. Brain Res Bull 54: 649–654.

Lehmann J, Feldon J. (2000) Long-term biobehavioral effects of maternal separation in the rat: consistent or confusing? Rev Neurosci 11: 383–408.

Lidow MS, Song ZM, Ren K. (2001) Long-term effects of short-lasting early local inflammatory insult. Neuroreport 12: 399–403.

Lin C, Al-Chaer ED. (2003) Long-term sensitization of primary afferents in adult rats exposed to neonatal colon pain. Brain Res 971: 73–82.

Liu D, Caldji C, Sharma S, et al. (2000) Influence of neonatal rearing conditions on stress-induced adrenocorticotropin responses and norepinepherine release in the hypothalamic paraventricular nucleus. J Neuroendocrinol 12: 5–12.

Liu J, Rovnaghi C, Garg S, et al. (2004) Hyperalgesia in young rats associated with opioid receptor desensitization in the forebrain. Eur J Pharmacol 491: 127–136.

Marsh D, Dickenson A, Hatch D, et al. (1999a). Epidural opioid analgesia in infant rats I: mechanical and heat responses. Pain 82: 23–32.

Marsh D, Dickenson A, Hatch D, et al. (1999b). Epidural opioid analgesia in infant rats II: responses to carrageenan and capsaicin. Pain 82: 33–38.

McLaughlin CR, Dewey WL. (1994) A comparison of the antinociceptive effects of opioid agonists in neonatal and adult rats in phasic and tonic nociceptive tests. Pharmacol Biochem Behav 49: 1017–1023.

McLaughlin CR, Lichtman AH, Viau V, et al. (1990) Tonic nociception in neonatal rats. Pharmacol Biochem Behav 36: 859–862.

Meaney MJ, Atiken DH, Bodnoff SR, et al. (1985) The effects of postnatal handling on the development of the glucocorticoid receptor systems and stress recovery in the rat. Prog Neuropsychopharmacol Biol Psychiatry 9: 731–734.

Meaney MJ, Aitken DH, Viau V, et al. (1989) Neonatal handling alters adrenocortical negative feedback sensitivity and hippocampal Type II glucocorticoid receptor binding in the rat. Neuroendocrinology 50: 597–604.

Mogil JS, Sternberg WF, Marek P, et al. (1996) The genetics of pain and pain inhibition. Proc Nat Acad Sci USA 93: 3048–3055.

Mogil JS, Chessler EJ, Wilson SG, et al. (2000) Sex differences in thermal nociception and morphine antinociception in rodents depend on genotype. Neurosci Biobehav Rev 24: 375–389.

Nandi R, Fitzgerald M. (2005) Opioid analgesia in the newborn. Eur J Pain 9: 105–108.

Palecek J, Paleckova V, Willis WD. (2002) The roles of pathways in the spinal cord lateral and dorsal funiculi in signaling nociceptive somatic and visceral stimuli in rats. Pain 96: 297–307.

Parker KJ, Buckmaster CL, Schatzberg AF, et al. (2004) Prospective investigation of stress inoculation in young monkeys. Arch Gen Psychiatry 61: 933–941.

Peng YB, Ling QD, Ruda MA, et al. (2003) Electrophysiological changes in adult rat dorsal horn neurons after neonatal peripheral inflammation. J Neurophysiol 90: 73–80.

Plotsky PM, Meaney MJ. (1993) Early, postnatal experience alters hypothalamic corticotropin-releasing factor (CRF) mRNA, median eminence CRF content and stress-induced release in adult rats. Brain Res Mol Brain Res 18: 195–200.

Porter FL, Porges SW, Marshall RE. (1988) Newborn pain cries and vagal tone: parallel changes in response to circumcision. Child Dev 59: 495–505.

Pryce CR, Feldon J. (2003) Long-term neurobehavioural impact of the postnatal environment in rats: manipulations, effects and mediating mechanisms. Neurosci Biobehav Rev 27: 57–71.

Rahman W, Fitzgerald M, Aynsley-Green A, et al. (1997) The effects of neonatal exposure to inflammation and/or morphine on neuronal responses and morphine analgesia in adult rats. In: Jensen TS, Turner JA, Wiesenfeld-

Hallin Z (eds). pp. 783–794. Proceedings of the 8th World Congress on Pain, pp. 783–794, IASP Press, Seattle, Washington DC.

Ren K, Blass EM, Zhou Q, et al. (1997) Suckling and sucrose ingestion suppress persistent hyperalgesia and spinal Fos expression after forepaw inflammation in infant rats. Proc Nat Acad Sci USA 94: 1471–1475.

Ren K, Anseloni V, Zou SP, et al. (2004) Characterization of basal and re-inflammation-associated long-term alteration in pain responsivity following short-lasting neonatal local inflammatory insult. Pain 110: 588–596.

Reynolds ML, Fitzgerald M. (1995) Long-term sensory hyperinnervation following neonatal skin wounds. J Comp Neurol 358: 487–498.

Ruda MA, Ling QD, Hohmann AG, et al. (2000) Altered nociceptive neuronal circuits after neonatal peripheral inflammation. Science 289: 628–631.

Saab CY, Park YC, Al-Chaer ED. (2004) Thalamic modulation of visceral nociceptive processing in adult rats with neonatal colon irritation. Brain Res 1008: 186–192.

Sanders RD, Patel N, Hossain M, et al. (2005). Isoflurane exerts antinociceptive and hypnotic properties at all ages in Fischer rats. Br J Anaesth 95: 393–399.

Schwetz I, Bradesi S, McRoberts JA, et al. (2004) Delayed stress-induced colonic hypersensitivity in male Wistar rats: role of neurokinin-1 and corticotropin-releasing factor-1 receptors. Am J Physiol Gastrointest Liver Physiol 286: G683–G691.

Shimada C, Kurumiya S, Noguchi Y, et al. (1990) The effect of neonatal exposure to chronic footshock on pain-responsiveness and sensitivity to morphine after maturation in the rat. Behav Brain Res 36: 105–111.

Smythe JM, McCormick CM, Rochford J, et al. (1994) The interaction between prenatal stress and neonatal handling on nociceptive response latencies in male and female rats. Physiol Behav 55: 971–974.

Sorkin LS, Westlund KN, Sluka KA, et al. (1992) Neural changes in acute arthritis in monkeys. IV. Time-course of amino acid release into the lumbar dorsal horn. Brain Res Brain Res Rev 17: 39–50.

Stam R, Ekkelenkamp K, Frankhuijzen AC, et al. (2002) Long-lasting changes in central nervous system responsivity to colonic distention after stress in rats. Gastroenterology 123: 1216–1225.

Sternberg WF, Ridgway CG. (2003) Effects of gestational stress and neonatal handling on pain, analgesia, and stress behavior of adult mice. Physiol Behav 78: 375–383.

Sternberg WF, Smith LD, Scorr L. (2004) Nociception and antinociception on the day of birth in mice: sex differences and test dependence. J Pain 5: 420–426.

Sternberg WF, Scorr L, Smith LD, et al (2005) Long-term effects of neonatal surgery on adulthood pain behavior. Pain 113: 347–353.

Teicher MH, Andersen SL, Polcari A, et al. (2003) The neurobiological consequences of early stress and childhood maltreatment. Neurosci Biobehav Rev 27: 33–44.

Teng CJ, Abbott FV. (1998) The formalin test: a dose-response analysis at three developmental stages. Pain 76: 337–347.

Walker C-D, Kudreikis K, Sherrard A, et al. (2003) Repeated neonatal pain influences maternal behavior, but not stress responsiveness in rat offspring. Dev Brain Res 140: 253–261.

Wang G, Ji Y, Lidow MS, et al. (2004a) Neonatal hind paw injury alters processing of visceral and somatic nociceptive stimuli in the adult rat. J Pain 5: 440–449.

Wang J, Peng X, Al-Chaer ED. (2004b) Sex-related differences in visceral sensitivity in adult rats with neonatal colon pain. Gastroenterology 126: A–161 (S1090).

6

Assessment of pain in neonates and infants

Bonnie J Stevens
Rebecca R Pillai Riddell
Timothy E Oberlander
Sharyn Gibbins

INTRODUCTION

Tremendous advances have been made in pain assessment over the past quarter century. However, assessing pain in newborn and older infants remains one of the most difficult challenges facing clinicians, researchers and parents. This challenge persists due to the infant's incapacity for verbal report, individual attitudes and beliefs, lingering misconceptions and insufficient knowledge in professional and lay care providers. Although there were few measures to assess pain in infants only a decade ago, a recent systematic review of infant pain assessment measures by Duhn and Medves (2004) indicates that there are now approximately three dozen univariate, multi-variate and composite measures for assessing pain in infants with varying degrees of psychometric testing, feasibility and clinical utility. This extremely rapid proliferation of measures addresses the dilemma of the lack of available infant pain measures. However, we still neither possess a single biologic measure or a small cadre of universally accepted, valid, reliable, feasible and clinically useful measures that would provide the basis for assessing all types of pain in infants.

Pain assessment is an essential pre-requisite to safe and efficacious management. Given there is no biologic gold standard for assessing pain in infants (Warnock and Lander 2004), physiological, biobehavioural and behavioural indicators need to be considered as surrogate markers for self-report. However, performing optimal pain assessment in infants constitutes more than careful observation of the quality and quantity of pain indicators using reliable and valid measures; attention to the developmental physiology of pain in infants, conceptual basis, the definition of types of pain in infants and the context in which pain is experienced complicate our task.

In this chapter, the conceptual basis of pain in infants, which serves as the foundation for pain measurement, will be reviewed. Types of pain in infants, including persistent acute and chronic pain and their associated measurement challenges will be described. Unidimensional and multidimensional measures will be categorized and evaluated and biomarkers will be highlighted using heart rate (HR) and cortisol responses as prototypic biomarkers. The criteria for evaluating pain and issues related to feasibility, clinical utility and clinical meaningfulness will be discussed. Special populations that present challenges to pain measurement including extremely low-birth-weight infants and infants at risk for neurological impairment will be described. Finally, the most pressing issues affecting infant pain management and future directions for enhancing pain assessment in infants will be discussed.

THE CONCEPTUALIZATION OF PAIN IN NEONATES AND INFANTS

Conceptual models

Pain is a subjective experience and, therefore, defies complete understanding of another's suffering. When assessing a patient in pain, acknowledging that pain is what the patient says it is, is strongly advocated (Agency for Health Care Policy & Research 1992). However, the question of how to assess pain in non-communicating individuals is paramount. Until an addendum was published in 2003, the International Association for the Study of Pain (IASP) codified a bias towards non-verbal populations' experiences of pain in their definition (IASP Task Force on Taxonomy 1994, 2003, Anand and Craig 1996). The 2003 addendum expanded the IASP pain definition by noting that 'the inability to communicate verbally in no way negates the possibility that an individual is experiencing pain and is in need of appropriate pain relieving treatment' (IASP Task Force on Taxonomy 2003). This revised definition equated the importance of non-verbal and verbal indicators, and allowed for a more inclusive definition of pain in infancy and across the lifespan in non-communicating populations. The integration of non-verbal communication into the current definition of pain emphasizes that we cannot simply extrapolate adult principles and frameworks to infants. Rather, we must acknowledge how an infant's developmental immaturity (both physical and psychological) impacts pain mechanisms and the crucial role of the caregiver.

Gate control theory (GCT) (Melzack and Wall 1965) reshaped how pain mechanisms were conceptualized. Subsequent research has substantiated many of the major principles of GCT (Sufka and Price 2002), and its conceptual value and utility remains strong (Dickenson 2002). Melzack commented that the most important contribution of the theory was that it forced scientists to accept the central role of the brain as an active component of pain transmission (Melzack 1999). The role that the brain plays in filtering, processing and modulating pain is fundamental to understanding pain assessment in the developing infant.

Much research attests to the infant's anatomical and functional requirements to transmit ascending pain signals (e.g. Anand and Hickey 1987, Fitzgerald

1991) but the brain's ability to modulate pain is much more limited due to immature pain descending pathways and limited cognitive capabilities (Mitchell and Boss 2002). Craig (1997) suggests a useful framework for understanding how an infant cognitively processes pain. Early stages in this developing process would suggest that the infant processes pain within the context of the current situation but is deficient in understanding the meaning or long-term consequences of the noxious distress. A higher order of processing whereby infants process their pain within the context of self-awareness and the ability to mentally travel through the past, present and future develops later. Thus, while infants are able to react to painful stimuli via afferent and efferent pathways, they have limited capacity to modulate the suffering of the pain experience by cognitive strategies such as distraction, attributing meaning to the pain or realizing there will be an end to the pain. Moreover, pain is so salient that it can pre-empt and preclude attention to other events such that it interferes with the important developmental processes where the infant discovers and learns about the external environment at a critical stage of life (Craig and Grunau 1993). The limited ability of an infant to moderate their pain experience places great importance on caregivers in accurately assessing pain and determining when they are suffering (Craig et al. 2000).

A sensitive appreciation of the infant in pain and their reliance on the caregiver is a fundamental starting point for conceptualizing infant pain assessment (Als et al. 1994). The sociocommunication model of infant pain asserts that infant pain should not be understood outside the context of the caregiver (see Chapter 22 for a more detailed description). The infant's experience of pain (i.e. their subjective perception of the pain) and expressions of pain (i.e. how an infant communicates their subjective experience to others) are strongly influenced by how the caregiver assesses and manages the pain. The infant in pain is assessed within the context of a dynamic, interactive process involving both the child and caregiver, each of whom are uniquely influenced by the greater spheres of family, community and culture. This model calls for an understanding of infant pain, cognizant of the larger contexts that influence both child and caregiver.

Types of pain in neonates and infants

Understanding the conceptualization of pain in infants provides researchers and clinicians with a broad context to base their assessment. From a more pragmatic perspective, a working taxonomy of pain classification is useful due to the differing underlying pathophysiologies and resultant differences in pain assessment and management (Jovey 2002). However, it is important not to view rigid boundaries within these categorizations, as exact delineations between types of pain are not clearly articulated for any age group.

Acute – procedural

Acute pain results from a specific nocioceptive event and is self-limited (American Pain Society 2001). The nature and frequency of acute pain in infancy has been well studied (Stevens et al. 2000a) and is now well accepted by infant caregivers (Craig et al. 2002, Pillai Riddell et al. 2004). The first acknowledgement of pain in infants was related to acute pain because of the ease of defining the noxious stimulus (e.g. a heel lance or immunization needle) and the resultant response. Careful examination of the behavioural (e.g. facial expression, body movements, flexion reflex and cry) and physiological (i.e. heart rate, respiratory rate, blood pressure, oxygen saturation, vagal tone, palmar sweating) indicators of acute procedural pain with consideration of the contextual factors that may influence these responses (e.g. sleep/wake state, stage of development, severity of illness) has resulted in a plethora of validated acute pain measures for term and preterm neonates and infants.

Acute – prolonged pain

Little research has been conducted to further our understanding of infant pain beyond acute procedural pain (Colleau 2001). However, a prolonged pain state is also clearly distinguishable because a clear stimulus (e.g. a surgical procedure, exposure to fire, exposure to multiple heelsticks) is readily discernible. More prolonged pain has a clearly definable beginning and an expected end point but is often seen as abating as a function of time since the noxious stimulus. Acute prolonged pain is also distinguishable from acute procedural pain because the longer time duration of the pain state results in a longer recovery period (e.g. greater fatigue, irritability, lower threshold for pain). Assessment of prolonged pain is challenging even in verbal populations because overt behaviours and the signs of sympathetic nervous system arousal (American Pain Society 2001) used as behavioural and physiologic pain indicators are often absent. Accordingly, assessing prolonged acute pain depends on observing behavioural activity or disruptions in functions over a period of hours rather than minutes (Debillon et al. 2001, Puchalski and Hummel 2002).

Chronic pain

The American Pain Society suggests that chronic pain occurs because healthcare professionals cannot appropriately remediate the underlying cause of acute pain. Chronic pain has been defined as a pathological pain state without apparent biological value that has persisted beyond the normal tissue healing time (i.e. usually 3 months) (Bonica 1953, Jovey 2002). These attributes suggest that the end of the pain state is not known. While health professionals can identify the concept of chronic pain in infancy (Pillai Riddell et al. 2006), there are no working definitions and/or validated assessment tools designed specifically for assessing chronic pain in infancy. As little can be easily generalized from research in either the acute infant pain domain or from research in chronic pain with older, verbal populations, foundational work to explore chronic pain in infancy is urgently required.

APPROACHES TO PAIN ASSESSMENT

The perception of pain is an inherent quality of life that appears early in ontogeny to serve as a signalling system for tissue damage (Anand and Craig 1996). Therefore, it is imperative for healthcare professionals to assess infant pain early and manage it appropriately. Unlike measurement that refers to the assignment of a numerical value to quantify the intensity or duration of pain, assessment is a complex process that places value on the significance of pain for the individual (Stevens et al. 2000b, Stevens and Gibbins 2002, Guinsburg et al. 2003, O'Rourke 2004). Assessment is influenced by personal beliefs, values, education and experience and, as such, is fraught with difficulty in non-verbal individuals.

Pain measures are classified as self-report, behavioural, physiological or biobehavioural. In light of the infants' inability to self-report, researchers and clinicians must use behavioural, physiological and biobehavioural indicators as proxies for pain. These indicators, either alone or in combination, form the basis for all infant pain measures. In infant pain, there is no validated single indicator pain measure. Therefore, all pain measures essentially consist of multiple indicators. However, these multiple indicator pain measures can be classified as unidimensional (Table 6.1) or multidimensional (Table 6.2) approaches, with composite measures (Table 6.3) being a subdivision within multidimensional measures that describe measures that encompass more than one type of indicator.

Unidimensional approach

Unidimensional pain measures include either one indicator (i.e. cry) or multiple indicators from one particular domain (e.g. facial actions within the behavioural domain).

Table 6.1 Unidimensional behavioural measures of infant pain

Measure	Age level	Indicators	Pain type	Psychometric properties
Baby Facial Action Coding system (Rosenstein and Oster 1988)	Term infants	Facial actions based on adaptation from adult work	Procedural	Interrater reliability (r = 0.65–0.85)
Infant Body Coding system (Craig et al. 1993)	Preterm infants 32 weeks gestational age (GA) to term infants	Hand movement Foot movement Arm movement Leg movement Head movement Torso movement	Procedural	Interrater reliability (r = 0.83) Face validity Content validity
Maximally Discriminative Facial Movement Coding System (Izard 1979)	Infants 0–2 years	Forehead and brow Eyes Nose ridge Mouth	Not clear	Interrater reliability (r = 0.83) Face validity Content validity Construct validity Convergent validity
Neonatal Facial Coding System (Grunau and Craig 1987)	Preterm infants >25 weeks GA to term infants	Brow bulge Eye squeeze Nasolabial furrow Open lips Horizontal mouth Vertical mouth Lips pursed Taut tongue Chin quiver Tongue protrusion	Procedural	Interrater reliability (r = 0.88) Intrarater reliability (r = 0.88) Content validity Face validity Construct validity Convergent validity Feasibility

Unidimensional behavioural indicators

Facial expression, cry and motor activity are the most widely used behavioural indicators of pain in preterm and term infants. The challenge with behavioural assessment in non-verbal individuals is distinguishing between pain and other states such as agitation or hunger. Multiple studies with preterm (Craig et al. 1993, Stevens et al. 1994, Harrison et al. 2002, Gibbins et al. 2003, Grunau et al. 2004, Holsti et al. 2004), term (Harrison et al. 2002, Gibbins et al. 2002, Stevens et al. 2004) and older (Johnston et al. 1993, 1996, Taddio et al. 1995) infants have used a heel lance or circumcision paradigm to examine changes in infants' behavioural responses to various levels of stimuli. Although severity of illness, co-existing morbidity, extremely low birth weight, or neurological, physical or pharmacologic impairment can influence infant pain expression, behavioural indicators are still recognized as the most valid indicators of pain for preterm, term and older infants (Hudson-Barr et al. 1998).

Facial expression is the most reliable and consistent behavioural indicator of infant pain across situations and populations. One of the most sensitive and specific examples of a unidimensional behavioural infant pain assessment measure is the Neonatal Facial Action Coding System (NFCS) (Grunau and Craig 1987, 1990) (see Table 6.4). The NFCS was adapted from the Facial Coding System (Ekman and Friesen 1978) and includes ten discrete facial actions (i.e. bulging brow, eyes squeezed tightly shut, deepening of the nasolabial furrow, open lips, pursed lips, mouth stretched vertically and horizontally, chin quiver, tongue protrusion and a taut tongue). Taut tongue and vertical mouth stretch, in particular, tend to be sensitive and specific to differentiation of the pain and no pain states (Craig et al. 2002). While the NFCS is time consuming for clinicians, recent research in clinical settings with less labour-intensive versions of NFCS (i.e. with fewer indicators) has shown high levels of reliability, construct validity and concurrent validity (Grunau et al. 1998, Pereira et al. 1999).

The role of facial expression in acute persistent or chronic pain in infants is unclear. Facial expression in response to procedural pain is reportedly diminished over time if the infant was less mature, had received

Table 6.2 Multidimensional pain measures in infants

Measure	Age level	Indicators	Pain type	Psychometric properties
Behavioral Pain Score (Robieux et al. 1991)	3 months–3 years	Facial expression Cry Body movement	Procedural	Discriminant validity (P < 0.01) as cited in Duhn and Medves 2004
Behavioral Pain Score (Pokela 1994)	28–42 weeks GA	Facial expression Body movement Response to handling Consolability Rigidity of body	Procedural	Discriminant validity (P < 0.0001) as cited in Duhn and Medves 2004
Children's and Infants' Postoperative Pain Scale (Büttner and Finke 2000)	Birth–4 years	Crying Facial expression Posture of the trunk Posture of the legs Motor restlessness	Prolonged (Post-operative)	Interrater reliability [less than 3 years old subsample] (r = 0.64–0.77) Internal consistency [less than 1 year old subsample] (r = 0.96) Content validity Construct and concurrent validity demonstrated in older subsample
Douleur Aigue du Nouveau-ne (DAN) (Carbajal et al. 1997, 2005, Bellieni et al. 2002)	25 weeks GA–full-term newborns	Facial expression Limb movement Vocalizations/ Attempts at vocalizations	Procedural	Internal consistency (r = 0.88) Interrater reliability (r = 0.91) Content validity Convergent and divergent validity across pain management conditions and pain conditions (P = 0.004–0.0001)
Modified Behavioral Pain Scale (MBPS) (Taddio et al. 1995)	2–6 months	Facial expression Cry Body movement	Procedural	Interrater reliability (ICC = 0.95) Internal consistency (r = 0.55–0.66) Test-rest reliability (r = 0.95) Content validity Construct validity (P < 0.01) Concurrent validity (r = 0.68–0.74)
FLACC Scale (Merkel et al. 1997, Manworren and Hynan 2003)	<3 years of age (work done with older age groups not reported)	Face Legs Activity Cry Consolability	Prolonged (Post-operative)	Interrater reliability (K = 0.61) Content validity Concurrent validity (P < 0.001)

many prior painful procedures or had been hospitalized for a long period of time (Grunau et al. 2001a, Johnston and Stevens 1996, Holsti et al. 2004). Due to the unpredictability of facial expression over time, it is important to combine facial expression for assessing prolonged pain.

Cry is a behavioural indicator of pain in infants (Michellson et al. 1977, 1983, Porter et al. 1988) that is frequently described in terms of presence or absence (Owens and Todt 1984), temporal characteristics, amplitude and/or pitch. The temporal domain of cry includes latency to cry, duration of expiratory and

Table 6.3 Composite pain measures in infants

Measure	Age level	Indicators	Pain stimulus	Psychometric properties
Clinical Scoring System (Barrier et al. 1989)	1–7 months	Infant sleep during the preceding hour Facial expression Cry Motor activity Excitability Flexion Sucking Tone Consolability	Prolonged (Postoperative)	Interrater reliability ($r = 0.79$–0.88) Content validity Discriminant validity ($P < 0.0001$)
Modified Postoperative Comfort Score (Guinsburg et al. 1998)	<32 weeks GA (postnatal age of 12 to 48 hours)	Sleep Facial expression Sucking Hyperreactivity Agitation Hypertonicity Toes/fingers flexion Consolability	Prolonged (Mechanical ventilation)	Convergent validity in bedside ($P < 0.00001$) and laboratory video coding ($P = 0.02$) Content validity Divergent validity shown between placebo and analgesic samples ($P < 0.05$)
Echelle Douleur Inconfort Nouveau-né (EDIN) (Debillon et al. 2001)	26–36 weeks GA	Facial expression Movement Sleep Consolability	Prolonged (Postoperative)	Interrater reliability ($r = 0.59$–0.74) Intrarater reliability Content validity Construct validity ($P < 0.000$)
Liverpool Infant Distress Scale (LIDS) (Horgan and Choonara 1996, Horgan et al. 2002)	Neonates	Facial expression Sleep pattern Cry quantity Cry quality Spontaneous movement Spontaneous excitability Flexion of fingers and toes Tone	Prolonged (Immediate postoperative period)	Internal consistency ($r = 0.84$–0.94) Interrater reliability ($r = 0.74$–0.88) Intrarater reliability ($r = 0.81$–0.96) Content validity Discriminant validity ($P = 0.004$–0.0000)
Modified Postoperative Comfort Score (Guinsburg et al. 1998)	Preterm infants	Sleep Facial expression Activity Tone Consolibility Cry Sociability	Prolonged (Postoperative)	Content validity Discriminant validity ($P < 0.0001$)
Neonatal Pain, Agitation and Sedation Scale (N-PASS) (Hummel et al. 2003)	<28 weeks–35 weeks GA (age correction for prematurity)	Crying/irritability Behaviour state Facial expression Extremities/tone Vital signs (heart rate, respiratory rate, blood pressure, oxygen saturation)	Prolonged (Mechanical ventilation or postoperative)	Preliminary reliability and validity testing in progress

Table 6.3 Composite pain measures in infants—*cont'd*

Measure	Age level	Indicators	Pain stimulus	Psychometric properties
Riley Infant Pain Scale (RIPS) (Schade et al. 1996)	<3 years or children unable to verbalize pain	Facial Body movement Sleep Verbal/vocal Consolability Response to movement/touch	Prolonged (Postoperative)	Interrater reliability (ICC = 0.53–0.83; lower for under 1 month age group) Internal consistency (r = 0.73–0.88) Content validity Discriminant validity (P < 0.001)
Pain Assessment Tool (PAT) (Hodgkinson et al. 1994)	27 weeks to full-term	Posture/tone Sleep pattern Expression Colour Cry Respirations Heart rate Oxygen saturations Blood pressure Nurse perception	Prolonged (Postoperative)	Interrater reliability (r = 0.85) Content validity Convergent validity (r = 0.38) Concurrent validity (r = 0.76) (Spence et al. 2005)
Scale for Use in Newborns (SUN) (Blauer and Gerstmann 1998)	24–40 weeks GA	Central nervous system state Breathing Movement Tone Face Heart rate Mean blood pressure	Procedural (Excluded postoperative)	Beginning indications of reliability Content validity Discriminant validity (p < 0.05–0.01)
Distress Scale for Ventilated Newborn Infants (DSVNI) (Sparshott 1996)		Facial expression Body movement Colour Heart rate Blood pressure Oxygenation Temperature		Face validity Content validity (as cited in 2nd edition of Duhn and Medves 2004)
The Comfort Scale (Ambuel et al. 1992, van Dijk et al. 2000)	Ventilated and non-ventilated <3 years	Alertness Calmness–agitation Respiratory response Crying (not scored in ventilated infants) Physical movement Muscle tone Facial tension	Prolonged (Postoperative)	Interrater reliability (K = 0.54–0.93) Internal consistency (r = 0.90–0.92) Content validity Convergent validity with clinician judgement (r = 0.89–0.96)
Crying, Requires increased oxygen, Increased vital signs, Expression, Sleeplessness, (CRIES) (Krechel and Bildner 1995)	Neonates 32–60 weeks	Crying Requires increased oxygen Increased vital signs Expression Sleeplessness	Prolonged (Postoperative)	Interrater reliability (r = 0.72) Content validity Concurrent validity (r = 0.49–0.73) Discriminant validity (P < 0.0001) Concurrent validity for 1st 24 hours (ICC = 0.34–0.65) (McNair et al. 2004)

Continued

Table 6.3 Composite pain measures in infants—*cont'd*

Measure	Age level	Indicators	Pain stimulus	Psychometric properties
Neonatal Infant Pain Scale (NIPS) (Lawrence et al. 1993)	Preterm and full–term	Facial expression Cry Breathing patterns Arm movement Leg movement State of arousal	Procedural	Interrater reliability ($r = 0.92$–0.97) Internal consistency (0.87–0.95) Content validity Concurrent validity ($r = 0.53$–0.83)
Pain Assessment in Neonates Scale (PAIN) (Hudson-Barr et al. 2002)	26–47 weeks GA	Facial expression Cry Breathing patterns Extremity movement State of arousal Oxygen saturation Increased heart rate	Procedural	Content validity Concurrent validity ($r = 0.93$)
Modified Infant Pain Scale (MIPS) (Bucholz et al. 1998)	4–30 weeks	Sleep during preceding hour Facial expression Quality of cry Spontaneous motor activity Excitability and responsiveness to stimulation Flexion of fingers and toes Sucking Overall tone Consolability Sociability Change in heart rate Change in blood pressure Fall in oxygen saturation	Prolonged (Postoperative)	Interrater reliability ($r = 0.85$) Content validity Convergent validity in dichotomous rating ($P < 0.0001$)
Premature Infant Pain Profile (PIPP) (Stevens et al. 1996)	Term and preterm neonates	Gestational age Behavioural state Heart rate Oxygen saturation Brow bulge Eye squeeze Nasolabial furrow	Procedural	Interrater reliability (ICC = 0.93–0.96) Intrarater reliability (ICC = 0.94–0.98) Internal consistency (alpha = 0.59–0.76) Content validity, construct validity (in preterm neonates, $P = 0.0001$–0.02; in term neonates, $P < 0.02$) Construct validity in clinical setting ($P < 0.0001$) Interrater reliability ($r = 0.94$–0.98) (Ballantyne et al. 1999) Concurrent validity with cry duration (Johnston et al. 1999a)

Table 6.3 Composite pain measures in infants—*cont'd*

Measure	Age level	Indicators	Pain stimulus	Psychometric properties
Cardiac Analgesic Assessment Scale (CAAS) (Suominen et al. 2004)	Birth upwards Mean age = 2.5 years	Pupillary size Heart rate Blood pressure Respiratory and motor response	Prolonged (Postoperative cardiac)	Interrater reliability (r = 0.86–1.0) Content validity Convergent validity (K = 0.33; P < 0.05 between pre–post bolus dose)
Napean Neonatal Intensive Care Unit Pain Assessment Tool (NNICUPAT) (Marceau 2003)	Ventilated infants 25–36 weeks GA	Facial expression Body movement Colour Saturation Respiration Heart rate Nurse perception of pain	Procedural	Pilot data Content validity Interrater reliability before and during procedure (r = 0.88) Interrater reliability after the procedure (r = 0.48) Preliminary concurrent validity during procedure (P < 0.01)
Bernese Pain Scale	27–41 weeks GA with or without mechanical ventilation	Alertness Duration of crying Time to calm Skin colour Eyebrow bulge with eye squeeze Posture Breathing pattern – changes of heart rate – oxygen saturation	Procedural	Pilot data Content validity Interrater reliability (r = 0.77–0.97) Construct validity (P < 0.0001) Concurrent validity (r = 0.086) Convergent validity (r = 0.907)

Table 6.4 Neonatal Facial Coding System (reprinted from Grunau and Craig 1987 with permission from The International Association for the Study of Pain)

Action	Description
Brow bulge	Bulging, creasing and vertical furrows above and between brows occurring as a result of the lowering and drawing together of the eyebrows
Eye squeeze	Identified by the squeezing or bulging of the eyelids. Bulging of the fatty pads about the infant's eyes is pronounced
Nasolabial furrow	Primarily manifested by the pulling upwards and deepening of the naso-labial furrow (a line or wrinkle which begins adjacent to the nostril wings and runs down and outwards beyond the lip corner)
Open lips	Any separation of the lips is scored as open lips
Stretch mouth (vertical)	Characterized by a tautness at the lip corners coupled with a pronounced downward pull on the jaw. Often stretch mouth is seen when an already wide open mouth is opened a fraction further by an extra pull at the jaw
Stretch mouth (horizontal)	This appears as a distinct horizontal pull at the corners of the mouth
Lip purse	The lips appear as if an 'oo' sound is being pronounced
Taut tongue	Characterized by a raised, cupped tongue with sharp tensed edges. The first occurrence of taut tongue is usually easy to see, often occurring with a wide open mouth. After this first occurrence, the mouth may close slightly. Taut tongue is scorable on the basis of the still visible tongue edges
Chin quiver	An obvious high-frequency up–down motion of the lower jaw

inspiratory cry, duration of pause between cries and regulation or rhythm of the cry bout. Amplitude is a measure of cry loudness, and pitch (measured as fundamental frequency) is the harmonic feature that includes variability, melody patterns, jitters, phonics and energy. Procedural-related cries are described as intense and high-pitched, which signals the need for intervention. The cry occurs immediately or very shortly after the painful stimulus and can usually be distinguished from cries due to hunger, anger or tiredness. Although less understood, postoperative or chronic pain cries have been described as longer in duration and occurring with shorter latency than procedural-related cries (Kirya and Werthermann 1978, Benini et al. 1993).

As with facial expression, differences in cry responses may be influenced by behavioural state, severity of illness, postnatal age and risk for neurologic impairment. Mature, healthy infants who are awake will elicit a robust cry in response to pain. Alternatively, preterm, acutely ill infants who are too immature or unwell may not cry and ventilated infants cannot cry in response to pain (Johnston and Strada 1986, Grunau and Craig 1987, Hadjistavropoulos et al. 1997, Stevens et al. 2005). Although cry can provide valuable information when it occurs, its absence cannot discount pain.

Body movements are also pain indicators across infancy. Reflexes that appear in fetal life are evident at the time of birth but decrease gradually over the postnatal period. Gross body movements are replaced by purposeful movements that localize pain (Franck 1986, Craig et al. 1993). The quality and quantity of movements is, however, dependent upon gestational age (GA). Preterm or acutely ill infants may lack sufficient energy to demonstrate body movements or may be restrained, medicated and/or unable to move. The Infant Body Coding System is a unidimensional measure that has been developed to examine body movements in response to pain (Craig et al. 1993). Many multidimensional measures include certain body movements (e.g. leg, arm and trunk movements) as one type of behavioural indicator (see Tables 6.2. and 6.3). Although all infants demonstrate withdrawal behaviours, the intensity and duration of the responses are related to GA and severity of illness. Unlike healthy full-term infants who respond vigorously to pain, extremely immature infants who experience multiple painful procedures may become limp and flaccid in response to repeated pain. Their movements are less organized and less observable than healthy term infants.

The flexion withdrawal reflex is a measure of nociceptive function in the central nervous system

(CNS) that parallels perceived pain in adults. The dorsal flexor reflex threshold can be assessed by applying von Frey filaments or hairs to the sole of the foot and recording the force required to elicit the withdrawal response. Infants have lower thresholds for the dorsal flexor withdrawal response and their reflexes are exaggerated compared to adults (Fitzgerald et al. 1988, Anand and Carr 1989, Andrews and Fitzgerald 1994). Infants have also demonstrated increased abdominal skin sensitivity during the first year of life when comparing infants with and without prenatally diagnosed unilateral hydronephrosis (Andrews et al. 2002) and wound sensitivity as a measure of analgesic effects following surgery (Andrews and Fitzgerald 2002).

Unidimensional physiological indicators and biomarkers

Having readily available and reliable markers of distress when assessing phenomena such as pain that is subjective and ambiguous is essential to the timely and appropriate recognition of pain in neonates and infants. Over the past two decades we have come to understand that physiological responses to a painful event should be accepted as evidence of pain reactivity, not just discounted as a 'surrogate measure' of pain in infants (Anand and Craig 1996). Whatever the physiologic repertoire available, the expression should be seen as sufficient to index pain reactivity. The specificity of whether the response is specific to pain continues to be a matter of investigation. However, what matters is what the reaction tells us about the infant's *capacity* to mount and regulate a response in the face of a painful event. In this sense 'pain biomarkers' could be regarded as a measure or index of reactivity or response and not a direct measure of 'infant pain' per se. Biomarkers of pain can then be broadly defined as the response of physiological processes within one or more systems that respond to a painful event (Fig. 6.1).

The neural substrate, related endocrine, immune and genetic components that comprise the pain system offer multiple potential biomarkers of pain. However, physiologic, contextual and developmental factors, as well as methodological factors related to the signal acquisition, processing and analysis frequently confound our use of biological responses to pain in neonates. It is beyond the scope of this chapter to adequately review the growing literature reporting on all biomarkers in pain research and the reader is referred to a number of prior publications (Goldman and Koren 2002, Oberlander and Saul 2002). Using heart rate (HR) and cortisol responses as prototypic biomarkers, what defines a suitable pain biomarker

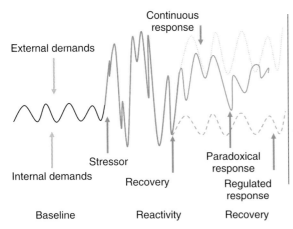

Figure 6.1 Hypothetical characteristic behaviours of stress/pain biomarkers extending from an undisturbed baseline condition to acute response phase (reactivity) to recovery (regulation of response) period (Oberlander 2005, unpublished).

will be explored and a number of contextual and methodological caveats related to the use of biomarkers as indices of neonatal pain reactivity will be reviewed.

Biomarkers are widely used in all areas of clinical work and health research. We might use biomarkers such as leukocyte count (WBC), temperature, or C reactive protein as indices of infection or inflammation or as an index reflecting a response to treatment. For the most part we are interested in whether they go up or down, but not typically in the magnitude or rate of change. These biomarkers reflect direct components of the system that responds to an outside stressor (i.e. bacterial invasion leading to infection). In contrast, the pain system involves more complex and interrelated responses that are much less easily quantified. Reactivity occurs at multiple levels of a highly diverse physiological system that includes central and peripheral neurons. Neurotransmitters, genes, inflammatory 'wound hormones' such as cortisol, β endorphins and growth hormone have been studied as indices of pain reactivity (Anand et al. 1987, Anand and Hickey 1992, Goldman and Koren 2002). Put simply, pain biomarkers can be characterized by cellular, molecular and physiological processes involved in pain and generalized stress responses.

Three uses of biomarkers can be identified. First, as *outcome measures*, biomarkers can quantify the effect of an analgesic intervention. Typically heart rate, stress hormones or catecholamine responses are blunted by interventions such as the use of EMLA (Lindh et al. 2000) or halothane (Anand and Hickey 1992). This has been demonstrated in multiple studies where HR and heart rate variability (HRV) responses have been used to assess the effects of analgesia during acute

heel lance pain or surgical procedures (Anand and Hickey 1992, Porges 1995).

Second, HR responses can be used as *predictors of health and development*. As a pain biomarker, measures of HRV have been widely used in study responses of multiple systems yielding measures of developmental vulnerability (Doussard-Roosevelt et al. 1997) and risk in low-birth-weight infants. In this sense, pain reactivity during NICU care is associated with later development. In former low-birth-weight infants (< 800 g and/or 25 weeks) where biobehavioural pain reactivity was studied at 32 weeks and followed to 8 months, low pain reactivity (pain-autonomic measures) at 32 weeks PCA was related to poorer motor function at 8 months corrected conceptual age (Grunau in press). In term infants, higher baseline vagal or parasympathetic modulation predicted greater cortisol response to a heel stick (i.e. reflected increased ability to react to stress) at 6 months of age (Gunnar et al. 1995).

Biomarkers have also been used as a *probe of CNS integrity* (Porges 1995). Commonly, HR or HRV either under basal or stress/pain conditions may reflect a component of brain injury. Compared with term-born neonates, preterm infants with intraventricular hemorrhage/periventricular leukomalacia (IVH/PVL) (25 weeks) studied at 33 weeks gestation, had reduced parasympathetic modulation during non-noxious stress (Hanna et al. 2000). Biomarkers may also be used to reflect the effects of early neonatal stressor pain exposure. In former low-birth-weight infants (≤28 weeks) at 8 months of age, patterns of basal and reactivity salivary cortisol responses to a visual challenge differed between extremely low gestational age (ELGA; ≤28 wks) and very low gestational age (VLGA; 29–32 weeks) and term-born infants (Grunau et al. 2004). Higher basal cortisol levels among ELGA infants were associated with greater cumulative neonatal pain exposure independent of illness severity and morphine exposure. Exposure to multiple painful events during the preterm period may contribute to 'resetting' subsequent basal arousal systems.

Ideally the biomarker should be a meaningful biological signal that reflects some component of the stress or pain system. In this sense, measures of the autonomic nervous system (ANS) function are well-suited contributors of biomarkers. The ANS mediates resources to meet between homeostasis (internal demands) and stress (external challenges) reactivity. Within relatively short times, the ANS is capable of demonstrating a response and recovery that can be quantified to yield measures of a magnitude, variability and direction of the signal (Fig. 6.2). As both a 'service' and 'response' system, the ANS plays a key

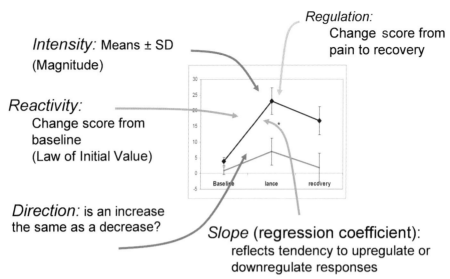

Figure 6.2 Quantifying components of the patterns of response to a painful event: hypothetical reactivity patterns comparing responses in Group A vs Group B. Patterns include measures of: *Intensity (magnitude), Reactivity, Regulation, Direction and Slope* (Oberlander 2005, unpublished).

part of the response to the needs of internal viscera (homeostasis) and external challenges (stress) and as such provides ample biomarker signals. The ANS is always 'on' and its components are plentiful; therefore, it can be easily studied via non-invasive signals. Perceptions and assumed threats to survival demand ANS activity which makes a *trade off* between competing needs. Effects are mediated via two branches: parasympathetic and sympathetic, and responses can be quantified to yield discrete continuous and bi-directional relationships between both branches (Grossman 1992, Porges 1995, Berntson et al. 1997).

Specific measures of ANS function can be derived from HR, particularly the variations that are linked to respiratory patterns (vagal tone), thus making it one of the most commonly used autonomic biomarkers. In this sense, HR may be regarded as a non-invasive 'window' into the central nervous system (Porges 1992). Moreover, systems that control autonomic aspects of cardiovascular function are closely linked to systems that modulate pain reactivity (Randich and Maixner 1984) and activation of vagal afferents can both facilitate and inhibit nociception (Malkik and Camm 1995). HR responses can be observed within seconds of a painful event, providing an 'immediate' or short-term measure of the stress response.

Salivary cortisol has also been widely used as a bio-marker of stress/pain responses of the hypothalamic–pituitary–adrenal (HPA) system (Walker et al. 2001). Cortisol, a steroid hormone, is the predominant glucocorticoid in humans and is a key component in regulating many homeostatic stress responses by mobilizing energy to meet the body's needs, such as elevating blood glucose levels. Because salivary cortisol reflects many precursor trophic and neuro-hormones in the brain (paraventricular nuclei of the hypothalamus, limbic system and pituitary), it has been widely studied as a biomarker of affective and behavioural responses to stress and pain (see Dickerson and Kemeny 2004 for a review). HPA and cortisol responses in particular, take minutes to observe and thus they are often described as the 'long-acting' component of a stress response.

While biomarkers may be readily and inexpensively obtained, decoding their complex and variable patterns into measurable and identifiable components is frequently challenging. Given that most biomarkers are a reflection of homeostatic physiologic systems, response patterns can be understood in terms of processes, which maintain function within a relatively narrow range. For the cardiovascular system, these responses represent a continuous feedback system between the CNS, the ANS and peripheral components. These functions maintain mean values of blood pressure and central venous volume within a narrow range reflected in vascular tone and changes in HR. Like all homeostatic functions, the greater increases and decreases of HR are thought to represent 'healthier' individuals (Porges 1992). The greater the organized patterns of rhythmic physiologic signals such as HR, the greater the capacity to respond to changing environmental demands. Therefore, quantifying variability in HR patterns provides measures of changes in ANS and CNS activity that may reflect behavioural indicators (i.e. reflecting neural capacities to mount a pain response) of pain.

Ideally a biomarker should be able to distinguish pain from other stressful or non-stressful events (i.e. it should have 100% sensitivity and 100% specificity). A static or slow-responding system is typically less suitable when compared with a dynamic one or one that has a limited range of responses (i.e. HR vs. WBC stress reactivity). Moreover, systems with inherent rhythms, such as the HPA diurnal pattern, may bias against observing an acute response to a painful event if one samples during a morning cortisol peak period. A predictable response pattern is easier to observe when the signal returns to a baseline compared with a response pattern that remains elevated (continuous response) or has an unpredictable or paroxysmal pattern following a stressful event (see Fig. 6.2). The cost and non-invasive accessibility of the signal also need to be considered when evaluating the utility of the biomarker.

Contextual variables inherent to the NICU care setting have important implications for the selection of appropriate biomarkers and interpreting response patterns. Health status of the infant, using measures of global illness severity (Goldstein et al. 1998) associated with preterm birth can alter the 'performance' of the biomarker. Reduced lung compliance associated with respiratory distress syndrome has been linked to attenuated HRV (Aarimaa et al. 1988, Ravenswaaij-Arts et al. 1995) and with lung recovery, HRV increases (Griffin et al. 1994). Mechanical ventilation has also been shown to increase respiratory-related changes in HRV (Ravenswaaif-Arts et al. 1995). As with spontaneous respiration, as the mechanical ventilation rate decreases, reflex sympathetic activation increases. Neurologic compromise from birth asphyxia and intraventricular haemorrhage also reduce HRV (Prietsch et al. 1994).

The administration of opioid analgesics may also influence biomarker response to a painful stimulus. In preterm and term infants, opioids clearly reduce HR responses to noxious events. In neonates undergoing surgery, opioids result in decreased cardiovascular responses to surgical stress (Anand and Hickey 1992). Responses to opioid analgesics, however, vary depending on the basal state of the infant. In a non-pain condition, opioids produce tachycardia and increased ventricular contractility by way of reflex sympathetic activation. These adverse side effects can be prevented by beta-adrenergic blockade (Vatner et al. 1975, Franz et al. 1982). In contrast, under conditions of high initial sympathetic activity such as pain or stress, opioids decrease blood pressure by a centrally mediated sympatholysis (Lowenstein et al. 1969).

The paraventricular nuclei of the hypothalamus (a key location for integration of neuroendocrine and autonomic responses) (Swanson and Sawchenko 1983) and the locus coeruleus (Aghajanian 1978) play essential roles in mediating inhibitory effects in the presence of pre-existing sympathetic activation. In addition, opioids binding to receptors in the vagal nuclei also mediate the increased parasympathetic outflow. These differing, contrary and context-based opioid-mediated effects conceivably have a confounding influence on the HR response to noxious events in the preterm infant in a NICU setting, thereby making it essential to account for these factors when interpreting an infant's clinical pain responses.

Considerable postnatal neural maturation may also have important influences on HRV responses in a NICU setting. Typically, mean HR among term-born infants increases to a maximum in the first 2 months of life and then decreases through infancy (Doussard-Roosevelt et al. 1997). In contrast, HRV undergoes opposite changes, and after the first 2 months of life is generally positively correlated with age (Izard et al. 1991, Finley and Nugent 1995, Massin and von Bernuth 1997). Among preterm infants, sympathetic control appears to dominate, while parasympathetic influences become predominant near term and beyond. In preterm infants, HRV increases with age but remains lower at term compared with term-born infants, suggesting continued maturational delay (Franz et al 1982, Porges 1992). Importantly, small-for-gestational-age infants may have a higher HR and lower HRV when compared with appropriate-for-gestational-age term-born infants (Spassov et al. 1994) suggesting that trends in maturation of cardiac autonomic control may be related to both gestational age and level of neurologic maturity.

Conceptual age is also another important modifier. Preterm infants (< 28 weeks) have been shown to be more responsive (i.e. their HR responses become increasingly more vigorous) (Porter et al. 1999b) to procedures as they progress towards term. Maximum HR response to a heel lance in infants born at 28 weeks, but studied at 4 weeks of extra-uterine life, was higher when compared with infants born at 32 weeks gestational age (Johnston et al. 1996).

Similarly, in a cross-sectional study of preterm infants ranging from 25–27 weeks to term, Craig et al. (1993) reported increasing HR responses to heel lance with increasing gestational age. In contrast, Johnston et al. (1996) found there were no differences in maximum HR in response to painful events among infants born at 28 gestational weeks of age studied at 2-week intervals over the succeeding 8 weeks of life. To what extent a higher mean HR in this study may have contributed to the lack of differences in response remains unknown.

The approach to quantifying patterns of response to a painful event needs to be considered. First, key characteristics should be identified: the amount of change from baseline, reactivity (*intensity*) in response to a painful event and the regulation phase (*recovery*) (Fig. 6.2). These characteristics can be quantified as a mean (SD) value or as a change score (simple time 1 minus time 2). As a reflection of capacity to up-regulate or down-regulate response, the *slope* of the response or recovery can be calculated using regression coefficients of the change from baseline to stress or stress to recovery (Linden et al. 1997).

In comparing responses between two or more groups, baseline condition matters in three key ways. First, not all baselines are the same. For example, HR responses of the same magnitude, but differing baseline value may represent differing levels of autonomic arousal that may influence pattern and extent of reactivity. In particular, an increase in HR from 100 to 160 beats per minute (bpm) (a change of 60 bpm) will not represent the same response as an increase from 150 to 210 bpm (also an increase of 60 bpm). In the latter instance, a ceiling effect may have occurred, where the infant is already in an aroused state at the outset of the noxious event and may demonstrate a smaller increase in sympathetic arousal and a smaller decrease in parasympathetic withdrawal (Grunau et al. 2001a).

The Law of Initial Value asserts that the size of a psychophysiologic response is dependent on the initial baseline level of the measure (Berntson et al. 1994). Typically HR and HRV responses are measured in relationship to a baseline value. If the starting or baseline levels between individuals or groups are similar, the observed changes can generally be considered comparable. However, if baseline measures are significantly different, the responses to painful events may also differ on the basis of differing baseline levels of cardiovascular function or autonomic arousal, and be less reflective of the noxious event itself. Thus, differing levels of arousal yield differing levels of response and may represent differing underlying control mechanisms.

HRV will vary depending on the length of the selected HR epoch as well as the proximity to the noxious event, limiting comparisons between studies. HRV increases as the length of the record increases (Saul et al. 1988) thus influencing the total HR variance and its spectral components. In past pain re-activity studies, epoch lengths have varied significantly from 30 seconds to 5 minutes (Porter et al. 1988, McIntosh et al. 1993, Oberlander et al. 1999b, 2000).

A recording of at least ten times the wavelength of the lowest frequency to be quantified has been recommended (Novak et al. 1997), but theoretically only one or two cycles must be included.

In general, most researchers compare mean differences in HR between groups in measures of beats per minute from a baseline period through to a recovery period. For some time it has been well recognized that typically HR shows an immediate increase following the noxious event (Owens 1984, Craig et al. 1993) and a decline in recovery following handling. A short decrease in HR has also been described 3–5 seconds after a vaccine, followed by the characteristic increase (Johnston and Strada 1986). This short-term decline in mean HR response has not been widely demonstrated, principally because the lengths of mean HR typically recorded as a pain measure are longer than a few seconds, and are dominated by the characteristic HR rise that occurs over the first few minutes following the noxious event. Other studies have compared differences in the magnitude of the HR response and the time to maximum HR response following a noxious event (Owens 1984).

While multiple biomarkers are easily available for use in studies of neonatal pain reactivity, no single biomarker characterizes all aspects of neonatal pain. The pain system has complex interrelationships with other reactivity systems and it remains impossible to make a single conclusion about 'the pain responses' based on the observation of one system. Typical contexts vary and may influence a marker to 'behave' differently under different contextual and illness conditions. Questions about how to quantify the acute response and regulation of that response, as well as the use of the biomarker in research need to be considered. How to use biomarkers modelled as outcome measures or developmental probes needs to be addressed when studying pain and developmental outcomes in this setting. Even when differences in biomarkers are statistically different from a baseline to pain condition, such differences may not be clinically meaningful. Similarly, it remains unclear what constitutes a biomarker 'behaviour' under conditions where acute pain occurs against a background of chronic or repetitive pain. Beyond being a direct index of risk or developmental outcome, pain reactivity, as illustrated by a biomarker response to an acute painful event, may also be considered a modifier or mediator of an interaction between early neonatal experience and health outcomes.

Multidimensional approach

The complex nature of pain suggests that comprehensive assessment from multiple dimensions may be warranted. This approach may also be justifiable given that correlations between behavioural and physiological indicators of pain from unidimensional measurement approaches are consistently reported to be low. A multidimensional measurement approach can be accomplished by simultaneously employing both subjective and objective data, by utilizing multiple dimensions within a particular measurement domain (e.g. multidimensional behavioural measures where facial actions, cry and body movements are all included in one scale) or by utilizing a composite measure which encompasses multiple domains that include a variety of self-report, physiologic, behavioural and contextual indicators.

Multidimensional behavioural infant pain measures have proliferated over the past decade (see Table 6.2). Although a composite measure offers more breadth of possible infant pain indicators, multidimensional measures provide greater depth of observation into a particular dimension of pain indicator (e.g. behavioural, physiological). For example, the Douleur Aiguë du Nouveau-né (DAN) (Carbajal et al. 1997) is a multidimensional behavioural measure designed to assess procedural pain in preterm and full-term infants (Table 6.5). After an intensive development process with hospitalized infants, three dimensions of infant pain behaviour, facial expressions, limb movements and vocal expression, were included in the DAN. The scores on each dimension sum to a maximum total of 10, with greater scores indicative of greater pain behaviour; a scoring feature which supports a common metric in many pain measures in infants and children. To increase utility in an intensive care setting, the scoring system of vocal expression includes special instructions for the intubated child. In addition to internal consistency and interrater reliability (Carbajal et al. 1997), this measure has demonstrated responsiveness to analgesic interventions in three randomized control trials (Bellieni et al. 2002, Carbajal et al. 2002, 2003). Moreover, strong concurrent validity with the Premature Infant Pain Profile has also been established (Carbajal et al. 2003, 2005). When interpreting the DAN, beyond the basic presence and absence of pain, the authors caution that interpretations of gradations of pain intensity should be limited until additional research is done in this area (Carbajal et al. 2002).

Although pain assessment has been significantly advanced with the advent of multiple new behavioural measures, trends in the development of these measures may have inadvertently limited our understanding of pain behaviour in infants (Warnock and Sandrin 2004). In particular, observation of a limited number of behaviours associated with a few painful

Table 6.5 DAN* Scale: a behavioural acute pain rating scale for neonates

Measure	Score
Facial expressions	
Calm	0
Snivels and alternates gentle eye opening and closing	1
Determine intensity of one or more of: eye squeeze, brow bulge, nasolabial furrow:	
Mild, intermittent with return to calm	2
Moderate	3
Very pronounced, continuous	4
Limb movements	
Calm or gentle movements	0
Determine intensity of one or more of the following signs: pedals, toes spread, legs tensed and pulled up, agitation of arms, withdrawal reaction:	
Mild, intermittent with return to calm	1
Moderate	2
Very pronounced, continuous	3
Vocal expression	
No complaints	0
Moans briefly: for intubated child, looks anxious or uneasy	1
Intermittent crying: for intubated child, gesticulations of intermittent crying	2
Long lasting crying, continuous howl; for intubated child, gesticulations of continuous crying	3

*Douleur Aiguë du Nouveau-né.
(Reprinted from Carbajal et al. *BMJ* 1999; **329**. Table 1. Reproduced with permission from the BMJ Publishing Group)

procedures (e.g. heel lance) over short time frames (e.g. a few seconds to a few minutes) may have pre-empted exploration of a broader array of pain indicators in infants across different pain paradigms and states. This approach has led to many similar or overlapping parameters amongst existing measures. Additional indicators that warrant further exploration include skin conductance (palmar sweating – Storm 2001) and neuroimaging techniques such as fMRI.

There has been a dramatic increase in the number of composite infant pain measures within the past 5 years (since the 2nd edition of this text) from 14 to 25 published measures (see Table 6.3). Indicators frequently extend beyond the traditional indicators and include indicators such as sleep patterns, behavioural state and consolability. Sleep patterns and consolability have generally received less attention than facial expression, cry and body movements, have little conceptual/theoretical clarity and, as such, are usually poorly defined (van Dijk et al. 2002). Behavioural state is more clearly defined and assists in establishing the context in which pain is experienced. An example of a composite measure utilizing behavioural state is the Premature Infant Pain Profile (PIPP) (Stevens et al. 1996). The PIPP is a seven-indicator four-point composite pain scale consisting of three behavioural (facial actions: brow bulge, eye squeeze, and nasolabial furrow), two physiologic (heart rate, oxygen saturation), and two contextual (gestational age, behavioural state) indicators of infant pain. The PIPP has demonstrated moderate internal consistency (0.59–0.76 item-total correlations), high

interrater (alpha = 0.95–0.97) and intrarater reliability (alpha = 0.89–0.91) (Stevens et al. 1996, Ballantyne et al. 1999) and construct validity (Ballantyne et al. 1999, McNair et al. 2004) (Fig. 6.3).

Several composite measures have been established as reliable and valid measures of infant pain. However, there continues to be debates on the merits of composite multidimensional approaches to measurement versus unidimensional approaches. Although it can be argued that composite scores provide the most comprehensive information about an infant's pain, data from the individual indicators frequently do not correlate highly especially across the broad age and developmental scope of infancy. Furthermore, the capacity of the observer to accurately assess multiple indicators simultaneously and the lack of well-defined observation periods often complicate the use of these

Premature Infant Pain Profile

Infant Study Number:_____
Date/Time: _____
Event: _____

Process	Indicator	0	1	2	3	Score
Chart	Gestational age	36 weeks and more	32–35 weeks, 6 days	28–31 weeks, 6 days	Less than 28 weeks	____
Observe infant 15 s	Behavioural state	Active/awake eyes open facial movements	Quiet/awake eyes open no facial movements	Active/sleep eyes closed facial movements	Quiet/sleep eyes closed no facial movements	____
Observe baseline Heart rate____ Oxygen saturation____ Observe infant 30s	Heart rate Max ____	0–4 beats/min increase	5–14 beats/min increase	15–24 beats/min increase	25 beats/min or more increase	____
	Oxygen saturation Min ____	0–2.4% decrease	2.5–4.9% decrease	5.0–7.4% decrease	7.5% or more decrease	____
	Brow bulge	None 0–9% of time	Minimum 10–39% of time	Moderate 40–69% of time	Maximum 70% of time or more	____
	Eye squeeze	None 0–9% of time	Minimum 10–39% of time	Moderate 40–69% of time	Maximum 70% of time or more	____
	Nasolabial furrow	None 0–9% of time	Minimum 10–39% of time	Moderate 40–69% of time	Maximum 70% of time or more	____
					Total score	____

Figure 6.3 PIPP (Stevens et al. 1996; Reproduced with permission from Lippincott Williams and Wilkins).
Scoring method for PIPP:
1. Familiarize yourself with each indicator and how it is scored
2. Score gestational age (from medical record) before you begin
3. Score behavioural state by observing the infant for 15 s immediately before the event
4. Record baseline heart rate and oxygen saturation
5. Observe the infant for 15 s immediately following the event, looking between the monitor and the infant. Score each indicator for the 30 s period of time, noting changes from baseline
6. Add all indicators to calculate the final score.

scales in both clinical and research endeavours. Future development, research and training utilizing user-friendly methods such as electronic and web-based training tools with real life practice sessions for users would go far in meeting this need.

CRITERIA FOR EVALUATION OF PAIN MEASURES

Psychometric properties of measurement

Support for subjective judgement as a valid approach to measurement derives ultimately from psycho-physics (McDowell and Newell 1996). Psychophysics is the study of how individuals perceive and make judgements about physical phenomena such as the brightness of light or the loudness of sound. To determine the relationship between the intensity of the stimulus and the individual's perception of it, psycho-physicists studied subjective judgements of stimuli that could be objectively measured on physical scales such as decibels or millimetres of mercury. In contrast to the psychophysicists, social and health scientists use subjective judgements as there frequently is no objective method of measuring the phenomenon of interest, especially if the phenomenon, such as pain, is inherently subjective. The adaptation of psycho-physical principles that attend to the quality of measurement are known as the psychometric proper-ties and include reliability, validity, sensitivity and specificity. As these properties are defined and dis-cussed in depth elsewhere (Stevens et al. 2000a), this material will not be repeated here.

Clinical utility, feasibility, clinical importance and clinically significant differences

The property of a measure that facilitates making decisions concerning a clinical practice is referred to as clinical utility. For a measure to possess clinical utility, it must be characterized by acceptance and convenience for the user. Clinically useful infant pain measures provide the user with the information they require to plan, implement and evaluate pain interventions and services. Clinical utility ensures that the needs of a particular infant, in a particular circum-stance and setting are met (Grunau et al. 1998). This construct is different from feasibility where the re-liability (i.e. concerned with precision and minimizing error) and validity (i.e. concerned with the degree to which the measure is assessing what it is designed to measure) of the measure are considered in light of whether the care provider can apply the measure effec-tively and efficiently at the bedside. Feasibility often involves evaluating the length of time for completion of the measure, the simplicity of scoring and inter-pretation, cost, format and training time (Stevens and

Gibbins 2002). Schiller evaluated the clinical utility of the PIPP (Stevens et al. 1996) and the CRIES (Krechel and Bildner 1995) measures in regards to time, cost, instructions, acceptability and format via a survey of NICU nurses following random assignment to instru-ment use and comparison of scores with a clinical pain expert. Both measures were rated as clinically useful, although the CRIES rated higher on comple-tion time and cost while the PIPP rated higher on acceptability (Schiller 1999). Clinical utility is the precursor to the determination of clinically significant differences. Clinical significance generally refers to the clinically meaningful differences in pain scores and outcomes to an individual. Conventionally, a 20% decrease in the pain score is thought to be clinically significant when the effectiveness of pharmacologic interventions is compared to placebo. In infants, this property is difficult to discern due to the lack of verbal capacity. In older children, Powell and colleagues reported that the minimum clinically significant difference (MCSD) in visual analogue scale (VAS) pain scores on children 8–15 years presenting in the hospital emergency department was 10 mm on a 100 mm VAS scale (Powell et al. 2001), which was comparable to adult reports (Rowbotham 2001). Shah et al., in soliciting opinions of parents and nurses on pain required prior to implementing a pain-relieving intervention, reported a MCSD of 15–20% (Shah et al. 2004). There is beginning consistency on the concept of clinical meaningfulness and the level of MCSD required in relation to pain outcomes; however, methods of evaluating the broader criteria of clinical utility and feasibility as they apply to infant pain measures warrant further attention.

PAIN ASSESSMENT IN VULNERABLE POPULATIONS OF NEONATES AND INFANTS

Extremely low/very-low-birth-weight neonates/infants

The survival of extremely low-birth-weight infants (ELBW; <1000 g) has improved over the last decade, and attention has shifted from sustaining life to improving the quality of life for infants and families (Vohr et al. 2000, Wood et al. 2000). Extremely low-birth-weight infants experience hundreds of painful procedures during their hospitalization and the long-term consequences of pain compel healthcare profes-sionals to identify pain early and manage it safely and effectively (Stevens et al. 2003). Existing pain measures have excluded ELBW infants, leaving clini-cians and researchers with limited guidance to manage pain. Extrapolation of behaviours from more mature infants negates the physiological and behavioural immaturity of ELBW infants. Inconsistencies with behavioural and physiological pain responses in ELBW infants and their inability to sustain responses over time may simply reflect poor regulation of their CNS development and not the presence or absence of pain.

Only a few researchers have examined indicators of pain for ELBW infants. Flexing and extending extremities, finger splaying, fisting and mouthing were movements consistent with pain; while startles, twitches, jitters and tremors were not associated with pain (Grunau et al. 2000, Holsti et al. 2004). Although these studies provide some description of ELBW infants' responses to pain, they were conducted when the infants were 32 weeks corrected age. The authors noted that the infants' responses to pain were affected by frequency of prior painful procedures, time since last painful procedure, duration of hospitalization and use of analgesics during the neonatal period. Future studies examining ELBW infants' responses to pain over time (beginning at the time of birth) may provide more information about this vulnerable population.

Infants with neurological impairments

To date very little is known about pain reactivity in neonates with a significant neurological injury (SNI) that can help guide us in developing pain assessment and management tools for infants in this setting. While there is an emerging sense that pain reactivity may be altered in older children with an SNI (Oberlander et al. 1999a), systematic differences in biobehavioural pain reactivity in neonates with an SNI have not been reported. In a single study of pain reactivity in preterm infants with and without cerebral parenchymal infarction (grade 4 intraventricular haemorrhage) or cystic periventricular leukomalacia, no differences were identified in facial action or measures of cardiac autonomic reactivity following an acute painful event (Oberlander et al. 2002). Moreover, few infant pain measures have been developed or validated with neonates who are at risk for or have demonstrated neurological impairment and we know little about attitudes of health professionals and parents towards the existence of pain in these babies or how their attitudes influence pain management. Recent results suggest these attitudes may not account for all behaviour by professionals. Professionals with experience in a NICU setting expressed the opinion that infants at risk for SNI have a reduced pain experience, when they were asked to complete questionnaires (Breau et al. 2006). However, in a second study, in which professionals were asked to rate video clips of infants experiencing a painful procedure, professionals' ratings of pain did not vary when presented with information suggesting the infants had low,

moderate or severe risk for future impairments based on current medical information (Breau et al. 2004). The authors suggest one interpretation of these contradictory results could be that reduced pain management for infants with greater risk for SNI (Stevens et al. 2003) may not be solely the reflection of opinions regarding pain expression in this group or the lack of tools for pain assessment. These results may also reflect opinions or beliefs about the use of pharmacological methods with this group resulting in the undermanagement of pain.

Thus, further research aimed at understanding the long-term effects of early pain for those at heightened risk for SNI should be approached from several directions; studies of pain assessment, pain management and the complex interactions among these and other perinatal factors that may affect long-term outcomes, against a backdrop of refined knowledge regarding expected development in a very diverse population. No one source of information will suffice.

Pain assessment in critically ill infants

Critical illness in infants has been defined either as severely ill infants in an intensive care environment requiring ventilation or by determining a severity of illness score, such as the Score for Neonatal Acute Physiology and SNAP Perinatal Extension (SNAP-II and SNAPPE-II) (Richardson et al. 2001) or the Clinical Risk Index for Babies (CRIB) (van Dijk et al. 2002). Stevens et al. (1994) demonstrated a significant interaction between severity of illness and behavioural state on physiologic pain response, implying that those who were in quiet sleep and most severely ill were most affected. Pain should also be assessed with the level of sedation (Ramsey 2000). One measure, the Neonatal Pain, Agitation and Sedation Scale (N-PASS) (Hummel et al 2003) uniquely combines the measurement of these constructs; however, there has been only minimal reporting of the psychometric properties of this measure. Other research has indicated that behavioural indicators such as 'tearing' and being 'too awake' were synonymous with pain in critically ill infants (van Dijk et al. 2002). Foster (2001) suggested that the expert judgement of the nurse is the key factor in assessing pain in critically ill children. However, Foster implies that judgement be articulated by expert nurses, leaving more novice nurses somewhat disadvantaged. Generally, there is a recognized difficulty in making observational differentiations between pain, agitation and sedation and the concepts require further exploration. On rare occasions, these infants receive muscle relaxants that preclude any behavioural responses; in these situations, physiological indicators may be useful in determining pain. A more in-depth description of management of infant pain in critically ill infants and those requiring palliative care can be found in Chapter 18.

ISSUES IN PAIN ASSESSMENT

Rapid maturation and malleability of the infant nervous system

Despite significant consistencies between the experience and expression of pain through different stages of life, it is crucial to recognize the much steeper trajectory of development in pain experience and expression through infancy. These changes reflect rapid maturation of the biological substrates underlying emotion, cognition, language and social relations (Craig 2002). Pain assessment tools may not have full generalizability to different age groups within infancy, such as between a premature baby, a full-term newborn and a 12-month-old infant. Researchers and clinicians must be cautious of the validation samples when selecting a pain assessment tool.

Moreover, this steep trajectory results in neuronal plasticity being highest during the postnatal period, suggesting that the nervous system is extremely malleable in response to noxious environmental influences (Porter et al. 1999b). For example, this was seen in a study comparing facial action in two same-aged samples of premature infants that had different levels of exposure to painful stimuli (Johnston and Stevens 1996). The infants who had more extensive pain experiences showed significantly less facial action. Caregivers must be cognizant that developmental capabilities (both physiological and psychological) may change after significant exposure to severe or repetitive pain insults.

Lack of specificity of the infant acute pain response

While most infant pain indicators are sensitive to painful events, they lack specificity to situations in which the infant is experiencing pain. This non-specificity is equally true for behavioural and physiological indicators. Thus, the utility of all indicators for acute pain is tempered by the lack of specificity and the inability to achieve validation of the pain assumption by infant self-report. Cues, such as an infant's cry, do not offer specific information about an infant's pain per se but rather offer information about the intensity of the distress (Craig et al. 2000).

Dissociation between physiological/behavioural and biochemical responses

In considering how pain is conceptualized, we might expect that infants would respond to tissue damage both behaviourally and physiologically in some con-sistent manner. However, reports that behavioural and physiological responses are either uncorrelated or weakly correlated ($r = 0.3$) across situations and studies are common (Stevens et al. 1994, Johnston et al. 1995). This dissociation in responsive systems suggests that physiologic systems are only loosely coupled to behavioural responsive systems (Barr 1998).

In the absence of self-report, this dissociation between physiologic and behavioural outcomes impedes both our judgement about pain intensity and our decision-making about the effectiveness of interventions as we are uncertain whether to rely most heavily on the behavioural, physiologic or a composite of pain indicators. An overall understanding of different behavioural and physiological indicators of pain leads many to assert that the assessment of infant pain should be multidimensional (an inherent strategy of composite measures), as no unitary measurement captures the phenomenon of infant pain completely (American Academy of Pediatrics 2001, American Pain Society 2001). Ensuring assessment across both types of assessment modalities will help overcome discrepancies between these two approaches and, at the very least, help decipher the presence of distress and the need for deeper investigation as to the presence of pain. However, the limitation of this approach is that the understanding of unique changes in individual pain indicators is often lost in the processes of summation and averaging of indicator scores.

Comprehending non-response in infant pain assessment

Some infants do not respond to tissue-damaging events (Johnston et al. 1999a). This phenomenon is especially perplexing because it is hard to distinguish between the absence of pain and the presence of so much pain that the infant cannot muster a response. Lack of response is puzzling for researchers, but even more problematic for clinicians, who may be withholding analgesics and other interventions based on non-response, when the infant actually is in pain. Non-responding (and limited responding) has been inversely related to time elapsed since an invasive procedure (Johnston et al. 1999c) and post-conceptual age (Craig et al. 1993). The reduced responding is hypothesized to be due to the limited energy available to maintain a vigorous pain response as these infants are using their metabolic resources primarily to maintain their precarious survival (Craig et al. 1993). In light of these factors, it is important to incorporate contextual factors such as an infant's medical history, age and how much time has been spent in potentially painful situations when making an assertion about the absence of pain.

Caregiver biases in assessing infant pain

Intrinsic to an acceptance of the dyadic interplay between caregiver and infants in pain is the problem of caregiver bias. In the case of infants, pain is not what the patient says but rather what the caregiver says. Who the caregiver is can also make a difference. Systematic differences in pain attributions between different groups of caregivers (parents, nurses, physicians) have been shown despite the presentation of the exact same infant pain behaviours (Pillai Riddell and Craig 2004).

Caregivers who are asked to make infant pain judgements are often faced with an ambiguous situation where distress is evident but pain in unclear. They are left to make educated guesses based on their personal experiences and/or medical/parental training. A caregiver's personal experiences with pain is more influential than the child's own experience with pain when they are making determinations about the utility of pain medication (Pillai Riddell et al. 2004). Moreover, archaic beliefs about pain tolerance, treatment or memory in infants all increase the possibility that an infant's pain signals and cues will be ignored. There is further speculation that under-assessing infant pain is a coping strategy used by health professionals that are put in a position where they need to put infants in pain as part of their daily job (Balda et al. 2000). When painful procedures are unavoidable, we need to assume that the infant will likely experience pain equal to or greater than what an average adult would experience when exposed to similar stimuli.

SUMMARY AND FUTURE DIRECTIONS

Great strides have been made in pain assessment over the past 5 years. However, there still remain large gaps in the infant assessment literature (e.g. persistent and chronic pain) that often preclude evidence-based optimal clinical pain management practices. We need no further measures to assess acute procedural pain in infants but rather we should validate existing measures and determine the clinical utility and feasibility of valid and reliable measures for practice. This is not to say that we should not be mindful of searching for novel indicators of pain such as biomarkers or indicators of cognitive pain perception but rather that we should turn our efforts away from finding novel recombinations of established indicators (such as facial activity, body movements and heart rates). We also need to focus on special populations of infants who have received less than adequate pain assessment and management as well as on the unresolved measurement issues across ages, populations and situations. Pain assessment remains the cornerstone of pain management and, as such, we must persevere, until we 'get it right'.

ACKNOWLEDGEMENTS

Bonnie Stevens' research is supported by operating grants from the Canadian Institutes for Health Research (CIHR) (MOP 37884, MOP 74539 CTP-79854). Rebecca Pillai Riddell's research is supported by a CIHR grant (MOP 74539) and a Postdoctoral Fellowship.

REFERENCES

Aarimaa T, Oja R, Antila K et al. (1988). Interaction of heart rate and respiration in newborn babies. Pediatric Res 24: 745–750.

Agency for Health Care Policy and Research. (1992). Acute pain management: Operative or medical procedures and trauma. Clinical practice guidelines (No AHCPR Pub No 92-0032). US Department of Health and Human Services, Rockville, MD.

Aghajanian GK. (1978). Tolerance of locus coeruleus neurones to morphine and suppression of withdrawal response by clonidine. Nature 276:186–188.

Als H, Lawhon G, Duffy F et al. (1994). Individualized developmental care for the very low-birth-weight preterm infant. Medical and neurofunctional effects. JAMA 272: 853–858.

Ambuel B, Hamlett KW, Marx CM et al. (1992). Assessing distress in pediatric intensive care environments: the COMFORT scale. J Pediatr Psychol 17: 95–109.

American Academy of Pediatrics Committee on Psychosocial Aspects of Child and Family Health, & Task Force on Pain in Infants, Children, and Adolescents. (2001). The assessment and management of acute pain in infants, children, and adolescents. Pediatrics 108: 793–797.

American Pain Society. (2001) Pediatric chronic pain: a position statement from the American Pain Society. Glenview, Illinois.

Anand KJS, Carr DB. (1989). The neuroanatomy, neurophysiology and neurochemistry of pain, stress, and analgesia in newborns and children. Pediatr Clin North Am 36: 795–815.

Anand KJ, Craig KD. (1996). New perspectives on the definition of pain. Pain 67: 3–6.

Anand KJS, Hickey PR. (1987). Pain and its effects in the human neonate and fetus. N Engl J Med 317: 1321–1329.

Anand KJ, Hickey PR. (1992). Halothane-morphine compared with high-dose sufentanil for anesthesia and postoperative analgesia in neonatal cardiac surgery. N Engl J Med 326: 1–9.

Anand KJ, Sippell WG, Aynsley-Green A. (1987). Randomised trial of fentanyl anaesthesia in preterm babies undergoing surgery: effects on the stress response. Lancet 1: 62–66.

Andrews K, Fitzgerald M. (1994). The cutaneous withdrawl reflex in human neonates: Sensitization, receptive fields and the effects of contra lateral stimulation. Pain 56: 95–102.

Andrews K, Fitzgerald M. (2002). Wound sensitivity as a measure of analgesic effects following surgery in human neonates and infants. Pain 99: 185–195.

Andrews K, Desai D, Dhillon H et al. (2002). Abdominal sensitivity in the first year of life: comparison of infants with and without prenatally diagnosed unilateral hydronephrosis. Pain 100: 35–46.

Balda R, Guinsburg R, Branco de Almeida M et al. (2000). The recognition of facial expression of pain in full-term newborns by parents and health professionals. Arch Pediatr Adolesc Med 154I: 1009–1016.

Ballantyne M, Stevens B, McAllister M et al. (1999). Validation of the premature infant pain profile in the clinical setting. Clin J Pain 15: 297–303.

Barr RG. (1998). Reflections on measuring pain in infants: dissociation in responsive systems and "honest signalling". Arch Dis Child Fetal Neonatal Ed 79: 152–156.

Barrier G, Attia J, Mayer M-N et al. (1989). Measurement of post-operative pain and narcotic administration in infants using a new clinical scoring system. Intensive Care Med (Suppl 1) 15: 537–539.

Bellieni C, Bagnoli F, Perrone S et al. (2002). Effect of multisensory stimulation on analgesia in term neonates: a randomized controlled trial. Pediatr Res 51: 460–463.

Benini F, Johnston CC, Faucher D et al. (1993). Topical anesthesia during circumcision in newborn infants. JAMA 270: 850–854.

Berntson GG, Uchino BN, Cacioppo JT. (1994). Origins of baseline variance and the law of initial values. Psychophysiology 31: 204–210.

Berntson GG, Bigger JT Jr, Eckberg DL et al. (1997). Heart rate variability: origins, methods, and interpretive caveats. Psychophysiology 34: 623–648.

Blauer T, Gerstmann D. (1998). A simultaneous comparison of three neonatal pain scales during common NICU procedures. Clin J Pain 14: 39–47.

Bonica J. (1953). The management of pain of cancer. J Michigan State Med Soc 52: 284–290.

Breau L, McGrath PJ, Stevens B et al. (2004). Healthcare professionals' perceptions of pain in infants at risk for neurologic impairment. BMC Pediatrics 4: 23.

Breau L, McGrath PJ, Stevens B et al. (2006). Judgments of pain in the neonatal intensive care setting: a survey of direct care staff's perceptions of pain in infants at risk for neurological impairment. Clin J Pain 22: 122–129.

Bucholz M, Karl HW, Pomietto M et al. (1998). Pain scores in infants: a modified infant pain scale versus visual analogue. J Pain Symptom Manage 15:117–124.

Büttner W, Finke W. (2000). Analysis of behavioural and physiological parameters for the assessment of postoperative analgesic demand in newborns, infants and young children: a comprehensive report on seven consecutive studies. Pediatr Anesthesia 10: 303–318.

Carbajal R, Paupe A, Hoenn E et al. (1997). DAN: une echelle comportementale d'evaluation de la douleur aigue du nouveau-ne. Archives de Pediatrie (4): 623–628.

Carbajal R, Lenclen R, Gajdos V et al. (2002). Crossover trial of analgesic efficacy of glucose and pacifier in very preterm neonates during subcutaneous injections. Pediatrics 110: 389–393.

Carbajal R, Veerapen S, Couderc S et al. (2003). Analgesic effect of breast feeding in term neonates: randomized controlled trial. BMJ 326: 13.

Carbajal R, Lenclen R, Jugie M et al. (2005). Morphine does not provide adequate analgesia for acute procedural pain among preterm neonates. Pediatrics 115: 1494–1500.

Colleau S. (2001). Easing the pain of seriously ill children: a progress report. Cancer Pain Release 14(3).

Craig KD. (1997). Implications of concepts of consciousness for understanding pain behaviour and the definition of pain. Pain Res Manage 2: 111–116.

Craig KD. (2002). Pain in infants and children: Sociodevelopmental variations on the theme. Pain (an updated review).

Craig K, Grunau RVE. (1993). Neonatal pain perception and behavioural measurement. In: Anand KJS, McGrath PJ (eds). Pain in neonates, pp. 67–105. Elsevier, Amsterdam.

Craig KD, Whitfield MF, Grunau R, et al. (1993). Pain in the preterm neonate: behavioural and physiological indices. Pain 52: 287–299.

Craig K, Gilbert-MacLeod C, Lilley C. (2000). Crying as an indicator of pain in infants. In: Barr RG, Hopkins B, Green JA (eds). Crying as a sign, a symptom, and a signal: clinical, emotional and developmental aspects of infant and toddler crying, pp. 23–40. MacKeith Press, London.

Craig KD, Korol CT, Pillai RR. (2002). Challenges of judging pain in vulnerable infants. Clin Perinatol 29: 445–458.

Debillon T, Zupan V, Ravault N, et al. (2001). Development and initial validation of the EDIN scale, a new tool for assessing prolonged pain in preterm infants. Arch Dis Child 85: F36–F40.

Dickenson AH. (2002). Gate Control Theory of pain stands the test of time. Br J Anaesth 88: 755–757.

Dickerson SS, Kemeny ME. (2004). Acute stressors and cortisol responses: a theoretical integration and synthesis of laboratory research. Psychol Bull 130: 355–391.

Doussard-Roosevelt JA, Porges SW, Scanlon JW et al. (1997). Vagal regulation of heart rate in the prediction of developmental outcome for very low birth weight preterm infants. Child Develop 68:173–186.

Duhn L, Medves J. (2004). A systematic integrative review of infant pain assessment tools. Adv Neonatal Care 4: 126–140.

Ekman P, Friesen WV. (1978). Facial action coding system: a technique for the measurement of facial movement. Consulting Psychologists Press, Palo Alto, CA.

Finley JP, Nugent ST. (1995). Heart rate variability in infants, children and young adults. J Auton Nerv Syst 51: 103–108.

Fitzgerald M. (1991). The developmental neurobiology of pain. Pain Research and Clinical Management. Proceedings of the VIth World Congress on Pain. Elsevier.

Fitzgerald M, Shaw A, MacIntosh N. (1988). Postnatal development of the cutaneous flexor reflex: Comparative study of preterm infants and newborn rat pups. Develop Med Child Neurol 30: 520–526.

Foster R. (2001). Nursing judgment: the key to pain assessment in critically ill children. J Soc Pediatr Nurs 6: 90–93.

Franck LS. (1986). A new method to quantitatively describe pain behavior in infants. Nurs Res 35: 28–31.

Franz DN, Hare DB, McCloskey KL. (1982). Spinal sympathetic neurons: possible sites of opiate-withdrawal suppression by clonidine. Science 215: 1643–1645.

Gibbins S, Stevens B, Hodnett E et al. (2002). Efficacy and safety of sucrose for procedural pain relief in preterm and term neonates. Nurs Res 51: 375–382.

Gibbins S, Stevens B, Asztalos E. (2003). Assessment and management of acute pain in high-risk neonates. Expert Opin Pharmacotherapy 4: 475–483.

Gibbins S, Maddalena P, Yamada J et al. (2005). The Premature Infant Pain Profile (PIPP): Testing the feasibility of an interactive teaching module for enhancing infant pain assessment (submitted to Advances in Neonatal Care).

Goldman RD, Koren G. (2002). Biologic markers of pain in the vulnerable infant. Clin Perinatol 29: 415–425.

Goldstein B, Fiser DH, Kelly MM et al. (1998). Decomplexification in critical illness and injury: relationship between heart rate variability, severity of illness, and outcome. Crit Care Med 26: 352–357.

Griffin MP, Scollan DF, Moorman JR. (1994). The dynamic range of neonatal heart rate variability. J Cardiovasc Electrophysiol 5: 112–124.

Grossman P. (1992). Respiratory and cardiac rhythms as windows to central and autonomic biobehavioral regulation: selection of window frames, keeping the panes clean and viewing the neural topography. Biol Psychol 34: 131–161.

Grunau RE. (In press). Biobehavioral reactivity to pain in preterm infants: a marker of neuromotor development?

Grunau R, Craig KD. (1987). Pain expression in neonates: facial action and cry. Pain 28: 395–410.

Grunau RVE, Craig K. (1990). Facial activity as a measure of neonatal pain expression. In: Tyler DC, Krane EJ (eds). Advances in pain therapy and research, Vol 15, pp. 147–156. Pediatric Pain. Raven Press, New York.

Grunau RE, Holsti L, Whitfield M et al. (2000). Are twitches, startles and body movements pain indicators in extremely low birth weight infants? Clin J Pain 16: 37–45.

Grunau RE, Oberlander TF, Whitfield MF et al. (2001a). Demographic and therapeutic determinants of pain reactivity in very low birth weight neonates at 32 weeks' post-conceptional age. Pediatrics 107: 105–112.

Grunau RE, Oberlander TF, Whitfield MF et al. (2001b). Pain reactivity in former extremely low birth weight infants at corrected age 8 months compared with term born controls. Infant Behav Develop 24: 41–55.

Grunau RE, Weinberg J, Whitfield MF. (2004). Neonatal procedural pain and preterm infant cortisol response to novelty at 8 months. Pediatrics 114: e77–84.

Grunau RVE, Obertander T, Holsti L et al. (1998). Bedside application of the Neonatal Facial Coding System in pain assessment of premature neonates. Pain 76: 277–286.

Guinsburg R, Kopelman B, Anand KJE et al. (1998). Physiological, hormonal and behavioral responses to a simple fentanyl dose in intubated and ventilated preterm neonates. J Pediatr 132 : 954–959.

Guinsburg R, de Almeida MF, de Araujo Peres C et al. (2003). Reliability of two behavioural tools to assess pain in preterm neonates. Sao Paulo Med J 121: 72–76.

Gunnar MR, Porter FL, Wolf CM et al. (1995). Neonatal stress reactivity: predictions to later emotional temperament. Child Develop 66: 1–13.

Hadjistavropoulos H, Craig K, Grunau RE et al. (1997). Judging pain in infants: Behavioural, contextual and developmental determinants. Pain 73: 319–324.

Hanna BD, Nelson MN, White-Traut RC et al. (2000). Heart rate variability in preterm brain-injured and very-low-birth-weight infants. Biol Neonate 77: 147–155.

Harrison D, Evans C, Johnston L et al. (2002). Bedside assessment of heel lance pain in the hospitalized infant. J Obstet Gynecol Neonatal Nurs 31: 551–557.

Hodgkinson K, Bear M, Thorn J et al. (1994). Measuring pain in neonates: evaluating an instrument and developing a common language. Aust J Adv Nurs 12: 17–22.

Holsti L, Grunau R, Oberlander T et al. (2004). Specific newborn individualized developmental care and assessment program movements are associated with acute pain in preterm infants in the neonatal intensive care unit. Pediatrics 114: 65–72.

Horgan M, Choonara I. (1996). Measuring pain in neonates: An objective score. Pediatr Nurs 8: 24–27.

Horgan M, Glenn S, Choonara I. (2002). Further development of the Liverpool Infant Distress Scale. J Child Health Care 6: 96–106.

Hudson-Barr DC, Duffey MA, Holditch-Davis D et al. (1998). Pediatric nurses' use of behaviors to make medication administration decisions in infants recovering from surgery. Res Nursing Health 21: 3–13.

Hudson-Barr D, Capper-Michel B, Lambert S et al. (2002). Validation of the Pain Assessment in Neonates (PAIN) scale with the Neonatal Infant Pain Scale (NIPS) Neonatal Network. J Neonatal Nurs 21: 15–21.

Hummel P, Puchalski M, Creech S et al. (2003). N-PASS: Neonatal pain, agitation and sedation scale – reliability and validity. Pediatric Academic Societies Annual Meeting, Seattle, Washington (Abstract).

IASP Task Force on Taxonomy. (1994). Classification of chronic pain, 2nd edn. In: Merskey H, Bogduk N (eds). pp. 209–214. IASP Press, Seattle, Washington.

IASP Task Force on Taxonomy. (2003). IASP pain terminology. Online. Available: http://www.iasp-pain.org/terms-p.html

Izard D. (1979). The Maximally Discriminative Facial Movement Coding System. University of Delaware, Newark, Delaware.

Izard CE, Porges SW, Simons RF et al. (1991). Infant cardiac activity: Developmental changes and relations with attachment. Develop Psychol 27: 432–439.

Johnston CC, Stevens B. (1996). Experience in a neonatal intensive care unit affects pain response. Pediatrics 98: 925–930.

Johnston CC, Strada ME. (1986). Acute pain response in infants: a multidimensional description. Pain 24: 373–382.

Johnston CC, Stevens B, Craig K et al. (1993). Developmental changes in pain expression in premature, full-term, two- and four-month-old infants. Pain 52: 201–208.

Johnston CC, Stevens B, Yang F et al. (1995). Differential response to pain by very premature neonates. Pain 61: 471–479.

Johnston CC, Stevens B, Yang F et al. (1996). Developmental changes in response to heelstick in preterm infants: a prospective cohort study. Dev Med Child Neurol 38: 438–445.

Johnston CC, Sherrard A, Stevens B et al. (1999a). Do cry features reflect pain intensity in preterm neonates? A preliminary study. Biol Neonate 76: 120–124.

Johnston CC, Stremler R, Horton L et al. (1999b). Effect of repeated doses of sucrose during heel stick procedure in preterm neonates. Biol Neonate 75: 160–166.

Johnston CC, Stevens BJ, Franck LS et al. (1999c). Factors explaining lack of response to heel stick in preterm newborns. J Obstet Gynecol Neonatal Nurs 28: 587–594

Jovey RD. (2002). Opioids, pain and addiction. In: Jovey RD (ed.) Managing pain: the Canadian healthcare professional's reference, pp. 63–77. Rogers Media, Toronto, Canada.

Kirya CA, Werthermann MW. (1978). Neonatal circumcision and penile dorsal nerve block. A painless procedure. J Pediatrics 92: 998–1000.

Krechel S, Bildner J. (1995). CRIES: a new neonatal postoperative pain measurement score: initial testing of validity and reliability. Paediatr Anaesth 5: 53–61.

Lawrence J, Alcock D, McGrath P et al. (1993). The development of a tool to assess neonatal pain. Neonat Network J Neonat Nurs 12: 59–66.

Linden W, Earle TL, Gerin W et al. (1997). Physiological stress reactivity and recovery: conceptual siblings separated at birth? J Psychosom Res 42: 117–135.

Lindh V, Wiklund U, Hakansson S. (2000). Assessment of the effect of EMLA during venipuncture in the newborn by analysis of heart rate variability. Pain 86: 247–254.

Lowenstein E, Hallowell P, Levine FH et al. (1969). Cardiovascular response to large doses of intravenous morphine in man. N Engl J Med 281: 1389–1393.

Malkik M, Camm AJ (eds). (1995). Heart rate variability, 1st edn. Future Publishing, Armonk, New York.

Manworren RC, Hynan LS. (2003). Clinical validation of FLACC: preverbal patient pain scale. Pediatr Nurs 29: 140–146.

Marceau J. (2003). Pilot study of a pain assessment tool in the Neonatal Intensive Care Unit. J Paediatr Child Health 39: 598–601.

Massin M, von Bernuth G. (1997). Normal ranges of heart rate variability during infancy and childhood. Pediatr Cardiol 18: 297–302.

McDowell I, Newell C. (1996). Measuring health: A guide to rating scales and questionnaires, 2nd ed. Oxford University Press, Oxford.

McIntosh N, van Veen L, Brameyer H. (1993). The pain of heel prick and its measurement in preterm infants. Pain 52: 71–74.

McNair C, Ballantyne M, Dionne K et al. (2004). Postoperative pain assessment in the neonatal intensive care unit. Arch Dis Childhood: Fetal Neonat Ed 89: 537–541.

Melzack R. (1999). Pain – an overview. Acta Anesthesiol Scand 43: 880–884.

Melzack R, Wall PD. (1965). Pain mechanisms: A new theory. Science 150: 971–979.

Merkel SI, Voepel-Lewis T, Shayevitz JR et al. (1997). The FLACC: a behavioral scale for scoring postoperative pain in young children. Pediatr Nurs 23: 293–297.

Michellson K, Sirvio P, Wasz-Hockert O. (1977). Pain cry in full term asphyxiated newborn infants correlated with late findings. Acta Paediatr Scand 66: 611(a).

Michellsson K, Jarvenpaa AL, Rinne A. (1983). Sound spectrographic analysis of pain cry in preterm infants. Early Hum Develop 8: 141–149.

Mitchell A, Boss BJ. (2002). Adverse effects of pain on the nervous systems of newborns and young children: A review of the literature. J Neurosci Nurs 34: 28–236.

Novak V, Saul JP, Eckberg DL. (1997). Task Force report on heart rate variability. Circulation 96: 1056–1057.

Oberlander TF, Saul JP. (2002). Methodological considerations for the use of heart rate variability as a measure of pain reactivity in vulnerable infants. Clin Perinatol 29: 427–443.

Oberlander TF, Gilbert CA, Chamber CT, et al. (1999a). Biobehavioral responses to acute pain in adolescents with a significant neurologic impairment. Clin J Pain 15: 201–209.

Oberlander TF, Grunau RE, Pitfield S et al. (1999b). The developmental character of cardiac autonomic responses to an acute noxious event in 4- and 8-month-old healthy infants. Pediatr Res 45: 519–525.

Oberlander TF, Grunau RE, Whitfield MF et al. (2000). Biobehavioral pain responses in former extremely low birth weight infants at four months' corrected age. Pediatrics 105: e6.

Oberlander TF, Grunau RVE, Fitzgerald C et al. (2002). Does parenchymal brain injury affect biobehavioral pain responses in very low birth weight infants at 32 weeks' postconceptional age? Pediatrics 110: 570–576.

O'Rourke D. (2004). The measurement of pain in infants, children and adolescents: From policy to practice. Phys Ther 84: 560–570.

Owens ME. (1984). Pain in infancy: conceptual and methodological issues. Pain 20: 213–230.

Owens ME, Todt EJ. (1984). Pain in infancy: neonatal reaction to a heel lance. Pain 20: 77–84.

Pereira AL, Guinsburg R, de Almeida MF et al. (1999). Validity of behavioural and physiologic parameters for acute pain assessment of term newborn infants. São Paulo Med J 117: 72–80

Pillai Riddell RR, Craig KD. (2004). Understanding caregivers' attributions of infant pain. J Pain 5: 106.

Pillai Riddell RR, Stevens BS, Yamada J et al. (2006). Understanding of chronic pain in infancy. Poster presentation, Annual Child Health Psychology Conference. Gainsville, Florida, May 2006.

Pillai Riddell R, Badali MA, Craig KD. (2004). Parental judgments of infant pain: Importance of perceived cognitive abilities, behavioural cues and contextual cues. Pain Res Clin Manage 9: 73–80.

Pokela M. (1994). Pain relief can reduce hypoxemia in distressed neonates during routine treatment procedures. Pediatrics 93: 379–383.

Porges SW. (1992). Vagal tone: a physiologic marker of stress vulnerability. Pediatrics 90: 498–504.

Porges SW. (1995). Cardiac vagal tone: a physiological index of stress. Neurosci Biobehav Rev 19: 225–233.

Porter FL, Porges SW, Marshall RE. (1988). Newborn cries and vagal tone: Parallel changes in response to circumcision. Child Develop 59: 495–505.

Porter FL, Grunau R, Anand KJS (1999a). Long-term effects of pain in infants. J Develop Behav Pediatr 20: 253–261.

Porter FL, Wolf CM, Miller JP. (1999b). Procedural pain in newborn infants: the influence of intensity and development. Pediatrics 104: e13.

Powell C, Kelly A, Williams A. (2001). Determining the minimum clinically significant difference in visual analogue pain score for children. Annals Emerg Med 37: 28–31.

Prietsch V, Knoepke U, Obladen M. (1994). Continuous monitoring of heart rate variability in preterm infants. Early Hum Develop 37: 117–131.

Puchalski M, Hummel P. (2002). The reality of neonatal pain. Adv Neonatal Care 2: 233–244.

Ramsey M. (2000). Measuring level of sedation in the intensive care unit. J Am Med Assoc 284: 441–442.

Randich A, Maixner W. (1984). Interactions between cardiovascular and pain regulatory systems. Neurosci Biobehav Rev 8: 343–367.

Ravenswaaij-Arts CM, Hopman JC, Kollee LA et al. (1995). The influence of artificial ventilation on heart rate variability in very preterm infants. Pediatr Res 37: 124–130.

Richardson DK, Corcoran JD, Escobar GJ et al. (2001). SNAP-II and SNAPPE-II: Simplified newborn illness severity and mortality risk scores. J Pediatr 138: 92–100.

Robieux K, Kumar R, Radhakrishnan S et al. (1991). Assessing pain and analgesia with a lidocaine-prilocain emulsion in infants and toddlers during venipuncture. J Pediatr 118: 971–973.

Rosenstein D, Oster H. (1988). Differential facial responses to four basic tastes in newborns. Child Dev 59: 1555–1568.

Rowbotham M. (2001). What is "clinically meaningful" reduction in pain? Pain 94: 131–132.

Saul JP, Albrecht P, Berger RD. (1988). Analysis of long term heart rate variability: methods, 1/f scaling and implications. Comput Cardiol 14: 419–422.

Schade JG, Joyce BA, Gerkensmeyer J et al. (1996). Comparison of three preverbal scales for postoperative pain assessment in a diverse pediatric sample. J Pain Symptom Manage 12: 348–359.

Shah V, Ipp M, Sam J et al. (2004). Eliciting the minimal clinically important difference in the pain response from parents of newborn infants and nurses. Pediatr Res 55: 519.

Shiller C. (1999). Clinical utility of two neonatal pain assessment measures. Master's thesis. Faculty of Nursing, University of Toronto.

Sparshott MM. (1996). The development of a clinical distress scale for ventilated newborn infants: identification of pain and distress based on validated behavioral scores. J Neonatal Nurs 2: 5–11.

Spassov L, Curzi-Dascalova L, Clairambault J et al. (1994). Heart rate and heart rate variability during sleep in small-for-gestational age newborns. Pediatr Res 35: 500–505.

Spence K, Gillies D, Harrison D et al. (2005). A reliable pain assessment tool for clinical assessment in the neonatal intensive care unit. J Obstet Gynecol Neonatal Nurs 34: 80–86.

Stevens B, Gibbins S. (2002). Clinical utility and clinical significance in the assessment and management of pain in vulnerable infants. Clin Perinatol 29: 459–468.

Stevens BJ, Johnston CC, Horton L. (1994). Factors that influence the behavioural pain responses of premature infants. Pain 59: 101–109.

Stevens B, Johnston C, Petryshen P et al. (1996). Premature Infant Pain Profile: development and initial validation. Clin J Pain 12: 13–22.

Stevens B, Johnston C, Gibbins S. (2000a). Pain assessment in neonates. In: Anand KS, Stevens BJ, McGrath PJ (eds). Pain in neonates, 2nd edn. pp. 101–130. Elsevier, Amsterdam and New York.

Stevens B, Gibbins S, Franck LS. (2000b). Treatment of pain in the neonatal intensive care unit. Pediatr Clin North Am 47: 633–650.

Stevens B, McGrath PJ, Gibbins S et al. (2003). Procedural pain in newborns at risk for neurologic impairment. Pain 105: 27–35.

Stevens B, Yamada J, Ohlsson A. (2004). Sucrose for analgesia in newborn infants undergoing painful procedures. Cochrane Database of Systematic Reviews (3):CD001069 Review.

Stevens B, Yamada J, Beyene J et al. (2005). Consistent management of repeated procedural pain with sucrose in preterm neonates: Is it effective and safe for repeated use over time? Clin J Pain 21: 543–548.

Storm H. (2001). Development of emotional sweating in preterms measured by skin conductance changes. Early Hum Develop 62: 149–158.

Sufka KJ, Price DD. (2002). Gate control theory reconsidered. Brain Mind 3: 277–290.

Suominen P, Caffin C, Linton S. (2004). The cardiac analgesic assessment scale (CAAS): a pain assessment tool for intubated and ventilated children after cardiac surgery. Paediatr Anaesth 14: 336–343.

Swanson LW, Sawchenko PE. (1983). Hypothalamic integration: organization of the paraventricular and supraoptic nuclei. Ann Rev Neurosci 6: 269–324.

Taddio A, Goldbach M, Ipp M et al. (1995). Effect of circumcision on pain responses during vaccination in male infants. Lancet 345: 291–292.

van Dijk M, Peters J, Bouwmeester N et al. (2002). Are postoperative pain instruments useful for specific groups of vulnerable infants? Clin Perinatol 29: 469–491.

Vatner SF, Marsh JD, Swain JA. (1975). Effects of morphine on coronary and left ventricular dynamics in conscious dogs. J Clin Invest 55: 207–217.

Vohr BR, Wright LL, Dusick AM et al. (2000). Neurodevelopmental and functional outcomes of extremely low birth weight infants in the National Institute of Child Health and Human Development Neonatal Research Network 1993–1994. Pediatrics 105: 1216–1226.

Walker C, Anand KJS, Plotsky PM. (2001). Development of the hypothalamic-pituitary-adrenal axis and the stress response. In: McEwen B, Goodman H (eds). Coping with the environment: neural and endocrine mechanisms, pp. 237–270. Oxford University Press, Oxford.

Warnock FF, Lander J. (2004). Foundations of knowledge about neonatal pain: Review article. J Pain Symptom Manage 27: 170–179.

Warnock F, Sandrin D. (2004). Comprehensive description of newborn distress behavior in response to acute pain (newborn male circumcision). Pain 107: 242–255.

Wood NS, Marlow N, Costeloe K et al. (2000). Neurologic and developmental disability after extremely preterm birth. EPICure study group. New Engl J Med 343: 378–384.

7

Infant colic – clinical implications and current controversies

Shuvo Ghosh
Ronald G Barr

INTRODUCTION

While the word 'colic' is derived from the Greek *kolikos*, the adjectival form of *kolon* (large intestine), and signifies pain of abdominal origin, the more specific term 'infant colic' (now often referred to as 'infant colic syndrome') has come to represent a particular group of symptoms during the first few months of life, with excessive crying at its core. Traditionally the aetiology of these symptoms has been presumed to be a gastrointestinal disturbance that causes pain, gas or discomfort. However, these same symptoms have been used frequently, if loosely, to describe a temperamental state ('being colicky') in a manner that runs counter to a specific painful origin. In recent years, a number of proposed reasons for infant colic and attendant management strategies have emerged, each with varying degrees of supportive evidence. Current theories about factors that may incite colic symptoms and new recommendations for the management and reduction of infant colic are a source of controversy.

Although the symptoms that comprise infant colic may indeed be a manifestation of any of several primary disturbances, the bulk of the present literature strongly suggests that infants with colic are generally free of organic pathology (Barr and Geertsma 2002, Lobo et al. 2004). Despite the circumstantial findings that suggest so, there is little evidence that infants with colic actually experience pain during crying episodes (Barr and Geertsma 2002). The behaviours exhibited in infant colic are present in normally developing infants, merely in lesser intensity or frequency. Effectively this means that for most infants, colic is a phenomenon within the spectrum of normative infant behaviour. Nevertheless, it is consistently one of the most common complaints raised by parents to infant healthcare providers and continues to present a difficult challenge in the clinical setting.

THE NORMAL CRYING SPECTRUM

In 1962, Brazelton published a seminal paper that helped to establish the typical pattern of infant crying behaviours (Brazelton 1962). Numerous subsequent studies have supported those initial findings (Gormally and Barr 1997). Normally, infants cry more during the first 3 months than at any other

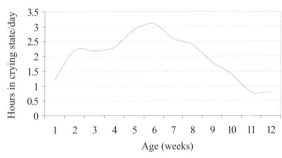

Figure 7.1 Example of a typical early infant crying curve. The period of peak crying levels tends to occur between 5 and 8 weeks of life with subsequent steady decreases. Levels usually reach a baseline by the age of 4 months.

age. The peak amount of crying occurs during the second month (Gormally and Barr 1997), with the start of this increase at 2 weeks and usually a return to baseline by 4 months. An example of a typical crying curve is given in Figure 7.1. There is an observable cluster of crying behaviour in the late afternoon and evening hours, although some infants cry more at various times of day, reflecting some variability in this diurnal pattern (St. James-Roberts and Plewis 1996). Those infants who do cry most in the evening hours typically tend to cry more during the rest of the day (St James-Roberts et al. 1993, Hill and Hosking 2000). Infants whose parents complain of 'colicky' behaviour and who fulfil the criteria for the standard definition of infant colic (see below) demonstrate longer and more unsoothable crying bouts, as well as increased facial activity while crying than their non-colicky counterparts (Barr et al. 1992, 2005). This usually leads such parents to perceive the crying as more intense, worrisome, urgent, and sick-sounding, with higher pitch and more harmonic distortion and 'breaks' in the cry (Lester et al. 1992, Stifter and Braungart 1992).

Parent perception of intensity is not necessarily associated with increased amounts of crying, but it may be affected by slightly different acoustical properties of the crying. Some evidence exists that the crying of infants with colic may have different acoustic structures in some circumstances that parents can detect (Zeskind and Barr 1997). However, there is little evidence of an acoustically distinct cry type (a 'colic' cry). Indeed, there has been considerable debate about whether there are cry types at all (pain cries, hunger cries, fatigue cries). Currently, the evidence is strongest that the infant cry is a graded signal, reflecting intensity of the stimulus and the infant's response, but not specific to the causal stimulus (Gustafson et al. 2000). Although not yet linked to infant colic per se, pain-induced autonomic nervous system activation could

contribute to differences in neural input to the vocal cords and result in increased cry pitch (Golub and Corwin 1985, Soltis 2004). In this way, a pain stimulus may contribute to changed caregiver behaviour response to crying or increased anxiety.

The normative crying pattern in infants (e.g. more crying in the morning versus evening) may also interact with individual differences in crying pattern when individual babies are considered. Some reports suggest that these differences may be due to differences in feeding experience as may occur among formula-fed infants (Hill and Hosking 2000) or among infants switched from breast to formula feeds (Barr et al. 1989, Lucas and St. James-Roberts 1982).

A great deal of normal infant behaviour, especially crying, is organized in a discontinuous pattern reflecting 'behavioural states' (Wolff 1987). Behavioural states typically have three determining properties (Wolff 1987):

1. Self-organization, in the sense that a behavioural state (like crying, sleeping, awake alert) is maintained until a pattern of events occurs that results in a shift to another state;
2. Relative stability, so that a state persists over a period of time (minutes rather than seconds); and
3. State-dependent responses; that is, when a stimulus experienced in one state results in a different response than the same stimulus experienced in another state.

Based on these properties, the organized crying state can be characterized by persistent cry vocalizations (ranging from whimpers to loud screams), resistance of limbs to passive movement, facial grimacing (sometimes accompanied by facial flushing), and diffuse motor activity (or rigid extension of the trunk) (Wolff 1984). The term 'fussing' can be characterized as a transitional state with intermittent vocalizing and less-intense, non-rhythmic motor activity than in the crying state (Wolff 1984). Intermittent crying is often a preliminary phase when an infant transitions from one behavioural state to another, with stops and starts of crying behaviour (including any part of the aforementioned characteristics) of varied intensity, that may or may not lead to full-blown, sustained, organized crying.

In infant colic, the features of vascular reactivity, vocalization, expression and motor movement are similar to such an organized state of crying. In this sense, it seems that much of the crying seen in infants with colic is a well-organized version of typical crying behaviour. Infants who are fussing or crying intermittently often have negative vocalizations as well, but not the full organization of the crying state. Such vocalizations (or those that mimic crying sounds) may become incorporated into the prolonged behavioural crying states seen in infants with colic. Moreover, soothing stimuli presented to infants who have not yet entered a sustained period of crying are much more likely to prevent the transition to fully organized crying, but may be ineffective when presented after an organized behavioural crying state has been established. This may be one explanation for the 'colic crying bout' that is sustained for long periods and recalcitrant to soothing (Barr et al. 2005).

During early postnatal life, the central nervous system undergoes a period of rapid growth and differentiation. This physiologic reorganization is likely reflected in the typical manifestations of infant colic and the crying state. Changing organizations in other states such as sleeping, wakefulness and alert activity (Wolff 1987) also emerge during the same period between 2 and 4 months of life. These processes may be, to some extent, interdependent. For example, the decline in infant crying behaviour after the early peak of 5–8 weeks probably represents one manifestation of increasingly stable wakefulness without crying (Ghosh and Barr 2004).

Maintaining a stable state of non-crying wakefulness is influenced by the maturity of cognitive, affective and motor functions of infants. Neuromaturation probably is reflected in the fact that infant states become less dependent on environmental factors. For example, during the first 3 months of life, infants grow increasingly responsive to the human voice and human figures (presented visually). Social smiling also becomes more pronounced after 6 weeks and is associated with increases in infant interaction with caregivers (Wolff 1987). Better hand control precedes self-soothing techniques such as thumb-sucking, a coordinated rhythmic motor action that may elicit a quiet awake state (Hopkins et al. 1988). The apparently 'spontaneous' remission of infant colic may be explained in part by neuromaturation that is manifested by more frequent achievement of stable waking states.

THE PAIN EXPERIENCE AND THE DEFINITION OF INFANT COLIC

Infant colic is a cluster of behaviours predominated by crying that occurs during the first 3 months of life. In a small percentage of cases, symptoms can persist into the fourth month or later. Early reports suggested this to occur in 30–48% of infants (Wessel et al. 1954, Illingworth 1955), but this number may be an overestimation. Nevertheless, the incidence of infant colic in the overall population lies somewhere between 10% and 40%, depending on how it is defined. Most

current definitions include crying as the core symptom. Some of this crying occurs in extended bouts when the infant is resistant to soothing. During such bouts, infants may present with behaviour that is often interpreted as a manifestation of pain: clenching of fists, flexing of legs over the abdomen, back arching, grimacing and facial reddening. At times the abdomen may seem distended or hard, and regurgitation/emesis and flatulence may accompany the bout of crying. In addition, some of these bouts can be described as 'paroxysmal' in that they have a sudden, unpredictable onset, with equally unpredictable amelioration, with no seeming relation to events in the infant's environment.

The paroxysmal nature of infant colic, sometimes accompanied by a pain-like facies, seems to support the possibility of pain, more specifically abdominal pain, as its source. Certain aetiologic factors have been hypothesized to induce abdominal pain and concomitant colic-like behaviour in infants, but thus far none are consistently associated with the organized crying state noted with infant colic. Yet this pain attribution persists because of the indisputable fact that colicky infants often appear to be experiencing some kind of distress that presents in an unpredictable manner (see Ch. 14).

Although the collection of characteristics for infant colic seem to comprise a distinct clinical phenomenon, they are in fact continuous with those seen in infants without colic and are usually described qualitatively (Ghosh and Barr 2004). Therefore, reliably determining whether or not an infant actually meets criteria for 'having colic' can be difficult clinically. In an attempt to better quantify the observed behaviour, Wessel et al. introduced criteria for colic most commonly referred to as the 'rule of threes' in 1954. These criteria are met when an infant cries for:

- ≥3 hours per day;
- ≥3 days per week;
- ≥3 weeks.

'Modified Wessel's criteria' (wherein the third criterion requiring crying for 3 or more weeks is dropped, and only criteria 1 and 2 are needed) are used in most studies of infant colic. Even though this modified Wessel's definition has proven useful in terms of comparing samples and in research, the relative arbitrariness in designating such rules is problematic. If strict adherence to the criteria is maintained, then infants who cry for a few minutes less than 3 hours per day would be considered not to have colic. However, since the evidence suggests that these infants are likely part of the same behavioural group as those who meet the standard criteria (St. James-Roberts et al. 1997, Lobo et al. 2004), the clinical relevance of such a definition of colic is limited.

Most cases of infant colic seem to represent behaviour at the high end of the spectrum of normal crying. Infant colic syndrome resembles normal crying behaviour, but with greater intensity, frequency and duration (Barr and Lessard 1999, Ghosh and Barr 2004). These behaviours are consistent in infants across cultures, for both term and preterm infants, and are unrelated to parenting style (Wessel et al. 1954, St. James-Roberts et al. 1994, 1998, Alvarez and St. James-Roberts 1996, Barr et al. 1996). Culturally different caregiver methods do not seem to affect the age-dependent, diurnal pattern of infant crying (Barr et al. 1991, St. James-Roberts et al. 1994). The same is true of prematurity. Infants born at 32 weeks manifest a crying curve that peaks at approximately 6 weeks corrected age rather than 6 weeks postnatally (Barr et al. 1996). While infants with colic are more likely to have unsoothable crying bouts than their typical counterparts, the frequency of such bouts is proportional to overall crying (St. James-Roberts et al. 1998).

Two other factors are relevant to the concept that infant colic represents the upper end of a continuous spectrum of crying behaviour. One is that only a very small number of infants with colic or their parents have concomitant organic disease processes. Only about 5% or fewer of cases in the primary care setting have identifiable pathology in the infant or a parent (Treem 1994). Psychosocial causes such as parental depression, poor caregiving style or inexperience have not been consistently associated with an increased prevalence of infant colic. While first-born infants are more often brought to a paediatrician with concerns about colic, no difference in crying amounts between first-born and later-born infants has been found (St. James-Roberts and Halil 1991). The other factor is that the physical and emotional outcomes for infants with colic do not differ from those of infants without colic, when controlled for general risk (Lehtonen et al. 2000, Castro-Rodriguez et al. 2001). Recent studies suggest that differences in long-term cognitive development occur only in children with excessive crying that is prolonged beyond 3 months of age (Rao et al. 2004); similarly, children who have persistent excessive crying up to 6 months of age may have an association with hyperactivity in middle childhood (8–10 years of age) (Wolke et al. 2002). However, neither of these patterns of crying are representative of infant colic limited to the first 3 months of life, as it is currently defined.

Other processes have been examined in regards to colic, to try to better understand the mechanism of excessive crying and the infant colic state. Studies have shown that infants with colic sleep less overall than infants without colic (Papousek and von Hofacker 1995, White et al. 2000). Differences during the day are accounted for by increased time spent crying; so only night-time sleep amounts are truly different (Kirjavainen et al. 2000, White et al. 2000). More recent studies find that excessively crying infants may have a disturbance that affects rapid eye movement and non-rapid eye movement sleep stage proportion, but only during evening hours, when crying occurs most (Kirjavainen et al. 2004). Furthermore, all-night sleep studies done at 2 months and at 7 months (after colic has resolved) show no differences in sleep structure between the two groups, implying that no physiological process is responsible for the slightly different sleep amounts (Kirjavainen et al. 2000). Similarly no contrast was noted in high, middle, or low frequencies in heart rate variability at 2 or 7 months of age (Kirjavainen et al. 2001). This suggests that neither the parasympathetic nor the sympathetic autonomic nervous system are aetiologically involved in the syndrome of infant colic. Support for this comes also from the finding that infants with colic have similar heart rate, vagal tone and salivary cortisol secretion as infants without colic, despite nearly twice as much daily crying (White et al. 2000).

Thus the common assumption that pain is the cause of infant colic simply remains unproven, with most evidence in the literature suggesting no such causality. Indeed, even the association of infant colic with increased physiologic stress has not been demonstrated. There may be increasing evidence for the opposite to be true, with decreased secretion of cortisol noted in infants with colic during periods of increased crying (Ghosh and Barr 2004). The usual attribution of the crying of colic to pain (so-called 'pain theory') behaviour is not well supported by available evidence, and other aetiologic factors associated with excessive crying have very low prevalence. A sampling of pathologic conditions sometimes associated with colic is shown in Table 7.1 (Miller and Barr 1991, Treem 1994, Ross Monographs 1997, Ghosh and Barr 2004).

THE POSSIBLE ROLE OF ALLODYNIA AND VISCERAL HYPERALGESIA

If evidence for pain as *the* aetiologic factor for infant colic is missing, it nevertheless remains possible that pain-relevant processes could, in principle, be implicated, although there is as yet no direct confirmatory evidence that they are. It is at least plausible to posit the idea that otherwise innocuous intestinal stimuli

Table 7.1 Organic conditions commonly associated with the etiology of infant colic[a]

Condition	Prevalence in primary care	Strength of association
Lactose intolerance	Variable but common	Extremely weak
Infantile migraine	Rare	Strong
Reflux oesophagitis	Rare	Moderate
Congenital glaucoma	Rare	Weak but possible
CNS abnormalities	Rare	Weak but possible
Maternal drug effects (e.g. Prozac)	Variable but uncommon	Strong
Isolated fructose intolerance	Rare	Strong
Bovine protein intolerance	≤ 5% of infants	Strong
Anomalous L coronary artery (from pulmonary artery)	Very rare	Strong

[a] all listed conditions account for approximately 5% of infants brought to primary care settings with the complaint of 'infant colic'

may cause discomfort in a subset of infants with colic or excessive crying. The hypersensitivity implied by this hypothesis might be due to altered mechanisms of afferent pathways, changes in the excitability of central neurons where afferent pathways project, or a series of developmental differences in the afferent–efferent loop (Grunau et al. 2001). The terms *visceral hyperalgesia* and *allodynia* are often used to describe these processes (see Ch. 14).

Hyperalgesia refers to a reduced pain threshold and/or a greater duration of response to a painful stimulus. Allodynia refers to painful experiences resulting from stimuli that usually do not cause pain. In the context of infant colic, normally occurring phenomena such as intestinal distension, mild gastro-oesophageal reflux or regurgitation, or motility changes might be experienced as painful or uncomfortable (allodynia) if these infants have visceral hyperalgesia. A similar explanation has been suggested for gastrointestinal syndromes in older children and adults with little evidence for organic disease, such as irritable bowel syndrome or recurrent paediatric abdominal pain (Mayer and Gebhart 1994).

Afferent pathways can become hypersensitive when repeated noxious stimuli or inflammation alter the sensitivity of the sensory system by the action of chemical mediators (Fitzgerald et al. 1989). Altered sensitivity affects the sensory information sent to secondary dorsal horn neurons. Additionally, it may affect reflex regulatory loops that control a variety of functions within the enteric nervous and gut effector cell systems, such as blood flow, peptide secretion and gut motility. Central hypersensitivity can last beyond the initial stimulus and becomes associated with

reduced thresholds and increases in the receptive field size of the dorsal horn neurons, allowing otherwise innocuous stimuli to excite previously unexcitable nociceptive pathways. If the dorsal horn cells are hyper-excitable, afferent hypersensitivity can also result. Notably, excitatory pathways in the spinal cord mature early, and continue to mature in the postnatal period, so these processes could play a role in even very young infants. Inhibitory processes tend to mature later in postnatal life: local inhibitory interneuronal connections in the substantia gelatinosa and the functional development of descending inhibitory signals from the brainstem occur as postnatal events in rat pups, and may do so in humans (Fitzgerald 2005).

Visceral hyperalgesia and allodynia in infant colic may be pertinent as processes that could explain why gastrointestinal distress remains a focus for clinicians and parents in some cases of excessive crying. They may provide a reason why apparent discomfort is noted in the absence of detectable pathology. The evening clustering of infant crying might be due to relatively increased sensory input to centrally hyper-excitable neurons during the daytime. Such pain experiences may persist long after an inciting stimulus has resolved. However, they can still be transient, which fits with the current opinion that infant colic does not have long-term effects on health and development. Later maturing descending cortical neuronal connections are likely to be important in governing dorsal horn neuronal excitability, particularly for pain perception (Owens et al. 1992). Such modulation consequentially inhibits excitatory tone so that resting activity and sensory responses in spinal dorsal horn neurons are reduced as the infant grows older.

The decline in crying behaviour and the overall developmental progression of infant colic syndrome could be secondary to modulation by increasing maturity of local inhibitory pathways because of inter-neuronal synaptogenesis in the spinal cord as well as progressively mature descending inhibitory systems from the brainstem and cortex. Finally, while cortical pain may play a role, as relative delay in the maturity of inhibitory connections also seems to occur in the cortex (Fitzgerald 2005), such mechanisms have not been clearly established for infants with colic.

ORGANIC PATHOLOGY IN INFANT COLIC

A number of pathophysiologic determinants of infant colic have been proposed, but those that are clinically identifiable have a low prevalence, especially in primary care settings. Infants with colic tend to have difficulty in calming, are resistant to soothing, and have episodes of crying that are hard to terminate once begun (Barr et al. 1991). The processes that underlie infant colic likely tend to maintain bouts of crying, rather than to initiate them.

Gastroenterologic pathology

Associations to dietary factors such as cow's milk protein or lactose have been proposed as possible stimuli to gastrointestinal pain episodes in infants with colic; as have disturbances of motility, gut hormones and differences in feeding behaviour. However, therapeutic success in dealing with any of these factors is difficult to distinguish from the pattern of normal crying behaviour in infants. Implication of these factors requires independent evidence of these processes other than the crying and associated behaviours themselves.

Protein intolerance

Hypersensitivity to bovine milk proteins in the diet has been implicated in infant colic. Some studies have reported the association of cow's milk with excessive crying (Leung and Lemay 2004) but true hypersensitivity with eosiniphilia and immunoglobulin E (IgE)-mediated responses has been reported in only a few cases (Harris et al. 1977, Stifter and Braungart 1992). If infants with colic had this condition, then modification of diet routinely ought to reduce the colicky behaviour; but in controlled studies this has not been convincingly demonstrated in more than a few infants (Forsyth et al. 1985). If this hypersensitivity were a common aetiology for infant colic, then formula-fed infants should frequently develop colic at much higher rates than breastfed infants due to the high concentration of potentially antigenic protein to which they are exposed. However, the prevalence, pattern and amount of crying associated with infant colic are similar in both breast- and formula-fed infants. Of note, however, is the fact that the most potentially antigenic bovine proteins, β-lactoglobulin and casein, are passed in breast milk (Estep and Kulczycki 2000) but in concentrations (up to 33 ng/mL) that are far lower than concentrations typically found in cow's milk formulas (greater than 1 mg/mL). Bovine immunoglobulin G (IgG), another possible antigenic protein, does pass in breast milk at comparable levels to cow's milk, and may be higher in the milk of mothers who report symptoms of infant colic (Clyne and Kulczycki 1991).

Protein intolerance usually causes additional symptoms such as vomiting and diarrhoea, that are not typically part of infant colic syndrome. A history of family atopy or other atopic manifestations are not differentially seen in infants with colic. Furthermore, no specific immunologic marker has been associated with colic symptoms. A very small number of infants have ever been studied and found to have increased plasma cell content in the lamina propria of small intestinal mucosa in response to a milk challenge in the presence of colic symptoms (Harris et al. 1977). Switching to hydrolyzed casein formula has not significantly reduced excessive crying (Forsyth 1989). In spite of these findings, hypersensitivity to bovine proteins probably does contribute to a small number of infant colic cases. Milk-protein allergy continues to be a controversial claim, and it is not clear whether it represents a specific mechanism for particular cases of colic, or if it is a mechanism that simply exacerbates the normal increase in crying during the first 3 months of life. For this reason, changing feeds is not recommended in the regular management of infant colic, since the yield for satisfactory outcomes (reduced crying) tends to be very low with this strategy. Only in the presence of other findings of protein intolerance, most importantly blood or mucus in stools, may it be worth considering this diagnosis. In such rare cases, mothers may be instructed to reduce dairy food intake if breast-feeding, and formula-fed infants may be switched to an alternative formula.

Carbohydrate intolerance

Intestinal gas has been considered a cause of infant colic, primarily because of the clinical association with abdominal distension, burping and flatus. The source of such gas would likely be intestinal, more particularly colonic, since the colon is the major site of abdominal gas. Colonic bacteria utilize a wide range of substrates to produce hydrogen and methane, but dietary carbohydrates result in the largest amount of gas.

Finding a link between the abdominal distress observed by parents and increased colonic gas would be a convenient explanation for infant colic. Incomplete lactose digestion unassociated with clinical disease has been proven by breath hydrogen testing under normal feeding conditions in healthy infants (Barr et al. 1984), and mild lactase insufficiency persists into the third month of life (Lifshitz et al. 1983). In theory this description fits a causative model for infant colic both in terms of the clinical symptomatology and timeline. Yet other findings suggestive of carbohydrate intolerance have never been clearly demonstrated in colicky infants, such as reducing substances in stool or changes in stool pH. Reducing lactose intake does not reduce crying (Barr et al. 1991), and there is no significant post-feed abdominal distension in infants with colic (Barr et al. 1992). One case of persistent excessive crying was shown to be due to fructose malabsorption (Wales et al. 1989) but that crying lasted beyond 4 months of life, with significant diarrhoea in the infant. No other convincing evidence exists that problems of carbohydrate absorption resulting in increased colonic gas play a significant role in the infant colic syndrome.

Motility

A pathogenetic relationship between infant colic and intestinal motility has not been established, but it is not unreasonable to suppose that some colicky infants may have abnormalities in gut motility. Most evidence for this explanation comes retrospectively after treatment of excessive crying episodes. Management of infant colic with dicyclomine hydrochloride, an anticholinergic drug, has been effective (Illingworth 1959, Weissbluth et al. 1984). Dicyclomine may have dual actions centrally and peripherally, causing decreased gastrointestinal spasm by directly relaxing smooth muscle fibres. Its effects in decreasing the amount of crying imply that motility may play a role in at least some cases of infant colic. Unfortunately, this drug has a dangerous side-effect profile including sudden infant death (Savino et al. 2002) or acute respiratory distress (Weissbluth et al. 1984, Lundell et al. 1998), making it unsuitable for use. More recent efforts in this domain have concentrated on cimetropium bromide, another anticholinergic drug, as an alternative. Its use is controversial, especially in North America, but there is evidence that cimetropium (a synthetic derivative of scopolamine) is more effective than placebo in the treatment of colic (Savino et al. 2002). Fennel seed oil (*Foeniculum vulgare*) also serves as an intestinal antispasmodic, and both the oil emulsion alone and a mixture of fennel, chamomile and balm mint in a herbal tea have been shown to

reduce colic symptoms (Weizman et al. 1993, Alexandrovich et al. 2003). In light of this, the possibility of a motility-related source for excessive crying cannot be completely ruled out, although no convincing data exist to show what motility difficulties may be present (Lobo et al. 2004).

Taste-mediated calming

Another potential source of infant colic relates to the proximate mechanisms for recruiting physiologic soothing systems in infants. Animal and human studies have shown that small amounts of sweet taste (particularly sucrose) applied to the tongue seem to initiate an intrinsic, centrally acting opioid system that has a quieting or calming effect (Shide and Blass 1989, Smith et al. 1990, Barr et al. 1999). The same process has been implicated in reduction of infant pain from noxious stimuli such as vaccinations or heel-stick blood draws (Barr et al. 1999). It seems that the calming effect of sucrose is specifically dependent on a normally functioning central opioid system, but some evidence is now emerging that endogenous opioids may not mediate pain reduction in the manner previously thought (Gradin and Schollin 2005). Nevertheless, changes in a central opioid-dependent calming system are plausibly associated with early increased crying, especially because the sucrose-induced calming effect is gradually reduced over the first 6 weeks of life, at the same time infant crying tends to increase. Infants with colic may have more pronounced changes in this system, as sucrose taste has been shown to be less effective in 6-week-old infants with colic compared to 6-week-old infants without colic (Barr et al. 1999). There is still much on-going research into the role of taste-induced calming and soothing processes (with or without the involvement of central or circulating opioids) that may turn out to be an important mediator of crying behaviour in infants.

Psychophysiologic factors

Behavioural interventions may modulate infant crying, and should be considered despite limited knowledge about which biologic processes they recruit. For example, behavioural factors (e.g. caregiving style, feeding patterns) may interact with gastrointestinal factors such as breast milk composition to affect crying. In human breast milk, protein and fat content are relatively low. In mammalian species, this type of milk composition correlates with low sucking rates, frequent feeding at short intervals, and continuous proximity to the food source in other mammalian species. Among humans, such feeding behaviour occurs in hunter-gatherer caregivers such as the !Kung San hunter-gatherers of Botswana. Small, frequent feeds may be reasonably thought to reduce infant crying due to reduction in hunger, by moderating the effects of previously described gastrointestinal factors, by more frequently eliciting taste-mediated calming and by increasing rhythmic sucking (a self-soothing behaviour). However, crying among !Kung San infants also has an early peak pattern in the first few months of life, and crying episodes occur with the same frequency as they do in North American infants; the only difference is that the duration of crying bouts is halved (Barr et al. 1991). This supports the concept that an early predisposition to increased crying exists but prolonged crying bouts and excessive crying are amenable to modification if not elimination by biologic and behavioural factors, including those associated with caregiving style (Barr et al. 2001).

Other research supports the potential for an association between infant colic and feeding problems (Miller-Lancar et al. 2004). Disorganized feeding behaviours and less responsiveness during feeding interactions have been observed, as well as more evidence of gastro-oesophageal reflux, in infants with colic. The organization of oral motor skills and regulation of crying behaviour may potentially occur synchronously in at least a sub-group of colicky infants.

MANAGEMENT OF INFANT COLIC: CONTINUING CONTROVERSIES

Overall, the recommendations and management plan for crying infants are similar whether or not they meet Wessel's or modified Wessel's criteria for infant colic. While early detection of organic disease is important, once significant pathology has been ruled out, a systematic approach is preferred. The indications and contraindications for several current treatment strategies follow.

Formula switching

In the absence of clinical symptoms such as persistent vomiting and/or diarrhoea, weight loss, blood and/or mucus in the stool, or persistence of crying behaviour beyond the usual period of increased crying, changing infant formulas is not typically recommended. If these symptoms are present in an infant receiving cow's milk formula, a limited trial of a bovine antigen-free formula may be attempted. Mothers of breastfeeding infants with colic who have these symptoms may try a diet in which their own intake is dairy-free.

Medications

There is no present indication for any pharmacologic intervention in the treatment of infant colic. While anticholinergics may play a role in the reduction of individual colic crises (fully organized crying bouts), further studies are required before any firm conclusions can be made in this regard. In Europe, cimetropium bromide has been used in infants with colic; equivalent use in North America has not been approved. Other medications implicated in colic treatment include alcohol, phenobarbitol and sodium bicarbonate (probably the active ingredient in 'gripe water'). Simethicone, a gas-neutralizing agent, has not been shown to provide any demonstrable benefit (Metcalf et al. 1994). Also, the safety profile of most of these medications in infants has yet to be established.

Movement and sound

Crib shakers, white noise (fans, dryers, continuous loop tapes or CDs) all provide stimulation analogous to that received with increased caregiver contact. Increased caregiver attention including swaddling, carrying and the promotion of rhythmic sucking may serve to calm infants. Mechanical intervention requires consideration of safety factors. Placing an infant on a clothes' dryer that is turned on is contraindicated due to the danger of serious injury from a fall.

Massage, manipulation and chiropractic care

To date, no strong evidence exists for massage or chiropractic intervention as effective treatment for infant colic (Canadian Paediatric Society 2002, Husereau et al. 2003). Such therapies are widely practiced because of the frustration emanating from the transient, unpredictable and mysterious nature of crying bouts in the infant colic syndrome. However, no studies show that chiropractic affects the natural course of crying patterns in the crying spectrum of normal infants.

'Crying out'

Allowing infants to cry without a caregiver response is not effective. Conceptualizing an operant condition/learning paradigm for management inevitably leads to the conclusion that responding to crying will 'spoil' the infant. There is little evidence to suggest that responding will result in negative consequences. In fact, leaving a crying infant alone for extended periods of time is difficult and probably a great stressor to families already experiencing difficulty with infant colic. Immediate responsivity likely activates multi-sensory channels that can partially soothe crying infants. Increased attempts at soothing with more contact and interaction are more likely to be associated with better outcomes, even if crying behaviour is not eliminated completely.

CONCLUSIONS

In part because of the connotations of the name and in part because of the associated clinical symptomatology, infant colic is still considered a manifestation of abdominal pain. A certain number of infants with colic may indeed experience gastrointestinal distress, due to either pathologic processes or hypersensitivity secondary to visceral hyperalgesia and allodynia. Though the complaint of infant colic is common, there is still no predominant aetiology that can explain the large majority of the cases. Until there is a better understanding of the mechanisms involved in excessive crying and associated behaviours, a variety of management strategies will continue to be attempted. The most important issue will continue to be appropriate reassurance and the prevention of secondary consequences such as caregiver anxiety and depression and the one truly tragic consequence of inappropriate caregiver responses to crying, shaken baby syndrome. Ongoing clinical surveillance of infants with early increased crying is also indicated to make sure the infant follows the known patterns of crying that subsides by 4–5 months. Excessive crying following that period, especially associated with other clinical symptomatology is much less frequent, but is more likely to have be a reflection of organic pathophysiology.

REFERENCES

Alexandrovich I, Rakovitskaya O, Kolmo E et al. (2003). The effect of fennel (*Foeniculum vulgare*) seed oil emulsion in infantile colic: a randomized, placebo-controlled study. Altern Ther Health Med 9: 58–61.

Alvarez M, St. James-Roberts I. (1996). Infant fussing and crying patterns in the first year in an urban community in Denmark. Acta Paediatr 85: 863–866.

Barr RG, Geertsma A. (2002). Colic: the pain perplex. In: Schecter NL, Berde CB, Yaster M (eds). Pain in infants, children, and adolescents, pp. 751–764. Lippincott Williams & Wilkins, Baltimore, MD.

Barr RG, Lessard J. (1999). Excessive crying. In: Bergman A (ed). 20 common problems in pediatrics, pp. 5–9. McGraw-Hill, New York.

Barr RG, Hanley J, Patterson DK et al. (1984). Breath hydrogen excretion of normal newborn infants in response to usual feeding patterns: evidence for "functional lactase insufficiency" beyond the first month of life. J Pediatr 104: 527–533.

Barr RG, Kramer MS, Pless IB et al. (1989). Feeding and temperament as determinants of early infant cry/fuss behavior. Pediatrics 84: 514–521.

Barr RG, Konner M, Bakeman R et al. (1991). Crying in Kung San infants: a test of the cultural specificity hypothesis. Dev Med Child Neurol 33: 601–610.

Barr RG, Rotman A, Yaremko J et al. (1992). The crying of infants with colic: a controlled empirical description. Pediatrics 90:14–21.

Barr RG, Chen S, Hopkins B et al. (1996). Crying patterns in preterm infants. Dev Med Child Neurol 38: 345–355.

Barr RG, Young SN, Wright JH et al. (1999). Differential calming response to sucrose taste in crying infants with and without colic. Pediatrics 103: 1–9.

Barr RG, Paterson JA, MacMartin LM et al. (2001). "Breastfeeding analgesia" for procedural pain in 2 month-old infants. Pediatr Res Supp 49: 313A.

Barr RG, Paterson J, MacMartin L et al. (2005). Prolonged and unsoothable crying bouts in infants with and without colic. J Dev Behav Pediatr 26: 1–10.

Brazelton TB. (1962). Crying in infancy. Pediatrics 29: 579–588.

Canadian Paediatric Society, Community Paediatrics Committee. (2002). Chiropractic care for children: controversies and issues. Pediatr Child Health 7: 85–89.

Castro-Rodriguez JA, Stern DA, Halonen M et al. (2001). Relation between infantile colic and asthma/atopy: a prospective study in an unselected population. Pediatrics 108: 878–882.

Clyne PS, Kulzcycki A. (1991). Human breast milk contains bovine IgG. Relationship to infant colic? Pediatrics 87: 439–444.

Estep DC, Kulczycki A. (2000). Colic in breast milk-fed infants: treatment by temporary substitution of Neocate infant formula. Acta Paediatrica 89: 795–802.

Fitzgerald M. (2005). The development of nociceptive circuits. Nat Rev Neurosci 6: 507–520.

Fitzgerald M, Millard C, McIntosh N. (1989). Cutaneous hypersensitivity following peripheral tissue damage in newborn infants and its reversal with topical anaesthesia. Pain 39: 31–36.

Forsyth BWC. (1989). Colic and the effect of changing formulas: a double-blind, multiple-crossover study. J Pediatr 115: 521–526.

Forsyth BWC, McCarthy PL, Leventhal JM. (1985). Problems of early infancy, formula changes, and mothers' beliefs about their infants. J Pediatr 106: 1012–1017.

Ghosh S, Barr RG. (2004). Colic and gas. In: Walker WA, Goulet O, Kleinman RE et al (eds). Pediatric gastrointestinal disease, pp. 210–224. BC Decker, Hamilton, Canada.

Golub HL, Corwin MJ. (1985). A physioacoustic model of the infant cry. In: Lester BM, Boukydis CFZ (eds). Infant crying: theoretical and research perspectives, pp. 59–82. Plenum Press, New York.

Gormally SM, Barr RG. (1997). Of clinical pies and clinical clues: proposal for a clinical approach to complaints of early crying and colic. Ambulatory Child Health 3: 137–153.

Gradin M, Schollin J. (2005). The role of endogenous opioids in mediating pain reduction by orally administered glucose among newborns. Pediatrics 115: 1004–1007.

Grunau RE, Oberlander TF, Whitfield MF et al. (2001). Demographic and therapeutic determinants of pain reactivity in very low birth weight neonates at 32 weeks' postconceptional age. Pediatrics 107: 105–112.

Gustafson GE, Wood RM, Green JA. (2000). Can we hear the causes of infants' crying? In: Barr RG, Hopkins B, Green JA (eds). Crying as a sign, a symptom, and a signal: clinical, emotional and developmental aspects of infant and toddler crying, pp. 8–22. MacKeith Press, London.

Harris MJ, Petts V, Penny R. (1977). Cow's milk allergy as a cause of infantile colic: immunofluorescent studies on jejunal mucosa. Acta Paediatr 13: 276–281.

Hill DJ, Hosking CS. (2000). Infantile colic and food hypersensitivity. J Pediatr Gastroenterol Nutr 30: S67–86.

Hopkins B, Janssen B, Kardaun O et al. (1988). Quieting during early infancy: evidence for a developmental change? Early Hum Dev 18: 111–124.

Husereau D, Clifford T, Aker P et al. (2003). Spinal manipulation for infantile colic. Canadian Coordinating Office for Health Technology Assessment Technology Report [42].

Illingworth RS. (1955). Crying in infants and children. BMJ 4905: 75–78.

Kirjavainen J, Karjavainen T, Huhtala V et al. (2000). Infants with colic have a normal sleep structure at 2 and 7 months of age. J Pediatr 137: 1–6.

Kirjavainen J, Jahnukainen T, Huhtala V et al. (2001). The balance of the autonomic nervous system is normal in colicky infants. Euro J Pediatr 90: 250–254.

Kirjavainen J, Lehtonen L, Kirjavainen T et al. (2004). Sleep of excessively crying infants: a 24 hour ambulatory sleep polygraphy study. Pediatrics 114: 592–600.

Lehtonen L, Gormally S, Barr RG. (2000). Clinical pies for etiology and outcome in infants presenting with early increased crying. In: Barr RG, Hopkins B, Green J (eds). Crying as a sign, a symptom, and a signal: clinical, emotional, and developmental aspects of infant and toddler crying, pp. 67–95. MacKeith Press, London.

Lester BM, Boukydis CFZ, Garcia-Coll CT et al. (1992). Infantile colic: acoustic cry characteristics, maternal perception of cry, and temperament. Infant Behav Develop 15: 15–26.

Leung AK, Lemay JF. (2004). Infantile colic: a review. J R Soc Health 124:162–166.

Lifshitz CH, O'Brian Smith E, Garza C. (1983). Delayed complete functional lactase sufficiency in breast-fed infants. J Pediatr Gastroenterol Nut 2: 478–482.

Lobo ML, Kotzer AM, Keefe MR et al. (2004). Current beliefs and management strategies for treating infant colic. J Pediatr Health Care 18: 115–122.

Lucas A, St. James-Roberts I. (1982).

Crying, fussing and colic behaviour in breast- and bottle-fed infants. Early Hum Develop 53: 9–18.

Lundell L, Dalenback J, Hattlebakk J et al. (1998). Outcome of open antireflux surgery as assessed in a Nordic multicentre prospective clinical trial. Nordic GORD-Study Group. Eur J Surg 164: 751–757.

Mayer EA, Gebhart GF. (1994). Basic and clinical aspects of visceral hyperalgesia. Gastroenterology 107: 271–293.

Metcalf TJ, Irons TG, Sher LD et al. (1994). Simethicone in the treatment of infant colic: a randomized placebo-controlled, multicenter trial. Pediatrics 94: 29–34.

Miller AR, Barr RG. (1991). Infantile colic: is it a gut issue? Pediatr Clin North Am 38: 1407–1423.

Miller-Lancar C, Bigsby R, High P et al. (2004). Infant colic and feeding difficulty. Arch Dis Childhood 89: 908–912.

Owens CM, Zhang D, Willis WD. (1992). Changes in the response states of primate spinothalamic cells caused by mechanical damage of the skin or activation of descending controls. J Neurophysiol 67: 1509–1527.

Papousek M, von Hofacker N. (1995). Persistent crying and parenting: search for a butterfly in a dynamic system. Early Develop Parent 4: 209–224.

Rao MR, Brenner RA, Schisterman EF et al. (2004). Long term cognitive development in children with prolonged crying. Arch Dis Childhood 89: 9889–9992.

Ross Monographs. (1997). Colic and excessive crying. Ross Products Division, Abbot Laboratories Columbus, OH.

St. James-Roberts I, Halil T. (1991). Infant crying patterns in the first year: normal community and clinical findings. J Child Psychol Psychiatry 32: 951–968.

St. James-Roberts I, Plewis I. (1996). Individual differences, daily fluctuations, and developmental changes in amounts of infant waking, fussing, crying, feeding and sleeping. Child Dev 67: 1–36.

St. James-Roberts I, Hurry J, Bowyer J. (1993). Objective confirmation of crying durations in infants referred for excessive crying. Arch Dis Childhood 68: 82–84.

St. James-Roberts I, Bowyer J, Varghese S et al. (1994). Infant crying patterns in Manali and London. Child Care Health Develop 20: 323–337.

St. James-Roberts I, Conroy S, Hurry J. (1997). Links between infant crying and sleep-waking at six weeks of age. Early Hum Dev 48: 143–152.

St. James-Roberts I, Conroy S, Wilsher K. (1998). Bases for maternal perceptions of infant crying. Arch Dis Childhood 24: 425–439.

Savino F, Brondello C, Cresi F et al. (2002). Cimetropium bromide in the treatment of crisis in infantile colic. J Pediatr Gastroenterol Nut 34: 417–419.

Shide DJ, Blass EM. (1989). Opioidlike effects of intraoral infusions of corn oil and polycose on stress reactions in 10-day-old rats. Behav Neurosci 103: 1168–1175.

Smith BA, Fillion TJ, Blass EM. (1990). Orally mediated sources of calming in 1-to 3-day old human infants. Dev Psychol 26: 731–737.

Soltis J. (2004). The signal functions of early infant crying. Behav Brain Sci 27: 443–458.

Stifter CA, Braungart J. (1992). Infant colic: a transient condition with no apparent effects. J Appl Dev Psychol 13: 447–462.

Treem WR. (1994). Infant colic: a pediatric gastroenterologist's perspective. Pediatr Clin North Am 41: 1121–1138.

Wales JKH, Primhak RA, Rattenbury J et al. (1989). Isolated fructose malabsorption. Arch Dis Childhood 65: 227–229.

Weissbluth M, Christoffel KK, Davis T. (1984). Treatment of infantile colic with dicyclomine hydrochloride. J Pediatr 104: 951–955.

Weizman Z, Alkrinawi S, Goldfarb D et al. (1993). Efficacy of herbal tea preparation in infantile colic. J Pediatr 122: 650–652.

Wessel MA, Cobb JC, Jackson EB et al. (1954). Paroxysmal fussing in infancy, sometimes called "colic". Pediatrics 14: 421–434.

White BP, Gunnar MR, Larson MC et al. (2000). Behavioral and physiological responsivity, sleep and patterns of daily cortisol production in infants with and without colic. Child Dev 71: 862–877.

Wolff PH. (1984). Discontinuous changes in human wakefulness around the end of the second month of life: a developmental perspective. In: Prechtl HFR (ed). Continuity of neural functions from prenatal to postnatal life, pp. 144–158. SIMP, Oxford.

Wolff PH. (1987). The development of

behavioral states and the expression of emotions in early infancy: new proposals for investigation. University of Chicago Press, Chicago, IL.

Wolke D, Rizzo P, Woods S. (2002). Persistent infant crying and hyperactivity problems in middle childhood. Pediatrics 109: 1054–1060.

Zeskind PS, Barr RG. (1997). Acoustic characteristics of naturally occurring cries of infants with "colic". Child Dev 68: 394–403.

Pharmacogenetics and pharmacogenomics of analgesic drugs

John N van den Anker
Dick Tibboel
Ron H van Schaik

INTRODUCTION

Safe and effective pain treatment in neonates and young infants requires thorough understanding of various developmental aspects of drug disposition and metabolism. In general, the phenotypic variation in drug disposition and metabolism is based on constitutional, genetic and environmental factors. Clearance of most medicines is decreased in neonates as compared to adults and older children. This can be attributed to the immaturity of renal function, i.e. decreased glomerular filtration rate and less effective tubular reabsorption and/or excretion, as well as to a maturational decreased capacity of drug metabolizing enzymes (van den Anker 1996, Rane 1999, Hines and McCarver 2002, McCarver and Hines 2002, Kearns et al. 2003). Moreover, as recently reviewed (Evans and McLeod 2003, Weinshilboum 2003), the disposition and action of many drugs are polygenically determined events whereby polymorphisms in drug-metabolizing enzymes, transporters and receptors cooperatively determine the spectrum of drug response (i.e. ranging from no effect – therapeutic failure to suprapharmacologic effect – drug toxicity). This chapter will focus on the importance of polymorphically expressed drug-metabolizing enzymes, receptors and regulatory proteins involved with antinociception in neonates and young infants.

ANALGESIC DRUGS

Codeine

Codeine, an oral pro-drug, is metabolized by CYP2D6 to morphine. CYP2D6 is a member of the cytochrome P450 superfamily, and is a major drug-metabolizing enzyme that contributes to the metabolism and biotransformation of many drugs (http://medicine.iupui.edu/flockhart/). To date, over 50 allelic variants encoding functional, reduced activity or non-functional gene products have been described for CYP2D6 (Daly et al. 1996) (http://www.imm.ki.se/CYPalleles/).

   Carriers of any two recessive loss-of-function alleles for CYP2D6 exhibit a so-called poor metabolizer (PM) phenotype while the remaining individuals are classified as ultra-rapid (UM), extensive (EM) or intermediate metabolizer (IM) phenotypes depending on their complement of alleles (Sachse et al. 1997, Griese et al. 1998, Gaedigk et al. 1999). In many instances, the PM phenotype for CYP2D6 exposes subjects to higher risks of dose-related drug toxicities or therapeutic failure when CYP2D6 is required to bioactivate a drug to a pharmacologically active moiety, such as codeine to morphine (May 1994). It is important to note that there is wide variability in the functional activity of the enzyme across the EM and IM phenotypes and that some subjects who are IMs have enzymatic activity that is only minimally superior to PMs. This is particularly important given that while only 2–5% of African-Americans exhibit the PM phenotype, nearly 30% of African-Americans exhibit the IM phenotype (Gaedigk et al. 2002). As a result, African-Americans, by virtue of their CYP2D6 genotype, are more likely (than Caucasians) to have compromised bioactivation of codeine, thereby potentially limiting its therapeutic utility. This assertion is supported in part by earlier work (Williams et al. 2002) that studied a largely Caucasian and Asian population following adenotonsillectomy and demonstrated that plasma morphine levels 1 hour after codeine administration were associated with CYP2D6 phenotype. The potential clinical importance of the IM phenotype for CYP2D6 has also been corroborated by recent studies which suggest that genotyping aids in the interpretation of clinical trials involving CYP2D6 substrates (Furman et al. 2004). Assessing CYP2D6 function at the allele level (i.e. associating each individual allelic variant with a specific functional level to derive a semi-quantitative measure of activity for various allele combinations) rather than at the genotype level may allow for calculation of a 'functional gene dose' and better prediction of serum drug concentrations for a given patient (Steimer et al. 2004).

The current knowledge regarding CYP2D6 pharmacogenetics in African-Americans and resultant CYP2D6 activity has important implications for the analgesic efficacy of codeine. Gaedigk et al. (2002) described 283 African-American subjects who were genotyped for CYP2D6 and phenotyped using urinary fractional recovery of dextromethorphan and its CYP2D6 catalyzed metabolite, dextrorphan. Overall, CYP2D6 activity was significantly reduced (P = 0.0001) when compared to Caucasian control subjects. This finding was associated with a greater frequency of the CYP2D6*17, *29 and *45/46 alleles in the African-Americans, resulting in a higher proportion of patients with an IM phenotype (Gaedigk et al. 2002). Gaedigk et al. (2002) examined the relative activity of the CYP2D6*29 allele using the COS-7 cell expression system and demonstrated that intrinsic clearance

(Cl_{int}) of dextromethorphan in microsomes expressing CYP2D6.29 protein was significantly less (47%) than cells expressing CYP2D6.2 protein. These in vitro findings are corroborated by in vivo data reported by Wennerholm et al. (2002), who demonstrated that CYP2D6*17 and *29 both caused changes in the disposition of four probe drugs in black Tanzanians and, specifically, that CYP2D6.17 exhibited altered substrate specificity when compared with CYP2D6.1 and .2. Together, these data suggest that for drugs that are substrates for CYP2D6, significant pharmacokinetic implications exist for African-American subjects consequent to pharmacogenetic differences that are associated with race and, in particular, the higher frequency of inheritance of the CYP2D6*17,*29 and *45/46 alleles.

As noted above, a review of pertinent literature supports a genotype–phenotype association for CYP2D6 that has the potential to produce clinically significant differences in enzyme activity and the dose – plasma concentration – effect profile for drugs that are substrates for this enzyme.

Finally, there are reports in the literature on the in vivo assessment of CYP2D6 activity in adults and children based on the metabolism of sparteine, dextromethorphan and, more recently, of tramadol with specific emphasis on the impact of CYP2D6 polymorphism on the phenotypic activity observed (Table 8.1) (Schmid et al. 1985, Jacq-Aigrain and Cresteil 1992, Paar et al. 1997, Kennedy et al. 2004, Allegaert et al. 2005b). However, observations on CYP2D6 activity in early neonatal life are still very limited and are mainly based on in vitro studies (Table 8.2), in part due to the ethical dilemma of administering 'probe drugs' to this specific population (Ladona et al. 1991, Treluyer et al. 1991, Jacqz-Aigrain and Cresteil 1992).

Tramadol

Tramadol (M) hydrochloride is a 4-phenyl-piperidine analogue of codeine. It acts as a centrally active analgesic, partially as a μ-receptor agonist and partially by its effects on the re-uptake monoamines. O-demethyl tramadol (M1) is produced by O-demethylation in the liver by CYP2D6 and has a much higher affinity for the μ-receptor compared to the parent drug. The other metabolite (N-demethyl tramadol, M2) produced after N-demethylation by CYP3A has no affinity for this receptor. CYP2D6 activity and M1 synthesis will therefore also have impact on the pharmacodynamics (i.e. analgesia) of this drug (Stamer et al. 2003, Grond and Sablotzki 2004).

Maturational aspects of plasma tramadol disposition in neonates, children and adults were documented

Table 8.1 Data on in vivo assessment of maturational CYP2D6 activity using either dextromethorphan or tramadol as test probe

Author	Population	Urine molar dextromethorphan/dextrorphan ratio		
		Number	Mean ratio (SD)	
Kennedy et al. (2004)	children	21	0.01 +/– 0.011	
Schmid et al. (1985)	adults, extensive metabolizer	245	0.01 +/– 0.022	
	adults, poor metabolizer	23	3.6 +/– 3.8	
Jacqz-Aigrain and Cresteil (1992)	adults, extensive metabolizers	144	0.01 +/– 0.03	
	adults, poor metabolizers	11	4.23 +/– 1.66	
Author	Population	Urine logarithmic molar tramadol/O-demethyl tramadol ratio		
		Number	Mean ratio	
Allegaert et al. (2005)	< 37 weeks PCA	8	1.5	
	37–41 weeks PCA	8	0.62	
	42–44 weeks PCA	5	0.65	
Paar et al. (1997)	adults	104	–0.101	
	adults, extensive metabolizer	71	–0.1	
	adults, poor metabolizer	9	0.45	

Table 8.2 Data on in vitro assessment of maturational CYP2D6 activity (assessed by dextrorphan production nmol/mg protein/h) compared to adult values

Author	Population	Activity
Ladona et al. (1991)	fetal, 14–24 weeks	0%
Treluyer et al. (1991)	fetal, 17–40 weeks	< 5%
	neonatal, < 24 hour	< 5%
	neonatal, day 1–7	5%
	neonatal, day 8–28	5–10%
Jacqz-Aigrain and Cresteil (1992)	fetal, 17–40 weeks	< 5%
	neonatal, < 24 hour	1–3%
	neonatal, day 1–7	10%
	neonatal, day 8–28	30%

recently, using a population pharmacokinetic approach. CYP2D6 activity was observed as early as 25 weeks postconceptual age (PCA), but a significant relationship between PCA and M1 metabolite formation was not demonstrated (Allegaert et al. 2005a).

In vivo assessment of CYP2D6 activity is mainly based on ratios of either tramadol (M/M1) or dextromethorphan (dextromethorphan/dextrorphan, DM/DX) in urine or plasma (Table 8.1) (Schmid et al. 1985, Paar et al. 1997, Abdel-Rahman et al. 2002, Park et al. 2005).

Data using tramadol disposition to assess CYP2D6 activity were reported by Paar et al. in adults and by Abdel-Rahman et al. in children (Paar et al. 1997, Abdel-Rahman et al. 2002). Paar et al. (1997) reported the urinary logarithmic M/M1 ratio in 104 adults, using 24-hour collections of urine after single oral administration of 50 mg tramadol. Based on a mean urinary retrieval of 31% of the initial dose, M, M1 and M2 contributed 38, 48 and 13% to overall tramadol retrieval, resulting in a phenotypic log M/M1 ratio of –0.101. These authors were also able to illustrate the relevance of CYP2D6 polymorphism on the renal M1 elimination since sparteine-poor metabolizers had a log M/M1 ratio of about 0.45 compared to –0.1 in extensive metabolizers.

The impact of CYP2D6 polymorphisms on phenotypic activity is not limited to adulthood since Abdel-Rahman et al. (2002) observed that M1 production was significantly higher in children with two versus one active allele.

Using the urinary DM/DX ratio, Kennedy et al. (2004) documented that the CYP2D6 activity in children is about equal to activity observed in adults (see Table 8.1) (Schmid et al. 1985, Jacqz-Aigrain and Cresteil 1992, Kennedy et al. 2004). Only recently, Park et al. (2005) reported on the ratio in single plasma samples collected 3 hours after oral administration of dextromethorphan. These authors observed a progressive decrease in median log DM/DX ratio (–1.67 in neonates, –2.37 in infants, –2.37 in children, –2.45 in adolescents, –2.44 in young and –2.47 in older adults), reflecting the maturational increase in CYPD6 activity.

CYP2D6 activity was observed even in extreme preterm neonates with a subsequent PCA-mediated maturational increase in metabolic activity (Allegaert et al. 2005a). At about term PCA, this activity seems to be equal to adult slow metabolizers (log M/M1 0.4 to 0.5) with subsequent maturation to reach adult activity level at 44 weeks PCA (log M/M1 = 0 to –0.1). When the relatively higher liver/body weight ratio in neonates as compared to adulthood is taken into account, this is also in line with the maturational trends observed by Treluyer et al. (1991) and Jacqz-Aigrain and Cresteil. (1992). Based on in vitro assessment of CYP2D6 activity, hereby using dextromethorphan as test probe, both authors observed CYP2D6 activity at about 30% of adult activity in hepatic tissue of 1 month old infants (PCA 44 weeks).

The present in vivo observations are of relevance for the pharmacodynamics of this specific drug and other moderate potent analgesics like codeine (Abdel-Rahman et al. 2002, Hines and McCarver 2002, Stamer et al. 2003, Grond and Sablotzki 2004). The relevance of both ontogeny and CYP2D6 polymorphism has been illustrated by the complex interaction of the disposition and pharmacodynamics of selective serotonin reuptake inhibitors (SSRIs) in early neonatal and paediatric life. Based on recent observations, neonates (< 44 weeks PCA) should be considered as phenotypic slow metabolizers. Dosages and treatment should be adjusted accordingly (Spencer 1993, Mhanna et al. 1997, Sallee et al. 2000, Stiskal et al. 2001).

In conclusion, using tramadol metabolism as marker, CYP2D6 activity was already observed at 25 PCA weeks and significant effects of PCA and postnatal age were documented, resulting in slow metabolizer phenotypic CYP2D6 activity at term age. However, interindividual variability in CYP2D6 activity was only partially explained by these maturational aspects. Polymorphisms therefore very likely contributed to the interindividual variability observed in early neonatal life.

Morphine

In 1806 morphine was isolated from opium by the pharmacist Serturner and is still one of the most commonly used drugs to achieve analgesia in adults, children and neonates. The analgesic effect of morphine is mediated by its interaction with receptors for endogenous opioids. Morphine acts on μ and κ receptors but the analgesic effect of morphine is mainly mediated by μ receptors as confirmed by loss of morphine analgesia in μ receptor knockout mice (Matthes et al. 1996, Loh et al. 1998, Rahman et al. 1998).

Variability in morphine analgesia can be due to genetic differences between individuals that play a role in determining bioavailability, disposition and metabolism of morphine (i.e. pharmacokinetics) and/or response to morphine (i.e. pharmacodynamics). These differences may be due to variations in genes responsible for drug metabolism, drug transport and drug targets, which in turn will determine the response to the drug.

The major pathway for morphine metabolism is by conjugation with glucuronic acid. Conjugation reactions lead to formation of covalent linkage between a functional group on a parent compound or phase I metabolite with endogenous substituents such as glucuronic acid, sulphate, glutathione, amino acid or acetate. Highly polar conjugated metabolites formed after these reactions are generally inactive. However, morphine is metabolized into an active conjugate morphine-6-glucuronide (M6G), which is a more potent analgesic than its parent compound (Portenoy et al. 1992, Faura et al. 1996). The UGT family of enzymes is primarily responsible for conjugation of morphine with glucuronic acid.

Metabolism and signal transduction

UDP-glucuronosyltransferases

The UDP-glucuronosyltransferases (UGTs) family serve a major role in the conjugation of potentially toxic drugs and endogenous compounds. UGTs catalyze the glucuronidation reaction resulting in addition of glucuronic acid to several lipophilic compounds. The resulting glucuronidated substrates are more polar than the parent compound and are readily eliminated through the biliary system and kidneys. UGT enzymes are classified on the basis of sequence homology into two gene subfamilies. UGT1 and UGT2 have been identified for mammalian UGT based on cDNA sequence (Mackenzie et al. 1997). The UGT1 cDNAs encode phenol and bilirubin metabolizing isoforms and a single gene encodes several human UGT1 isoforms. The UGT2 gene subfamily encodes the odorant and steroid-metabolizing isoforms. In contrast to UGT1, UGT2 isoenzymes are encoded by several independent genes. The UGT2 genes are further divided into the UGT2A gene subfamily that encodes olfactory-specific isoforms, and the UGT2B gene subfamily that encodes steroid-metabolizing isoforms in the liver. Since glucuronidation is an essential pathway for the elimination of morphine in addition to many compounds, genetic polymorphism in UGTs has toxicological and physiological importance.

The UGT2B7 gene was isolated by Carrier et al. (2000). It is located on chromosome 4 and has six exons spanning about 16 kb (Carrier et al. 2000, Riedy et al. 2000). It has smaller introns than other UGT2B genes. In addition to being expressed in the liver, UGT2B7 is also expressed in other organs including the intestines, kidneys and brain (Fisher et al. 2000, Yamada et al. 2003). The UGT2B7 acts on a broad range of substrates and is responsible for glucuronidation of steroids, zidovudine, retinoids, morphine and epirubicin (Coffman et al. 1997, Barbier et al. 2000, Samokyszyn et al. 2000, Innocenti et al. 2001, Turgeon et al. 2001). Furthermore, it is the only isoform known to conjugate morphine (Coffman et al. 1997, Carrier et al. 2000).

Polymorphisms in UGT genes have the potential to alter the enzymatic activity of UGT2B7, thus affecting the rate of glucuronidation contributing to the variability in pharmacokinetics of the substrate. Unlike many glucuronidated metabolites the metabolite of morphine, M6G, is more potent than the parent compound. Thus functional mutations in UGT2B7 genes might have important clinical consequences in terms of analgesia related to variability in morphine metabolism. Many investigators have studied metabolism of morphine and variations in UGT2B7 genes. These studies involved either patients with cancer or healthy individuals.

A missense polymorphism, 802C/T, is described in exon 2 resulting in the formation of variant UGT2B7 H268Y (Jin et al. 1993). This UGT2B7 variant was demonstrated to glucuronidate many endogenous compounds and xenobiotics (Jin et al. 1993). However, in a study of 175 Norwegian cancer patients receiving chronic oral morphine therapy, variant H268Y did not appear to have functional effects on morphine and its metabolite levels (Holthe et al. 2003). This group also identified six novel variants in the promoter region of UGT2B7. The frequency of variants appears to be related to the ethnicity of individuals studied. Bhasker et al. (2000) demonstrated that the 268H allele frequency was over tenfold more prevalent compared to 268Y in the Japanese while these alleles occurred with about the same frequency in a Caucasian population.

In a study of morphine pharmacogenetics by Sawyer et al. (2003), variation in the UGT2B7 gene was studied in a group of patients receiving patient-controlled analgesia with morphine. Among 60 patients phenotyped by M6G/morphine plasma ratios, the UGT2B7 gene was sequenced in six patients with the highest and six patients with the lowest M6G/morphine ratios. This study identified the −161C/T variant in the UGT2B7 promoter area that was in com-

plete linkage disequilibrium with the known variant 802C/T in exon 2. Patients homozygous for −161C and 802C alleles (C/C variation) had significantly lower levels of metabolites of morphine, namely M6G and morphine-3-glucuronide (M3G) indicating that inter-individual differences in morphine glucuronidation may be the result of genetic variation in UGT2B7. However it was not clear if the potential functional variant was at the −161 or 802 position (Sawyer et al. 2003).

Duguay et al. (2004) described a polymorphism −79 G/A in the UGT2B7 gene that was thought to have functionality from in vitro studies. However in a human study of Norwegian individuals with cancer on chronic morphine treatment, morphine and its metabolite levels were not significantly different from non-carrier individuals in individuals who were heterozygous for the mutation.

Opioid receptors

The powerful effect of morphine is mediated through the μ-opioid receptors, which are located on plasma membrane of neurons and other peripheral cells. Three classical opioid receptors, μ, κ and δ, have been studied extensively. Opioid receptor-like 1 (ORL-1) receptors have been discovered recently. Each receptor has a unique distribution in the brain, spinal cord and periphery. The analgesic effect of morphine is produced by binding with receptors for endogenous opioids mainly mediated by μ receptors (Matthes et al. 1996, Loh et al. 1998, Rahman et al. 1998). Kozac et al. (1994) located the μ-opioid receptor gene, OPRM1 to chromosome 10. Large differences in the clinical response to morphine have been postulated by some researchers due to polymorphisms in the μ-opioid receptor gene.

Lotsch et al. (2002) researched pharmacogenetics as a basis for variability in the clinical response to morphine therapy. Pupillary diameter was used as a measure of central effect of morphine in a two-way crossover study. Diameter of the pupil was measured every 20 minutes for 18 hours after administration of morphine or its active metabolite M6G. The opioid effect was compared in six individuals with single nucleotide polymorphism (SNP) A118G. Morphine dosing was individualized to get similar effects in all participants. The response to morphine was not affected by presence of the polymorphism. However the potency of M6G to constrict the pupil was significantly lower in heterozygous carriers of A118G and the potency was even lower in participants homozygous for A118G. Based on this study Hollt (2002) suggested that M6G does not contribute to the action of morphine to a major extent, as the effect of morphine was not affected by the A118G polymorphism while the effect of M6G was lowered by the presence of the studied polymorphism. This was also indicated by a 20 times decreased potency of M6G over morphine in constricting the pupil. The differences in potencies may be due to lower blood–brain barrier permeability of M6G compared to morphine, as the receptor affinities for both morphine and M6G are comparable (Wu et al. 1997).

μ-opioid receptors appear to be not only the site of action of opioids for pain control but also substances of abuse such as heroin. Many studies have looked at associations of polymorphisms in the μ-opioid receptor gene and occurrence of substance abuse. Bond et al. (1998) described five SNPs in the coding region of OPRM1 gene by sequencing DNA from 113 former heroin addicts and 39 individuals with no history of addiction. The most prevalent SNP was a nucleotide substitution at position 118 (118A-G), present in about 10% of the study population followed by C17T polymorphism in 6.6% of the study population. Allele frequencies were significantly different among the ethnic groups studied for both A118G and C17T. For A118G polymorphism there was no significant difference for allele frequency in both groups while the C17T variant was present in a higher proportion in the opioid-dependent group at a marginal significance level (P = 0.054). The variant A118G receptor did not show altered binding affinity to most opioids. However it bound to β-endorphin about three times more potently than the most common allelic form of the receptor. β-endorphin is an endogenous opioid that activates the μ-opioid receptor. Furthermore β-endorphin is approximately three times more potent at the A118G variant receptor in agonist-induced activation of G protein-coupled potassium channels. It was suggested that SNPs in the μ-opioid receptor gene may have implications for therapeutics and vulnerability to develop addiction based on altered binding affinity of β-endorphin to the 118A-G receptor.

G protein-coupled receptors

G protein-coupled receptors (GPCRs) represent pharmaceutical targets for numerous medicinal compounds. GPCR activation is determined not only by the initiation of signalling cascades but also by regulatory mechanisms that control the extent and duration of their signals. The balance of activation and desensitization dictate the ultimate physiological response to both endogenous and exogenous receptor stimuli. Therefore these mechanisms may play a particularly relevant role during chronic exposure to agonists such as opiates that use either direct or indirect GPCR signalling mechanisms to mediate their effects. Therefore, the regulation of GPCRs may have bearing on the neuronal adaptations that underlie the reinforcing properties of opiates (Bohn et al. 2004).

GPCR signalling can be regulated by several different means. Feedback regulation of components of the signalling cascades occurs downstream of receptor activation, resulting in overall decreased cellular activity that can, in turn, affect several other receptor signalling systems. A more proximal regulatory mechanism of GPCR signalling affects G protein activity. A family of proteins known as 'regulators of G protein signalling' or RSG proteins, directly target the activity of G proteins, thereby limiting the potential for GPCR activation (Dohlman and Thorner 1997, De Vries et al. 2000). By increasing GTP activity, RSG proteins have a net effect of decreasing GPCR signalling. The most proximal means of specifically regulating GPCR signalling is by directly targeting the receptor; this is mediated by a process of homologous desensitization. Specific GPCR kinases (GRKs) and arrestin proteins mediate the homologous desensitization of numerous GPCRs upon agonist activation (Ferguson et al. 1998, Luttrell and Lefkowitz 2002). The non-visual system GRKs have a vast tissue distribution and are widely expressed throughout the central nervous system (Erdtman-Vourliotis et al. 2001). Likewise, the non-visual system arrestins, β-arrestin-1 and -2, are ubiquitously expressed and are also present in most brain structures (Gurevich et al. 2002). GPCR desensitization is initiated by the phosphorylation of the activated receptor by GRKs (Premont et al. 1995). The receptor can then bind β-arrestins, which prevents the receptor from activating more G proteins despite the continued presence of agonist (Pitcher et al. 1998). This process represents a prominent mechanism for GPCR desensitization. It is crucial that GPCR signalling can be halted, as many neurotransmitters act at GPCRs and the response to such agonists must be carefully controlled.

The regulation of GPCRs is also relevant when exogenous agonists are administered. Opiates lead to GPCR activation, particularly of the μ-opioid receptors. Therefore, the regulation of these receptors could have bearings on opiate actions, especially when these drugs are used for extended time periods when receptor desensitization becomes prominent.

Opioid receptor regulation

The analgesic actions of morphine are mediated predominantly via μ-opioid receptors, as suggested by extensive pharmacological studies and also demonstrated by the lack of morphine analgesia observed in knockout mice that are deficient in μ-opioid receptor (Mansour et al. 1995, Matthes et al. 1996). These mice also experience no response to morphine in locomotor activity, hypothermia, respiratory depression, inhibition of gastrointestinal motility, induction of tolerance, dependence, withdrawal or addiction (Loh et al. 1998). Overall, this GPCR activity is the site of morphine's actions for mediating all of these physiological manifestations. Therefore, the desensitization of the μ-opioid receptor presents a critical point of regulation that could potentially dictate the extent of morphine effects on each of these physiological parameters, including the addictive properties associated with its use.

Classically, GPCRs are desensitized and internalized after prolonged agonist stimulation (Ferguson et al. 1998). The μ-opioid receptor follows this classical paradigm when high-efficacy agonists, such as etorphine or enkephalin derivatives, are presented. However, the μ-opioid receptor fails to internalize upon morphine stimulation (Whistler and von Zastrow 1998, Zhang et al. 1998). Alternatively, overexpression of GRK2 promotes morphine-induced receptor internalization (Zhang et al. 1998). In addition, morphine does not induce pronounced receptor phosphorylation nor is it as efficacious at inducing β-arrestin-2 interactions unless GRK2 is overexpressed, demonstrating that the cellular complement of desensitizing elements can determine the receptor's fate (Zhang et al. 1998). Chronic morphine treatments differentially affect certain neuronal populations; some populations display μ-opioid receptor desensitization, whereas other brain regions do not (Noble and Cox 1996).

Morphine-induced antinociception

Of all the genetically altered strains of mice tested in the hot-plate antinociception paradigm, the only strain in which significant differences were observed regarding morphine sensitivity is the β-arrestin-2-knockout strain. Specifically, in the absence of β-arrestin-2, μ-opioid receptor desensitization is impaired (Bohn et al. 2000). Furthermore, this attenuated desensitization could be correlated with enhanced and prolonged morphine-induced antinociception. The mice also display dramatically attenuated tolerance after acute or chronic morphine treatment (Bohn et al. 1999, 2000, 2002). This observation indicates that opiate tolerance may be the behavioural manifestation of receptor desensitization. When the desensitization mechanism is disrupted, the tolerance to

the drug is no longer observed. However, a provocative finding is that even when tolerance to morphine has been abolished, physical dependence still persists in these mice (Bohn et al. 2000). This observation indicates that although some aspects of the μ-opioid receptor signalling may be enhanced, others may not be affected, such as the μ-opioid receptor-mediated signalling, that leads to the development of dependence (Bohn et al. 2004). Therefore, the β-arrestin-2 knockout mice represent an interesting model system in which the removal of a GPCR regulatory element has led to profound changes in some responses to morphine (i.e. enhanced analgesia and abolished antinociceptive tolerance), while maintaining the same response to morphine in another respect (i.e. no difference in the degree of physical dependence) (Bohn et al. 2004).

The GRK/β-arrestin system is likely the most prominent μ-opioid receptor regulator and in the absence of β-arrestin-2, the contributions of PKC can be more readily revealed. Importantly, these observations demonstrate that two different systems (spinal and supraspinal) involved in pain perception can use different regulatory pathways to mediate the actions of a single drug, morphine, at the μ-opioid receptor.

A further indication of the degree of importance of β-arrestin-2 in the regulation of morphine responsiveness is that the β-arrestin-2 heterozygous mice demonstrate almost identically altered responses as the β-arrestin-2 knockout mice (Bohn et al. 1999, 2000, 2003). Therefore, deficiency in one allele or pharmacological inhibition of half of the β-arrestin-2 activity could potentially result in a similar phenotype observed after full ablation of the gene. This could have great therapeutic implications because most pharmacological inhibitors do not result in complete elimination of molecular function.

Morphine induces antinociception by activating μ-opioid receptors in spinal and supraspinal regions of the CNS. β-arrestin-2, a G-protein-coupled receptor-regulating protein, regulates the μ-opioid receptor in vivo (Bohn et al. 2004). Mice lacking β-arrestin-2 experience enhanced morphine-induced analgesia and do not become tolerant to morphine as determined in the hot-plate test, a paradigm that primarily assesses supraspinal pain responsiveness. Using the warm water tail-immersion paradigm, which primarily assesses spinal reflexes to painful thermal stimuli, the knockout mice showed greater basal nociceptive thresholds and markedly enhanced sensitivity to morphine. However, after a delayed onset, they do develop tolerance, although to a lesser degree than the wild-type mice (Bohn et al. 2004). These data provide in vivo evidence that the μ-opioid receptor is differentially regulated in diverse regions of the CNS.

Catechol-O-methyltransferase

The catechol-O-methyltransferase (COMT) enzyme is one of the enzymes that metabolizes the catechol-amines dopamine, epinephrine and norepinephrine, thereby acting as a key modulator of dopaminergic and adrenergic/noradrenergic neurotransmission (Mannisto and Kaakkola 1999, Rakvag et al. 2005). The involvement of catecholamines in pain modulation is known from clinical and experimental studies (Rakvag et al. 2005). The neuronal content of enkephalins is reduced by chronic activation of dopaminergic neurotransmission (George and Kertesz 1987, Chen et al. 1993, Steiner and Gerfen 1999). An up-regulation of μ-opioid receptors in various regions of the brain follows the reduction of enkephalin content.

An abundant functional polymorphism of the COMT gene that codes the substitution of valine (Val) by methionine (Met) at codon 158 (Val[158]Met) is associated with a difference in thermostability leading to a three- to four-fold reduction in the activity of the COMT enzyme. The alleles are codominant so that individuals with the Val/Val genotype have the highest activity of COMT, those with the Met/Met genotype have the lowest activity of COMT, and heterozygous individuals are intermediate. Different levels of COMT activity conferred by Val[158]Met genotypes may therefore have important influences on functions regulated by these neurotransmitters, including μ-opioid system responses.

In animal models, the chronic activation of dopaminergic neurotransmission at D2 receptors, a situation parallel to that encountered in Met/Met homozygotes, reduces the neuronal content of enkephalin peptides and induces compensatory increases in regional μ-opioid receptor concentrations in various brain regions (George and Kertesz 1987, Chen et al. 1993, Steiner and Gerfen 1999). Reductions in D2 receptor-mediated neurotransmission, similar to that achieved by the higher levels of COMT activity in Val/Val homozygotes, results in opposite effects on the μ-opioid system.

Zubieta et al. (2003) hypothesized that enhanced activation of dopaminergic neurotransmission in individuals with the low-activity COMT enzyme would result in lower levels of enkephalins, and consequently more pain due to decreased endogenous analgesia. They confirmed that individuals with the COMT Met/Met genotype had higher sensory and affective ratings of pain following an experimental pain stimulus and also had higher regional density of μ-opioid receptors (Zubieta et al. 2003).

Responses to pain and other stressors are regulated by interactions between multiple brain areas and neuro-chemical systems. Individuals homozygous for the Met[158] allele of the COMT polymorphism showed diminished regional μ-opioid system responses to pain compared with heterozygotes (Val[158]Met). These effects were accompanied by higher sensory and affective ratings of pain and a more negative internal affective state. Opposite effects were observed in Val[158] homozygotes. The COMT Val[158]Met polymorphism thus influences the human experience of pain and may underlie inter-individual differences in the adaptation and responses to pain.

SUMMARY

Until 1987, neonates and young infants were believed to be unable to experience pain. Since then the use of analgesic agents in this specific patient population has increased exponentially. Research has primarily concentrated on the development of pain assessment instruments and clinical trials investigating the safety and efficacy of several analgesics in neonates and young infants.

However, safe and effective pain treatment in neonates and young infants requires thorough understanding of the influence of growth and development on the disposition and actions of drugs used for pain relief. In addition, research into the pharmacogenetics and pharmacogenomics of transporters, receptor systems and cell signalling will further elucidate the developmental events that affect the treatment of pain in neonates and young infants. The increasing amount of knowledge on the regulation of genes involved in the disposition and action of analgesic drugs in animals and adults is, however, still far from being implemented in daily neonatal and paediatric clinical practice. To date no high-volume prospective data are available on the distribution of the different polymorphisms in neonates treated for different kinds of pain around the world. Moreover, the impact of disease on the disposition and action of analgesic drugs in this vulnerable patient population has never been evaluated. Finally, the consequences of race and ethnicity as they relate to the appropriate (most effective and safe) choice of analgesic drugs need to be elucidated. The incorporation of this important and crucial information into dosing regimens of different pain medicines in this young age group will result in a more personalized pain management.

ACKNOWLEDGEMENTS

Supported in part by grant 1 U10HD45993-02 (J.N.A.), NIH/NICHD and by grant 1 K24 RR19729-02 (J.N.A.), NIH/NCRR.

REFERENCES

Abdel-Rahman SM, Leeder JS, Wilson JT et al. (2002). Concordance between tramadol and dextromethorphan parent/metabolite ratios: the influence of CYP2D6 and non-CYP2D6 pathways on biotransformation. J Clin Pharmacol 42: 24–29.

Allegaert K, Anderson B, Verbesselt R et al. (2005a). Tramadol disposition in the very young: an attempt to assess in vivo cytochrome P4502D6 activity. Br J Anaesth 95: 231–239.

Allegaert K, van den Anker JN, Verbesselt R et al. (2005b). O-demethylation of tramadol in the first months of life. Eur J Clin Pharmacol 61: 837–842.

Barbier O, Turgeon D, Girard C et al. (2000). 3'-azido-3'-deoxythimidine (AZT) is glucuronidated by human UDP-glucuronosyltransferase 2B7 (UGT2B7). Drug Metab Dispos 28: 497–502.

Bhasker CR, McKinnon W, Stone A et al. (2000). Genetic polymorphisms of UDP-glucuronosyltransferase 2B7 (UGT2B7) at aminoacid 268: ethnic diversity of alleles and potential clinical significance. Pharmacogenetics 10: 679–685.

Bohn LM, Lefkowitz RJ, Gainetdinov RR et al. (1999). Enhanced morphine analgesia in mice lacking beta-arrestin 2. Science 286: 2495–2498.

Bohn LM, Gainetdinov RR, Lin FT et al. (2000). Mu-opioid receptor desensitization by beta-arrestin-2 determines morphine tolerance but not dependence. Nature 408: 720–723.

Bohn LM, Lefkowitz RJ, Caron MG. (2002). Differential mechanisms of morphine antinociceptive tolerance revealed in (beta)arrestin-2 knock-out mice. J Neurosci 22: 10494–10500.

Bohn LM, Gainetdinov RR, Sotnikova TD et al. (2003). Enhanced rewarding properties of morphine but not cocaine, in β-arrestin-2 knock-out mice. J Neurosci 23: 10265–10273.

Bohn LM, Gainetdinov PR, Caron MG. (2004). G protein-coupled receptor kinase/β-arrestin systems and drugs of abuse. Neuromolecular Med 5: 41–50.

Bond C, Laforge KS, Tian M et al. (1998). Single-nucleotide polymorphism in the human mu opioid receptor gene alters beta endorphin binding and activity: possible implications for opioid addiction. Proc Nat Acad Sci 95: 9608–9613.

Carrier JS, Turgeon D, Journault K et al. (2000). Isolation and characterization of the human UGT2B7 gene. Biochem Biophys Res Commun 272: 616–621.

Chen JF, Aloyo VJ, Weiss B. (1993). Continuous treatment with the D2 dopamine receptor agonist quinpirole decreases D2 dopamine receptors, D2 dopamine receptor messenger RNA and proenkephalin messenger RNA, and increases μ-opioid receptors in mouse striatum. Neuroscience 54: 669–680.

Coffman BL, Rios GR, King CD et al. (1997). Human UGT2B7 catalyzes morphine glucuronidation. Drug Metab Dispos 25: 1–4.

Daly A, Brockmöller J, Broly F et al. (1996). Nomenclature for human CYP2D6 alleles. Pharmacogenetics 6: 193–201.

De Vries L, Zheng B, Fischer T et al. (2000). The regulator of G protein signaling family. Annu Rev Pharmacol Toxicol 40: 235–271.

Dohlman HG, Thorner J. (1997). RSG proteins and signaling by heterotrimeric G proteins. J Biol Chem 272: 3871–3874.

Duguay Y, Baar C, Skorpen F et al. (2004). A novel functional polymorphism in the uridine diphosphate-glucuronosyltransferase 2B7 promoter with significant impact on promoter activity. Clin Pharmacol Ther 75: 223–233.

Erdtman-Vourliotis M, Mayer P, Ammon S et al. (2001). Distribution of G-protein-coupled receptor kinase (GRK) isoforms 2,3,5 and 6 mRNA in the rat brain. Brain Res Mol Brain Res 95: 129–137.

Evans WE, McLeod HL. (2003). Pharmacogenomics - drug disposition, drug targets and side effects. N Engl J Med 348: 538–549.

Faura CC, Moore A, Horga JF. (1996). Morphine and morphine 6 glucuronide plasma concentration and effect on cancer pain. J Pain Symptom Manage 112: 95–102.

Ferguson SS, Zhang J, Barak LS et al. (1998). Molecular mechanism of G protein-coupled receptor desensitization and resensitization. Life Sci 62: 1561–1565.

Fisher MB, Vandenbranden M, Findlay K et al. (2000). Tissue distribution and interindividual variation in human UDP-glucuronosyltransferase activity: relationship between UGT1A1 promoter genotype and variability in a liver bank. Pharmacogenetics 10: 727–739.

Furman KD, Grimm DR, Mueller T et al. (2004). Impact of CYP2D6 inter-mediate metabolizer alleles on single-dose desipramine pharmacokinetics. Pharmacogenetics 14: 279–284.

Gaedigk A, Gotschall RR, Forbes NS et al. (1999). Optimization of cytochrome P4502D6 (CYP2D6) phenotype assignment using a genotyping algorithm based on allele frequency data. Pharmacogenetics 9: 669–682.

Gaedigk A, Bradford LD, Marcucci KA et al. (2002). Unique CYP2D6 activity distribution and genotype-phenotype discordance in black Americans. Clin Pharmacol Ther 72: 76–89.

George SR, Kertesz M. (1987). Met-enkephalin concentrations in striatum respond reciprocally to alterations in dopamine neurotransmission. Peptides 8: 487–492.

Griese E, Zanger UM, Brudermanns U et al. (1998). Assessment of the predictive power of genotypes for the in vivo catalytic function of CYP2D6 in a Caucasian population. Pharmacogenetics 8: 15–26.

Grond S, Sablotzki A. (2004). Clinical pharmacology of tramadol. Clin Pharmacokinet 43: 879–923.

Gurevich EV, Benovic JL, Gurevich VV. (2002). Arrestin2 and arrestin3 are differentially expressed in the rat brain during postnatal development. Neuroscience 109: 421–436.

Hines RN, McCarver DG. (2002). The ontogeny of human drug-metabolizing enzymes: Phase I oxidative enzymes. J Pharmacol Exp Ther 300: 355–360.

Hollt V. (2002). A polymorphism (A118G) in the mu-opioid receptor gene affects the response to morphine-6-glucuronide in humans. Pharmacogenetics 12: 1–2.

Holthe M, Rakvag TN, Klepstad P et al. (2003). Sequence variations in the UDP-glucuronosyltransferase 2B7 (UGT2B7) gene: identification of 10 novel single nucleotide polymorphisms (SNPs) and analysis of their relevance to morphine glucuronidation in cancer patients. Pharmacogenomics J 3: 17–26.

Innocenti F, Iyer L, Ramirez J et al. (2001). Epirubicin glucuronidation is catalysed by human UDP-glucuronosyltransferase 2b7. Drug Metab Dispos 29: 686–692.

Jacqz-Aigrain E, Cresteil T. (1992). Cytochrome P450-dependent metabolism of dextromethorphan: fetal and adult studies. Dev Pharmacol Ther 18: 161–168.

Jin C, Miners JO, Lillywhite KJ et al. (1993). Complementary deoxyribonucleic acid cloning and expression of a human liver uridine diphosphate-glucuronosyltransferase glucuronidating carboxylic acid-containing drugs. J Pharmacol Exp Ther 264: 475–479.

Kearns GL, Abdel-Rahman SM, Alander SW et al. (2003). Developmental pharmacology – drug disposition, action, and therapy in infants and children. New Engl J Med 349: 1157–1167.

Kennedy MJ, Abdel-Rahman SM, Kashuba AD et al. (2004). Comparison of various urine collection intervals for caffeine and dextromethorphan phenotyping in children. J Clin Pharmacol 44: 708–714.

Kozak CA, Filie J, Adamson MC et al. (1994). Murine chromosomal location of the mu and kappa opioid receptor gene. Genomics 21: 659–661.

Ladona MG, Lindstrom B, Thyr C et al. (1991). Differential foetal development of the O- and N-demethylation of codeine and dextromethorphan in man. Br J Clin Pharmacol 32: 295–302.

Loh HH, Liu HC, Cavalli A et al. (1998). Mu-opioid receptor knockout in mice: effects on ligand-induced analgesia and morphine lethality. Brain Res Mol Brain Res 54: 321–326.

Lotsch J, Skarke C, Grösch S et al. (2002). The polymorphism A118G of the human mu-opioid receptor gene decreases the pupil constrictory effect of morphine-6-glucuronide but not that of morphine. Pharmacogenetics 12: 3–9.

Luttrell LM, Lefkowitz RJ. (2002). The role of beta-arrestins in the termination and transduction of G-protein-coupled receptor signals. J Cell Sci 115: 455–465.

Mackenzie PI, Owens IS, Burchell B et al. (1997). The UDP glycosyltransferase gene superfamily: recommended nomenclature update based on evolutionary divergence. Pharmacogenetics 7: 255–269.

Mannisto PT, Kaakkola S. (1999). Catechol-O-methyltransferase (COMT): biochemistry, molecular biology, pharmacology, and clinical efficacy of the new selective COMT inhibitors. Pharmacol Rev 51: 593–628.

Mansour A, Watson SJ, Akil H. (1995). Opioid receptors: past, present and future. Trends Neurosci 18: 69–70.

Matthes HW, Maldonado R, Simonin F et al. (1996). Loss of morphine-induced analgesia, reward effect and withdrawal symptoms in mice lacking the mu-opioid-receptor gene. Nature 383: 759–760.

May D. (1994). Genetic differences in drug disposition. J Clin Pharmacol 34: 881–887.

McCarver DG, Hines RN. (2002). The ontogeny of human drug-metabolizing enzymes: phase II conjugation enzymes and regulatory mechanisms. J Pharmacol Exp Ther 300: 361–366.

Mhanna MJ, Bennet JB, Izatt SD. (1997). Potential fluoxetine chloride (Prozac) toxicity in a newborn. Pediatrics 100: 158–159.

Noble F, Cox BM. (1996). Differential desensitization of mu- and delta-opioid receptors in selected neural pathways following chronic morphine treatment. Br J Pharmacol 117: 161–169.

Paar WD, Poche S, Gerloff J et al. (1997). Polymorphic CYP2D6 mediates O-demethylation of the opioid analgesic tramadol. Eur J Clin Pharmacol 53: 235–239.

Park J, Kim K, Park P et al. (2005). Effect of age on the activity of cytochrome P450 2D6 using dextromethorphan phenotyping in humans. Clin Pharmacol Ther 77: P24.

Pitcher JA, Freedman NJ, Lefkowitz RJ. (1998). G protein-coupled receptor kinases. Annu Rev Biochem 67: 653–692.

Portenoy RK, Thaler HT, Inturrisi CE. (1992). The metabolite morphine-6-glucuronide contributes to the analgesia produced by morphine infusion in patients with pain and normal renal function. Clin Pharmacol Ther 51: 422–431.

Premont RT, Inglese J, Lefkowitz RJ. (1995). Protein kinases that phosphorylate activated G protein-coupled receptors. FASEB J 9: 175–182.

Rahman W, Dashwood MR, Fitzgerald M et al. (1998). Postnatal development of multiple opioid receptors in the spinal cord and development of spinal morphine analgesia. Brain Res Dev Brain Res 108: 239–254.

Rakvag TT, Klepstad P, Baar C et al. (2005). The Val[158]Met polymorphism of the human catechol-O-methyltransferase (COMT) gene may influence morphine requirements in cancer pain patients. Pain 116: 73–78.

Rane A. (1999). Phenotyping of drug metabolism in infants and children: potentials and problems. Pediatrics 104: 640–643.

Riedy M, Wang JY, Miller AP et al. (2000). Genomic organization of the UGT2b gene cluster on human chromosome 4q13. Pharmacogenetics 10: 251–260.

Sachse C, Brockmöller J, Bauer S et al. (1997). Cytochrome P450 2D6 variants in a Caucasian population: allele frequencies and phenotypic consequences. Am J Hum Genet 60: 284–295.

Sallee FR, DeVane CL, Ferrell RE. (2000). Fluoxetine-related death in a child with cytochrome P-450 2D6 genetic deficiency. J Child Adolesc Psychopharmacol 10: 27–34.

Samokyszyn VM, Gall WE, Zawada G (2000). 4-hydroxyretinoic acid, a novel substrate for human liver microsomal UDP-glucuronosyltransferases and recombinant UGT2B7. J Biol Chem 85: 4819–4826.

Sawyer MB, Innocenti F, Das S et al. (2003). A pharmacogenetic study of uridine diphosphate glucuronosyl-transferase 2B7 in patients receiving morphine. Clin Pharmacol Ther 73: 566–574.

Schmid B, Bircher J, Preisig R et al. (1985). Polymorphic dextromethorphan metabolism: co-segregation of oxidative O-demethylation with debrisoquin hydroxylation. Clin Pharmacol Ther 38: 618–624.

Spencer MJ. (1993). Fluoxetine hydrochloride (Prozac) toxicity in a neonate. Pediatrics 92: 721–722.

Stamer UM, Lehnen K, Hothker F et al. (2003). Impact of CYP2D6 genotype on postoperative tramadol analgesia. Pain 105: 231–238.

Steimer W, Zopf K, von Amelunxen S et al. (2004). Allele-specific change of concentration and functional gene dose for the prediction of steady-state serum concentrations of amitriptyline and nortriptyline in CYP2C19 and CYP2D6 extensive and intermediate metabolizers. Clin Chem 50: 1623–1633.

Steiner H, Gerfen CR. (1999). Enkephalin regulates acute D2 dopamine receptor antagonist-induced immediate-early gene expression in striatal neurons. Neuroscience 88: 795–810.

Stiskal JA, Kulin N, Koren G et al. (2001). Neonatal paroxetine withdrawal syndrome. Arch Dis Child Fetal Neonatal Ed 84: F134–F135.

Treluyer JM, Jacqz-Aigrain E, Alvarez F et al. (1991). Expression of CYP2D6 in developing human liver. Eur J Biochem 202: 583–588.

Turgeon D, Carrier JS, Levesque E et al. (2001). Relative enzyme activity, protein stability and tissue distribution of human steroid metabolizing

UGT2B subfamily members. Endocrinology 142: 778–787.

van den Anker JN. (1996). Pharmacokinetics and renal function in preterm infants. Acta Paediatr 85: 1393–1399.

Weinshilboum R. (2003). Inheritance and drug response. New Engl J Med 348: 529–537.

Wennerholm A, Dandara C, Sayi J et al. (2002). The African-specific CYP2D6*17 allele encodes an enzyme with changed substrate specificity. Clin Pharmacol Ther 71: 77–88.

Whistler JL, von Zastrow M. (1998). Morphine-activated opioid receptors elude desensitization by beta-arrestin. Proc Natl Acad Sci USA 95: 9914–9919.

Williams DG, Patel A, Howard RF. (2002). Pharmacogenetics of codeine metabolism in an urban population of children and its implications for analgesic reliability. Br J Anaesth 89: 839–845.

Wu D, Kang YS, Bickel U et al. (1997). Blood brain barrier permeability to morphine-6-glucuronide is markedly reduced compared with morphine. Drug Metab Dispos 25: 768–771.

Yamada H, Ishii K, Ishii Y et al. (2003). Formation of highly analgesic morphine-6-glucuronide following physiologic concentration of morphine in human brain. J Toxicol Sci 28: 395–401.

Zhang J, Ferguson SS, Barak LS et al. (1998). Role for G protein-coupled receptor kinase in agonist-specific regulation of mu-opioid receptor responsiveness. Proc Natl Acad Sci USA 95: 7157–7162.

Zubieta JK, Heitzeg MM, Smith YR et al. (2003). COMT val[158]met genotype affects μ-opioid neurotransmitter responses to pain stressor. Science 299: 1240–1243.

9

Pharmacokinetics and pharmacodynamics of analgesic drugs

Brian J Anderson
Nicholas H G Holford

INTRODUCTION

Therapeutic catastrophes in neonates such as the grey baby syndrome attributable to chloramphenicol and phocomelia due to thalidomide have shaped modern drug development. Unmonitored off-label use of medicines in neonates and infants, extrapolated from adult data, has resulted in significant morbidity that could have been avoided or minimized by investigation in this population. A surge of interest in developmental pharmacology, methods for scaling paediatric pharmacokinetic (PK) parameters from adult and individual drug studies in children of all ages is improving current drug management in the first year of life. This chapter examines pharmacokinetic and pharmacodynamic (PD) changes after birth, explores common size models and reviews the pharmacology of analgesic drugs commonly used in early infancy.

DEVELOPMENTAL PHARMACOLOGY

Absorption

The rate at which most drugs are absorbed when given by the oral route is slower in neonates and young infants than in older children. The time (Tmax) at which maximum concentration (Cmax) is achieved is prolonged (Fig. 9.1). Gastric emptying and intestinal motor motility mature through infancy and normal adult rates may not be reached until 6–8 months (Grand et al. 1976, Gupta and Brans 1978, Carlos et al. 1997, Liang et al. 1998). Many of the effects of the immature gastrointestinal system are either not characterized or the effect of immaturity is uncertain. Immature conjugation and transport of bile salts into the intestinal lumen may affect lipophilic drug blood concentrations (Poley et al. 1964, Suchy et al. 1981), but these effects have not been quantified. The role of altered intestinal microflora in neonates and its effect on drugs is uncertain (Linday et al. 1987).

The larger relative skin surface area, increased cutaneous perfusion and thinner stratum corneum in neonates increase absorption and exposure of topically applied drugs (e.g. local anaesthetic creams). Neonates have reduced levels of methaemoglobin reductase and fetal haemoglobin is more readily oxidized compared to adult haemoglobin. This, combined with increased

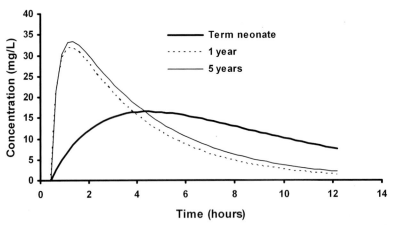

Figure 9.1 Simulated mean predicted time–concentration profiles for a term neonate, a 1-year-old infant and a 5-year-old child given acetaminophen elixir. (Reproduced from Anderson BJ et al. Anesthesiology 2002; 96:1336–1345, with permission.)

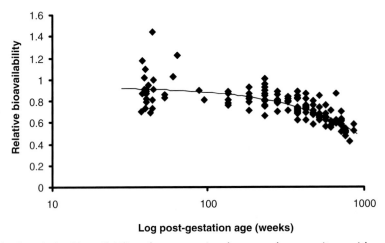

Figure 9.2 Changes in the relative bioavailability of an acetaminophen capsule suppository with age. (Adapted from Anderson BJ et al. Anesthesiology 2002; 96:1336–1345, with permission.)

absorption through the neonatal epidermis, resulted in reluctance to use lidocaine-prilocaine cream (EMLA) in this age group. These fears are unfounded if the cream is used as a single dose but may cause harm with repeat dosing (Taddio et al. 1995, 1997).

We might expect the reduced muscle bulk, skeletal muscle blood flow and inefficient muscular contractions in neonates (Greenblatt and Koch-Weser 1976) to decrease intramuscular absorption. This is not necessarily the case (Sheng et al. 1964, Kafetzis et al. 1979), partly because of size issues (see below) and the higher density of skeletal muscle capillaries (Carry et al. 1986).

The rectal route is associated with erratic and variable absorption. Age, formulation, rectal contents, rectal contractions (with consequent expulsion) and depth of rectal insertion all affect absorption and

relative bioavailability (van Hoogdalem et al. 1991a, 1991b). The rectal route has the potential to partially reduce first-pass hepatic extraction by draining into the inferior and middle haemorrhoidal veins. Age influences the relative bioavailability of some drugs, but this may not be always attributable to first-pass effects (Fig. 9.2).

The onset time of inhaled analgesic gases and vapours is generally more rapid in infants than in adults (Salanitre and Rackow 1969). Developmental changes of both the lung architecture and mechanics in these early years play a role. The greater fraction of the cardiac output distributed to the vessel-rich tissue group (i.e. a clearance factor) and the lower tissue/blood solubility (i.e. a volume factor) also affect the more rapid wash-in of inhalational anaesthetics in the younger age group (Lerman 1992). Solubility has considerable effects on the uptake of inhalational agents in children. Solubility determines the volume of distribution. An inhalational agent with a greater volume of distribution will take longer to reach a steady-state concentration when delivered at a constant rate. The solubilities in blood of halothane, isoflurane, enflurane and methoxyflurane are 18% less in neonates than in adults. The solubilities of these same agents in the vessel-rich tissue group in neonates are approximately one half of those in adults (Lerman et al. 1986). This may be due to the greater water content and decreased protein and lipid concentration in neonatal tissues. Age has little effect on the solubility of the less-soluble agents such as nitrous oxide (Malviya and Lerman 1990). Infants, with their decreased solubility, would be expected to have a shorter time to reach a predetermined fraction exhaled/fraction inhaled (F_E/F_I) ratio because of a smaller volume of distribution.

Distribution

Body composition

Total body water constitutes 85% of the body weight in the preterm neonate and 75% in term neonates. This decreases to approximately 60% at 5 months and remains relatively constant from this age on (Friis-Hansen 1961). The major component contributing to this reduction in body water is the decrease in extracellular fluid (ECF). ECF constitutes 45% of the body weight at birth and 26% at 1 year. There is a further ECF reduction during childhood until adulthood where it contributes 18%. The percentage of body weight contributed by fat is 3% in a 1.5 kg premature neonate and 12% in a term neonate; this proportion doubles by 4–5 months of age. 'Baby fat' is lost when the infant starts walking and protein mass increases (20% term neonate, 50% adult). Relative body proportions change dramatically over the first few years of life and may affect volumes of distribution of drugs.

Plasma proteins

Acidic drugs (e.g. barbiturates) tend to bind mainly to albumin while basic drugs (e.g. diazepam, amide local anaesthetic agents) bind to globulins, lipoproteins and glycoproteins. Plasma protein binding of many drugs is decreased in the newborn infant relative to adults, but the clinical impact of this decrease is minor for most drugs. Reduced clearance in this age group has greater effect (Anderson et al. 1997). Protein binding changes are important for the rare case of a drug with more than 95% protein binding, a high extraction ratio and a narrow therapeutic index that is given parenterally (e.g. lidocaine IV) or a drug with

a narrow therapeutic index that is given orally and has a very rapid equilibration half-time (Benet and Hoener 2002).

Blood–brain barrier (BBB)

The BBB is a lipid membrane interface between the endothelial cells of the brain blood vessels and the ECF of the brain. Brain uptake of drugs is dependent on lipid solubility and blood flow. It was postulated that BBB permeability to water-soluble drugs such as morphine changes with maturation. This concept originated from a study (Way et al. 1965) demonstrating that neonates less than 4 days of age developed ventilatory depression following intramuscular morphine 0.05 mg/kg. This dose should depress ventilation minimally in adults. Ventilatory depression in neonates following intramuscular pethidine (meperidine) 0.5 mg/kg was similar to that expected in adults (Way et al. 1965). This finding is consistent with pethidine, unlike morphine, being lipid soluble and therefore crossing the immature or mature BBB equally (Way et al. 1965). However, the increased neonatal respiratory depression observed after morphine could be due to pharmacokinetic age-related changes. For example, the volume of distribution of morphine is reduced in term neonates (Bouwmeester et al. 2004) and we might expect initial concentrations of morphine to be higher in neonates than in adults. Respiratory depression is the same in children from 2–570 days of age at the same morphine concentration (Lynn et al. 1993). The role of transporters across the BBB for morphine has only recently been explored (Tunblad et al. 2005) in non-human species. Direct demonstration of the developmental changes in transporter activity and their impact on drug transport across the BBB remain speculative.

Drug metabolism

The liver is the primary organ for clearance of most drugs. Non-polar, lipid-soluble drugs are converted to more polar and water-soluble compounds. Water-soluble drugs are excreted unchanged in the kidneys by glomerular filtration and/or renal tubular secretion. Many of these processes are immature in the neonate and mature to reach adult levels within the first year of life, although there may be exceptions to this rule (e.g. N-acetyltransferase) (Pariente-Khayat et al. 1997). These developmental changes are predicted by age and are independent of size (represented by body weight). Clearance increases with gestation, but birth may be a major stimulus for the maturation of drug metabolism (Hines and McCarver 2002, McCarver and Hines 2002). Maturation of clearance in neonates may be described by both postconception age (PCA) and postnatal age (PNA). We believe that PCA is a more physiologically appropriate covariate to explain the time course of changes in clearance. We are not aware of any direct demonstration that clearance changes as a consequence of being born.

Hepatic elimination

Phase 1 reactions Phase 1 metabolic processes involve oxidative, reductive or hydrolytic reactions that are commonly catalyzed by the mixed function oxidase system. The cytochrome P450 (CYP) is the major enzyme system for oxidation of drugs. There are distinct patterns associated with isoform-specific developmental expression of CYPs. Some appear to be switched on by birth, while for others birth is necessary but not sufficient for the onset of expression (Hines and McCarver 2002, Koukouritaki et al. 2004). CYP2E1 activity surges after birth, CYP2D6 becomes detectable soon thereafter, the CYP3A4 and CYP2C family appear during the first week, whereas CYP1A2 is the last to appear (Kearns et al. 2003). Neonates are dependent on the immature CYP3A4 for bupivacaine clearance and CYP1A2 for ropivacaine clearance, dictating reduced epidural infusion rates in this age group (Berde 1992, Anderson and Hansen 2004).

Phase 2 reactions Knowledge of maturation of phase 2 enzymes remains incomplete (McCarver and Hines 2002). Some phase 2 pathways are mature at birth (sulphate conjugation), while others are not (acetylation, glycination, glucuronidation). The individual isoforms of glucuronosyltransferase (UGT) mature at different rates. Morphine is largely metabolized by uridine-5′-diphosphate UGT2B7 to morphine-3-glucuronide and morphine-6-glucuronide (de Wildt et al. 1999b). In vitro studies using liver microsomes from fetuses aged 15–27 weeks indicated that mor-

phine glucuronidation was approximately 10–20% of that seen with adult microsomes (Pacifici et al. 1982, 1989). Morphine glucuronidation has been demonstrated in premature infants as young as 24 weeks. Clearance increases after birth with a maturation half-time of approximately 3 months (Bouwmeester et al. 2004) (Fig. 9.3). The neonate can use sulphate conjugation as an alternative route for substrates such as morphine or acetaminophen before glucuronidation develops. Clearance increases in early life as hepatic glucuronidation enzyme pathways mature. The sulphate pathway is the dominant metabolic route for acetaminophen in infancy (Alam et al. 1977).

Renal elimination

Drugs and their metabolites are excreted by the kidneys by two processes: glomerular filtration and tubular secretion. Glomerular filtration rate (size normalized using predicted body surface area) is at adult values at 5–6 months (West et al. 1948, Arant 1978). Proximal tubular secretion reaches adult levels by 7 months of age (West et al. 1948, Arant 1978).

Extrahepatic elimination

Many drugs are metabolized at extrahepatic sites. Remifentanil is rapidly broken down by non-specific esterase in tissue and erythrocytes. Clearance is increased in younger children but this may be attributable to size (see below) and maturation profiles are unknown. A rate constant representing hydrolysis by plasma esterases of propacetamol (a prodrug of acetaminophen) to acetaminophen was size related, but not age related (Anderson et al. 2005). The ester group of local anaesthetics is metabolized by plasma pseudocholinesterase, which is reduced in neonates. The in vitro plasma half-life of 2-chloroprocaine in

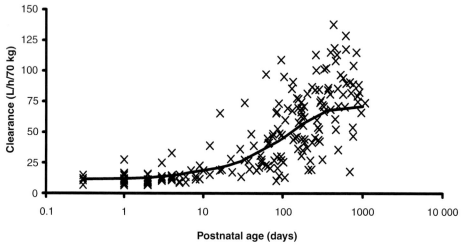

Figure 9.3 Maturation of morphine clearance with age. Total body morphine clearance is 80% that of 'adult' values by 6 months. (Data from Bouwmeester et al. 2004.)

umbilical cord blood is twice that in maternal blood (Zsigmond and Downs 1971), but there are no in vivo studies examining the effects of age.

Polymorphisms of metabolic enzymes

Polymorphisms of the genes encoding for metabolic enzymes contribute to a large degree of inter-individual PK variability (de Wildt et al. 1999a). Polymorphism of CYP2D6, for example, is inherited as an autosomal recessive trait. Homozygous individuals are deficient in the metabolism of a variety of important groups of drugs – β-adrenoreceptor blocking agents, anti-depressants, neuroleptic agents and opioids. Poor metabolizers have reduced morphine production from codeine (Williams et al. 2001). Tramadol is also metabolized by O-demethylation in the liver (CYP2D6) to O-demethyl tramadol (M1) and the M1 metabolite has a μ-opioid affinity approximately 200 times greater than tramadol; CYP2D6 iso-enzyme activity is important for the analgesic effect attributable to tramadol.

PHARMACODYNAMICS

Pharmacokinetics is what the body does to the drug, while pharmacodynamics is what the drug does to the body. The precise boundary between these two processes is ill defined and often requires a link describing movement of drug from the plasma to the biophase and its target. Drugs may exert effects at non-specific membrane sites by interference with transport mechanisms, by enzyme inhibition or induction or by activation or inhibition of receptors.

Developmental changes

There are few data describing age-related pharmaco-dynamic changes despite recognition that the number, affinity and type of receptors or the availability of natural ligands changes with age. Opioid receptors are not fully developed in the newborn rat and mature into adulthood (Freye 1996), but human neonatal increased sensitivity to morphine is attributable to PK rather than PD differences. Correlations between the opioid drug plasma concentrations and validated pain scores are weak (Suri et al. 1997, Olkkola and Hamunen 2000).

Gamma-aminobutyric acid (GABA) is the neuro-transmitter at most inhibitory synapses in the human central nervous system. The $GABA_A$ receptor complex is the site of action for benzodiazepines, barbiturates and numerous anaesthetic agents (Franks and Lieb 1994). At birth the cerebellum only contains one-third the number of $GABA_A$ receptors found in an adult and these are comprised of subunits with reduced binding affinity for benzodiazepines (Brooks-Kayal

and Pritchett 1993). Major changes in receptor binding and subunit expression occur during post-natal development (Chugani et al. 2001). $GABA_A$ receptor complex, identified by positron emission tomography, was more prevalent at 2 years and the values then decreased exponentially to 50% of peak values by 17 years (Chugani et al. 2001). These changes are consistent with age-related minimal alveolar concentration (MAC) changes of inhalational anaesthetics (Marshall et al. 2000). The MAC (%) of isoflurane, for example, is 1.3 in a premature neonate, 1.4 at term, 1.9 at 6–12 months and 1.6 at 17 years.

The sigmoid Emax model

The relation between drug concentration and effect may be described by a hyperbolic curve according to the equation:

$$Effect = E0 + (Emax \times Ce^N)/(EC_{50}^N + Ce^N)$$

where E0 is the baseline response, Emax is the maximum effect change, Ce is the concentration in the effect compartment, EC_{50} is the concentration producing 50% Emax and N is the Hill coefficient defining the steepness of the concentration–response curve (Holford and Sheiner 1981). At low concen-trations this non-linear relationship may approach linearity (Fig. 9.4).

Efficacy is the maximum response on a dose– or concentration–response curve and is measured by Emax. EC_{50} can be used as a measure of potency relative to another drug provided N and Emax for the two drugs are the same.

The time course of drug effect

Immediate effects

A simple situation in which drug effect is directly related to concentration does not mean that drug effects parallel the time course of concentration. This occurs only when the concentration is low in relation to EC_{50}. In this situation the plasma half-life of the drug may correlate closely with the half-life of drug effect. Many drugs, however, have a short half-life but a long duration of effect. If the initial concen-tration is very high in relation to the EC_{50}, then drug concentrations 5 half-lives later, when we might expect minimal concentration, may still exert consid-erable effect. This is because of the shape of the Emax model. Low concentrations may still be about the EC_{50} concentration, for example, and so exert effect. This is common for drugs that act on enzymes (e.g. NSAIDs).

Delayed effects

Delayed effect model A plasma concentration– effect plot can form a counter-clockwise hysteresis loop

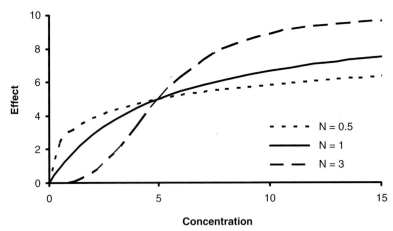

Figure 9.4 The sigmoid Emax model.

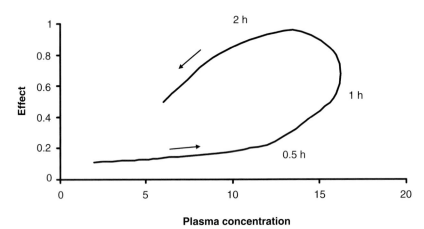

Figure 9.5 The counter-clockwise hysteresis loop.

(Fig. 9.5) because of this delay in effect. Hull et al. (1978) and Sheiner et al. (1979) introduced the effect compartment concept for muscle relaxants. The effect compartment concentration is not the same as the blood or serum concentration and is not a real measurable concentration. A single first-order parameter (Teq, $T_{1/2}$keo) describes the equilibration half-time. It is assumed that the concentration in the central compartment is the same as that in the effect compartment at equilibrium, but that a time delay exists before the drug reaches the effect compartment. The concentration in the effect compartment is used to describe the concentration–effect relationship.

Physiological substance turnover model Many drug actions are mediated through synthesis or elimination of a physiological substance (Holford 1992). The concentration at the site of drug effect either stimulates or inhibits the rate of production or elimination of the physiological substance (response variable). Warfarin, for example, inhibits the recycling of vitamin K epoxide to the active vitamin K form that is involved in the production of prothrombin complex. Turnover models provide a reasonable description of the mechanism of delayed action for many drugs (Jonkers et al. 1989).

SIZE MODELS

Weight is commonly used to determine dose in children. The variation of weight at any given age is considerable, being least at 1 year (+25% to –20% at 10 kg; from 3rd to 97th centile) and reaching a maximum at about 13 years (+45% to –26% at 40 kg) (Lack and Stuart Taylor 1997). Body weight is used commonly, although it is now widely recognized that there is a non-linear relationship between weight and drug elimination capacity.

Linear size models for young children have led to the idea that there is an enhanced capacity of children to metabolize drugs due to proportionally larger livers and kidneys than their adult counterparts (Tenenbein 2000). This idea arises because clearance, expressed per kg of body weight, is larger in children than adults. Developmental and physiological changes during growth such as an increased relative

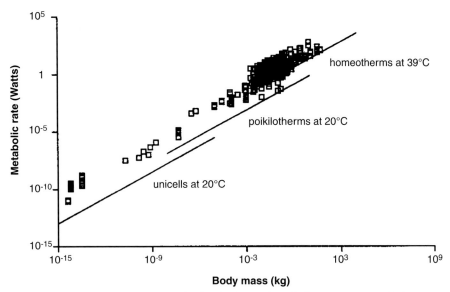

Figure 9.6 A comparison of the temperature-standardised relation for whole-organism metabolic rate as a function of body mass. The 'allometric $^3/_4$ power model' fits for unicells, poikilotherms and homeotherms, uncorrected for temperature, are also shown. (Adapted from Gillooly JF et al. Effects of size and temperature on metabolic rate. Science 2001; 293: 2248–2251, with permission.)

liver size or increased hepatic blood flow have been invoked (Tenenbein 2000) to explain the higher clearance per kg.

Dawson, in 1940, reviewed evidence that smaller species are generally more tolerant of drug treatment than larger species and concluded that adjustment of drug dose using a body weight exponent of less than 1 was justified. Body surface area (BSA) was subsequently proposed in 1950 to be a more satisfactory index of drug requirements than body weight or age, particularly during infancy and childhood (Crawford et al. 1950). Drug dosage rules for children, based on BSA, have been described which use percentage of an adult dose to calculate an appropriate child's dose (Catzel and Olver 1981, Lack and Stuart Taylor 1997). Another size model using an exponent of weight ($W^{3/4}$) has also been proposed (Holford 1996). The latter, which may be termed the 'allometric $^3/_4$ power model' has been found to be useful in normalizing a large number of physiological (Peters 1983) and pharmacokinetic variables (Boxenbaum 1982, Ritschel et al. 1992). The per kilogram, surface area and allometric $^3/_4$ power models are but three of numerous different approaches which have been described as a means of predicting physiological function from body size.

The allometric model

Most body size relations take the form:

$$y = a \cdot W^b$$

where y is the biological characteristic to be predicted, W is the body mass and a and b are empirically derived constants. In all species studied, including humans, the log of basal metabolic rate (BMR) plotted against the log of body weight produces a straight line with a slope of $^3/_4$ (Kleiber 1932, Brody et al. 1934, Stahl 1967, Peters 1983). This exponential function is the same for homeotherms, poikilotherms and unicellular organisms (Peters 1983). Mass- and temperature-compensated resting metabolic rates of microbes, ectotherms, endotherms (including those in hibernation), and plants in temperatures ranging from 0°C to 40°C are similar (Gillooly et al. 2001) (Fig. 9.6).

West et al. (1997) have used fractal geometric concepts to explain this phenomenon. This group analyzed organisms in terms of the geometry and physics of a network of linear tubes required to transport resources and wastes through the body. Such a system, they reasoned, must have three key attributes. The network must reach all parts of a three-dimensional body; a minimum amount of energy should be required to transport the materials in a fluid medium; and the terminal branches of the networks should all be the same size, as cells in most species are roughly similar sizes (Williams 1997). The $^3/_4$ power law for metabolic rates was derived from a general model that describes how essential materials are transported through space-filled fractal networks of branching tubes (West et al. 1997). These design principles are independent of detailed dynamics and explicit models and should apply to virtually all organisms (Banavar 1999, West et al. 1999).

This allometric $^3/_4$ power model may be used to scale metabolic processes such as drug clearance (CL) as follows:

$$CL_i = CL_{std} \cdot \left(\frac{W_i}{W_{std}} \right)^{3/4}$$

where CL_i is the clearance in the individual of weight W_i and CL_{std} is the clearance in a standardized individual with weight W_{std} (Holford 1996).

When applied to physiological volumes (V), the power parameter is 1:

$$V_i = V_{std} \cdot \left(\frac{W_i}{W_{std}} \right)^1$$

This index has been demonstrated for blood volume, vital capacity and tidal volume (Guyton 1947, Adolph 1949, Stahl 1967, Prothero 1980, West et al. 1997). The volume of distribution in the central compartment (V_c), volume of distribution by area (V_{beta}) and volume of distribution at steady state (V_{dss}) also show direct proportionality to body weight (Mahmood 1998).

Time-related indices (T) such as heart rate, respiratory rate or drug half-times have a power of $^1/_4$ (Dedrick et al. 1970, McMahon 1980, Peters 1983, Ritschel et al. 1992, Gronert et al. 1995, West et al. 1997).

$$T_i = T_{std} \cdot \left(\frac{W_i}{W_{std}} \right)^{1/4}$$

The pharmacokinetic time scale originated from an imaginary concept of 'physiologic time'. Most mammals have the same number of heartbeats and breaths in their life span. The difference between small and large animals is that smaller animals have faster physiologic processes and consequently a shorter life span. (Ritschel et al. 1992). A power function of $^1/_4$ can be derived for pharmacokinetic half-times based on basic pharmacokinetics applied to allometric predictions of clearance and volume:

$$T_{1/2} = \ln(2) \cdot \frac{V}{CL} \propto \ln(2) \cdot \frac{W^1}{W^{3/4}} = \ln(2) \cdot W^{1/4}$$

The surface area model

The original surface area model proposed by Du Bois and Du Bois (1916) was predicted from nine adults of diverse body shape. These nine individuals included a tall thin adult male, a fat adult woman, and a 36-year-old cretin with the 'physical development of a boy of 8 years'. The youngest individual from this group was 12 years old. It is now common practice to use the

Du Bois and Du Bois formula to predict surface area from weight (W) and height (H):

$$BSA = W(kg)^{0.425} \cdot H(cm)^{0.725} \cdot 0.007184$$

This formula belongs to the same class of allometric models that include those using weight alone.

Nomograms determined from this formula are often used. Surface area can also be estimated from an allometric model with a power parameter of $^2/_3$ (Boxenbaum and DiLea 1995, Holford 1996). This 'allometric $^2/_3$ power model' assumes metabolic rate is scaled by geometric descriptors of body size (Williams 1997). The surface area formula assumes that adults and children are geometrically similar. However, infants are not morphologically similar to adults – infants have short stumpy legs, relatively big heads and large body trunks. The surface area formula is inaccurate in children with a predicted surface area of less than 1.3 m^2 (an average 12-year-old) by direct photometric measurement (Mitchell et al. 1971).

When a standard surface area of 1.9 m^2 is used with the allometric $^2/_3$ power surface area model, clearances agree quite well with the $^3/_4$ power model except at body weights below 7 kg. When the allometric surface area is used, clearance is over-predicted by more than 10% at body weights below 20 kg (Mitchell et al. 1971). The mass of empirical evidence suggests that the appropriate scaling factor is significantly different from 0.67 and is compatible with the theoretically expected value of 0.75 (Kleiber 1961, Schmidt-Nielsen 1984, West et al. 1997, 1999).

The linear per kilogram model

The linear per kilogram model is the poorest model when used for interspecies scaling of metabolic processes such as total body clearance, but remains the most commonly used in humans. In humans, under-prediction of clearance of more than 10% occurs at body weights less than 47 kg when compared to the allometric $^3/_4$ power model. This discrepancy increases as size decreases and approaches 50% for a newborn human of 3.5 kg. Because clearance is reduced in this age group for developmental reasons, use of the linear per kilogram model may get close to the right answer for the wrong reason.

Figure 9.7 shows clearance changes with weight for a hypothetical drug using the three different models. Age-related clearance increases throughout infancy and reaches adult values at approximately 1 year using an allometric $^3/_4$ power model. The linear per kilogram model shows an increased clearance compared to adults at approximately 1 year (10 kg). This apparent increased clearance in infants has been interpreted to mean that children have an enhanced capacity to

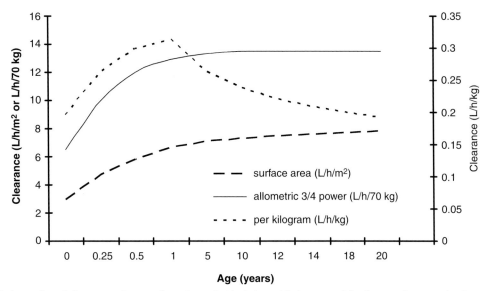

Figure 9.7 Age-related clearance changes for a hypothetical drug. All three models show an increase in clearance over the first year of life due to maturation of metabolic pathways. Clearance expressed using the linear per kilogram model then decreases with age after 1 year to reach adult levels in adolescence. This course is not evident with the allometric $^3/_4$ power and surface area models. (Reproduced from Anderson and Meakin, Paediatr Anaesth 2002; 12: 205–219, with permission from Blackwell Publishing.)

metabolize drugs but is more likely to be an artefact due to the use of the linear per kilogram model.

The $^1/_4$ power family of allometric models forms a better basis for size scaling than either the surface area or per kilogram models. Once size is scaled then deviations from predictions based on allometry are noticeable. The cause of these deviations can then be sought. The prime example of such a deviation is the reduced clearance in neonates, attributable to immaturity of hepatic and renal clearance systems.

COMMON ANALGESIC DRUGS

Acetaminophen (paracetamol)

Mechanism of action

Acetaminophen is widely used in the management of pain, but is lacking in anti-inflammatory effects. Analgesia is mediated through inhibition of prostaglandin synthesis within the central nervous system (COX III, COX 2b). Analgesic effect also involves an inhibitory action on spinal nitric oxide mechanisms (Piletta et al. 1991, Bjorkman et al. 1994, Bjorkman 1995) and serotonergic pathways (Courade et al. 2001).

Analgesic pharmacodynamics

Acetaminophen is believed to be an effective antipyretic at serum concentrations of 10–20 mg/L (Peterson and Rumack 1978), and these concentrations have been extrapolated to those that provide analgesia. However, the paper by Rumack (Peterson and Rumack 1978), which is often cited as the source for these antipyretic

serum concentrations of 10–20 mg/L, makes reference to an unpublished source. There are few data examining acetaminophen analgesia in neonates. These data suggest poor analgesic effect after painful procedures (van Lingen et al. 1999a, 2001), after circumcision (Howard et al. 1994) or during heel prick (Shah et al. 1998). This is in contrast to documented analgesic effect in infants and children (Rod et al. 1989, Korpela et al. 1999, Anderson et al. 2001). It is unclear why poor analgesic effect is reported in neonates, but it may be attributable to inadequate serum concentrations, type of pain stimulus or assessment tools for the discrimination of pain.

Korpela et al. (1999) have calculated a rectal dose after day-stay surgery at which 50% of the children did not require a rescue opioid to be 35 mg/kg. Time delays of approximately 1 hour between peak concentration and peak effect are reported (Arendt Nielsen et al. 1991, Nielsen et al. 1992). Pain fluctuations, pain type and placebo effects complicate interpretation of clinical studies. Anderson et al. (2001) obtained population parameter estimates (population parameter variability) of Emax 5.17 (64%) and EC_{50} 9.98 (107%) mg/L (the greatest possible pain relief (visual analogue scale (VAS) 0–10) would equate to an Emax of 10). The equilibration half-time (Teq) of the analgesic effect compartment was 53 (217%) min. A target effect compartment concentration of 10 mg/L was associated with a pain reduction of 2.6/10 (using a VAS 0–10) (Anderson et al. 2001).

Pharmacokinetics

Bioavailability Acetaminophen has low first-pass metabolism and the hepatic extraction ratio is 0.11–0.37 in adults (Rawlins et al. 1977). The relative bioavailability of rectal compared with oral acetaminophen formulations (rectal/oral) has been reported as 0.52 (range 0.24–0.98) (Audenaert et al. 1995) and even as low as 0.3 (Dange et al. 1987). The relative bioavailability is higher in neonates and approaches unity. The relative bioavailability of rectal formulations appears to be age related (see Fig. 9.2) (Anderson and Meakin 2002).

Rate of absorption Acetaminophen has a pKa of 9.5 and in the alkaline medium of the duodenum acetaminophen is non-ionized. Consequently, absorption of the non-ionized form from the duodenum to the systemic circulation is rapid in children. Brown et al. (1992) have reported rapid absorption ($T_{1/2}$abs 2.7, se 1.2 min; Tlag 4.2, se 0.4 min) parameters in febrile children given elixir orally. Similar absorption half-lives have been estimated in children given acetaminophen as an elixir before tonsillectomy ($T_{1/2}$abs 4.5 min, CV 63%, Tlag 0) (Anderson et al. 2001). Absorption in infants under the age of 3 months was delayed 3.68 times, consistent with delayed gastric emptying in young infants (Anderson et al. 2000a). Oral absorption was considerably delayed in premature neonates in the first few days of life (see Fig. 9.2) (Anderson et al. 2002).

Rectal absorption Rectal absorption is slow and erratic with large variability (Gaudreault et al. 1988, Birmingham et al. 1997). For example, absorption parameters for the triglyceride base were $T_{1/2}$abs 1.34 h (CV 90%), Tlag 0.14 h (31%). The absorption half-life for rectal formulations was prolonged in infants under

3 months (1.51 times greater) compared to those seen in older children (Anderson et al. 2000c).

Clearance Several studies confirm sulphate metabolism to be the dominant route of elimination in neonates (Levy et al. 1975b, Miller et al. 1976, van Lingen et al. 1999a). Glucuronide/sulphate ratios range from 0.12 in premature neonates of 28–32 weeks postconception, 0.28 in those at 32–36 weeks postconception (van Lingen et al. 1999b) to 0.34 in term neonates 0–2 days old (Miller et al. 1976). Ratios of 0.75 in children 3–9 years, 1.61 in those aged 12 years and 1.8 in adults are reported (Miller et al. 1976). Approximately 4% of acetaminophen is excreted in urine unmetabolized and the amount is dependent on urine flow (Miners et al. 1992).

A total body clearance in full-term neonates of 4.9 (CV 38%) L/h/70kg after enteral acetaminophen has been reported using an allometric $^3/_4$ power model (Anderson et al. 2000c). This clearance is approximately 40% that of older children (2–15 years). Clearance over the first year of life reaches 80% of that seen in older children by 6 months. Further investigation using published data from premature neonates (Anderson et al. 2002) confirmed this trend in the very young. Clearance increased from 28 weeks postconception (0.74 L/h/70 kg) with a maturation half-life of 11.3 weeks to reach 10.9 L/h/70 kg by 60 weeks (Fig. 9.8).

Volume of distribution The population distribution volumes in children are similar to those reported in adults (56–70 L) (Prescott 1996). The volume of distribution for acetaminophen in mammals (Prescott 1996), including humans, is 49–70 L/70 kg as we would expect from the allometric size model with a power function of 1. The volume of distribution

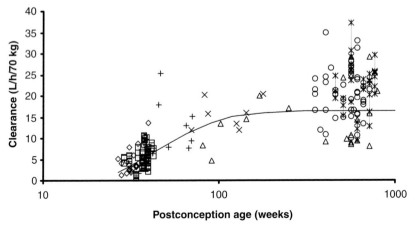

Figure 9.8 Individual predicted acetaminophen clearances determined after intravenous administration and standardized to a 70-kg person are plotted against postconception age. Children given multiple doses have clearance estimates from each occasion linked by a fine line. The solid line represents the non-linear relation between clearance and age. (Reproduced from Anderson BJ et al. Paediatr Anaesth 2005; 15: 282–292 with permission.)

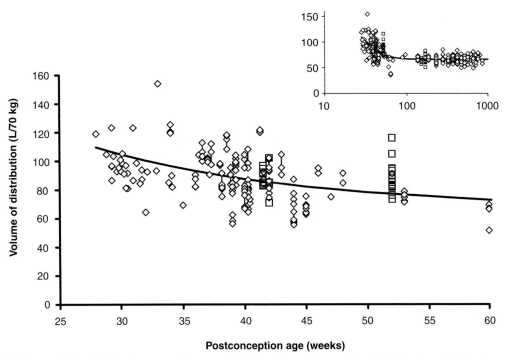

Figure 9.9 Volume of distribution changes with age up to 60 weeks postconception. Individual predicted volumes, standardized to a 70-kg person are plotted against age. The solid line demonstrates the non-linear relationship between volume of distribution and age. The figure inset includes older children and shows the V_{std} of 66.6 L/70 kg reached out of infancy. The x-axis (postconception age in weeks) of the inset figure uses a log scale. (Reproduced from Anderson BJ et al. Anaesthesiology 2002; 96: 1336–1345, with permission.)

decreases exponentially with a maturation half-life of 11.5 weeks from 109.7 L/70 kg at 28 weeks postconception to 72.9 L/70 kg by 60 weeks (Fig. 9.9). Fetal body composition and water distribution alter considerably during the third trimester and over the first few months of life, probably reflecting neonatal body composition and the rapid changes in body water distribution in early life.

Parenteral formulation Propacetamol (N-acetylparaaminophenoldiethyl aminoacetic ester) is a watersoluble prodrug of acetaminophen that can be administered intravenously over 15 min. It is rapidly hydroxylated into acetaminophen (1 g propacetamol = 0.5 g acetaminophen) (Granry et al. 1997, Anderson et al. 2005). An alternative intravenous acetaminophen formulation is now available that does not require hydrolysis and is associated with less pain on injection.

Toxicity

The toxic metabolite of acetaminophen, N-acetyl-p-benzoquinone imine (NAPQI) is formed by the cytochrome P450s CYP2E1, 1A2 and 3A4 (Slattery et al. 1996). This metabolite binds to intracellular hepatic macromolecules to produce cell necrosis and damage. Infants less than 90 days old have decreased

expression of CYP2E1 activity in vitro compared with older infants, children and adults (Johnsrud et al. 2003). CYP3A4 appears during the first week, whereas CYP1A2 is the last to appear (Kearns et al. 2003). Neonates can produce hepatotoxic metabolites (e.g. NAPQI), but the lower activity of cytochrome P450 in neonates and higher glutathione stores may explain the low incidence of acetaminophen-induced hepatotoxicity seen in neonates (Levy et al. 1975a, Roberts et al. 1984).

Non-steroidal anti-inflammatory drugs

Mechanism of action

The non-steroidal anti-inflammatory drugs (NSAIDs) are a heterogeneous group of compounds that share common antipyretic, analgesic and anti-inflammatory effects. NSAIDs act by reducing prostaglandin biosynthesis through inhibition of cyclo-oxygenase (COX) which exists as two major isoforms (COX-1 and COX-2) (Mitchell et al. 1993). The prostanoids produced by COX-1 isoenzyme protect the gastric mucosa, regulate renal blood flow and induce platelet aggregation. NSAID-induced gastrointestinal toxicity, for example, is generally believed to occur through blockade of COX-1 activity, whereas the anti-inflammatory effects of NSAIDs are thought to occur primarily through inhibition of the inducible isoform, COX-2. Some of the NSAIDs may also inhibit the lipo-oxygenase pathway by an action on hydroperoxy fatty acid peroxidase.

Pharmacodynamics

The NSAIDs are commonly used in children for antipyresis and analgesia. The anti-inflammatory properties of the NSAIDs have, in addition, been used in such diverse disorders as juvenile idiopathic arthritis, renal and biliary colic, dysmenorrhoea, Kawasaki disease and cystic fibrosis (Konstan et al. 1991, 1995, Oermann et al. 1999, Scott et al. 1999a). The NSAIDs indometacin and ibuprofen are also used to treat delayed closure of patent ductus arteriosus (PDA) in premature infants (Van Overmeire et al. 2000).

Analgesia There are no linked PK–PD studies investigating NSAID analgesia in neonates or infants. Pain relief attributable to NSAIDs has been compared to pain relief from other analgesics or analgesic modalities, e.g. caudal blockade (Ryhanen et al. 1994, Splinter et al. 1997), acetaminophen (Walson et al. 1989, Baer et al. 1992, Watcha et al. 1992, Van Esch et al. 1995, Bertin et al. 1996, Bennie et al. 1997, Johnson et al. 1997, Goyal et al. 1998, Davies and Skjodt 2000, Romsing et al. 2001, Tawalbeh et al. 2001, Figueras Nadal et al. 2002, Pickering et al. 2002, Purssell 2002) and morphine (Munro et al. 1994, Vetter and Heiner 1994, Gunter et al. 1995, Morton and O'Brien 1999, Oztekin et al. 2002) in children. These data confirm that NSAIDs in children are effective analgesic drugs, improving the quality of analgesia, but they do not quantify the effect. It is not possible to develop an understanding of the dose–effect relationship from these data, nor is it possible to determine if equipotent doses are being compared. The effectiveness of these medications in neonates, infants and children is unknown. NSAID concentration–response relationships have been described for adults (Mandema and Stanski 1996, Suri et al. 1997, Boni et al. 1999a). Mandema and Stanski (1996) studied patients ($n = 522$) given a single oral or intramuscular administration of placebo or a single intramuscular dose of 10, 30, 60 or 90 mg ketorolac for postoperative pain relief after ortho-paedic surgery. Pain relief was found to be a function of drug concentration (Emax model), time (waxing and waning of placebo effect), and an individual random effect. The Emax, EC_{50} and Teq were 8.5 (with a possible maximum of 10), 0.37 mg/L and 24 minutes respectively.

PDA closure Both indometacin and ibuprofen are used to expedite PDA closure in premature neonates

by inhibiting prostaglandin synthesis, namely PGE2 (Van Overmeire et al. 2000, 2001, Shaffer et al. 2002). Smyth et al. suggested a serum concentration of 0.4 mg/L 24 h after the last dose of indometacin in 35 infants (gestational age 25–34 weeks; postnatal age 1–77 days) was associated with PDA closure (Smyth et al. 2004). Shaffer et al. (2002) examined factors affecting PDA closure after indometacin treatment in poor responders – neonates <1000 g and/or ≥10 days postnatal age. Closure appears dependent on a critical pre-dose serum concentration of 1.9 mg/L in neonates <10 days of age and 1.4 mg/L in neonates ≥10 days age. Dose and duration of treatment were increased in the older group, which was assumed to be due to increased clearance.

Pharmacokinetics

Pharmacokinetic age-related changes and covariate effects are poorly documented for many of the NSAIDs (Litalien and Jacqz-Aigrain 2001). There is a paucity of data in infants less than 6 months of age.

NSAIDs are rapidly absorbed in the gastrointestinal tract after oral administration in children. Time to maximal concentration is generally 1–2 h, but de-pends on formulation and concomitant food intake (Troconiz et al. 2000). The relative bioavailability of oral preparations approaches 1 compared to intra-venous. The rate and extent of absorption after rectal administration of NSAIDs such as ibuprofen, diclofenac, flurbiprofen, indometacin and nimesulide are less than oral routes (van Hoogdalem et al. 1991b).

NSAID PK is usually described using a one-compartment, first-order elimination model. Clearance is reduced in neonates and increases with age. The linear per kilogram model has been used to describe ibuprofen clearance. Clearance increases from 2.06 ml/h/kg at 22–31 weeks PCA (Aranda et al. 1997), 9.49 ml/h/kg at 28 weeks PCA (Van Overmeire et al. 2001) to 140 ml/kg/min at 5 years (Scott et al. 1999a). Similar data are reported for indometacin (Olkkola et al. 1989, Wiest et al. 1991, Smyth et al. 2004).

The apparent volume of distribution (V/F) is small in adults (<0.2 L/kg, suggesting minimal tissue binding) but is larger in children, e.g. ketorolac V/F in children 4–8 years is twice that of adults (Olkkola and Maunuksela 1991, Forrest et al. 1997). Premature neonates (22–31 weeks gestational age) given intra-venous ibuprofen had a V/F of 0.62 (SD 0.04) L/kg (Aranda et al. 1997). Van Overmeire et al. (2001) report a dramatic reduction in ibuprofen central volume (Vc/F) following closure of the PDA in prema-ture neonates (0.244 vs. 0.171 L/kg). The NSAIDs, as a group, are weakly acidic, lipophilic and highly protein bound. Compared to adults the bound fraction is high in children (e.g. etodolac, 93.9 vs. 95.5%) (Boni et al. 1999b) and premature neonates (e.g. ibuprofen, 94.9 vs. 98.7%) (Aranda et al. 1997). The impact of this reduced protein binding is probably minimal with routine dosing because NSAIDs cleared by the liver have a low hepatic extraction ratio (Benet and Hoener 2002). In addition, they have a long equilibration time between plasma and effect compartments (Benet and Hoener 2002).

NSAIDs undergo extensive phase 1 and phase 2 enzyme biotransformation in the liver, with subsequent excretion into urine or bile. The impact of enterohepatic circulation in neonates is unknown. Hepatic NSAID elimination is dependent on the free fraction of NSAID within the plasma and the intrinsic enzyme activities of the liver. Renal elimination is not an important elimination pathway for the commonly used NSAIDs. Pharmacokinetic parameter estimate variability is large, partly attributable to covariate effects of age, size and pharmacogenomics. Ibuprofen, for example, is metabolized by the CYP2C9 and CYP2C8 subfamilies (Gal et al. 1990, Touw 1997). It is known that considerable variation exists in the expression of CYP2C activities among individuals, and functional polymorphism of the gene coding for CYP2C9 has been described (Hamman et al. 1997). CYP2C9 activity is low immediately after birth, subsequently increasing progressively to peak activity at a young age, when expressed as mg/kg/h (Tanaka 1998).

NSAID elimination is all too frequently described only in terms of half-life, which is therefore confounded by volume of distribution. The plasma half-lives of NSAIDs in adults range from 0.25 to >70 h, indicating wide differences in clearance. Elimination half-lives are longer in neonates than children. An elimination half-life of 30.5 (SD 4.2) h was reported in premature infants receiving ibuprofen within the first 12 hours of life (Aranda et al. 1997), in contrast with 1.6 (SD 0.7) h in infants and children aged 3 months to 10 years (Kelley et al. 1992). Clearance increases from birth, but reported estimates are confounded by age and weight (Wiest et al. 1991). There are no longitudinal studies describing postnatal maturation from different gestational ages. Clearance (L/h/kg) is generally increased in childhood compared to adult values both for the established NSAIDs (Korpela and Olkkola 1990, Bertin et al. 1991, Olkkola and Maunuksela 1991, Brown et al. 1992, Ugazio et al. 1993, Gonzalez-Martin et al. 1997, Kauffman et al. 1999) and for the newer COX-2 inhibitors (Stempak et al. 2002), as we might expect when the per kilogram model is used.

Many NSAIDs exhibit stereoselectivity. Ketorolac, for example, is supplied and administered as a racemic mixture that contains a 1:1 ratio of the R(+) and S(−) stereoisomers. Pharmacologic activity resides almost exclusively with the S(−) stereoisomer. Clearance of the S(−) enantiomer was four times that of the R(+) enantiomer (6.2 vs. 1.4 ml/min/kg) in children 3–18 years (Kauffman et al. 1999) and the apparent volume of distribution of the S(−) enantiomer was greater than that of the R(+) form (0.82 vs. 0.50 L/kg). Because of the greater clearance and shorter half-life of S(−)-ketorolac, pharmacokinetic predictions based on racemic assays may overestimate the duration of pharmacologic effect. Selective glucuronidation of the S(−) enantiomer suggests that stereoselective metabolism may also be a contributing factor (Kauffman et al. 1999). Ibuprofen stereoselectivity is also reported in premature neonates (<28 weeks gestation). R- and S-ibuprofen half-lives were about 10 h and 25.5 h, respectively. The mean clearance of R-ibuprofen (CLR = 12.7 mL/h) was about 2.5-fold higher than for S-ibuprofen (CLS = 5.0 mL/h) (Gregoire et al. 2004).

There is relatively little transfer from maternal to fetal blood. Excretion of NSAIDs into breast milk of lactating mothers is low. Infant exposure to ketorolac via breast milk is estimated to be 0.4% of the maternal exposure (Brocks and Jamali 1992).

Drug interactions

NSAIDs undergo drug interactions through altered clearance and competition for active renal tubular secretion with other organic acids. High protein binding among the NSAIDs has been used to explain drug interactions with oral anticoagulant agents, oral hypoglycaemics, sulfonamides, bilirubin and other protein-bound drugs. An influential paper by Aggeler et al. (1967) showed that warfarin administered with phenylbutazone increased plasma warfarin concentrations and prothrombin time in normal volunteers. Phenylbutazone displaces warfarin from its albumin-binding sites in vitro but this observation should not be extrapolated to explain changes in prothrombin time. The observed effect is due to changes in drug metabolic clearance and not from changes in protein binding (Benet and Hoener 2002).

Ibuprofen reduced the glomerular filtration rate by 20% in premature neonates, affecting aminoglycoside clearance, and this effect appears independent of gestational age (Allegaert et al. 2004, 2005b). No significant difference in the change in cerebral blood volume, change in cerebral blood flow, or tissue oxygenation index was found between administration of ibuprofen or placebo in neonates (Naulaers et al. 2005).

Safety issues

The most common adverse events in NSAID recipients are nausea, dizziness and headache. NSAIDs have potential to cause gastrointestinal irritation, blood clotting disorders, renal impairment, neutrophil dysfunction and bronchoconstriction (Kam and See 2000, Simon et al. 2002) – effects postulated to be related to COX-1/COX-2 ratios, although this concept may be an oversimplification (Lipsky et al. 2000, Brater et al. 2001, McCrory and Lindahl 2002).

Renal effects The effect of short-term treatment with NSAIDs on healthy kidneys is negligible in adults (Lesko and Mitchell 1995, 1997, 1999) and children (Szer et al. 1991, Houck et al. 1996, Flato et al. 1998). Renal dysfunction also occurs in children compromised by dehydration, hypovolaemia, hypotension or pre-existing renal disease (Ray et al. 1988, van Biljon 1989, Buck and Norwood 1996, Forrest et al. 1997, Primack et al. 1997, Moghal et al. 1998). NSAIDs may potentiate the toxicity of other drugs such as aminoglycosides and cyclosporin (Sheiner et al. 1994, Kovesi et al. 1998) and may reduce renal blood flow in preterm neonates (Shah and Ohlsson 2006).

Gastrointestinal effects Adverse gastrointestinal (GI) effects are significant in adults, particularly in those with peptic ulcer disease, *H. pylori* or advanced age (Bombardier et al. 2000, Feldman and McMahon 2000, Silverstein et al. 2000). The risk of acute GI bleeding in children given short-term ibuprofen was estimated to be 7.2/100 000 (CI 2–18/100 000) (Lesko and Mitchell 1995, 1999) and was not different from those children given acetaminophen. The incidence of clinically significant gastropathy is comparable to adults in children given NSAIDs for juvenile idiopathic arthritis (JIA) (Dowd et al. 1995, Keenan et al. 1995), but gastro-duodenal injury may be very much higher (75%) depending on assessment criteria (e.g. abdominal pain, anaemia, endoscopy) (Mulberg et al. 1993). Similar data for neonates are not available.

Bleeding propensity The commonly used NSAIDs such as ketorolac, diclofenac, ibuprofen and ketoprofen have reversible antiplatelet effects, which are attributable to the inhibition of thromboxane synthesis. This side effect is of concern during the perioperative period (Souter et al. 1994, Rusy et al. 1995). Bleeding time is usually slightly increased, but it remains within normal limits in children with normal coagulation systems (Bean-Lijewski and Hunt 1996, Niemi et al. 1997, 2000). Neonates given prophylactic idometacin to induce PDA closure did not have an increased frequency of intraventricular haemorrhage (Ment et al. 1994).

Opioid analgesic drugs

Morphine

Morphine is obtained from the poppy, *Papaver somniferum*, and is the most commonly used opioid in neonates, infants and children. Morphine's main analgesic effect is by µ-receptor activation (Matthes et al. 1996, Sora et al. 1997, Loh et al. 1998). Morphine (named after the Greek God of dreams, Morpheus) is soluble in water, but lipid solubility is poor compared with other opioids. Morphine's low oil/water partition coefficient of 1.4 and its pKa of 8 (10–20% unionized drug at physiologic pH) contribute to delayed onset of peak action with slow penetration into the brain. Morphine is available as elixir, immediate-release tablets, slow-release tablets or granules and parenteral formulations, as the sulphate or hydrochloride salt.

Pharmacodynamics Target analgesic plasma concentrations are believed to be 10–20 ng/ml after major surgery in neonates and infants (Kart et al. 1997b, Lynn et al. 1998, Bouwmeester et al. 2001, 2004). The concentration required for sedation during mechanical ventilation may be higher. Mean morphine concentrations of 125 ng/ml were required to produce adequate sedation in 50% of neonates (Chay et al. 1992). The large pharmacokinetic and pharmacodynamic variability means that morphine is often titrated to effect using small incremental doses (0.02 mg/kg) in neonates and infants suffering postoperative pain (Anderson et al. 1999). The effect compartment equilibration half-time (Teq) for morphine is ~17 min in adults (Inturrisi and Colburn 1986) and can be predicted for younger age groups, based on allometric modelling (Table 9.1) (Anderson et al. 2002).

The principal metabolites of morphine, morphine-3-glucuronide (M3G) and morphine-6-glucuronide (M6G), have pharmacologic activity. M6G has greater analgesic potency than morphine (Osborne et al. 2000, Murthy et al. 2002) and also respiratory depressive effects (Osborne et al. 1992, Thompson et al. 1995). It has been suggested that M3G antagonizes morphine and M6G has antinociceptive and respiratory depressive effects (Smith et al. 1990, Gong et al. 1992) and contributes to the development of tolerance.

Pharmacokinetics Morphine is mainly metabolized by the hepatic enzyme uridine-5′-diphosphate glucuronosyl transferase-2B7 (UGT2B7) into M3G and M6G (Coffman et al. 1997, Faura et al. 1998). M6G/morphine ratios increase with age from 0.8 in neonates to 4.2 in children (Smith et al. 1990, Barrett et al. 1996). These ratio changes are attributed to the maturation of hepatic and renal clearance with age, but the clinical effect of these ratio changes is probably minimal in the neonate. Reduced morphine clearance and receptor numbers (opioid, GABA, acetylcholine) in the neonate are postulated to have greater impact on pain perception (Coyle and Campochiaro 1976).

Morphine sulphation is a minor metabolic pathway (Choonara et al. 1990, McRorie et al. 1992). Clearance

Table 9.1 Morphine clearance changes with age

Age	Vd (L/70 kg)	CL (L/h/kg)	CL$_{std}$ (L/h/70 kg)	Teq (min)
24–27 weeks		0.136	3.378 (47)	
28–31 weeks		0.193	5.07 (49)	
Term neonate	84	0.44	14.5	8
3 months	131	1.14	43.1	
6 months	136	1.43	57.3	
1 year	136	1.57	67.8	10
3 year	136	1.51	71.1	
Adult	136	1.01	71.1	17

Note: The increased clearance (L/h/kg) observed during infancy is a size artifact. Clearance reaches adult levels (equivalent to hepatic blood flow) using an allometric size model (L/h/70 kg) by the end of infancy. Data from Bouwmeester et al. (2003). Premature neonatal data from Scott et al. (1999b). Predictions using the allometric model are similar to those observed by Lynn et al. (1998) and McRorie et al. (1992). The effect compartment equilibration half-time (Teq) adult data are from Inturrisi and Colburn (1986) and the predictions based on allometric modelling (Anderson and Meakin 2002). Vd = volume of distribution at steady state.

is perfusion limited with a high hepatic extraction ratio. Oral bioavailability is ~35% due to this first pass effect. The metabolites are cleared renally and partly by biliary excretion (McRorie et al. 1992). Some recirculation of morphine occurs due to gastro-intestinal β-glucuronidase activity (Koren and Maurice 1989). Impaired renal function leads to M3G and M6G accumulation (Choonara et al. 1989).

Fetuses are capable of metabolizing morphine from 15 weeks' gestation (Pacifici et al. 1982, 1989). Morphine clearance matures with postconceptual age (Kart et al. 1997a, Faura et al. 1998) reaching adult values at 6–12 months (Anderson et al. 1997, van Lingen et al. 2002). The increased clearance observed in children, when expressed per kilogram, is a size artifact and not attributable to this age group's increased liver size (Table 9.1 and Figure 9.3). Pharmacokinetics in children have been described: volume of distribution 136 L/70 kg (%CV, 59.3), formation clearance to M3G 64.3 (58.8) L/h/70 kg, formation clearance to M6G 3.63 (82.2) L/h/70 kg, morphine clearance by other routes 3.12 L/h/70 kg, elimination clearance of M3G 17.4 (43.0) L/h/70 kg, elimination clearance of M6G 5.8 (73.8) L/h/70 kg. The volume of distribution increased exponentially with a maturation half-life of 26 days from 83 L/70 kg at birth; formation clearance to M3G and M6G in-creased with a maturation half-life of 88.3 days from 10.8 and 0.61 L/h/70 kg respectively at birth. Metabolite clearance increased with age (maturation half-life 129 days) similar to that described for glomerular filtration rate (GFR) maturation in infants. M3G elimination clearance is greater than GFR,

suggesting tubular secretion and non-renal elimination (Bouwmeester et al. 2003).

Morphine pharmacokinetic parameters show large inter-individual variability contributing to the range of morphine serum concentrations observed during constant infusion. Clinical circumstances, such as type of surgery and concurrent illness (McRorie et al. 1992, Pokela et al. 1993, Lynn et al. 1998) also influence morphine pharmacokinetics. Protein binding of morphine is low (from 20% in premature neonates (Bhat et al. 1992, McRorie et al. 1992) to 35% in adults) (Olsen 1975) but has minimal impact on disposition changes with age.

Side effects and tolerance Respiratory depression may occur at concentrations of 20 ng/ml and is similar in children aged from 2 to 570 days at the same morphine concentration (Lynn et al. 1993). Intrathecal dosing causes similar respiratory depression at similar cerebrospinal fluid (CSF) concentrations in children 4 months to 15 years (Nichols et al. 1993). Hypo-tension, bradycardia and flushing reflect morphine's histamine-releasing property and are associated with rapid intravenous bolus administration (Anand et al. 2000). The incidence of vomiting in postoperative children is related to morphine dose. Doses above 0.1 mg/kg were associated with a greater than 50% incidence of vomiting (Weinstein et al. 1994, Anderson et al. 2000b).

Withdrawal symptoms are observed in neonates after cessation of continuous morphine infusion for greater than 2 weeks and possibly shorter periods if doses >40 µg/kg/h are administered. Prevention strategies include the use of neuraxial analgesia, nurse-controlled sedation management protocols, ketamine or naloxone infused concurrently with morphine infusion and the use of alternate agents (e.g. methadone) with lower potential for tolerance (Suresh and Anand 1998, 2001).

Fentanyl

Fentanyl offers greater haemodynamic stability than morphine (Hickey et al. 1985, Yaster et al. 1987,), rapid onset (Teq = 6.6 min) and short duration of effect. Its relative increased lipid solubility and small molecular conformation enables efficient penetration of the BBB and redistribution.

Pharmacodynamics Fentanyl is a potent μ-receptor agonist with a potency 70–125 times that of morphine. A plasma concentration of 15–30 ng/ml is required to provide total intravenous anaesthesia in adults, while the IC_{50}, based on EEG evidence, is 10 ng/ml (Wynands et al. 1983, Scott and Stanski 1987). The intra-operative use of fentanyl 3 μg/kg in infants did not result in respiratory depression or hypoxaemia in a placebo controlled trial (Barrier et al. 1989). Only three out of 2000 non-intubated infants and children experienced short apnoeic episodes after fentanyl 2–3 μg/kg for the repair of facial lacerations (Billmire et al. 1985). Fentanyl has similar respiratory depression in infants and adults when the plasma concentrations are similar (Hertzka et al. 1989).

Pharmacokinetics Fentanyl is metabolized by oxidative N-dealkylation (CYP3A4) into nor-fentanyl and hydroxylized (Tateishi et al. 1996, Labroo et al. 1997). All metabolites are inactive and a small amount of fentanyl is renally eliminated unmetabolized (Jacqz-Aigrain and Burtin 1996). Fentanyl clearance is 70–80% of adult values in term neonates and, standardized to a 70-kg person, reaches adult values (approx. 50 L/h/70 kg) within the first 2 weeks of life (Koehntop et al. 1986, Gauntlett et al. 1988, Anderson et al. 1997). The increased clearance observed in infancy, when expressed per kilogram, is most likely an artifact of the linear per kg model rather than a postulated increase in hepatic blood flow in this age group. Volume of distribution at steady state (Vss) for fentanyl is ~5.9 L/kg in term neonates and decreases with age to 4.5 L/kg during infancy, 3.1 L/kg during childhood, and 1.6 L/kg in adults (Johnson et al. 1984). Fentanyl clearance may be impaired with decreased hepatic blood flow, e.g. from increased intra-abdominal pressure in neonatal omphalocele repair (Gauntlett et al. 1988).

Fentanyl is widely distributed with short duration of effect due to redistribution to deep, lipid-rich compartments. Fentanyl redistributes slowly from lipid-rich tissues after discontinuation of therapy, resulting in prolonged periods of sedation and respiratory depression (Koehntop et al. 1986). The context-sensitive half-time after 1 h infusion is ~20 min but, after 8 h is 270 min (Hughes et al. 1992).

Side effects Tolerance to synthetic opioids develops more rapidly (3–5 days) compared to morphine (2 weeks) and heroin (>2 weeks) (Arnold et al. 1991, Franck et al. 1998, Chana and Anand 2001). Fentanyl also has a propensity for muscular rigidity (Taddio 2002). Other drugs metabolized by CYP3A4 (e.g. cyclosporin, erythromycin) may compete for clearance and increase fentanyl plasma concentrations (Touw 1997, Tanaka 1998).

The respiratory depression caused by fentanyl (hours) may outlast its analgesic effect (35–45 min) due to the prolonged context-sensitive half-life and/or recirculation of fentanyl bound to the stomach's acid medium (up to 20% of an IV dose) or delayed release from peripheral compartments (Stoeckel et al. 1979, Bjorkman et al. 1990).

Non-opioid analgesics

Tramadol

Tramadol is a moderately potent analgesic (Bamigbade and Langford 1998, Turturro et al. 1998). It is an analogue of codeine and its analgesic effect is mediated through norepinephrine re-uptake inhibition, both increased release and decreased re-uptake of serotonin in the spinal cord and a weak μ-opioid receptor effect (Poulsen et al. 1996, Bamigbade and Langford 1998, De Witte et al. 2001, Stamer and Stuber 2001).

Pharmacodynamics Tramadol's affinity for opioid receptors is ~6000 times weaker than morphine, but the active o-demethyltramadol (+)-M1 metabolite has an affinity ~200 times greater than tramadol (Poulsen et al. 1996), thus mediating tramadol-attributed opioid effects. Both the μ-receptor effect and reduced serotonin uptake in descending spinal cord pathways may contribute to its emetic effect. A serum tramadol concentration above 100 ng/ml is associated with satisfactory postoperative analgesia after dental surgery (Payne et al. 2002). A higher target tramadol concentration of 300 μg/L has been suggested in adult patients given fentanyl 5 μg/kg intra-operatively or 600 (590) μg/L in adults not given other supplementary analgesics (Grond and Sablotzki 2004).

Pharmacokinetics The (+)-M1 is formed via the genetically polymorphic CYP2D6 iso-enzyme system responsible for codeine metabolism (Poulsen et al. 1996) and individuals may be classified as extensive or poor metabolizers of tramadol. Higher concentrations of the (+)-M1 metabolite and greater analgesic efficacy of tramadol are reported in extensive metabolizers with reduced nausea, vomiting and tiredness amongst poor metabolizers (Poulsen et al. 1996). CYP2D6 activity has been observed in premature neonates as early as 25 weeks PCA (Allegaert et al. 2005a).

Tramadol clearance in neonates has been described using a two-compartment, zero-order input, first-order elimination linear model (Allegaert et al. 2005a). Clearance increased from 25 weeks postconception age (PCA) (5.52 L/h/70 kg) to reach 84% of the mature values (24 (CV 43.6%) L/h/70 kg) by 44 weeks PCA (standardized to a 70 kg person using allometric '1/4 power' models). The mature value is similar to that described by others in older children and adults (Murthy et al. 2000, Payne et al. 2002). Central volume of distribution decreased from 25 weeks PCA (256 L/70 kg) to reach 120% of its mature value by 87 weeks PCA. Formation clearance to M1 contributed to 43% of the tramadol clearance (Allegaert et al. 2005a).

Side effects Tramadol's adverse effect profile includes nausea, vomiting, constipation, dizziness, somnolence, fatigue, sweating and pruritus. Tramadol has a greatly reduced potential for sedation, respiratory depression (<0.5% in children and neonates) (Bosenberg and Ratcliffe 1998) and dependence compared to conventional opioids (Broome et al. 1999). Tramadol is associated with a high incidence of postoperative nausea and vomiting (PONV) in adults and children (up to 50%) limiting its usefulness (Pang et al. 1999, 2000, van den Berg et al. 1999, Torres et al. 2001). PONV is generally managed with the anti-emetic, ondansetron. Ondansetron is a serotonin antagonist (anti 5-HT$_3$) and the CYP2D6 iso-enzyme is also involved in the metabolism of ondansetron. Thus, concurrent use results in a mutual reduction of effect – tramadol less potent as an analgesic and ondansetron less effective as an anti-emetic. Tramadol does not cause histamine release, but its use has been associated with seizures (Tobias 1997, Gibson 1996).

Ketamine

The analgesic properties of ketamine are mediated by multiple mechanisms at central and peripheral sites. The contribution from N-methyl-D-aspartate (NMDA) receptor antagonism and interactions with cholinergic, adrenergic, serotonergic, opioid pathways and local anaesthetic effects remain to be fully elucidated.

Pharmacodynamics Ketamine is available as a mixture of two enantiomers – the S(+)-enantiomer has four times the potency of the R(–)-entantiomer (Geisslinger et al. 1993). S(+)-ketamine has approximately twice the potency of the racemate. The metabolite norketamine has a potency one-third that of its parent (Leung and Baillie 1986). Plasma concentrations associated with hypnosis and amnesia during surgery are 0.8–4 µg/ml; awakening usually occurs at concentrations lower than 0.5 µg/ml. Pain thresholds are elevated at 0.1 µg/ml (Grant et al. 1983).

Pharmacokinetics Ketamine has high lipid solubility with rapid distribution. Ketamine undergoes N-demethylation to form norketamine. Racemic ketamine elimination is complicated by R(–)-ketamine inhibiting the elimination of S(+)-ketamine (Ihmsen et al. 2001). Clearance in children is similar to adult rates (80 L/h/70 kg, i.e. liver blood flow) within the first 6 months of life, when corrected for size using allometric models (Cook and Davis 1993, Anderson et al. 1997). Clearance in the neonate is reduced (26 L/h/70 kg) (Cook and Davis 1993, Hartvig et al. 1993). Vss decreases with age, from 3.46 L/kg at birth, to 3.03 L/kg in infancy, 1.18 L/kg at 4 years age, and 0.75 L/kg in adulthood (Cook and Davis 1993). There is a high hepatic extraction ratio and the relative bioavailability of nasal and rectal formulations were 50% and 30% respectively (Pedraz et al. 1989, Malinovsky et al. 1996).

Side effects Psycholergic emergence reactions can cause distress, but are not problematic under 5 years of age. These can be ameliorated by the benzodiazepines. An antisialagogue may be required to diminish copious secretions (Hollister and Burn 1974). Tolerance in children was described following the repeated use of ketamine (Byer and Gould 1981).

CONCLUSIONS

Neonates and infants are very different from adults. Their psychology, social structure, behaviour and disease spectrum are different. Growth and developmental aspects account for major pharmacokinetic differences between children and adults. Body size accounts for most of the pharmacokinetic differences between older children and adults. Additional differences in neonates and infants are largely attributable to developmental changes, which can be described by gestational age. Pharmacodynamic factors that may influence the clinical response to analgesics in early life remain poorly defined.

REFERENCES

Adolph EF. (1949). Quantitative relations in the physiological constitutions of animals. Science 109: 579–585.

Aggeler PM, O'Reilly RA, Leong L et al. (1967). Potentiation of anticoagulant effect of warfarin by phenylbutazone. New Engl J Med 276: 496–501.

Alam SN, Roberts RJ, Fischer LJ. (1977). Age-related differences in salicylamide and acetaminophen conjugation in man. J Pediatr 90: 130–135.

Allegaert K, Cossey V, Langhendries JP, et al. (2004). Effects of co-administration of ibuprofen-lysine on the pharmacokinetics of amikacin in preterm infants during the first days of life. Biol Neonate 86: 207–211.

Allegaert K, Anderson BJ, Verbesselt R, et al. (2005a). Tramadol disposition in the very young: an attempt to assess in vivo cytochrome P-450 2D6 activity. Br J Anaesth 95: 231–239.

Allegaert K, Cossey V, Debeer A, et al. (2005b). The impact of ibuprofen on renal clearance in preterm infants is independent of the gestational age. Pediatr Nephrol 20: 740–743.

Anand KJS, Stevens BJ, McGrath PJ. (2000). Systemic analgesic therapy. Elsevier, Amsterdam.

Anderson BJ, Hansen TG. (2004). Getting the best from pediatric pharmacokinetic data. Paediatr Anaesth 14: 713–715.

Anderson BJ, Meakin GH. (2002). Scaling for size: some implications for paediatric anaesthesia dosing. Paediatr Anaesth 12: 205–219.

Anderson BJ, McKee AD, Holford NH. (1997). Size, myths and the clinical pharmacokinetics of analgesia in paediatric patients. Clin Pharmacokinet 33: 313–327.

Anderson BJ, Persson M, Anderson M. (1999). Rationalising intravenous morphine prescriptions in children. Acute Pain 2: 59–67.

Anderson BJ, Pearce S, McGann JE, et al. (2000a). Investigations using logistic regression models on the effect of the LMA on morphine induced vomiting after tonsillectomy. Paediatr Anaesth 10: 633–638.

Anderson BJ, Ralph CJ, Stewart AW, et al. (2000b). The dose–effect relationship for morphine and vomiting after day-stay tonsillectomy in children. Anaesth Intensive Care 28: 155–160.

Anderson BJ, Woollard GA, Holford NH. (2000c). A model for size and age changes in the pharmacokinetics of paracetamol in neonates, infants and children. Br J Clin Pharmacol 50: 125–134.

Anderson BJ, Woollard GA, Holford NH. (2001). Acetaminophen analgesia in children: placebo effect and pain resolution after tonsillectomy. Eur J Clin Pharmacol 57: 559–569.

Anderson BJ, van Lingen RA, Hansen TG, et al. (2002). Acetaminophen developmental pharmacokinetics in premature neonates and infants: a pooled population analysis. Anesthesiology 96: 1336–1345.

Anderson BJ, Pons G, Autret-Leca E, et al. (2005). Pediatric intravenous paracetamol (propacetamol) pharmacokinetics: a population analysis. Paediatr Anaesth 15: 282–292.

Aranda JV, Varvarigou A, Beharry K, et al. (1997). Pharmacokinetics and protein binding of intravenous ibuprofen in the premature newborn infant. Acta Paediatr 86: 289–293.

Arant BS Jr. (1978). Developmental patterns of renal functional maturation compared in the human neonate. J Pediatr 92: 705–712.

Arendt Nielsen L, Nielsen JC, Bjerring P. (1991). Double-blind, placebo controlled comparison of paracetamol and paracetamol plus codeine – a quantitative evaluation by laser induced pain. Eur J Clin Pharmacol 40: 241–247.

Arnold JH, Truog RD, Scavone JM, et al. (1991). Changes in the pharmacodynamic response to fentanyl in neonates during continuous infusion. J Pediatr 119: 639–643.

Audenaert SM, Wagner Y, Montgomery CL, et al. (1995). Cardiorespiratory effects of premedication for children. Anesth Analg 80: 506–510.

Baer GA, Rorarius MG, Kolehmainen S, et al. (1992). The effect of paracetamol or diclofenac administered before operation on postoperative pain and behaviour after adenoidectomy in small children. Anaesthesia 47: 1078–1080.

Bamigbade TA, Langford RM. (1998). Tramadol hydrochloride: an overview of current use. Hosp Med 59: 373–376.

Banavar JR. (1999). Size and form in efficient transportation networks. Nature 399: 130–132.

Barrett DA, Barker DP, Rutter N, et al. (1996). Morphine, morphine-6-glucuronide and morphine-3-glucuronide pharmacokinetics in newborn infants receiving diamorphine infusions. Br J Clin Pharmacol 41: 531–537.

Barrier G, Attia J, Mayer MN, et al. (1989). Measurement of post-operative pain and narcotic administration in infants using a new clinical scoring system. Intensive Care Med 15:, S37–39.

Bean-Lijewski JD, Hunt RD. (1996). Effect of ketorolac on bleeding time and postoperative pain in children: a double-blind, placebo-controlled comparison with meperidine. J Clin Anesth 8: 25–30.

Benet LZ, Hoener BA, et al. (2002). Changes in plasma protein binding have little clinical relevance. Clin Pharmacol Ther 71: 115–121.

Bennie RE, Boehringer LA, McMahon S, et al. (1997). Postoperative analgesia with preoperative oral ibuprofen or acetaminophen in children undergoing myringotomy. Paediatr Anaesth 7: 399–403.

Berde C. (1992). Convulsions associated with pediatric regional anesthesia. Anesth Analg 75: 164–166.

Bertin L, Rey E, Pons G, et al. (1991) Pharmacokinetics of tiaprofenic acid in children after a single oral dose. Eur J Clin Pharmacol 41: 251–253.

Bertin L, Pons G, d'Athis P, et al. (1996) A randomized, double-blind, multicentre controlled trial of ibuprofen versus acetaminophen and placebo for symptoms of acute otitis media in children. Fundam Clin Pharmacol 10: 387–392.

Bhat R, Abu-Harb M, Chari G, et al. (1992). Morphine metabolism in acutely ill preterm newborn infants. J Pediatr 120: 795–799.

Billmire DA, Neale HW, Gregory RO. (1985). Use of i.v. fentanyl in the outpatient treatment of pediatric facial trauma. J Trauma 25: 1079–1080.

Birmingham PK, Tobin MJ, Henthorn TK, et al. (1997). Twenty-four-hour pharmacokinetics of rectal acetaminophen in children: an old drug with new recommendations. Anesthesiology 87: 244–252.

Bjorkman R. (1995). Central antinociceptive effects of non-steroidal anti-inflammatory drugs and paracetamol. Experimental studies in the rat. Acta Anaesthesiol Scand Suppl 103: 1–44.

Bjorkman S, Stanski DR, Verotta D, et al. (1990). Comparative tissue concentration profiles of fentanyl and alfentanil in humans predicted from tissue/blood partition data obtained in rats. Anesthesiology 72: 865–873.

Bjorkman R, Hallman KM, Hedner J, et al. (1994). Acetaminophen blocks spinal hyperalgesia induced by NMDA and substance P. Pain 57: 259–264.

Bombardier C, Laine L, Reicin A, et al. (2000). Comparison of upper gastrointestinal toxicity of rofecoxib and naproxen in patients with rheumatoid arthritis. VIGOR Study Group. N Engl J Med 343: 1520–1528.

Boni J, Korth-Bradley J, McGoldrick K, et al. (1999a). Pharmacokinetic and pharmacodynamic action of etodolac in patients after oral surgery. J Clin Pharmacol 39: 729–737.

Boni JP, Korth-Bradley JM, Martin P, et al. (1999b). Pharmacokinetics of etodolac in patients with stable juvenile rheumatoid arthritis. Clin Ther 21: 1715–1724.

Bosenberg AT, Ratcliffe S. (1998). The respiratory effects of tramadol in children under halothane an anaesthesia. Anaesthesia 53: 960–964.

Bouwmeester NJ, Anand KJS, van Dijk M, et al. (2001). Hormonal and metabolic stress responses after major surgery in children aged 0–3 years: a double-blind, randomized trial comparing the effects of continuous versus intermittent morphine. Br J Anaesth 87: 390–399.

Bouwmeester NJ, van den Anker JN, Hop WC, et al. (2003). Age- and therapy-related effects on morphine requirements and plasma concentrations of morphine and its metabolites in postoperative infants. Br J Anaesth 90: 642–652.

Bouwmeester NJ, Anderson BJ, Tibboel D, et al. (2004). Developmental pharmacokinetics of morphine and its metabolites in neonates, infants and young children. Br J Anaesth 92: 208–217.

Boxenbaum H. (1982). Interspecies scaling, allometry, physiological time, and the ground plan of pharmacokinetics. J Pharmacokinet Biopharm 10: 201–227.

Boxenbaum H, DiLea C. (1995). First-time-in-human dose selection: allometric thoughts and perspectives. J Clin Pharmacol 35: 957–966.

Brater DC, Harris C, Redfern JS, et al. (2001). Renal effects of COX-2-selective inhibitors. Am J Nephrol 21: 1–15.

Brocks DR, Jamali F. (1992). Clinical pharmacokinetics of ketorolac tromethamine. Clin Pharmacokinet 23: 415–427.

Brody S, Proctor RC, Ashworth US. (1934). Basal metabolism, endogenous nitrogen, creatinine, and sulphur excretions as functions of body weight. Univ Mo Agric Exp Sta Res Bull 220: 1–40.

Brooks-Kayal AR, Pritchett DB. (1993). Developmental changes in human gamma-aminobutyric acidA receptor subunit composition. Ann Neurol 34: 687–693.

Broome IJ, Robb HM, Raj N, et al. (1999). The use of tramadol following day-case oral surgery. Anaesthesia 54: 289–292.

Brown RD, Wilson JT, Kearns GL, et al. (1992). Single-dose pharmacokinetics of ibuprofen and acetaminophen in febrile children. J Clin Pharmacol 32: 231–241.

Buck ML, Norwood VF. (1996). Ketorolac-induced acute renal failure in a previously healthy adolescent. Pediatrics 98: 294–296.

Byer DE, Gould AB Jr. (1981). Development of tolerance to ketamine in an infant undergoing repeated anesthesia. Anesthesiology 54: 255–256.

Carlos MA, Babyn PS, Marcon MA, et al. (1997). Changes in gastric emptying in early postnatal life. J Pediatr 130: 931–937.

Carry MR, Ringel SP, Starcevich JM. (1986). Distribution of capillaries in normal and diseased human skeletal muscle. Muscle Nerve 9: 445–454.

Catzel P, Olver R. (1981). Paediatric prescriber. Blackwell, Oxford.

Chana SK, Anand KJ. (2001). Can we use methadone for analgesia in neonates? Arch Dis Child Fetal Neonatal Ed 85: F79–81.

Chay PC, Duffy BJ, Walker JS. (1992). Pharmacokinetic–pharmacodynamic relationships of morphine in neonates. Clin Pharmacol Ther 51: 334–342.

Choonara IA, McKay P, Hain R, et al. (1989). Morphine metabolism in children. Br J Clin Pharmacol 28: 599–604.

Choonara I, Ekbom Y, Lindstrom B, et al. (1990). Morphine sulphation in children. Br J Clin Pharmacol 30: 897–900.

Chugani DC, Muzik O, Juhasz C, et al. (2001). Postnatal maturation of human GABAA receptors measured with positron emission tomography. Ann Neurol 49: 618–626.

Coffman BL, Rios GR, King CD, et al. (1997). Human UGT2B7 catalyzes morphine glucuronidation. Drug Metab Dispos 25: 1–4.

Cook RD, Davis PJ. (1993). Pediatric anesthesia pharmacology. In: Lake CL (ed). Pediatric cardiac anesthesia. Appleton & Lange, East Norwalk, pp. 134.

Courade JP, Chassaing C, Bardin L, et al. (2001). 5-HT receptor subtypes involved in the spinal antinociceptive effect of acetaminophen in rats. Eur J Pharmacol 432: 1–7.

Coyle JT, Campochiaro P. (1976). Ontogenesis of dopaminergic–cholinergic interactions in the rat striatum: a neurochemical study. J Neurochem 27: 673–678.

Crawford JD, Terry ME, Rourke GM. (1950). Simplification of drug dosage calculation by application of the surface area principle. Pediatrics 5: 783–790.

Dange SV, Shah KU, Deshpande AS, et al. (1987). Bioavailability of acetaminophen after rectal administration. Indian Pediatr 24: 331–332.

Davies NM, Skjodt NM. (2000). Choosing the right nonsteroidal anti-inflammatory drug for the right patient: a pharmacokinetic approach. Clin Pharmacokinet 38: 377–392.

Dawson WT. (1940). Relations between age and weight and dosages of drugs. Ann Intern Med 13: 1594–1613.

de Wildt SN, Kearns GL, Leeder JS, et al. (1999a). Cytochrome P450 3A: ontogeny and drug disposition. Clin Pharmacokinet 37: 485–505.

de Wildt SN, Kearns GL, Leeder JS, et al. (1999b). Glucuronidation in humans. Pharmacogenetic and developmental aspects. Clin Pharmacokinet 36: 439–452.

De Witte JL, Schoenmaekers B, Sessler DI, et al. (2001). The analgesic efficacy of tramadol is impaired by concurrent administration of ondansetron. Anesth Analg 92: 1319–1321.

Dedrick RL, Bishoff KB, Zaharko DZ. (1970). Interspecies correlation of plasma concentration history of methotrexate. Cancer Chemother Rep Part I 54: 95–101.

Dowd JE, Cimaz R, Fink CW. (1995). Nonsteroidal antiinflammatory drug-induced gastroduodenal injury in children. Arthritis Rheum 38: 1225–1231.

Du Bois D, Du Bois EF. (1916). Clinical calorimetry: tenth paper. A formula to estimate the approximate surface area if height and weight be known. Arch Intern Med 17: 863–871.

Faura CC, Collins SL, Moore RA, et al. (1998). Systematic review of factors affecting the ratios of morphine and its major metabolites. Pain 74: 43–53.

Feldman M, McMahon AT. (2000). Do cyclooxygenase-2 inhibitors provide benefits similar to those of traditional nonsteroidal anti-inflammatory drugs, with less gastrointestinal toxicity? Ann Intern Med 132: 134–143.

Figueras Nadal C, Garcia de Miguel MJ, Gomez Campdera A, et al. (2002). Effectiveness and tolerability of ibuprofen-arginine versus paracetamol in children with fever of likely infectious origin. Acta Paediatr 91: 383–390.

Flato B, Vinje O, Forre O. (1998). Toxicity of antirheumatic and anti-inflammatory drugs in children. Clin Rheumatol 17: 505–510.

Forrest JB, Heitlinger EL, Revell S. (1997). Ketorolac for postoperative pain management in children. Drug Saf 16: 309–329.

Franck LS, Vilardi J, Durand D, et al. (1998). Opioid withdrawal in neonates after continuous infusions of morphine or fentanyl during extracorporeal membrane oxygenation. Am J Crit Care 7: 364–369.

Franks NP, Lieb WR. (1994). Molecular and cellular mechanisms of general anaesthesia. Nature. 367: 607–614.

Freye E. (1996). Development of sensory information processing – the ontogenesis of opioid binding sites in nociceptive afferents and their significance in the clinical setting. Acta Anaesthesiol Scand Suppl 109: 98–101.

Friis-Hansen B. (1961). Body water compartments in children: changes during growth and related changes in body composition. Pediatrics 28: 169–181.

Gal P, Ransom JL, Schall S, et al. (1990). Indomethacin for patent ductus arteriosus closure. Application of serum concentrations and pharmacodynamics to improve response. J Perinatol 10: 20–26.

Gaudreault P, Guay J, Nicol O, et al. (1988). Pharmacokinetics and clinical efficacy of intrarectal solution of acetaminophen. Can J Anaesth 35: 149–152.

Gauntlett IS, Fisher DM, Hertzka RE, et al. (1988). Pharmacokinetics of fentanyl in neonatal humans and lambs: effects of age. Anesthesiology 69: 683–687.

Geisslinger G, Hering W, Thomann P, et al. (1993). Pharmacokinetics and pharmacodynamics of ketamine enantiomers in surgical patients using a stereoselective analytical method. Br J Anaesth 70: 666–671.

Gibson TP. (1996). Pharmacokinetics, efficacy, and safety of analgesia with a focus on tramadol HCl. Am J Med 101: 47S–53S.

Gillooly JF, Brown JH, West GB, et al. (2001). Effects of size and temperature on metabolic rate. Science 293: 2248–2251.

Gong QL, Hedner J, Bjorkman R, et al. (1992). Morphine-3-glucuronide may functionally antagonize morphine-6-glucuronide induced antinociception and ventilatory depression in the rat. Pain 48: 249–255.

Gonzalez-Martin G, Maggio L, Gonzalez-Sotomayor J, et al. (1997). Pharmacokinetics of ketorolac in children after abdominal surgery. Int J Clin Pharmacol Ther 35: 160–163.

Goyal PK, Chandra J, Unnikrishnan G, et al. (1998). Double blind randomized comparative evaluation of nimesulide and paracetamol as antipyretics. Indian Pediatr 35: 519–522.

Grand RJ, Watkins JB, Torti FM. (1976). Development of the human intestinal tract: a review. Gastroenterology 70: 790–810.

Granry JC, Rod B, Monrigal JP, et al. (1997). The analgesic efficacy of an injectable prodrug of acetaminophen in children after orthopaedic surgery. Paediatr Anaesth 7: 445–449.

Grant IS, Nimmo WS, McNicol LR, et al. (1983). Ketamine disposition in children and adults. Br J Anaesth 55: 1107–1111.

Greenblatt DJ, Koch-Weser J. (1976). Intramuscular injection of drugs. N Engl J Med 295: 542–546.

Gregoire N, Gualano V, Geneteau A, et al. (2004). Population pharmacokinetics of ibuprofen enantiomers in very premature neonates. J Clin Pharmacol 44: 1114–1124.

Grond S, Sablotzki A. (2004). Clinical pharmacology of tramadol. Clin Pharmacokinet 43: 879–923.

Gronert GA, Fung DL, Jones JH, et al. (1995). Allometry of pharmacokinetics and pharmacodynamics of the muscle relaxant metocurine in mammals. Am J Physiol 268: R85–91.

Gunter JB, Varughese AM, Harrington JF, et al. (1995). Recovery and complications after tonsillectomy in children: a comparison of ketorolac and morphine. Anesth Analg 81: 1136–1141.

Gupta M, Brans Y. (1978). Gastric retention in neonates. Pediatrics 62: 26–29.

Guyton AC. (1947). Measurement of the respiratory volumes of laboratory animals. Am J Physiol 150: 70–77.

Hamman MA, Thompson GA, Hall SD. (1997). Regioselective and

stereoselective metabolism of ibuprofen by human cytochrome P450 2C. Biochem Pharmacol 54: 33–41.

Hartvig P, Larsson E, Joachimsson PO. (1993). Postoperative analgesia and sedation following pediatric cardiac surgery using a constant infusion of ketamine. J Cardiothorac Vasc Anesth 7: 148–153.

Hertzka RE, Gauntlett IS, Fisher DM, et al. (1989). Fentanyl-induced ventilatory depression: effects of age. Anesthesiology 70: 213–218.

Hickey PR, Hansen DD, Wessel DL, et al. (1985). Pulmonary and systemic hemodynamic responses to fentanyl in infants. Anesth Analg 64: 483–486.

Hines RN, McCarver DG. (2002). The ontogeny of human drug-metabolizing enzymes: phase I oxidative enzymes. J Pharmacol Exp Ther 300: 355–360.

Holford NHG. (1992). Population pharmacodynamic models. In: Van Boxtel CJ, Holford NHG, Danhof M (eds). The in vivo study of drug action. Elsevier, Amsterdam, pp. 61–69.

Holford NHG. (1996). A size standard for pharmacokinetics. Clinical Pharmacokinet 30: 329–332.

Holford NH, Sheiner LB. (1981). Understanding the dose–effect relationship: clinical application of pharmacokinetic-pharmacodynamic models. Clin Pharmacokinet 6: 429–453.

Hollister GR, Burn JM. (1974). Side effects of ketamine in pediatric anesthesia. Anesth Analg 53: 264–267.

Houck CS, Wilder RT, McDermott JS, et al. (1996). Safety of intravenous ketorolac therapy in children and cost savings with a unit dosing system. J Pediatr 129: 292–296.

Howard CR, Howard FM, Weitzman ML. (1994). Acetaminophen analgesia in neonatal circumcision: the effect on pain. Pediatrics 93: 641–646.

Hughes MA, Glass PS, Jacobs JR. (1992). Context-sensitive half-time in multicompartment pharmacokinetic models for intravenous anesthetic drugs. Anesthesiology 76: 334–341.

Hull CJ, Van Beem HB, McLeod K, et al. (1978). A pharmacodynamic model for pancuronium. Br J Anaesth 50: 1113–1123.

Ihmsen H, Geisslinger G, Schuttler J. (2001). Stereoselective pharmacokinetics of ketamine: R(–)-ketamine inhibits the elimination of S(+)-ketamine. Clin Pharmacol Ther 70: 431–438.

Inturrisi CE, Colburn WA. (1986). Pharmacokinetics and pharmacodynamics of opioids.

In: Foley KM, Inturrisi CE (eds). Advances in pain research and therapy. Opioid analgesics in the management of clinical pain. Raven Press, New York, pp. 441–452.

Jacqz-Aigrain E, Burtin P. (1996). Clinical pharmacokinetics of sedatives in neonates. Clin Pharmacokinet 31: 423–443.

Johnson KL, Erickson JP, Holley FO, et al. (1984). Fentanyl pharmacokinetics in the paediatric population. Anesthesiology 61: A441.

Johnson GH, Van Wagoner JD, Brown J, et al. (1997). Bromfenac sodium, acetaminophen/oxycodone, ibuprofen, and placebo for relief of postoperative pain. Clin Ther 19: 507–519.

Johnsrud EK, Koukouritaki SB, Divakaran K, et al. (2003). Human hepatic CYP2E1 expression during development. J Pharmacol Exp Ther 307: 402–407.

Jonkers R, van Boxtel CJ, Koopmans RP, et al. (1989). A nonsteady-state agonist antagonist interaction model using plasma potassium concentrations to quantify the beta-2 selectivity of beta blockers. J Pharmacol Exp Ther 249: 297–302.

Kafetzis DA, Sinaniotis CA, Papadatos CJ, et al. (1979). Pharmacokinetics of amikacin in infants and pre-school children. Acta Paediatr Scand 68: 419–422.

Kam PC, See AU. (2000). Cyclo-oxygenase isoenzymes: physiological and pharmacological role. Anaesthesia 55: 442–449.

Kart T, Christrup LL, Rasmussen M. (1997a). Recommended use of morphine in neonates, infants and children based on a literature review: Part 1 – Pharmacokinetics. Paediatr Anaesth 7: 5–11.

Kart T, Christrup LL, Rasmussen M. (1997b). Recommended use of morphine in neonates, infants and children based on a literature review: Part 2 – Clinical use. Paediatr Anaesth 7: 93–101.

Kauffman RE, Lieh-Lai MW, Uy HG, et al. (1999). Enantiomer-selective pharmacokinetics and metabolism of ketorolac in children. Clin Pharmacol Ther 65: 382–388.

Kearns GL, Abdel-Rahman SM, Alander SW, et al. (2003). Developmental pharmacology – drug disposition, action, and therapy in infants and children. N Engl J Med 349: 1157–1167.

Keenan GF, Giannini EH, Athreya BH. (1995). Clinically significant gastropathy associated with nonsteroidal antiinflammatory drug use in children with juvenile rheumatoid arthritis. J Rheumatol 22: 1149–1151.

Kelley MT, Walson PD, Edge JH, et al. (1992). Pharmacokinetics and pharmacodynamics of ibuprofen isomers and acetaminophen in febrile children. Clin Pharmacol Ther 52: 181–189.

Kleiber M. (1932). Body size and metabolism. Hilgardia 6: 315–333.

Kleiber M. (1961). The fire of life: an introduction to animal energetics. Wiley, New York.

Koehntop DE, Rodman JH, Brundage DM, et al. (1986). Pharmacokinetics of fentanyl in neonates. Anesth Analg 65: 227–232.

Konstan MW, Hoppel CL, Chai BL, et al. (1991). Ibuprofen in children with cystic fibrosis: pharmacokinetics and adverse effects. J Pediatr 118: 956–964.

Konstan MW, Byard PJ, Hoppel CL, et al. (1995). Effect of high-dose ibuprofen in patients with cystic fibrosis. N Engl J Med. 332: 848–854.

Koren G, Maurice L. (1989). Pediatric uses of opioids. Pediatr Clin North Am 36: 1141–1156.

Korpela R, Olkkola KT. (1990). Pharmacokinetics of intravenous diclofenac sodium in children. Eur J Clin Pharmacol 38: 293–295.

Korpela R, Korvenoja P, Meretoja OA. (1999). Morphine-sparing effect of acetaminophen in pediatric day-case surgery. Anesthesiology 91: 442–447.

Koukouritaki SB, Manro JR, Marsh SA, et al. (2004). Developmental expression of human hepatic CYP2C9 and CYP2C19. J Pharmacol Exp Ther 308: 965–974.

Kovesi TA, Swartz R, MacDonald N. (1998). Transient renal failure due to simultaneous ibuprofen and aminoglycoside therapy in children with cystic fibrosis. N Engl J Med 338: 65–66.

Labroo RB, Paine MF, Thummel KE, et al. (1997). Fentanyl metabolism by human hepatic and intestinal cytochrome P450 3A4: implications for interindividual variability in disposition, efficacy, and drug interactions. Drug Metab Dispos 25: 1072–1080.

Lack JA, Stuart Taylor ME. (1997). Calculation of drug dosage and body surface area of children. Br J Anaesth 78: 601–605.

Lerman J. (1992). Pharmacology of inhalational anaesthetics in infants and children. Paediatr Anaesth 2: 191–203.

Lerman J, Schmitt Bantel BI, Gregory GA, et al. (1986). Effect of age on the solubility of volatile anesthetics in human tissues. Anesthesiology 65: 307–311.

Lesko SM, Mitchell AA. (1995). An assessment of the safety of pediatric ibuprofen. A practitioner-based randomized clinical trial. JAMA 273: 929–933.

Lesko SM, Mitchell AA. (1997). Renal function after short-term ibuprofen use in infants and children. Pediatrics 100: 954–957.

Lesko SM, Mitchell AA. (1999). The safety of acetaminophen and ibuprofen among children younger than two years old. Pediatrics 104: e39.

Leung LY, Baillie TA. (1986). Comparative pharmacology in the rat of ketamine and its two principal metabolites, norketamine and (Z)-6-hydroxynorketamine. J Med Chem 29: 2396–2399.

Levy G, Garrettson LK, Soda DM. (1975a). Evidence of placenta transfer of acetaminophen. Pediatrics 55: 895.

Levy G, Khanna NN, Soda DM, et al. (1975b). Pharmacokinetics of acetaminophen in the human neonate; formation of acetaminophinglycuronide and sulfate in relation to plasma bilirubin concentration and D-glucoric acid excretion. Pediatrics 55: 818–825.

Liang J, Co E, Zhang M, et al. (1998). Development of gastric slow waves in preterm infants measured by electrogastrography. Am J Physiol 274: G503–508.

Linday L, Dobkin JF, Wang TC, et al. (1987). Digoxin inactivation by the gut flora in infancy and childhood. Pediatrics 79: 544–548.

Lipsky PE, Brooks P, Crofford LJ, et al. (2000). Unresolved issues in the role of cyclooxygenase-2 in normal physiologic processes and disease. Arch Intern Med 160: 913–920.

Litalien C, Jacqz-Aigrain E. (2001). Risks and benefits of nonsteroidal anti-inflammatory drugs in children: a comparison with paracetamol. Paediatr Drugs 3: 817–858.

Loh HH, Liu HC, Cavalli A, et al. (1998). mu Opioid receptor knockout in mice: effects on ligand-induced analgesia and morphine lethality. Brain Res Mol Brain Res 54: 321–326.

Lynn AM, Nespeca MK, Opheim KE, et al. (1993). Respiratory effects of intravenous morphine infusions in neonates, infants, and children after cardiac surgery. Anesth Analg 77: 695–701.

Lynn A, Nespeca MK, Bratton SL, et al. (1998). Clearance of morphine in postoperative infants during intravenous infusion: the influence of age and surgery. Anesth Analg 86: 958–963.

Mahmood I. (1998). Interspecies scaling: predicting volumes, mean residence time and elimination half-life. Some suggestions. J Pharm Pharmacol 50: 493–499.

Malinovsky JM, Servin F, Cozian A, et al. (1996). Ketamine and norketamine plasma concentrations after i.v., nasal and rectal administration in children. Br J Anaesth 77: 203–207.

Malviya S, Lerman J. (1990). The blood/gas solubilities of sevoflurane, isoflurane, halothane, and serum constituent concentrations in neonates and adults. Anesthesiology 72: 793–796.

Mandema JW, Stanski DR. (1996). Population pharmacodynamic model for ketorolac analgesia. Clin Pharmacol Ther 60: 619–635.

Marshall J, Rodarte A, Blumer J, et al. (2000). Pediatric pharmacodynamics of midazolam oral syrup. Pediatric Pharmacology Research Unit Network. J Clin Pharmacol 40: 578–589.

Matthes HW, Maldonado R, Simonin F, et al. (1996). Loss of morphine-induced analgesia, reward effect and withdrawal symptoms in mice lacking the mu-opioid-receptor gene. Nature 383: 819–823.

McCarver DG, Hines RN. (2002). The ontogeny of human drug-metabolizing enzymes: phase II conjugation enzymes and regulatory mechanisms. J Pharmacol Exp Ther 300: 361–366.

McCrory CR, Lindahl SG. (2002). Cyclooxygenase inhibition for postoperative analgesia. Anesth Analg 95: 169–176.

McMahon TA. (1980). Scaling physiological time. Lect Math Life Sci 13: 131–133.

McRorie TI, Lynn AM, Nespeca MK, et al. (1992). The maturation of morphine clearance and metabolism. Am J Dis Child 146: 972–976.

Ment L, Oh W, Ehrenkranz RA, et al. (1994). Low-dose indomethacin in prevention of intraventricular hemorrhage: a multicenter randomized trial. Pediatrics 93: 543–550.

Miller RP, Roberts RJ, Fischer LJ. (1976). Acetaminophen elimination kinetics in neonates, children, and adults. Clin Pharmacol Ther 19: 284–294.

Miners JO, Osborne NJ, Tonkin AL, et al. (1992). Perturbation of paracetamol urinary metabolic ratios by urine flow rate. Br J Clin Pharmacol 34: 359–362.

Mitchell D, Strydon NB, Van Graun CH, et al. (1971). Human surface area: comparison of the dubois formula with direct photometric measurement. Pfugers Arch 325: 188–190.

Mitchell JA, Akaraserreenont P, Thiemermann C, et al. (1993). Selectivity of nonsteroidal antiinflammatory drugs as inhibitors of constitutive and inducible cyclooxygenase. Proc Natl Acad Sci USA 90: 11693–11697.

Moghal NE, Hulton SA, Milford DV. (1998). Care in the use of ibuprofen as an antipyretic in children. Clin Nephrol 49: 293–295.

Morton NS, O'Brien K. (1999). Analgesic efficacy of paracetamol and diclofenac in children receiving PCA morphine. Br J Anaesth 82: 715–717.

Mulberg AE, Linz C, Bern E, et al. (1993). Identification of nonsteroidal antiinflammatory drug-induced gastroduodenal injury in children with juvenile rheumatoid arthritis. J Pediatr 122: 647–649.

Munro HM, Riegger LQ, Reynolds PI, et al. (1994). Comparison of the analgesic and emetic properties of ketorolac and morphine for paediatric outpatient strabismus surgery. Br J Anaesth 72: 624–628.

Murthy BV, Pandya KS, Booker PD, et al. (2000). Pharmacokinetics of tramadol in children after i.v. or caudal epidural administration. Br J Anaesth 84: 346–349.

Murthy BR, Pollack GM, Brouwer KL. (2002). Contribution of morphine-6-glucuronide to antinociception following intravenous administration of morphine to healthy volunteers. J Clin Pharmacol 42: 569–576.

Naulaers G, Delanghe G, Allegaert K, et al. (2005). Ibuprofen and cerebral oxygenation and circulation. Arch Dis Child Fetal Neonatal Ed 90: F75–76.

Nichols DJ, Yaster M, Lynn AM, et al. (1993). Disposition and respiratory effects of intrathecal morphine in children. Anesthesiology 79: 733–738.

Nielsen JC, Bjerring P, Arendt Nielsen L, et al. (1992). Analgesic efficacy of immediate and sustained release paracetamol and plasma concentration of paracetamol. Double blind, placebo-controlled evaluation using painful laser stimulation. Eur J Clin Pharmacol 42: 261–264.

Niemi TT, Taxell C, Rosenberg PH. (1997). Comparison of the effect of intravenous ketoprofen, ketorolac and diclofenac on platelet function in volunteers. Acta Anaesthesiol Scand 41: 1353–1358.

Niemi TT, Backman JT, Syrjala MT, et al. (2000). Platelet dysfunction after intravenous ketorolac or propacetamol. Acta Anaesthesiol Scand 44: 69–74.

Oermann CM, Sockrider MM, Konstan MW. (1999). The use of anti-inflammatory medications in cystic fibrosis: trends and physician attitudes. Chest 115: 1053–1058.

Olkkola KT, Hamunen K. (2000). Pharmacokinetics and pharmacodynamics of analgesic drugs. In: Anand KJ, Stevens B, McGrath P (eds). Pain in neonates 2nd revised and enlarged edition. Elsevier, Amsterdam, pp. 135–158.

Olkkola KT, Maunuksela EL. (1991). The pharmacokinetics of postoperative intravenous ketorolac trimethamine in children. Br J Clin Pharmacol 31: 182–184.

Olkkola KT, Maunuksela EL, Korpela R. (1989). Pharmacokinetics of postoperative intravenous indomethacin in children. Pharmacol Toxicol 65: 157–160.

Olsen GD. (1975). Morphine binding to human plasma proteins. Clin Pharmacol Ther 17: 31–35.

Osborne R, Thompson P, Joel S, et al. (1992). The analgesic activity of morphine-6-glucuronide. Br J Clin Pharmacol 34: 130–138.

Osborne PB, Chieng B, Christie MJ. (2000). Morphine-6 beta-glucuronide has a higher efficacy than morphine as a mu-opioid receptor agonist in the rat locus coeruleus. Br J Pharmacol 131: 1422–1428.

Oztekin S, Hepaguslar H, Kar AA, et al. (2002). Preemptive diclofenac reduces morphine use after remifentanil-based anaesthesia for tonsillectomy. Paediatr Anaesth 12: 694–699.

Pacifici GM, Sawe J, Kager L, et al. (1982). Morphine glucuronidation in human fetal and adult liver. Eur J Clin Pharmacol 22: 553–558.

Pacifici GM, Franchi M, Giuliani L, et al. (1989). Development of the glucuronyltransferase and sulphotransferase towards 2-naphthol in human fetus. Dev Pharmacol Ther 14: 108–114.

Pang WW, Mok MS, Lin CH, et al. (1999). Comparison of patient-controlled analgesia (PCA) with tramadol or morphine. Can J Anaesth 46: 1030–1035.

Pang WW, Mok MS, Huang S, et al. (2000). Intraoperative loading attenuates nausea and vomiting of tramadol patient-controlled analgesia. Can J Anaesth 47: 968–973.

Pariente-Khayat A, Rey E, Gendrel D, et al. (1997). Isoniazid acetylation metabolic ratio during maturation in children. Clin Pharmacol Ther 62: 377–383.

Payne KA, Roelofse JA, Shipton EA. (2002). Pharmacokinetics of oral tramadol drops for postoperative pain relief in children aged 4 to 7 years – a pilot study. Anesth Prog 49: 109–112.

Pedraz JL, Calvo MB, Lanao JM, et al. (1989). Pharmacokinetics of rectal ketamine in children. Br J Anaesth 63: 671–674.

Peters HP. (1983). Physiological correlates of size. In: Beck E, Birks HJB, Conner EF (eds). The ecological implications of body size. Cambridge University Press, Cambridge, pp. 48–53.

Peterson RG, Rumack BH. (1978). Pharmacokinetics of acetaminophen in children. Pediatrics 62: 877.

Pickering AE, Bridge HS, Nolan J, et al. (2002). Double-blind, placebo-controlled analgesic study of ibuprofen or rofecoxib in combination with paracetamol for tonsillectomy in children. Br J Anaesth 88: 72–77.

Piletta P, Porchet HC, Dayer P. (1991). Central analgesic effect of acetaminophen but not of aspirin. Clin Pharmacol Ther 49: 350–354.

Pokela ML, Olkkola KT, Seppala T, et al. (1993). Age-related morphine kinetics in infants. Dev Pharmacol Ther 20: 26–34.

Poley JR, Dower JC, Owen CA Jr, et al. (1964). Bile acids in infants and children. J Lab Clin Med 63: 838–846.

Poulsen L, Arendt-Nielsen L, Brosen K, et al. (1996). The hypoalgesic effect of tramadol in relation to CYP2D6. Clin Pharmacol Ther 60: 636–644.

Prescott LF. (1996). Paracetamol (acetaminophen). A critical bibliographic review. Taylor and Francis Publishers, London.

Primack WA, Rahman SM, Pullman J. (1997). Acute renal failure associated with amoxicillin and ibuprofen in an 11-year-old boy. Pediatr Nephrol 11: 125–126.

Prothero JW. (1980). Scaling of blood parameters in animals. Comp Biochem Physiol A67: 649–657.

Purssell E. (2002). Treating fever in children: paracetamol or ibuprofen? Br J Community Nurs 7: 316–320.

Rawlins MD, Henderson BD, Hijab AR. (1977). Pharmacokinetics of paracetamol (acetaminophen) after

intravenous and oral administration. Eur J Clin Pharmacol 11: 283–286.

Ray PE, Rigolizzo D, Wara DR, et al. (1988). Naproxen nephrotoxicity in a 2-year-old child. Am J Dis Child 142: 524–525.

Ritschel WA, Vachharajani NN, Johnson RD, et al. (1992). The allometric approach for interspecies scaling of pharmacokinetic parameters. [Review]. Comp Biochem Physiol C 103: 249–253.

Roberts I, Robinson MJ, Mughal MZ, et al. (1984). Paracetamol metabolites in the neonate following maternal overdose. Br J Clin Pharmacol 18: 201–206.

Rod B, Monrigal JP, Lepoittevin L, et al. (1989). [Treatment of postoperative pain in children in the recovery room. Use of morphine and propacetamol by the intravenous route]. Cah Anesthesiol 37: 525–530.

Romsing J, Ostergaard D, Senderovitz T, et al. (2001). Pharmacokinetics of oral diclofenac and acetaminophen in children after surgery. Paediatr Anaesth 11: 205–213.

Rusy LM, Houck CS, Sullivan LJ, et al. (1995). A double-blind evaluation of ketorolac tromethamine versus acetaminophen in pediatric tonsillectomy: analgesia and bleeding. Anesth Analg 80: 226–229.

Ryhanen P, Adamski J, Puhakka K, et al. (1994). Postoperative pain relief in children. A comparison between caudal bupivacaine and intramuscular diclofenac sodium. Anaesthesia 49: 57–61.

Salanitre E, Rackow H. (1969). The pulmonary exchange of nitrous oxide and halothane in infants and children. Anesthesiology 30: 388–394.

Schmidt-Nielsen K. (1984). Scaling: why is animal size so important? Cambridge University Press, Cambridge.

Scott JC, Stanski DR. (1987). Decreased fentanyl and alfentanil dose requirements with age. A simultaneous pharmacokinetic and pharmacodynamic evaluation. J Pharmacol Exp Ther 240: 159–166.

Scott CS, Retsch-Bogart GZ, Kustra RP, et al. (1999a). The pharmacokinetics of ibuprofen suspension, chewable tablets, and tablets in children with cystic fibrosis. J Pediatr 134: 58–63.

Scott CS, Riggs KW, Ling EW, et al. (1999b). Morphine pharmacokinetics and pain assessment in premature newborns. J Pediatr 135: 423–429.

Shaffer CL, Gal P, Ransom JL, et al. (2002). Effect of age and birth weight on indomethacin pharmacodynamics

in neonates treated for patent ductus arteriosus. Crit Care Med 30: 343–348.

Shah SS, Ohlsson A. (2006). Ibuprofen for the prevention of patent ductus arteriosis in preterm and/or low bi weight infants. Cochrane Database Syst Rev 1: CD004213.

Shah V, Taddio A, Ohlsson A. (1998). Randomised controlled trial of paracetamol for heel prick pain in neonates. Arch Dis Child Fetal Neonatal Ed 79: F209–211.

Sheiner LB, Stanski DR, Vozeh S, et al. (1979). Simultaneous modeling of pharmacokinetics and pharmacodynamics: application to D-tubocurarine. Clin Pharmacol Ther 25: 358–371.

Sheiner PA, Mor E, Chodoff L, et al. (1994). Acute renal failure associated with the use of ibuprofen in two liver transplant recipients on FK506. Transplantation 57: 1132–1133.

Sheng KT, Huang NN, Promadhattavedi V. (1964). Serum concentrations of cephalothin in infants and children and placental transmission of the antibiotic. Antimicrob Agent Chemother 10: 200–206.

Silverstein FE, Faich G, Goldstein JL, et al. (2000). Gastrointestinal toxicity with celecoxib vs nonsteroidal anti-inflammatory drugs for osteoarthritis and rheumatoid arthritis: the CLASS study: A randomized controlled trial. Celecoxib Long-term Arthritis Safety Study. JAMA 284: 1247–1255.

Simon AM, Manigrasso MB, O'Connor JP. (2002). Cyclo-oxygenase 2 function is essential for bone fracture healing. J Bone Miner Res 17: 963–976.

Slattery JT, Nelson SD, Thummel KE. (1996). The complex interaction between ethanol and acetaminophen. Clin Pharmacol Ther 60: 241–246.

Smith MT, Watt JA, Cramond T. (1990). Morphine-3-glucuronide – a potent antagonist of morphine analgesia. Life Sci 47: 579–585.

Smyth JM, Collier PS, Darwish M, et al. (2004). Intravenous indometacin in preterm infants with symptomatic patent ductus arteriosus. A population pharmacokinetic study. Br J Clin Pharmacol 58: 249–258.

Sora I, Takahashi N, Funada M, et al. (1997). Opiate receptor knockout mice define mu receptor roles in endogenous nociceptive responses and morphine-induced analgesia. Proc Natl Acad Sci USA 94: 1544–1549.

Souter AJ, Fredman B, White PF. (1994). Controversies in the perioperative use of nonsterodial antiinflammatory drugs. Anesth Analg 79: 1178–1190.

Splinter WM, Reid CW, Roberts DJ, et al. (1997). Reducing pain after inguinal hernia repair in children: caudal anesthesia versus ketorolac tromethamine. Anesthesiology 87: 542–546.

Stahl WR. (1967). Scaling of respiratory variables in mammals. J Appl Physiol 22: 453–600.

Stamer UM, Stuber F. (2001). Analgesic efficacy of tramadol if coadministered with ondansetron. Anesth Analg 93: 1626.

Stempak D, Gammon J, Klein J, et al. (2002). Single-dose and steady-state pharmacokinetics of celecoxib in children. Clin Pharmacol Ther 72: 490–497.

Stoeckel H, Hengstmann JH, Schuttler J. (1979). Pharmacokinetics of fentanyl as a possible explanation for recurrence of respiratory depression. Br J Anaesth 51: 741–745.

Suchy FJ, Balistreri WF, Heubi JE, et al. (1981). Physiologic cholestasis: elevation of the primary serum bile acid concentrations in normal infants. Gastroenterology 80: 1037–1041.

Suresh S, Anand KJ. (1998). Opioid tolerance in neonates: mechanisms, diagnosis, assessment, and management. Semin Perinatol 22: 425–433.

Suresh S, Anand KJS. (2001). Opioid tolerance in neonates: a state of the art review. Paediat Anaesth 11: 511–521.

Suri A, Estes KS, Geisslinger G, et al. (1997). Pharmacokinetic–pharmacodynamic relationships for analgesics. Int J Clin Pharmacol Ther 35: 307–323.

Szer IS, Goldenstein-Schainberg C, Kurtin PS. (1991). Paucity of renal complications associated with nonsteroidal antiinflammatory drugs in children with chronic arthritis. J Pediatr 119: 815–817.

Taddio A. (2002). Opioid analgesia for infants in the neonatal intensive care unit. Clin Perinatol 29: 493–509.

Taddio A, Shennan AT, Stevens B, et al. (1995). Safety of lidocaine-prilocaine cream in the treatment of preterm neonates. J Pediatr 127: 1002–1005.

Taddio A, Stevens B, Craig K, et al. (1997). Efficacy and safety of lidocaine-prilocaine cream for pain during circumcision. N Engl J Med 336: 1197–1201.

Tanaka E. (1998). Clinically important pharmacokinetic drug–drug interactions: role of cytochrome P450 enzymes. J Clin Pharm Ther 23: 403–416.

Tateishi T, Krivoruk Y, Ueng YF, et al. (1996). Identification of human liver cytochrome P-450 3A4 as the enzyme responsible for fentanyl and sufentanil N-dealkylation. Anesth Analg 82: 167–172.

Tawalbeh MI, Nawasreh OO, Husban AM. (2001). Comparative study of diclofenac sodium and paracetamol for treatment of pain after adenotonsillectomy in children. Saudi Med J 22: 121–123.

Tenenbein M. (2000). Why young children are resistant to acetaminophen poisoning. J Pediatr 137: 891–892.

Thompson PI, Joel SP, John L, et al. (1995). Respiratory depression following morphine and morphine-6-glucuronide in normal subjects. Br J Clin Pharmacol 40: 145–152.

Tobias JD. (1997). Seizure after overdose of tramadol. South Med J 90: 826–827.

Torres LM, Rodriguez MJ, Montero A, et al. (2001). Efficacy and safety of dipyrone versus tramadol in the management of pain after hysterectomy: a randomized, double-blind, multicenter study. Reg Anesth Pain Med 26: 118–124.

Touw DJ. (1997). Clinical implications of genetic polymorphisms and drug interactions mediated by cytochrome P-450 enzymes. Drug Metabol Drug Interact 14: 55–82.

Troconiz IF, Armenteros S, Planelles MV, et al. (2000) Pharmacokinetic-pharmacodynamic modelling of the antipyretic effect of two oral formulations of ibuprofen. Clin Pharmacokinet 38: 505–518.

Tunblad K, Hammarlund-Udenaes M, Jonsson EN. (2005). Influence of probenecid on the delivery of morphine-6-glucuronide to the brain. Eur J Pharm Sci 24: 49–57.

Turturro MA, Paris PM, Larkin GL. (1998). Tramadol versus hydrocodone-acetaminophen in acute musculoskeletal pain: a randomized, double-blind clinical trial. Ann Emerg Med 32: 139–143.

Ugazio AG, Guarnaccia S, Berardi M, et al. (1993). Clinical and pharmacokinetic study of nimesulide in children. Drugs 46: 215–218.

van Biljon G. (1989). Reversible renal failure associated with ibuprofen in a child. A case report. S Afr Med J 76: 34–35.

van den Berg AA, Halliday E, Lule EK, et al. (1999). The effects of tramadol on postoperative nausea, vomiting and headache after ENT surgery. A placebo-controlled comparison with equipotent doses of nalbuphine and pethidine. Acta Anaesthesiol Scand 43: 28–33.

Van Esch A, Van Steensel Moll HA, Steyerberg EW, et al. (1995). Antipyretic efficacy of ibuprofen and acetaminophen in children with febrile seizures. Arch Pediatr Adolesc Med 149: 632–637.

van Hoogdalem E, de Boer AG, Breimer DD. (1991a). Pharmacokinetics of rectal drug administration, Part I. General considerations and clinical applications of centrally acting drugs. Clin Pharmacokinet 21: 11–26.

van Hoogdalem EJ, de Boer AG, Breimer DD. (1991b). Pharmacokinetics of rectal drug administration, Part II. Clinical applications of peripherally acting drugs, and conclusions. Clin Pharmacokinet 21: 110–128.

van Lingen RA, Deinum HT, Quak CM, et al. (1999a). Multiple-dose pharmacokinetics of rectally administered acetaminophen in term infants. Clin Pharmacol Ther 66: 509–515.

van Lingen RA, Deinum JT, Quak JM, et al. (1999b). Pharmacokinetics and metabolism of rectally administered paracetamol in preterm neonates. Arch Dis Child Fetal Neonatal Ed 80: F59–63.

van Lingen RA, Quak CM, Deinum HT, et al. (2001). Effects of rectally administered paracetamol on infants delivered by vacuum extraction. Eur J Obstet Gynecol Reprod Biol 94: 73–78.

van Lingen RA, Simons SH, Anderson BJ, et al. (2002). The effects of analgesia in the vulnerable infant during the perinatal period. Clin Perinatol 29: 511–534.

Van Overmeire B, Smets K, Lecoutere D, et al. (2000). A comparison of ibuprofen and indomethacin for closure of patent ductus arteriosus. N Engl J Med 343: 674–681.

Van Overmeire B, Touw D, Schepens PJ, et al. (2001). Ibuprofen pharmacokinetics in preterm infants with patent ductus arteriosus. Clin Pharmacol Ther 70: 336–343.

Vetter TR, Heiner EJ. (1994). Intravenous ketorolac as an adjuvant to pediatric patient-controlled analgesia with morphine. J Clin Anesth 6: 110–113.

Walson PD, Galletta G, Braden NJ, et al. (1989). Ibuprofen, acetaminophen, and placebo treatment of febrile children. Clin Pharmacol Ther 46: 9–17.

Watcha MF, Ramirez Ruiz M, White PF, et al. (1992). Perioperative effects of oral ketorolac and acetaminophen in children undergoing bilateral myringotomy. Can J Anaesth 39: 649–654.

Way WL, Costley EC, Way EL. (1965). Respiratory sensitivity of the newborn infant to meperidine and morphine. Clin Pharmacol Ther 6: 454–461.

Weinstein MS, Nicolson SC, Schreiner MS. (1994). A single dose of morphine sulfate increases the incidence of vomiting after outpatient inguinal surgery in children. Anesthesiology 81: 572–577.

West JR, Smith HW, Chasis H. (1948). Glomerular filtration rate, effective renal blood flow, and maximal tubular excretory capacity in infancy. J Pediatr 32: 10–18.

West G, Brown J, Enquist B. (1997). A general model for the origin of allometric scaling laws in biology. Science 276: 122–126.

West GB, Brown JH, Enquist BJ. (1999). The fourth dimension of life: fractal geometry and allometric scaling of organisms. Science 284: 1677–1679.

Wiest DB, Pinson JB, Gal PS, et al. (1991). Population pharmacokinetics of intravenous indomethacin in neonates with symptomatic patent ductus arteriosus. Clin Pharmacol Ther 49: 550–557.

Williams N. (1997). Fractal geometry gets the measure of life's scales. Science 276: 34.

Williams DG, Hatch DJ, Howard RF. (2001). Codeine phosphate in paediatric medicine. Br J Anaesth 86: 413–421.

Wynands JE, Townsend GE, Wong P, et al. (1983). Blood pressure response and plasma fentanyl concentrations during high- and very high-dose fentanyl anesthesia for coronary artery surgery. Anesth Analg 62: 661–665.

Yaster M, Koehler RC, Traystman RJ. (1987). Effects of fentanyl on peripheral and cerebral hemodynamics in neonatal lambs. Anesthesiology 66: 524–530.

Zsigmond EK, Downs JR. (1971). Plasma cholinesterase activity in newborns and infants. Can Anaesth Soc J 18: 278–285.

Evidence for systemic morphine and fentanyl analgesia

Anna Taddio

INTRODUCTION

Opioids are the mainstay of systemic analgesia treatment in hospitalized infants and have become increasingly utilized in an attempt to decrease pain in this population (Barker and Rutter 1995, Johnston et al. 1997, Porter et al. 1997). The increased utilization of opioid analgesics is due to the combined effects of many factors, including an increased awareness that neonates feel pain and an ethical obligation to treat the pain with analgesics. In addition, there is a growing body of evidence demonstrating that untreated neonatal pain can lead to altered reactivity to pain that persists throughout infancy and childhood (Taddio and Katz 2005), further justifying mitigation of pain with pharmacologic interventions. These factors have been outlined in recent international consensus statements promoting the routine use of analgesics in this population (American Academy of Pediatrics 2000, Anand 2001).

In this chapter, the clinical use of opioid analgesia in the neonate and young infant will be reviewed. A review of the clinical pharmacology of morphine and fentanyl are specifically provided with an emphasis on data from recently conducted clinical trials. The conclusion will summarize the literature and provide some directions for future research.

CLINICAL PHARMACOLOGY OF OPIOID ANALGESICS

Pharmacokinetics and pharmacodynamics

Opioid analgesics bind to three major groups of membrane receptors in the spinal cord and brain: mu, kappa and delta. Stimulation of receptors leads to a decrease in neuronal firing and nociceptive input to the brain, and a diminution of the biologic responses to pain including; cardiorespiratory (e.g. hypertension, tachycardia, hypoxemia), endocrine (e.g. hypothalamic–pituitary–adrenocortical (HPA) activation), metabolic (e.g. hyperglycaemia), immune system and coagulation/haemostasis changes (Anand 1993). In addition to these mechanisms of action, opioids can produce analgesia by interacting with local receptors in peripheral tissues (Stein 1995).

Morphine, a naturally occurring phenanthrene alkaloid isolated from opium, is the prototype opioid analgesic, an agonist at mu and kappa receptors. The onset of action following intravenous doses is 5 minutes, and peak effects occur after 10–30 minutes. The duration of action is between 3 and 8 hours (Koren and Maurice 1989). In adults, morphine is metabolized primarily to two active compounds, morphine-3-glucuronide (M3G) and morphine-6-glucuronide (M6G) that are renally excreted with the parent compound. M3G, the major metabolite, is an opioid antagonist and respiratory stimulant, particularly among preterm neonates (Bhat et al. 1990). M6G, a minor metabolite, has potent opioid agonist and respiratory depressant activity (Gong et al. 1991).

Other opioids that share a similar pharmacodynamic profile to morphine are referred to as 'morphine-like agonists'. Fentanyl is a synthetic morphine-like agonist. Together, morphine and fentanyl are the most commonly used opioids in neonates. Relative to morphine, fentanyl has an increased lipid solubility that facilitates more efficient and rapid penetration of the blood–brain barrier. Fentanyl has a potency of approximately 50–100-fold that of morphine. Its peak effect occurs within 5–15 minutes, and its duration of action is less than 2 hours (Koren and Maurice 1989). The pharmacokinetic half-life of fentanyl does not correspond well with its biologic half-life (Koren and Maurice 1989) due to redistribution from 'deep compartments' such as muscle, stomach and fat. Redistribution from these deep compartments may result in delayed episodes of respiratory depression (Singleton et al. 1987). Fentanyl is a high hepatic extraction drug, almost entirely metabolized by N-dealkylation and hydroxylation to inactive metabolites (Jacqz-Aigrain and Burtin 1996). Fentanyl may be preferable to morphine in clinical situations necessitating a short onset and duration of action, and haemodynamic stability (fentanyl does not stimulate histamine release). Fentanyl appears to be less sedating than morphine, induces tolerance more rapidly, and is more likely to cause muscular rigidity (see Adverse effects, p. 148).

The most rapid and extreme physiological changes occur during the neonatal period, resulting in dramatic alterations in drug disposition and large intra- and inter-individual variability (recently reviewed by Kearns et al. (2003)). Infants have proportionately less fat and muscle but more water content. Protein concentrations and binding capacity are lower. Moreover, metabolic and excretory functions are diminished (Davis et al. 1989). Together, these physiologic differences lead to decreases in protein binding, metabolism and excretion, and increases in elimination half-life (time for drug concentration in blood to decrease by one-half) of opioid analgesics in neonates, with more pronounced deficiencies in preterm infants. A correlation between clearance and/or half-life of opioid analgesics and corresponding gestational age,

birthweight or postnatal age has been demonstrated in some studies (Kart et al. 1997a, Santeiro et al. 1997, Lynn et al. 2000, Saarenmaa et al. 2000). It should be recognized, however, that certain disease states and clinical conditions have the potential to further modify drug disposition in the neonate by changing volume of distribution or clearance parameters. Examples include dehydration, surgery, cardiac disease, hypoxaemia, hypotension, infection (such as necrotizing enterocolitis), mechanical ventilation, extracorporeal membrane oxygenation (ECMO) or concurrent administration of inducing and inhibiting drugs (Gauntlett et al. 1988, Hartley and Levene 1995, Lynn et al. 1998, Bouwmeester et al. 2003, Peters et al. 2005).

The net result of physiologic differences between neonates and adults is that morphine hepatic glucuronidation is proportionately lower in neonates (Pacifici et al. 1982), and a greater fraction of the parent drug is renally excreted. However, neonates utilize an additional minor metabolic pathway, namely sulphate conjugation, to excrete morphine (Kart et al. 1997a). Some enterohepatic recirculation of morphine occurs due to β-glucuronidase activity in the gut (Koren and Maurice 1989) which may contribute to a decrease in morphine clearance. The half-life and the duration of action of morphine are prolonged in neonates, mainly due to a decrease in metabolic capacity and therefore total body clearance. Clearance approaches adult values by 2–6 months of age (Kart et al. 1997a, Bouwmeester et al. 2004). Values for volume of distribution, although previously reported to be similar across all ages (Kart et al. 1997a), were recently found to increase with age in the first 6 months of life (Bouwmeester et al. 2004). The metabolic clearance of fentanyl is diminished in newborn infants compared to older populations, but increases dramatically within the first weeks of life (Saarenmaa et al. 2000). In addition, fentanyl has a larger volume of distribution and longer half-life in the neonate (Jacqz-Aigrain and Burtin 1996). The pharmacokinetic parameters and usual starting analgesic doses of both morphine and fentanyl in neonates and adults are shown in Table 10.1 (Kart et al. 1997a). A recent review and pharmacokinetic meta-analysis suggested an alternative dosing strategy for morphine based on the development of morphine pharmacokinetics. For these calculations, it was assumed that the effective analgesic plasma morphine concentration is 15 ng/ml (Kart et al. 1997b). Although valid scoring methods for the assessment of pain and sedation are available, it is difficult to accurately diagnose and quantify pain and stress in neonates and infants. Regardless of dosing method

Table 10.1 Pharmacokinetic parameters and usual analgesic doses of morphine and fentanyl in neonates versus adults

	Vd (L/kg)	Pr (%)	CL (ml/min/kg)	$t_{1/2}$ (h)	Usual dose*
Morphine					
Neonate (Kart et al. 1997a)	PT + FT: 2.8	PT + FT: 18–22 (McRorie et al. 1992, Bhat et al. 1990)	PT: 2.2 FT: 8.1	PT: 9.0 FT: 6.5	SD: 50–100 µg/kg MD: 5–30 µg/kg/h
Infant (McRorie et al. 1992, Lynn et al. 1998)	4.8–5.5	18–21	10.5–48.9	2.8	As above
Adult (Burns et al. 1992, Lugo and Kern 2002)	3.2	35 (Mather 1983)	54	2–3.5	SD: 10 mg
Fentanyl					
Neonate (Gauntlett et al. 1988)	PT: FT: 5.1–11.2		PT: 12.12–13.03 FT: 0–17.94	PT: 6.0–32.0 FT: 5.28–13.45	SD: 1–3 µg/kg MD: 0.5–2 µg/kg/h
Infant (Johnson et al. 1984)	4.45		18.1	3.88	As above
Adult: (Bussche and Noorduin 1986)	4.0	84	11.6	3.7	SD: 0.1 mg

Vd = volume of distribution at steady state, Pr = protein binding, CL = total body clearance, $t_{1/2}$ = half-life, PT = preterm, FT = full-term, *SD = single intravenous dose, MD = intravenous maintenance infusion dose.

employed, dose regimens must always be individually titrated to each infant's requirements due to the large inter-individual variability in pharmacokinetics and dynamics.

Analgesia is believed to occur after a minimum concentration of opioid is achieved in the serum, and this concentration is referred to as the minimum effective analgesic concentration (MEAC) (Yaster and Nichols 2001). The MEAC may differ within the same patient from day to day and thus, maintaining adequate analgesia requires continuous assessments of pain (Yaster and Nichols 2001). In adults, the MEAC of morphine generally ranges from 10–50 ng/ml (Yaster and Nichols 2001). Few investigators have attempted to characterize the minimum concentration of morphine required for analgesia and sedation in neonates. Chay et al. (1992) determined that a concentration of morphine of 125 ng/ml was required to produce adequate sedation in 50% of ventilated infants (full-term and preterm) and that concentrations above 300 ng/ml were associated with adverse effects.

In a study by Hartley et al. (1993) a mean plasma concentration of 94 ng/ml was efficacious in ventilated premature neonates. Of note, these morphine concentrations are higher than those reported to be analgesic in children (i.e. 4–65 ng/ml) (Kart et al. 1997b). It has been suggested that lower concentrations of M6G and immaturity of opioid receptors (decreased receptor concentrations and/or receptor affinity) in the neonatal brain explain the increased concentration of morphine required in this population. However, another explanation for the discrepancy in morphine requirements between neonates and children is wide variability in study designs employed by investigators. These include variability in patient characteristics (i.e. clinical state, severity of pain), assessment tools and assay method for morphine analysis (Kart et al. 1997b).

For example, in the study by Chay et al. (1992), sedation and analgesia were measured, and it is possible that higher concentrations of morphine are needed to achieve sedation compared to analgesia (Kart et al. 1997b). Morphine plasma concentration was not correlated with analgesia or respiratory depression in a recent study of postoperative pain in full-term neonates (Bouwmeester et al. 2003) and in a study of 0–1-year-old infants (Lynn et al. 2000). Similarly, a concentration–response relationship has not been demonstrated for morphine when administered in preterm infants for analgesia during acute pain (Scott et al. 1999, Carbajal et al. 2005).

The serum MEAC of fentanyl ranges from 0.5–2.5 ng/ml in adults (Yaster and Nichols 2001). In a study by Saarenmaa et al. (2000), the steady-state serum fentanyl concentration was significantly correlated with pain scores in newborn infants 26–42 weeks gestational age undergoing mechanical ventilation. Infants received a bolus dose followed by an infusion rate of 1.5 µg/kg/hour; the mean serum fentanyl concentration was 2.5 ng/ml after 24–48 hours. The MEAC, however, was not specified. In another study by Roth and colleagues (1991), a mean plasma concentration of 1.7 and 2.1 ng/ml was adequate and well tolerated when fentanyl was used as a sedative in infants <34 weeks gestation and ≥34 weeks gestation, respectively. The mean infusion rate was 0.64 and 0.75 µg/kg/hour, respectively. Plasma fentanyl concentrations required for adequate sedation have been noted to increase over time, possibly due to tolerance (Arnold et al. 1991).

Clinical trials

Opioid analgesics have been increasingly utilized in neonates over the last two decades for the management of moderate to severe procedural pain, postoperative pain, disease-related pain, and as sedatives to reduce the stress of intensive care in mechanically ventilated infants. At first glance, there appear to be substantial data supporting their place in neonatal clinical medicine. However, closer examination of published trials reveals many unanswered questions about their clinical pharmacology in this population. There are insufficient data regarding the concentration–response relationship of opioids. Determination of the concentration–response relationship is complex, usually requiring multiple blood samples that are correlated with response, and is neither feasible nor reliable for this population. There are potential confounding effects of developmental state and medical condition. Equally important are conflicting data regarding the clinical effectiveness of opioids. The lack of a universally accepted method of pain assessment across populations of neonates and infants has contributed to a lack of precision in the determination of pharmacodynamic response. Most recently, opioids have not been demonstrated to improve long-term neurological outcomes in hospitalized preterm neonates, running counter to the belief that minimizing stress in preterm infants was an important part of preventing the development of neurologic injury (Anand et al. 2004). A more detailed review of the clinical trials utilizing morphine or fentanyl analgesia in neonates is provided below.

Procedural pain

Opioid analgesics are clinically warranted for use in neonates undergoing noxious medical procedures. Clinical trials have investigated the clinical effectiveness of morphine or fentanyl for noxious medical procedures including percutaneous venous catheter placement, heel lancing, endotracheal intubation and endotracheal suctioning. A summary of the results is shown in Table 10.2. While initial studies demonstrated decreased pain, some recent studies have demonstrated non-significant effects. Differences in study methodologies, including statistical power, variation in the procedure evaluated, outcome measure(s) used and time course for evaluation of response have inevitably contributed to some of the observed variability in results. In addition, some studies have included infants maintained on morphine infusions, while others have included infants given a single bolus dose prior to the noxious event, and it is unclear whether supplemental bolus doses are appropriate for infants already stabilized on opioid infusions. Moreover, it is important to note that most of the available data are limited to infants receiving ventilatory support. It has been suggested that non-ventilated infants receive one-quarter to one-half the usual opioid dose, however, the safety and efficacy of this practice has not been rigorously evaluated. Finally, the analgesia achieved after combined use of opioid analgesics and other sedatives or analgesic agents has not been evaluated.

Based on these cumulative data, the effectiveness of morphine for procedural pain has now been called into question. Future studies are needed to determine what factors influence apparent opioid effectiveness in neonates undergoing procedural pain so that rational guidelines may be developed for their optimal use in clinical practice.

Postoperative pain

Operative procedures are performed in newborn infants for the management of specific congenital anomalies as well as for urgent medical conditions. In two separate landmark studies, opioid analgesics were shown to decrease the stress response and improve clinical outcome when used during operative procedures in newborns (Anand et al. 1987, Anand and Hickey 1992).

Continuous intravenous opioid infusions are the standard of care for moderate and severe postoperative pain in the newborn and young infant (Kost-Byerly 2002). Nevertheless, there are many unanswered questions pertaining to the clinical use of opioids in this setting. For example, the optimal dosing titration and weaning methods have not yet been

Table 10.2 Selected neonatal studies evaluating morphine or fentanyl for procedural pain

Reference	Design	Sample	Drug regimen	Outcomes	Comments
Carbajal et al. 2005	DB RCT Heel lance N = 42	GA: 23–32 wks (mean = 27 wks) BW: 0.96 kg PNA: NR Wt. at study: NR	Morphine (M) 100 µg/kg IV LD, then IV infusion of either: 10 (23–26 wks GA), 20 (27–29 wks GA), or 30 µg/kg/h (30–32 wks GA), OR Placebo (P)	No difference in DAN, PIPP for M vs. P at baseline before study, at 2–3 h after LD, or 20–28 h after infusion	N = 42 ventilated Plasma M level not correlated with DAN or PIPP No difference in hypotension for M vs. P: at baseline, 2 vs. 0, 2–3 h after LD, 3 vs. 0, 20–28 h after infusion, 1 vs. 0
Scott et al. 1999	Prospective observational study Heel lance N = 48	GA: 24–39 wks BW: NR PNA: NR Wt. at study: NR	Morphine (M) 50 µg/kg IV LD, then IV infusion (mean, 24 µg/kg/h × 80 hours) THEN No treatment (NT)	↓NFCS in M vs. NT at swab and heel lance	N = 46 ventilated Plasma M level not correlated with NFCS Adverse events NR
Moustogiannis et al. 1996	Non-randomized CT Percutaneous venous catheter N = 19	GA: mean 28.5–30 wks BW: mean 1007–1054 g PNA: mean 5–7.8 d Wt. at study: mean 1070–1365 g	Morphine (M) 0.05 mg/kg or 0.1 mg/kg IV (?bolus) OR No treatment (NT)	↓ HR and skin blood flow for M vs. NT No difference in BP, RR, O_2 satn, number of successful attempts	N = 12 ventilated; most in M group Mean BP did not change in M group
Cordero et al. 1991	RCT Broviac catheter N = 29	GA: mean 27–28 wks BW: 600–1350 g PNA: 5–30 d Wt at study: 620–1320 g	Lidocaine 1% 5 mg/kg SC + Fentanyl 2 µg/kg IV (F) OR Lidocaine 1% 5 mg/kg SC + Secobarbital 1 mg/kg IV (S)	↓O_2 satn in S vs. F; ↑FiO_2 in S vs. F; ↑ blood glucose in S vs. F No difference in HR, BP, epinephrine, norepinephrine	N = 23 ventilated No. of successful attempts NR Study treatment blinding and adverse events NR

Continued

Table 10.2 Selected neonatal studies evaluating morphine or fentanyl for procedural pain—cont'd

Reference	Design	Sample	Drug regimen	Outcomes	Comments
Anand et al. 2004	DB RCT Tracheal suctioning N = 898	GA: 23–32 wks BW: 1.0 kg PNA: <4 days old Wt at study: NR	Morphine (M) 100 μg/kg IV LD, then IV infusion of either: 10 (23–26 wks GA), 20 (27–29 wks GA), or 30 μg/kg/h (30–32 wks GA), OR Placebo (P)	No difference in composite outcome (death, IVH, PVL) for M vs. P ↓PIPP at 24 h (not at 72 h) for M vs. P ↓HR, RR and ↑O$_2$ satn for M vs. P at some timepoints for M vs. P	N = 898 ventilated ↑Hypotension, ventilation time, and time to full-volume nasogastric feeds for M vs. P
Simons et al. 2003	DB RCT Tracheal suctioning N = 150	GA: 29 wks BW: 1.2 kg PNA: 9 h Wt at study: NR	Morphine (M) 100 μg/kg IV LD, then IV infusion of 10 μg/kg/h OR Placebo (P)	No difference in PIPP, NIPS, VAS for M vs. P (assessments made twice daily) ↓IVH for M vs. P No difference in poor neurologic outcome (IVH, PVL, death) or comorbidities (chronic lung disease, sepsis, PDA, necrotizing enterocolitis) for M vs. P	N = 150 ventilated No difference in duration of ventilation, NICU stay for M vs. P
Lemyre et al. 2004	DB RCT Endotracheal intubation N = 132	GA: 27–28 wks BW: 0.9–1 kg PNA: 3–8 days Wt at study: NR	Morphine (M) 200 μg/kg IV LD OR Placebo (P)	↑duration of hypoxemia for M vs. P Similar HR, BP, duration of procedure, number of attempts	No difference in ventilator support over 24 h
Taddio et al. 2006	DB RCT Percutaneous central venous catheter N = 132	GA: 27.5–30 wks BW: 0.9–1.45 kg PNA: 30.6 wks Wt at study: 1.1–1.44 kg	Tetracaine (T) OR Morphine (M) 100 mg/kg IV over 20 min OR Tetracaine + Morphine (TM) OR No treatment	↓Brow bulge for TM and M vs. T and NT ↓HR for TM, M and T vs. NT	N = 130 ventilated ↑Ventilation rate for M vs. non-M ↑Erythema for T vs. non-T No difference in hypotension

BP, blood pressure; BW, birthweight; CT, controlled trial; DAN, Douler Aiguë Nouveau-né; DB, double-blind; FiO$_2$, fraction of inspired oxygen; GA, gestational age; HR, heart rate; IV, intravenous; IVH, intraventricular heamorrhage; LD, loading dose; N, total sample size; NFCS, neonatal facial coding system; NICU, neonatal intensive care unit; NIPS, Neonatal Infant Pain Scale; NR, not reported; O$_2$ satn, oxygen saturation; PDA, patent ductus arteriosus; PIPP, premature infant pain profile; PNA, postnatal age; PVL, periventricular leucomalacia; RCT, randomized controlled trial; RR, respiratory rate; SC, subcutaneous; VAS, visual analogue scale; Wt at study, weight at time of study.

determined. Infusion doses have been recommended over intermittent bolus doses in order to maintain stable plasma concentrations and minimize the risk of under- and over-analgesia associated with troughs and peaks (Farrington et al. 1993). Few studies, however, have documented the effects of bolus dosing versus continuous infusions. In one study of continuous versus intermittent 'as needed' morphine after surgery in 0–1-year-old infants, infusions resulted in improved analgesia and a higher total morphine dose, but no difference in safety (Lynn et al. 2000). In another study of fentanyl (2 µg/kg 2-hourly bolus dosing versus 1 µg/kg/h continuous infusion), bolus dosing was associated with a similar efficacy, but a higher incidence of apnoea (Vaughn et al. 1996). In a recent comparison of continuous morphine infusions (10 µg/kg/h) versus intermittent dosing (i.e., 30 µg/kg 3-hourly) for postoperative pain, no differences were demonstrated in efficacy or safety after major abdominal or thoracic surgery (Van Dijk et al. 2002). Moreover, there was no consistent correlation between physiological responses to pain and behavioural responses to pain (Bouwmeester et al. 2001).

Recent studies have suggested different infusion doses according to gestational age to account for maturation of drug elimination pathways (Kart et al. 1997b). Using pre-existing pharmacokinetic data, one group of investigators targeted doses in order to achieve plasma concentrations of 20 ng/ml (Lynn et al. 2000). To date, plasma concentrations have not been shown to correlate with analgesia (Bouwmeester et al. 2003). In addition, there are no published guidelines for the use of opioids in non-intubated infants, and local practices regarding extubation during concurrent analgesia are highly variable.

Apart from these issues, there are no published studies investigating the potential opioid-sparing effects of combination interventions (including non-steroidal anti-inflammatory drugs or acetaminophen) for postoperative pain. The prevention of adverse effects, including tolerance and withdrawal reactions by use of either specific dosing regimens, opioid-sparing regimens or opioid antagonists, requires further investigation.

Sedation during mechanical ventilation
Opioid analgesics have been increasingly used for sedation and analgesia in ventilated preterm infants (Saarenmaa et al. 1999) because of pharmacological effects that promise to be of benefit in the infant's short-term and long-term trajectories. Acute benefits include: reduction of stress; promotion of blood pressure stability; ventilator synchrony (by decreasing spontaneous respirations and promoting synchronized

breathing with the ventilator); and improved oxygenation. In the long term, reduced stress, as well as reduced fluctuations in oxygenation and blood pressure are believed to minimize the risk of neurologic injury and death (Barker and Rutter 1996).

Several randomized placebo-controlled trials have investigated the effects of opioids on pain and long-term outcomes in ventilated preterm infants. Anand et al. (1999) found that preterm infants who received morphine infusions (vs. placebo dextrose) in the first days of life had significantly less pain during tracheal suctioning and improved long-term neurological outcomes (defined as a reduced risk of death and of major neurological morbidity). A third group of infants who received midazolam had significantly worse outcomes compared to morphine, but no difference in pain. In contrast, Quinn and colleagues (1993) and Dyke et al. (1995) demonstrated a decrease in pain but no difference in long-term outcomes using morphine for an average duration of 2 days. Similarly, Lago et al. (1998) and Orsini et al. (1996) demonstrated reduced behavioural stress, but not neonatal complications with fentanyl administration in the first 3–5 days of life.

Two large trials examining the effects of preemptive morphine analgesia were recently carried out. In the first study by Simons et al. (2003) involving 150 preterm neonates (mean gestational age, 29 weeks), morphine infusions (100 µg/kg bolus, followed by 10 µg/kg/h for 7 days) were associated with no differences compared to placebo on pain during acute procedures (i.e. tracheal suctioning). In addition, morphine was associated with a decreased incidence of intraventricular haemorrhage, but not overall neurological outcome. In the second multi-centre study by Anand et al. (2004), 898 infants were randomized to morphine or placebo. After a bolus dose of 100 µg/kg, morphine infusions of 10, 20 or 30 µg/kg/h were administered for up to 14 days to infants of 23–26 weeks, 27–29 weeks and 30–32 weeks gestational age respectively. Unlike the previous study, morphine reduced pain during acute procedures (i.e. tracheal suctioning). However, it did not affect neurological outcome and was associated with significant adverse effects, including hypotension, increased time to full-feeding and a longer duration of ventilation. Moreover, administration of additional doses of morphine (i.e. open-label) was associated with worse outcomes, although this may have been due to underlying illness in those infants. Based on their findings, the authors questioned whether the pain from ventilation is significant enough to warrant opioid analgesia. They suggested that if opioids are indicated, lower doses and variations in the doses are administered, according to the clinical situation. Alternatively, sedative agents may be tried.

In a recent meta-analysis including all available controlled trials to date (Bellu et al. 2005), it was concluded that infants given morphine during mechanical ventilation demonstrated less pain compared to a placebo. No statistically significant differences in long-term outcomes, including mortality, neuro-developmental outcomes and ventilation duration, however, were reported, and morphine was associated with an increased time to full enteral feeding.

Based on these data, the role of systemic opioid analgesia, particularly morphine, in ventilated preterm infants is unclear. It is important to note, however, that the effects of morphine infusions were primarily assessed for acute procedural pain rather than ongoing sedation. Moreover, it is not known if the results of previous studies with morphine can be extrapolated to fentanyl, which has a slightly different pharmacologic profile. At the present time, clinicians will have to use their best clinical judgement. This involves identifying infant parameters that predict benefit (i.e. sedation and analgesia) versus risk (i.e. hypotension) and treating only infants where the benefits outweigh the risks. There are currently insufficient data to support an expectation of improved clinical outcome.

Adverse effects of opioids

Opioid analgesics are associated with potentially serious and life-threatening adverse effects, including: respiratory depression; glottic and chest wall rigidity; hypotension; bradycardia; urinary retention; ileus; and seizures. Continuous monitoring and frequent assessment of vital signs can prevent the development of significant adverse events. Fortunately, the effects can be reversed by opioid antagonists, such as naloxone (0.01–0.1 mg/kg). Small doses of naloxone are usually administered first and repeated if necessary (owing to its relatively short duration of action). Fentanyl-induced muscle rigidity can be reversed by administration of a muscle relaxant such as pancuronium (in a dosage of 0.015 mg/kg) (Hickey et al. 1985) or naloxone (0.01 mg/kg, repeatedly administered until the rigidity subsides) (Wells et al. 1994). It must be remembered that when opioid antagonists such as naloxone are used, the analgesic effects of opioids will be reversed as well.

The risk of opioid-induced adverse effects can be minimized by rational drug selection and dosing. For example, morphine should be avoided in preterm infants with blood pressure instability because it can contribute to hypotension (Hall et al. 2005). Morphine may cause bronchospasm in infants with reactive airways disease. In addition, opioid co-administration with benzodiazepines, such as midazolam, should be avoided because this drug combination increases the risk of hypotension and respiratory depression (Yaster et al. 1990).

Opioids act on brainstem respiratory centres and decrease all phases of respiration (rate, depth, volume, and tidal exchange) (Koren and Maurice 1989), which can lead to apnoea and respiratory arrest. There is also retention of CO_2 owing to a decrease in responsiveness of the respiratory centre. Respiratory depression and CO_2 retention result in cerebral vasodilation and an increase in cerebrospinal fluid (CSF) pressure unless ventilatory support can maintain CO_2 within normal limits. One study found that neonates were more susceptible than adults to the respiratory depressant action of morphine when the same 'mg per kg' dose was used. It was speculated that this was due to a greater permeability of the neonatal blood–brain barrier to morphine (Way et al. 1965). However, higher systemic exposure may also be used to explain the results of that study. In a more recent study of the respiratory effects of intravenous morphine infusions, concentrations above 20 ng/ml were associated with respiratory depression (defined as hypercarbia or a shift in end-tidal CO_2 curve). In addition, there was no difference in the susceptibility to respiratory depression in neonates compared to infants and children (Lynn et al. 1993). In a separate study of fentanyl-induced ventilatory depression, no differences were observed between infants (0–1 year), children and adults (Hertzka et al. 1989). Opioids also cause rigidity of thoracic and abdominal muscles and glottic closure (Scamman 1983, Lajarrige et al. 1993). Muscle rigidity prevents inflation of the chest, impairing oxygen–carbon dioxide exchange, and leads to increased ventilatory requirements, hypercapnia and convulsions (Pokela et al. 1992, Van Lemmen and Semmekrot 1996).

Opioid analgesia may increase the level of ventilatory support that is required in ventilated infants (Purcell-Jones et al. 1987, Orsini et al. 1996, Vaughn et al. 1996). Infants with impaired pulmonary function, neurologic disease or a history of prematurity may be at higher risk of clinically significant respiratory depression (Acute Pain Management Guideline Panel 1992, Vaughn et al. 1996). In non-intubated neonates, there is the potential for apnoea necessitating intubation (Purcell-Jones et al. 1987). Apnoea has been reported in non-intubated infants who received morphine doses of 50–100 µg/kg (Tholl et al. 1994). Administration of a single dose of 100 µg/kg was not associated with apnoea in two other reports in a total of 26 spontaneously breathing neonates (Purcell-Jones et al. 1987, Pokela et al.

1993). Apnoea was a frequent adverse effect of post-operative fentanyl analgesia in non-intubated neonates that had been extubated in the operating room: the incidence was 100% (4/4) for infants treated with fentanyl bolus dosing (2 μg/kg every 2 hours) and 30% (3/10) for infants treated with continuous infusions (1 μg/kg/h) (Vaughn et al. 1996). Hypoxaemic events were reported in 100% (6/6) of infants given intravenous bolus dose injections to manage postoperative pain (Haberkern et al. 1996).

Opioids can cause hypotension and bradycardia (Bovill et al. 1984). Certain subgroups of infants, such as hypovolaemic infants, may be at increased risk for hypotension. Hypotension is less likely to occur following administration of synthetic opioids such as fentanyl, compared to morphine (which releases histamine). It is important to note that mild decreases in blood pressure and heart rate may be expected in highly stressed infants because of a decrease in stress and/or sedative effect induced by the drugs (Gauntlett et al. 1988, Rutter and Evans 2000). In two separate studies in preterm ventilated neonates, systemic (and cerebral) blood flow was not significantly altered by morphine, when given in a dose of either 100 μg/kg infused quickly, or 100 μg/kg/h given over 2 hours (Sabatino et al. 1997, Rutter and Evans 2000). Similarly, administration of a slow bolus infusion of 3 μg/kg of fentanyl did not affect either general or cerebral haemodynamics in preterm newborn infants (Hamon et al. 1996). Moreover, duct closure was not inhibited by morphine (Rutter and Evans 2000).

Opioid analgesics decrease intestinal secretions and peristalsis, resulting in constipation and ileus. Opioid analgesics also cause bladder spasm and urinary retention through their effects on smooth muscle and sphincter tone. Decreased gastrointestinal motility can postpone enteral feeding (Saarenmaa et al. 1999) and increase serum bilirubin concentration (Roth et al. 1991). Fentanyl has been associated with significantly less effects on gastrointestinal motility than morphine (Saarenmaa et al. 1999).

Abnormal seizure-like movements, as well as electrically recorded seizures, have been reported in neonates who received either morphine or fentanyl (Koren et al. 1985, Da Silva et al. 1999). Risk factors appear to include rapid infusion rates and high plasma concentrations (Koren et al. 1985). The effect of a test dose of naloxone on seizure activity may be observed to determine if seizures are opioid-induced (Da Silva et al. 1999).

In adults, opioids are frequently associated with nuisance-type adverse effects, including nausea, pruritis and vomiting. The frequency of these adverse effects in neonates is not well documented. In one trial of morphine for postoperative pain in 0–1-year-old infants, 30% (25/83) of infants experienced either emesis or pruritis or both adverse effects (Lynn et al. 2000); the incidence of emesis and pruritis was 19% (5/26), and 4% (1/26), respectively, in another study including infants of the same age range (Lynn et al. 1998). In another study of postoperative pain in infants 3–12 months old, the incidence of pruritis was 67% (4/6) (Haberkern et al. 1996). Pruritis may manifest itself as agitation due to excessive body movements made in an attempt to alleviate the symptom. Unfortunately, this side effect can be mistakenly interpreted as pain and lead to increases in the opioid dose and adverse effects. Some authors have recommended using either diphenhydramine or low-dose naloxone to treat pruritis (Haberkern et al. 1996, Yaster and Nichols 2001).

It is important to note that opioid-induced adverse effects may be caused by medication errors (Gill et al. 1996). Vigilance on the part of medical, nursing and pharmacy staff are needed to ensure that dosage regimens are appropriate and that infants are adequately monitored.

Continuous opioid administration may lead to the development of acute opioid tolerance (Mao et al. 1995, Kissin et al. 2000) and opioid-induced facilitation of nociceptive processing (Crain and Shen 1995, Celerier et al. 1999, Li et al. 2001) thereby increasing the requirements for postoperative analgesia and enhancing postoperative pain. Strategies to maximize pain relief and minimize the development of acute opioid tolerance and opioid-induced hypersensitivity include co-administration of NMDA receptor antagonists such as low-dose ketamine (Celerier et al. 2000, Laulin et al. 2002) and dextromethorphan and ultra low-dose opioid antagonists such as naloxone and naltrexone (Gan et al. 1997, Crain and Shen 2000). However, there are no studies in neonates or infants that address acute opioid tolerance, opioid-induced facilitation of nociceptive processing and their reversal by opioid antagonists or NMDA receptor antagonists.

Opioid tolerance in neonates requires dose escalation to maintain analgesia and sedation. The rate of development of tolerance is variable between infants, but may be as short as a few days after the beginning of therapy. Tolerance is believed to develop more rapidly with continuous infusions of opioids (rather than intermittent doses) and with the use of synthetic opioids (e.g. fentanyl) (Suresh and Anand 1998). According to various authors, the development of tolerance to fentanyl in neonates occurs after a cumulative fentanyl dose of 1.6–2.5 mg/kg, or after 5–9 days of continuous infusion therapy (Arnold et al. 1990, Katz et al. 1994). It has been suggested that the risk of developing opioid tolerance may be reduced by instituting other comfort measures concurrently that supplement opioid analgesia/sedation such as noise reduction (Grehn 1998), or by switching opioids and using sedatives (if appropriate) (Suresh and Anand 1998).

Abrupt discontinuation of opioid analgesics may be accompanied by withdrawal reactions in infants that are physiologically dependent. The main body systems affected in opioid withdrawal include the central nervous system, autonomic system and gastrointestinal system. In one retrospective study of the frequency of adverse effects following opioid use in neonates for ≥3 days, the most frequently observed symptoms were irritability, hypertonicity, diaphoresis, hyperthermia and vomiting with feeds (Norton 1988). Forty-eight percent of 18 neonates given morphine and 84% of 15 neonates who received fentanyl experienced withdrawal reactions. Withdrawal reactions were correlated with dose and duration of infusion and lasted from 1 to 11 days. Fentanyl was associated with a longer duration of withdrawal (mean, 3.9 days) compared to morphine (2.3 days).

Some authors have suggested tapering schedules for discontinuation of opioids; the rationale being that gradual removal of the drug will prevent withdrawal reactions. At present, there are no experimental data supporting one tapering method over another and individual patient needs should be considered. In general, more aggressive tapering schedules are advised for patients who have received short-term therapy compared to those taking opioids for longer durations. For short-term therapy, opioid doses are decreased by approximately 25% to 50% of the dose per day and the drug is discontinued within 2–3 days. Doses are decreased by 10–20% of the original dose per day for long-term therapy, and infusion regimens may be switched to intermittent dosing regimens before discontinuation. An approach to weaning opioid infusions was recently published by Anand and colleagues (1999). The same opioid that was used therapeutically is usually used during the weaning process. Continual observation and evaluation of withdrawal reactions is necessary throughout the tapering period. Many NICUs have implemented tapering protocols to facilitate the process (Grehn 1998). They use objective tools to monitor symptoms (Suresh and Anand 1998) and tailor opioid dosing requirements accordingly. Withdrawal reactions are managed with opioids. Non-pharmacological interventions, as described in Chapter 12, are added to supplement their effects. Non-opioid medications are less frequently used to manage withdrawal reactions (Yaster et al. 1996, Suresh and Anand 1998).

Long-term effects of opioid analgesia

Several investigative teams have attempted to determine whether opioid analgesia in the neonatal period is associated with long-term effects, both positive and negative, in the neonate. Morphine infusions in ventilated preterm neonates have not been associated with improved neurological outcomes (Anand et al. 2004). In addition to neurological outcomes, researchers have identified parental attachment and imprinting as potential targets of disruption by opioid analgesics. These concerns stemmed from studies of the ontogeny of various neurotransmitter systems in the nervous system demonstrating extensive postnatal development with increased plasticity in the neonate compared to the adult. Briefly, human studies have shown that infants born to opioid-abusing mothers may have cognitive and behavioural problems (although these data are confounded by other risk factors associated with drug abuse). Animal studies have demonstrated altered receptor number, analgesia and tolerance in the adult following exposure in early life.

It should be noted, however, that it is possible that non-medical opioid exposure in the neonatal period may lead to different pharmacological effects from when it is used for painful conditions (Rahman et al. 1997). In a study that investigated long-term neurologic and behavioural outcomes in newborn infants exposed to opioids during clinical care (for 56 hours to 5 days), no adverse effects were observed. Infants who received morphine ($n = 57$) were not different from those who did not ($n = 30$) in intelligence quotient (IQ), motor impairment or behaviour problems. In fact, there was a trend for better scores in the morphine-exposed group (MacGregor et al. 1998).

Finally, iatrogenic pain is commonplace in newborn infants, and there is accumulating evidence that untreated neonatal pain has long-lasting effects on pain responsivity in infancy and childhood (Taddio and Katz 2005). Furthermore, it has been hypothesized that the clinical use of opioids in infants undergoing noxious procedures is protective against any future changes in pain responsivity. This hypothesis is supported by studies in which analgesics administered prior to noxious procedures have led to a reduction in the magnitude of long-term changes in pain behaviours (Oberlander et al. 2000, Grunau et al. 2001a, 2001b, Peters et al. 2003). These data are further discussed in Chapter 4.

CONCLUSIONS

Newborn infants have the capacity to perceive pain and there is accumulating evidence that untreated pain and stress may have long-lasting effects on subsequent pain responses later in infancy (Taddio and Katz 2005). There is an ethical obligation to optimally manage pain in infants and, at present, opioid analgesics are justified for the management of moderate and severe pain in this population. There remain some unanswered questions, however, regarding optimal utilization of these drugs in the clinical setting. For instance, there are unresolved issues regarding the most appropriate dosing regimen for individual infants. In addition, recent studies do not support the routine use of opioids in neonates that are ventilated or undergoing procedural pain.

This is in contrast to clear documentation of the adverse effects of opioid analgesia, including hypotension and respiratory depression. Clearly, more research is needed to determine the factors that impact on analgesic effectiveness and methods to maximize the benefit to risk ratio. Hopefully, these initiatives will lead to improved pain management in infants and improved outcome.

ACKNOWLEDGEMENT

Dr. Taddio is supported by a Canadian Institutes of Health Research New Investigator Award.

REFERENCES

Acute Pain Management Guideline Panel. (1992). Acute pain management in infants, children, and adolescents: operative and medical procedures. Quick reference guide for clinicians. AHCPR Pub MD; No. 92-0020.

American Academy of Pediatrics (Committee on Fetus and Newborn; Committee on Drugs; Section on Anesthesiology; and Section on Surgery) Canadian Paediatric Society (The Fetus and Newborn Committee). (2000). Prevention and management of stress and pain in the newborn infant. Pediatrics 105: 454–461.

Anand KJS. (1993). Relationships between stress responses and clinical outcome in newborns, infants, and children. Crit Care Med 21: S358–S359.

Anand KJS. (2001). International Evidence-Based Group for Neonatal Pain. Consensus statement for the prevention and management of pain in the newborn infant. Arch Ped Adolesc Med 155: 173–180.

Anand KJS, Hickey PR. (1992). Halothane-morphine compared with high dose sufentanil for anesthesia and post-operative analgesia in neonatal cardiac surgery. New Engl J Med 326: 1–9.

Anand KJS, Sippell WG, Aynsley-Green A. (1987). Randomized trial of fentanyl anaesthesia in preterm babies undergoing surgery: effects on the stress response. Lancet 1: 243–248.

Anand KJS, McIntosh N, Lagercrantz H, et al. (1999). Analgesia and sedation in preterm neonates who require ventilatory support. Arch Ped Adolesc Med 153: 331–338.

Anand KJS, Whit Hall R, Desai N, et al. (2004). Effects of morphine analgesia in ventilated preterm neonates: primary outcomes from the NEOPAIN randomized trial. Lancet 363: 1673–1682.

Arnold JH, Truog RD, Orav EJ, et al. (1990). Tolerance and dependence in neonates sedated with fentanyl during extracorporeal membrane oxygenation. Anesthesiology 73: 1136–1140.

Arnold JH, Truog RD, Scavone JM, et al. (1991). Changes in the pharmaco-dynamic response to fentanyl in neonates during continuous infusion. J Pediatr 119: 639–643.

Barker DP, Rutter N. (1995). Exposure to invasive procedures in neonatal intensive care unit admissions. Arch Dis Child (Fetal and Neonatal Edition) 72: F47–F48.

Barker DP, Rutter N. (1996). Stress, severity of illness, and outcome in ventilated preterm infants. Arch Dis Child 75: F187–F190.

Bellu R, deWaal KA, Zanini R. (2005). Opioids for neonates receiving mechanical ventilation. The Cochrane Library Volume (3).

Bhat R, Chari G, Gulati A, et al. (1990). Pharmacokinetics of a single dose of morphine in preterm infants during the first week of life. J Pediatr 117: 477–481.

Bouwmeester NJ, Anand KJS, Van Dijk M. (2001). Hormonal and metabolic stress responses after major surgery in children aged 0–3 years: a double-blind, randomized trial comparing the effects of continuous versus intermittent morphine. Br J Anaesth 873: 390–399.

Bouwmeester NJ, Hop WCJ, Van Dijk M. (2003). Postoperative pain in the neonate: age-related differences in morphine requirements and metabolism. Intens Care Med 29: 2009–2015.

Bouwmeester NJ, Anderson BJ, Tibboel D, et al. (2004) Developmental pharmacokinetics of morphine and its metabolites in neonates, infants and young children. Br J Anaesth 92: 208–217.

Bovill JG, Sebel PS, Stanley TH. (1984). Opioid analgesics in anesthesia: with special reference to their use in cardiovascular anesthesia. Anesthesiology 61: 731–755.

Burns AM, Shelly MP, Park GR. (1992). The use of sedative agents in critically ill patients. Drugs 43: 507–515.

Bussche GV, Noorduin H. (1986). Alfentanil and sufentanil: towards a more specific use of narcotics in anesthesia. Drug Develop Res 8: 341–346.

Carbajal R, Lenclen R, Jugie M, et al. (2005). Morphine does not provide adequate analgesia for acute procedural pain in preterm neonates. Pediatrics 115: 1494–1500.

Celerier E, Laulin J, Larcher A, et al. (1999). Evidence for opiate-activated NMDA processes masking opiate analgesia in rats. Brain Res 847: 18–25.

Celerier E, Rivat C, Jun Y, et al. (2000). Long-lasting hyperalgesia induced by fentanyl in rats: preventive effect of ketamine. Anesthesiology 92: 465–472.

Chay PCW, Duffy BJ, Walker JS. (1992). Pharmacokinetic–pharmacodynamic relationships of morphine in neonates. Clin Pharmacol Ther 51: 334–342.

Cordero L, Gardner DK, O'Shaughnessy R. (1991). Analgesia versus sedation during broviac catheter placement. Am J Perinatol 8: 284–287.

Crain SM, Shen KF. (1995). Ultra-low concentrations of naloxone selectively antagonize excitatory effects of morphine on sensory neurons, thereby increasing its antinociceptive potency and attenuating tolerance/dependence during chronic cotreatment. Proc Natl Acad Sci USA 92: 10540–10544.

Crain SM, Shen KF. (2000). Antagonists of excitatory opioid receptor functions enhance morphine's analgesic potency and attenuate opioid tolerance/dependence liability. Pain 84: 121–131.

Da Silva O, Alexandrou D, Knoppert D, et al. (1999). Seizure and electroencephalographic changes in the newborn period induced by opiates and corrected by naloxone infusion. J Perinatol 19: 120–123.

Davis PJ, Killian A, Stiller RL, et al. (1989). Pharmacokinetics of alfentanil in newborn premature infants and older children. Develop Pharmacol Ther 13: 21–27.

Dyke MP, Kohan R, Evans S. (1995). Morphine increases synchronous ventilation in preterm infants. J Paed Child Health 31: 176–179.

Farrington EA, McGuinness GA, Johnson GF. (1993). Continuous intravenous morphine infusion in postoperative newborn infants. Am J Perinatol 10: 84–87.

Gan TJ, Ginsberg B, Glass PS, et al. (1997). Opioid-sparing effects of a low-dose infusion of naloxone in patient-administered morphine sulfate. Anesthesiology 87: 1075–1081.

Gauntlett IS, Fisher DM, Hertzka RE, et al. (1988). Pharmacokinetics of fentanyl in neonatal humans and lambs: effects of age. Anesthesiology 69: 683–687.

Gill AM, Cousins A, Nunn AJ, et al. (1996). Opiate-induced respiratory depression in pediatric patients. Ann Pharmacother 30: 125–129.

Gong Q-L, Hedner T, Hedner J, et al. (1991). Antinociceptive and ventilatory effects of the morphine metabolites: morphine-6-glucuronide and morphine-3-glucuronide. Euro J Pharmacol 193: 47–56.

Grehn LS. (1998). Adverse responses to analgesia, sedation, and neuromuscular blocking agents in infants and children. AACN Clin Issues 9: 36–48.

Grunau RE, Oberlander TF, Whitfield MF, et al. (2001a). Demographic and therapeutic determinants of pain reactivity in very low birth weight neonates at 32 weeks' postconceptional age. Pediatrics 107: 105–112.

Grunau RE, Oberlander TF, Whitfield MF, et al. (2001b). Pain reactivity in former extremely low birth weight infants at corrected age 8 months compared with

term born controls. Infant Behav Develop 24: 41–55.

Haberkern CM, Lynn AM, Geiduschek JM, et al. (1996). Epidural and intravenous bolus morphine for postoperative analgesia in infants. Can J Anaesth 43: 1203–1210.

Hall RW, Kronsberg SS, Barton BA, et al. (2005). Morphine, hypotension, and adverse outcomes among preterm neonates: who's to blame? Secondary results from the NEOPAIN trial. Pediatrics 115: 1351–1359.

Hamon I, Hascoet JM, Debbiche A, et al. (1996). Effects of fentanyl administration on general and cerebral haemodynamics in sick newborn infants. Acta Paediatrica 85: 361–365.

Hartley R, Levene MI. (1995). Opioid pharmacology in the newborn. In: Aynsley-Green A, Ward Platt MP, Lloyd-Thomas AR (eds). Stress and pain in infancy and childhood. Balliere's Clinical Paediatrics 3: 467–493.

Hartley R, Green M, Quinn M, et al. (1993). Pharmacokinetics of morphine infusion in premature neonates. Arch Dis Child 69: 55–58.

Hertzka RE, Gauntlett IS, Fisher DM, et al. (1989). Fentanyl-induced ventilatory depression: effects of age. Anesthesiology 70: 213–218.

Hickey PR, Hansen DD, Wessel DL, et al. (1985). Blunting of stress responses in the pulmonary circulation of infants by fentanyl. Anesth Analg 64: 1137–1142.

Jacqz-Aigrain E, Burtin P. (1996). Clinical pharmacokinetics of sedatives in neonates. Clin Pharm 31: 423–443.

Johnson KL, Erickson JP, Holley FO, et al. (1984). Fentanyl pharmacokinetics in the pediatric patient. Anesthesiology 62: A441.

Johnston CC, Collinge JM, Henderson S, et al. (1997). A cross-sectional survey of pain and analgesia in Canadian neonatal intensive care units. Clin J Pain 13: 308–312.

Kart T, Christrup LL, Rasmussen M. (1997a). Recommended use of morphine in neonates, infants and children based on a literature review: part I-pharmacokinetics. Paediatr Anaesth 7: 5–11.

Kart T, Christrup LL, Rasmussen M. (1997b). Recommended use of morphine in neonates, infants and children based on a literature review: part 2-clinical use. Paediatr Anaesth 7: 93–101.

Katz R, Kelly HW, Hsi A. (1994). Prospective study on the occurrence of

withdrawal in critically ill children who receive fentanyl by continuous infusion. Crit Care Med 22: 763–767.

Kearns GL, Abdel-Rahman SM, Alander SW, et al. (2003). Developmental pharmacology – drug disposition, action, and therapy in infants and children. N Engl J Med 349: 1157–1167.

Kissin I, Bright CA, Bradley EL Jr. (2000). The effect of ketamine on opioid-induced acute tolerance: can it explain reduction of opioid consumption with ketamine-opioid analgesic combinations? Anesth Analg 91: 1483–1488.

Koren G, Maurice L. (1989). Pediatric use of opioids. Pediatr Clin North Am 36: 1141–1156.

Koren G, Butt W, Chinyanga H, et al. (1985). Postoperative morphine infusion in newborn infants: assessment of disposition characteristics and safety. J Pediatr 107: 963–967.

Kost-Byerly S. (2002). New concepts in acute and extended postoperative pain management in children. Anesthesiol Clin North America 20: 115–135.

Lago P, Benini F, Agosto C. (1998). Randomised controlled trial of low dose fentanyl infusion in preterm infants with hyaline membrane disease. Arch Dis Child 79: F194–F197.

Lajarrige C, Adafer M, Mouthemy G, et al. (1993). Effet du fentanyl sur la ventilation du premature. Arch Fr Pediatr 50: 271–274.

Laulin JP, Maurette P, Corcuff JB, et al. (2002). The role of ketamine in preventing fentanyl-induced hyperalgesia and subsequent acute morphine tolerance. Anesth Analg 94: 1263–1269.

Lemyre B, Doucette J, Kalyn A, et al. (2004). Morphine for elective endotracheal intubation in neonates: a randomized trial. BMC Pediatrics 4: 20.

Li X, Angst MS, Clark JD. (2001). Opioid-induced hyperalgesia and incisional pain. Anesth Analg 93: 204–209.

Lugo RA, Kern SE. (2002). Clinical pharmacokinetics of morphine. J Pain Palliat Care Pharmacother 16: 5–18.

Lynn AM, Nespeca M, Opheim KE, et al. (1993). Respiratory effects of intravenous morphine infusions in neonates, infants, and children after cardiac surgery. Anesth Analg 77: 695–701.

Lynn A, Nespeca MK, Bratton SL, et al. (1998). Clearance of morphine in postoperative infants during intravenous infusion: the influence of age and surgery. Anesth Analg 86: 958–963.

Lynn AM, Nespeca M, Bratton SL, et al. (2000). Intravenous morphine in postoperative infants: intermittent bolus dosing versus targeted continuous infusions. Pain 88: 89–95.

MacGregor R, Evans D, Sugden D, et al. (1998). Outcome at 5–6 years of prematurely born children who received morphine as neonates. Arch Dis Child 79: F40–F43.

McRorie TI, Lynn AM, Nespeca MK, et al. (1992). The maturation of morphine clearance and metabolism. Am J Dis Child 146: 972–976.

Mao J, Price DD, Mayer DJ. (1995). Mechanisms of hyperalgesia and morphine tolerance: a current view of their possible interactions. Pain 62: 259–274.

Mather LE. (1983). Pharmacokinetic and pharmacodynamic factors influencing the choice, dose and route of administration of opiates for acute pain. Clin Anesth 1: 17–40.

Moustogiannis AN, Raju TNK, Roohey T, et al. (1996). Intravenous morphine attenuates pain induced changes in skin blood flow in newborn infants. Neurol Res 18: 440–444.

Norton SJ. (1988). After effects of morphine and fentanyl analgesia: a retrospective study. Neonatal Network 7(3): 25–28.

Oberlander TF, Grunau RE, Whitfield MF, et al. (2000). Biobehavioral pain responses in former extremely low birth weight infants at four months' corrected age. Pediatrics 105(1): e6. Online. Available: http://www.pediatrics.org/cgi/content/full/105/1/e6

Orsini AJ, Leef KH, Costarino A. (1996). Routine use of fentanyl infusions for pain and stress reduction in infants with respiratory distress syndrome. J Pediatr 129: 140–145.

Pacifici GM, Sawe J, Kager L, et al. (1982). Morphine glucuronidation in human fetal and adult liver. Eur J Clin Pharmacol 22: 553–558.

Peters JWB, Koot HM, deBoer JB, et al. (2003). Major surgery within the first 3 months of life and subsequent biobehavioral pain responses to immunization at later age: a case comparison study. Pediatrics 111: 129–135.

Peters JWB, Anderson BJ, Simons SHP, et al. (2005). Morphine pharmacokinetics during venoarterial

extracorporeal membrane oxygenation in neonates. Intens Care Med 31: 257–263.

Pokela M-L, Ryhanen PT, Koivisto ME, et al. (1992). Alfentanil-induced rigidity in newborn infants. Anesth Analg 75: 252–257.

Pokela M-L, Olkkola KT, Seppala T, et al. (1993). Age-related morphine kinetics in infants. Develop Pharmacol Ther 20: 26–34.

Porter FL, Wolf CM, Gold J, et al. (1997). Pain and pain management in newborn infants: a survey of physicians and nurses. Pediatrics 100: 626–632.

Purcell-Jones G, Dormon F, Sumner E. (1987). The use of opioids in neonates. A retrospective study of 933 cases. Anaesthesia 42: 1316–1320.

Quinn MW, Wild J, Dean HG, et al. (1993). Randomised double-blind controlled trial of effect of morphine on catecholamine concentrations in ventilated pre-term babies. Lancet 342: 324–327.

Rahman W, Fitzgerald M, Aynsley-Green A, et al. (1997). The effects of neonatal exposure to inflammation and/or morphine on neuronal responses and morphine analgesia in adult rats. In: Jensen TS, Turner JA, Wiesenfeld-Hallin Z. (eds). Proceedings of the 8th World Congress on Pain, Progress in pain research and management. IASP Press, Seattle 8: 783–794.

Roth B, Schlunder C, Houben F. (1991). Analgesia and sedation in neonatal intensive care using fentanyl by continuous infusion. Develop Pharmacol Ther 17: 121–127.

Rutter N, Evans N. (2000). Cardiovascular effects of an intravenous bolus of morphine in the ventilated preterm infant. Arch Dis Child 83: F101–F103.

Saarenmaa E, Huttunen P, Leppaluoto J, et al. (1999). Advantages of fentanyl over morphine in analgesia for ventilated newborn infants after birth: a randomized trial. J Pediatr 134: 144–150.

Saarenmaa E, Neuvonen P, Fellman V. (2000). Gestational age and birth weight effects on plasma clearance of fentanyl in newborn infants. J Pediatr 136: 767–770.

Sabatino G, Quartulli L, DiFabio S, et al. (1997). Hemodynamic effects of intravenous morphine infusion in ventilated preterm babies. Early Human Develop 47: 263–270.

Santeiro ML, Christie J, Stromquist C, et al. (1997). Pharmacokinetics of

continuous infusion fentanyl in newborns. J Perinatol 17: 135–139.

Scamman FL. (1983). Fentanyl-O2-N2O rigidity and pulmonary compliance. Anesth Analg 62: 332–334.

Scott CS, Riggs W, Ling EW, et al. (1999). Morphine pharmacokinetics and pain assessment in premature newborns. J Pediatr 135: 423–429.

Simons SHP, van Dijk M, van Lingen A. (2003). Routine morphine infusion in preterm newborns who received ventilatory support. JAMA 290: 2419–2427.

Stein C. (1995). The control of pain in peripheral tissue by opioids. New Engl J Med 1332: 1685–1690.

Singleton MA, Rosen JI, Fisher DM. (1987). Plasma concentrations of fentanyl in infants, children and adults. Can J Anaesth 35(2): 152–155.

Suresh S, Anand KJS. (1998). Opioid tolerance in neonates: mechanisms, diagnosis, assessment, and management. Semin Perinatol 22(5): 425–433.

Taddio A, Katz J. (2005). The effects of early pain experience in full-term and preterm neonates on subsequent pain responses later in infancy and childhood. Pediatr Drugs 7(4): 245–257.

Taddio A, Lee C, Yip A, et al. (2006). Intravenous morphine and topical tetracaine for treatment of pain in neonates undergoing central line placement. JAMA 295: 793–800.

Tholl DA, Wager MS, Sajous CH, et al. (1994). Morphine use and adverse effects in a neonatal intensive care unit. Am J Hosp Pharm 51: 2801–2803.

Van Dijk M, Bouwmeester NJ, Duivenvoorden HJ, et al. (2002). Efficacy of continuous versus intermittent morphine administration after major surgery in 0–3-year-old infants; a double-blind randomized controlled trial. Pain 98: 305–313.

Van Lemmen RJ, Semmekrot BA. (1996). Muscle rigidity causing life-threatening hypercapnia following fentanyl administration in a premature infant. Eur J Pediatr 155: 1067.

Vaughn PR, Townsend SF, Thilo EH, et al. (1996). Comparison of continuous infusion of fentanyl to bolus dosing in neonates after surgery. J Pediatr Surg 31: 1616–1623.

Way WL, Costley EC, Way EL. (1965). Respiratory sensitivity of the newborn infant to meperidine and morphine. Clin Pharmacol Ther 6: 454–461.

Wells S, Williamson M, Hooker D. (1994). Fentanyl-induced chest wall rigidity in a neonate: a case report. Heart Lung 23: 196–198.

Yaster M, Nichols DG. (2001). Pain management in the critically ill child. Indian J Pediatr 68: 749–769.

Yaster M, Nichols DG, Deshpande JK, et al. (1990). Midazolam-fentanyl intravenous sedation in children: case report of respiratory arrest. Pediatrics 86: 463–467.

Yaster M, Berde C, Billet C. (1996). The management of opioid and benzodiazepine dependence in infants, children, and adolescents. Pediatrics 98: 135–140.

Central and peripheral regional analgesia and anaesthesia

Navil Sethna
Santhanam Suresh

INTRODUCTION

All invasive medical procedures, no matter how minor, produce tissue damage and activate a nociceptive process coupled with physiological and psychological stress responses. Untreated or inadequately treated pain is now widely recognized to adversely affect the well-being of the infant, hinder recovery after surgery, and probably affect long-term life experiences (Anand et al. 1985, 1987, Grunau et al. 1994, Porter et al. 1999). This has led to a growing interest in improving management of pain in children of all ages, including premature infants.

Central (neuroaxial) and peripheral regional anaesthetic techniques have a significant but limited place in the practice of pain management in infants and children. Regional anaesthetic techniques presumably afford many of the same advantages for paediatric patients as they do in the adult patient. However, there are few controlled clinical trials evaluating the advantages and adverse effects in neonates and infants compared to conventional analgesic strategies. The safe and successful performance of peripheral and central neural block techniques in infants and toddlers demands specific knowledge of anatomical, pharmacological and psychological domains of development. A thorough knowledge of the developmental differences and sufficient prior skills practice of the regional neural block in adults greatly enhance the safe and successful application of these techniques in the paediatric population. In this chapter, we will discuss peripheral and central anaesthetic techniques available to practitioners who care for this population, along with scientific information supporting their use (Bosenberg et al. 1992, Wolf et al. 1998, Sethna and Berde 2002).

LIMITATIONS OF GENERAL ANAESTHESIA IN THE NEONATE

In the past 30 years, significant advances in perinatal medicine and understanding of reproductive processes have led to a marked increase in the incidence of premature infants (Guyer et al. 1995). The emergence of a large population of premature and former premature infants presenting for surgical procedures led to rising concerns about the risk of postoperative apnoea and oxygen desaturation from respiratory depressant medications in the management of perioperative pain and renewed interest in paediatric regional anaesthesia, particularly spinal anaesthesia in high-risk premature infants (Abajian et al. 1984). The incidence of postoperative apnoea ranges from 11 to 37% following general anaesthesia whereas the incidence is insignificant and the frequency and severity of oxygen desaturation and bradycardia are considerably diminished when spinal anaesthesia is employed alone (Harnik et al. 1986, Kurth et al. 1987, Welborn et al. 1991, Cote et al. 1995, Krane et al. 1995, Somri et al. 1998, William et al. 2001).

The occurrence of postoperative apnoea and periodic breathing in former premature infants recovering from minor surgical procedures after general anaesthesia has been recognized relatively recently. Several reports have investigated the incidence, risk factors, and possible ways to reduce the potential for apnoea after general anaesthesia, including possible benefits of regional anaesthesia as a safe alternative to general anaesthesia (Steward 1982, Liu et al. 1983, Kurth et al. 1987, Welborn et al. 1990). All these reports are limited by small samples of infants, considerable differences in the definition of apnoea, the degree of complicated medical history, the type of impedance pneumography monitoring (continuous versus standard pneumography and nursing observation), and institutional clinical practices. A recent study pooled eight of the prospective studies on the incidence of postoperative apnoea after general anaesthesia in a combined analysis. The likelihood of apnoea occurring in premature and former premature infants undergoing herniorrhaphy under general anaesthesia was found to be inversely related to both gestational and postconceptional age. Anaemia (haemoglobin <30%) was a significant risk factor, particularly in infants of postconceptional age of 34 weeks and greater. However, the influence of other risk factors such as a history of necrotizing enterocolitis, neonatal apnoea, respiratory distress syndrome, bronchopulmonary dysplasia, or operative use of opioids and/or muscle relaxants could not be determined from this small sample size (Cote et al. 1995).

The frequency of prolonged postoperative apnoea (defined as apnoea ≥ 15 seconds) after general anaesthesia occurs in approximately 70% of premature infants <42 weeks postconceptional age and decreases to approximately 5% by postconceptual age 50–60 weeks (Kurth et al. 1987, Malviya et al. 1993). Most apnoeic episodes occur within 2 hours of general anaesthesia but the initial episode of apnoea may occur as late as 12 hours following general anaesthesia and may persist for 24–48 hours in some premature infants less than 42 weeks postconceptional age. The risk of postoperative apnoea can be reduced by the use of intravenous caffeine (10 mg/kg) intraoperatively, judicious use of opioids and other central nervous system depressants, and unsupplemented spinal or caudal anaesthesia (Welborn et al. 1989, 1990, 1991, Krane et al. 1995, Craven et al. 2003).

Although general anaesthesia with inhaled agents such as halothane may blunt the nociceptive processing, it incompletely blocks the noxious neural traffic from reaching the central nervous system. The use of high-dose opioid anaesthesia, which may more effectively suppress the perioperative nociception and metabolic–endocrine responses, is limited by attendant respiratory depression (Anand et al. 1987, Anand and Hickey 1992).

ADVANTAGES AND LIMITATIONS OF REGIONAL ANAESTHESIA AND ANALGESIA

Regional anaesthetic techniques are currently going through a renaissance in paediatric anaesthesia practice and are regaining the degree of prominence held at the turn of the 20th century. Their use is now considered basic to paediatric anaesthesia practice. Regional anaesthesia is defined as a state of temporary inhibition of specific sensory nerve fibres (and in most instances motor and autonomic fibres as well) by local anaesthetic without interruption of consciousness. In contrast, regional analgesia is a state of partial or complete pain relief while maintaining general motor and autonomic function. Most regional anaesthetic techniques employ local anaesthetic agents as the primary nerve-blocking agent which stabilizes neuronal membranes and prevents nerve conduction by inhibiting ionic fluxes required for the initiation and conduction of impulses. Opioids and other adjuvant analgesics (such as clonidine, ketamine) that act by a different mode of action may be added to local anaesthetics to enhance analgesia through additive or synergistic mechanisms. While preservative-free ketamine S (+)-isomer is commercially available in Europe for epidural use, its spinal/epidural use is not universally accepted due to lack of adequate preclinical neurotoxicity data (Eisenach et al. 1998, de Beer and Thomas 2003, Eisenach and Yaksh 2003).

Analogous to adult clinical practice, the most important application for neural axis anaesthesia and analgesia is management of intra- and postoperative pain in children undergoing abdominal and thoracic operations, particularly those children who are at high risk for respiratory compromise from concurrent disease processes or who receive opioids for pain relief. In general, the benefits of paediatric regional anaesthesia and analgesia likely include perioperative modification of neuroendocrine stress responses, effective pain control, rapid recovery, and shortened hospital stay (Bosenberg et al. 1992, McNeely et al. 1997a, Wolf et al. 1998, Wilson et al. 2001). The presumed mechanisms by which regional anaesthesia produces pain control and modification of the neuroendocrine response is by hindering the passage of the noxious neural signals to the spinal dorsal horn neurons (peripheral nerve blocks) or modifying the signals at the level of the nerve roots and dorsal horn cells (epidural and spinal blocks) (Suresh et al. 2002). Combining caudal epidural anaesthesia with general anaesthesia for lower abdominal and lower extremity procedures significantly suppresses the neuroendocrine responses (ACTH, beta-endorphin, epinephrine, norepinephrine, ADH, hyperglycaemia and cortisol) compared to general anaesthesia alone. Similarly, combining lumbar or thoracic epidural anaesthesia with general anaesthesia and extending the epidural analgesia after major abdominal procedures has favourably modified neuroendocrine responses both intra- and postoperatively (Giaufre et al. 1985, Murat et al. 1988, Wolf et al. 1993).

Possible benefits of unsupplemented spinal or epidural anaesthesia in conscious premature infants are reduced frequency of postoperative apnoea and elimination of the need for tracheal intubation in premature infants with chronic respiratory disease (Welborn et al. 1991, Krane et al. 1995, Somri et al. 1998, Bouchut et al. 2001b). Systematic review of regional versus general anaesthesia in high-risk premature and former premature infants undergoing inguinal herniorrhaphy in early infancy identified a total population of only 108 patients in randomized and quasi-randomized controlled trials (Craven et al. 2003). Regrettably, these trials were of inadequate quality and the overall results found no evidence that spinal anaesthesia is more effective than general anaesthesia with respect to the incidence of postoperative morbidity. However, when data were reanalyzed after excluding infants who received respiratory depressant agents simultaneously with spinal anaesthesia, there was a statistically significant reduction in the incidence of postoperative apnoea in the group that received spinal anaesthesia compared to the group that received general anaesthetic, implying the immature brainstem is susceptible to analgesic-induced respiratory depressant effects (Craven et al. 2003).

Major disadvantages of these anaesthetic techniques are technical difficulties, failure to achieve adequate surgical anaesthesia, need for significant sedation in vigorous and active infants, and apnoea from inadvertent high spinal and epidural anaesthesia (Frumiento et al. 2000).

ADVERSE EFFECTS AND COMPLICATIONS OF REGIONAL ANAESTHETIC TECHNIQUES

Accidental intravascular injection of local anaesthetics during the performance of central and peripheral nerve blocks (e.g. circumcision) has been reported. Small doses may produce central nervous system excitation and seizures and large doses may produce dysrhythmias and cardiac arrest (Ved et al. 1993, Fried et al. 1994, Tanaka et al. 2001). Inadvertent intravascular injection of air and venous air embolism have also been reported during identification of the epidural space (Guinard and Borboen 1993, Schwartz and Eisenkraft 1993, Sethna and Berde 1993). Accidental injection of local anaesthetics into the cerebrospinal fluid results in high spinal anaesthesia that may result in respiratory difficulties, apnoea or cardiovascular compromise (Desparmet 1990, Afshan and Khan 1996). Needle- and catheter-induced injury of the spinal cord and major nerves is a potential complication but is extremely rare in skilful hands. A recent epidemiological survey in a large series of children receiving central and peripheral regional anaesthetic techniques did not find major neurological complications (Giaufre et al. 1996). While infection at the site of indwelling epidural catheters is very rare, the catheter entry site should be inspected daily for evidence of skin infection. Despite the presence of significant bacterial colonization with short-term (2–5 days) indwelling caudal and epidural catheter tips in two recent prospective studies, serious local and systemic infection did not ensue. In both these studies, the culture results and risk of infection may have been influenced by prophylactic administration of antibiotics during most of the surgical patients (Strafford et al. 1995, McNeely et al. 1997b, Kost-Byerly et al. 1998). Nevertheless, a few sporadic cases of serious infectious complications have been reported in children and infants (Emmanuel 1994, Larsson et al. 1997, Meunier et al. 1997). These reports underscore the importance of strict aseptic technique, avoidance of local tissue trauma, daily inspection of skin catheter entry site and use of styleted epidural needles and closed infusion systems. All epidural catheter entry sites should be inspected daily for contamination and evidence of skin infection particularly in caudally placed epidural catheters because of the potential for soiling from urine and faecal matter in infants and toddlers. Motor weakness of lower extremities can develop from epidural infusions with local anaesthetics, although this complication often is not problematic in premature and term infants who are not ambulating. The occurrence of muscle weakness is less of an issue during infusion of low concentrations of local anaesthetic and usually resolves with adjustment of the dose.

PHARMACOLOGY OF LOCAL ANAESTHETICS

Since local anaesthetics are the predominant agents utilized for most regional anaesthesia techniques, it is appropriate to review some specific issues related to the pharmacology of local anaesthetics in neonates and infants. Available data on the absorption, distribution and metabolism of local anaesthetics are limited in infants and insufficiently evaluated in newborn and premature infants.

The pKa values of the commonly used local anaesthetics are close to the physiologic pH of 7.4. This results in considerable amounts of these agents existing in the ionized form and being distributed throughout body water compartments. The extra-cellular space is larger in neonates and infants than in adults (40% compared to 20% of the body weight) and consequently the peak plasma levels of initial doses of local anaesthetics are relatively low compared to adults.

Infants under 6 months of age have lower serum concentrations of albumin and alpha-1-acid glyco-protein. The concentration of alpha-1-glycoprotein is 50% lower in premature neonates compared to term neonates (Lerman et al. 1989). Low protein binding of amide-type anaesthetics such as bupivacaine and lidocaine may result in dramatic increases in the con-centration of free (unbound) drug that can potentially predispose these patients to central nervous system and cardiovascular system toxicity (Frawley et al. 2000).

Hepatic degradation of amide-type local anaesthe-tics involves aromatic hydroxylation, N-dealkylation and amide hydrolysis. Hepatic clearance is slower in newborn infants and approaches adult functional capacity by 3–6 months of life. Bupivacaine and lidocaine, the most commonly used amide local anaesthetics, have prolonged elimination half-lives in infants under the age of 6 months. Therefore, admin-istration of repeated doses or continuous infusions of local anaesthetics should be administered at lower dose ranges (see section on epidural anaesthesia and analgesia) (Tucker 1986, Sethna and Berde 2002). This was emphasized early in the use of continuous epidural infusions with reports of bupivacaine toxicity during continuous infusions (Agarwal et al. 1992, McCloskey et al. 1992). Single enantiomers, levobupi-vacaine and ropivacaine, were recently introduced for use in infants and children as safer alternatives to racemic bupivacaine. Both enantiomers provide a wider range of safety for systemic toxicity with equivalent analgesic efficacy to racemic bupivacaine and lesser motor block (Santos and DeArmas 2001). Ropivacaine

is less cardiotoxic at equivalent plasma concentrations of racemic bupivacaine and has a higher threshold for central nervous toxicity from the unbound plasma concentration in healthy subjects (Knudsen et al. 1997, Bardsley et al. 1998). A few population pharmaco-kinetic studies of ropivacaine in infants (0–12 months) have evaluated both the total and unbound plasma (the primary determinant systemic toxicity) concen-trations (Habre et al. 2000, Wulf et al. 2000, McCann et al. 2001, Rapp et al. 2004, Bosenberg et al. 2005). The mean and range of peak and unbound plasma concentrations of ropivacaine observed over a period of 5.7 hours after a single injection via the caudal route were well below the toxic concentration. The apparent unbound fraction clearance increases and the elimination of half-life decreases with age in infants during the first year of life. The terminal half-life ranges from 6.7 hours at 1 month of age to 2.2 hours at 9 months of age with an inter-individual variability of 39% (coefficient of variation) (Rapp et al. 2004). A recent pharmacokinetic study of ropivacaine infusion in 45 term infants under 1 year of age (median age 116 days, range 0–362 days) demon-strated a low clearance of unbound ropivacaine in neonates (mean 33 ml/ min/kg) compared to infants above the age of one month; mean 80, 124 and 163 ml/min/kg in the age groups of 1–3, 3–6 and 6–12 months respectively (Bosenberg et al. 2005). The plasma concentration of unbound ropivacaine reached a steady-state level after a 24-hour infusion period in all infants including neonates. At the termination of the infusion period of 48–72 hours the unbound ropivacaine concentrations were higher in neonates (median 0.1 mg/L, range 0.04–0.2) than infants older than 1 month (median 0.03 mg/L, range 0.003–0.1) but were below the threshold concen-tration for central nervous system toxicity in adults (≥0.4 mg/L) and none of the infants clinically mani-fested adverse effects of systemic toxicity. Nevertheless, caution is advised with the use of ropivacaine infusion in the first week of life due to a large variability in hepatic metabolism and the limited data in this age group.

There is only one published pharmacokinetic trial that examined a single injection of levobupivacaine via the caudal route in 48 children younger than 2 years and 11 infants under the age of 3 months (range un-specified) (Chalkiadis et al. 2004). After administra-tion of levobupivacaine 2 mg/kg, the time to peak plasma concentration ranged 5–60 minutes (median 30 minutes) and reached significantly later in infants younger than 3 months. The peak venous plasma concentration ranged between 0.4 and 2 μg/ml (mean 0.9 ± 0.4). Although the maximum plasma concentra-tion of levobupivacaine was within the acceptable safe range for racemic bupivacaine, this is a preliminary study with limited blood sampling time of 60 minutes and so further trials are needed to fully characterize the pharmacokinetic profile of levobupivacaine in early infancy.

CENTRAL (NEURAL AXIS) ANAESTHESIA AND ANALGESIA

Cardiovascular and respiratory responses to neural axis anaesthesia

Despite the variability in the doses used by different investigators and the achievement of high spinal sensory anaesthesia/analgesia of T4–T6, in most infant trials haemodynamic instability and respiratory compromise have not been observed (Dohi et al. 1979, Abajian et al. 1984, Harnik et al. 1986, Oberlander et al. 1995). Similarly, children younger than 5 years of age have been shown to tolerate sympatholysis from mid-thoracic epidural anaesthesia well. Cardiac output, blood pressure and heart rate are maintained at a relatively stable level (Payen et al. 1987, Larousse et al. 2002). Presently, there is no satisfactory explanation for the cardiovascular stability observed in infants in the face of high thoracic sympathectomy. A recent study in former premature infants undergoing herniorrhaphy with spinal anaesthesia suggests that the autonomic reflex responses to thoracic spinal anaesthesia (C7–T4 level) was most likely due to decrease of parasympathetic modulation of the cardiac function. The expected decreases in heart rate and blood pressure from the peripheral and cardiac sympatholysis were offset by the diminished cardiac vagal activity (Oberlander et al. 1995). Minute ventilation is also maintained within normal range during high thoracic sensory block (T2–T4) in premature infants. The tidal volume exchange is maintained near normal range by compensatory increase in the diaphragm muscle activity that offsets any potential ventilatory compromise from loss of intercostal and accessory muscle function (Pascucci et al. 1990).

Epidural anaesthesia and analgesia

As with adults, in children the administration of a local anaesthetic to the epidural space is accomplished at various sites along the epidural space. The epidural space is accessed via the (1) saccrococcygeal hiatus (caudal epidural block), (2) lumbar intervertebral spaces (lumbar epidural block), and (3) thoracic intervertebral spaces (thoracic epidural block). In infants and young children, the caudal and lumbar routes are utilized to advance epidural catheters to the thoracic epidural space (Bosenberg et al. 1988, Gunter and Eng 1992, Gunter 2000). Advancement of an epidural catheter to a considerable length is not always reliable

due to potential for the catheter to kink, coil, migrate through the intervertebral foramina or to be misplaced into the subarachnoid or vascular space (van Niekerk et al. 1990, Blanco et al. 1996). As with adults, the most reliable approach to place an epidural catheter is to access the epidural space directly at the appropriate intervertebral space so that only a short length of the catheter is threaded and optimal analgesia is possible through administration of minimal effective concentrations and doses of local anaesthetics (Fig. 11.1). However, in an anaesthetized child direct access to the epidural space in the thoracic region can be fraught with potential neurological complications (Rose 2003).

An alternative approach is to advance the epidural catheters from either the caudal or lumbar route to the thoracic epidural space but this approach could be associated with a high failure rate ranging from 15% with the caudal to 83% with the lumbar approach (van Niekerk et al. 1990, Blanco et al. 1996). The reliability of the lumbar approach can be improved by accessing the lumbar epidural space in the midline at L5–S1 (modified Taylor approach) and insertion of a Crawford needle (rather than a Tuohy needle) at a shallow angle.

The success rate of achieving the desired thoracic segments with this modified Taylor approach is a high 93% and is comparable to the success rate reported with the caudal-to-thoracic approach in experienced hands (Bosenberg et al. 1988, 1992, Gunter 2000). This modified technique may offer several technical advantages over the access from other lumbar intervertebral spaces because the L5–S1 intervertebral space is large, easy to identify (prominent L5 and less prominent S1 spinous processes), least likely to be distorted by spine deformity and allows a shallow insertion of a Crawford needle for easy alignment with the long axis of the spine thereby facilitating easy advancement of the epidural catheter. It may also be associated with a lower incidence of infection compared to the caudal-to-thoracic approach in view of a lower incidence of bacterial colonization of the indwelling epidural catheters at the lumbar compared to the caudal site (McNeely et al. 1997b, Kost-Byerly et al. 1998, Gunter 2000).

Although advancing the epidural catheter from the lumbar-to-thoracic route is relatively as safe as the caudal-to-thoracic approach compared to direct placement of the epidural catheter at the thoracic intervertebral spaces in an anesthetized child, unlike the caudal approach it carries the potential of inadvertent spinal tap. Therefore, the caudal approach is widely accepted as the practical and safe route for a single injection of local anaesthetic and advancing the caudal-to-thoracic catheter. Though the caudal route is

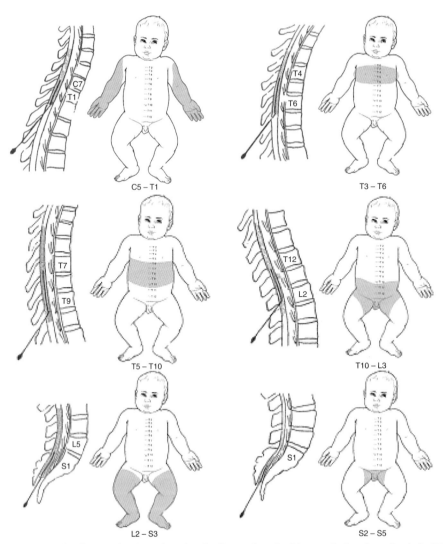

C5 – T1

T3 – T6

T5 – T10

T10 – L3

L2 – S3

S2 – S5

Figure 11.1 Segmental epidural anaesthesia and analgesia. (Reproduced with permission from Buckely PF In: Loeser JD et al. (eds). Textbook of Bonica's management of pain, 2000, Ch 102, p. 1946 with permission from Lippincott Williams and Wilkins.)

associated with a higher incidence of cutaneous bacterial colonization relative to the lumbar site in infants and toddlers, the incidence of epidural infection of short-term (2–5 days) indwelling catheters has not been shown to be higher (McNeely et al. 1997b, Kost-Byerly et al. 1998).

Considering the higher failure rate with both the advancement of caudal-to-thoracic and lumbar-to-thoracic catheters (7–83%) several approaches are proposed to improve the reliability and safety of epidural catheter placement.

1. The use of a radiographic guide either by fluoroscopy or epidurography. This approach is time-consuming, expensive, not readily available and is associated with very rare but potentially

serious adverse reaction to contrast media and radiation exposure.

2. The use of an electrical nerve stimulation-guided technique; although this requires some technical expertise and special equipment it is probably the most economical and less time-consuming than other approaches. The setup consists of a commercially available open tip, single-orifice wire-reinforced epidural catheter (Arrow Flextip Plus, Arrow International, Inc., Reading, USA), Johans ECG adaptor and a nerve stimulator. After placement of the epidural catheter it is filled with saline, the anode lead of the stimulator is connected to an electrode over a limb for grounding and the cathode lead is connected to the ECG adaptor at the hub of the epidural

catheter. The nerve stimulator is adjusted to deliver a frequency of 1 Hz and a pulse of 200 ms and is gradually increased from zero until segmental muscle contractions of the torso or limb are visible (Tsui et al. 1998). Electrical current transmitted via the saline-filled epidural catheter is capable of stimulating the neural tissue adjacent to the catheter tip. The threshold current necessary to elicit motor response depends on the proximity of the catheter tip to the neural tissue. In general, magnitudes of the current required to elicit a motor response within the epidural space, subarachnoid space, subdural space and proximity to a nerve root are 1–10 mA, 0.2 mA, 0.3 mA and 0.5 mA, respectively (Tamai et al. 2004, Tsui et al. 2005). These suggested current thresholds are derived from experience with the low-resistance epidural catheters (wire reinforced).

The first trial in children ($n = 21$) aged 5 weeks to 2.5 years showed usefulness of the electrical stimulation test in verifying the proper placement of the epidural catheters advanced from the caudal-to-thoracic epidural space with a 90% success rate as determined clinically by the satisfactory postoperative epidural analgesia. The average time required to verify correct placement of the epidural catheter was 14 minutes (range 5–25 minutes) (Tsui et al. 2001). A second trial in a smaller number of older children ($n = 10$) 1–4 years of age confirmed the findings of the previous study on the efficacy of epidural nerve stimulator guidance in improving the success rate of placement of caudal-to-thoracic epidural catheters (Tamai et al. 2004). Interestingly, the electrical nerve stimulation seems to offer no advantage over the standard method of direct epidural catheter placement and verification of the correct placement with the use of epidural test dose in children (Goobie et al. 2003).

3. The use of ultrasound imaging has the advantage of real-time visualization of the epidural space, exact depth, needle advancement and catheter location. It also has the potential for identifying anatomical variations and screening of anatomical details relevant to the spine (Rapp and Grau 2004). A pilot study in infants compared the estimation of epidural catheter length required to reach the target cranial spinal segments from the lumbar approach using ultrasound imaging versus clinical measurement of the desired catheter length using cutaneous landmarks. The epidural catheter was visualized in nine of the 12 infants, all less than 6 months old. The entire length of the catheter was visualized only in five infants but

the tip of the catheter was not visualized distinctly (Chawathe et al. 2003). As the resolution of ultrasound imaging technology designed for regional block techniques improves so will the reliability of visualizing the epidural catheter. This technique is evolving; training and experience in viewing images is imperative for successful and time-saving application. It also has the potential for improving the safety of both the peripheral and central nerve blocks relative to other methods of confirmation of accurate placement of block needles and catheters.

4. Direct placement of an epidural catheter in the extrapleural paravertebral space before the closure of a unilateral thoracotomy incision may offer a safer alternative approach to thoracic epidural catheter placement (see blow).

Caudal-epidural analgesia

Caudal-epidural anaesthesia and analgesia is the most widely used regional technique in awake and anaesthetized infants and children and is accomplished either by injection of a single or repeated doses and by continuous infusion of local anaesthetics. The merits of each technique are summarized in Tables 11.1 and 11.2. A major disadvantage of a single-dose caudal-epidural anaesthesia is limited duration of analgesia of approximately 60 minutes. It also requires large anaesthetic volumes and provides a variable short-lived duration of postoperative analgesia (Table 11.1). These limitations are circumvented by either addition of an adjuvant agent such as opioids or clonidine to enhance the quality and prolong the duration of analgesia, or placement of an indwelling epidural catheter for continuous infusion of local anaesthetics and to extend postoperative analgesia (Table 11.2) (Bosenberg 1998, van Niekerk et al. 1990, Gunter and Eng 1992, De Negri et al. 2001).

Continuous epidural infusion is commonly used as an adjunct to general anaesthesia (balanced anaesthesia) to effectively control pain, avoid the need for systemic opioids, allow early tracheal extubation, and for continuation of the infusion for management of postoperative pain. Such a combination technique is appealing where postoperative intensive care support is scarce (Bosenberg 1998). The safety and efficacy of various infusion regimens have been investigated in children of different ages but only limited data are available in neonates and infants (Table 11.3). As with adults, the addition of adjuvant analgesics such as opioids, clonidine (an alpha 2-adrenergic agonist) and ketamine (NMDA receptor antagonist) to epidural local anaesthetic infusions have the benefit of reducing the effective dose of local anaesthetics and

Table 11.1 Caudal-epidural anaesthesia with a single-dose injection of local anaesthetics in awake infants (Touloukian et al. 1971, Hassan 1977, Spear et al. 1988, Gunter et al. 1991)*

Postnatal age at the time of surgery	Local anaesthetic concentration and dose	Sensory spinal segment levels	Anaesthetic duration (minutes)	Advantages and disadvantages
17 ± 13 weeks	Bupivacaine 0.375% 3.75 mg/kg	T5 ± 2	89 ± 8	A prospective study Technical failure occurred in 1 out of 20 infants 5 out of 20 infants required supplementation
7 ± 4 months	Bupivacaine 0.25% with epinephrine 1:200 000 2.5–3.25 mg/kg	T10–T1	Maximum 90	A retrospective study 4 out of 7 infants required supplementation
4–120 weeks	Lidocaine 1.5% or mepivacaine 1.5% 7–11 mg/kg	T6	60	Prospective study 17 out of 70 infants required supplementation
3.9 ± 4.9 weeks	Lidocaine 0.5–1% 4.8 ± 1 mg/kg	T10	60	Retrospective study 2 out of 14 infants required supplementation

*These four reports of a single-dose injection of local anaesthetics were selected from among the many trials of caudal anaesthesia in children of all ages because of their inclusion of neonates and infants only.
(From Regional Anesthesia and Analgesia 1998 with permission)

thereby decreasing the potential risks of systemic toxicity (Wolf et al. 1991, Cook et al. 1995, De Negri et al. 2001). Varying opinions exist among paediatric practitioners regarding the relative risks and benefits of opioids and other adjuvant agents administered either exclusively or in combination with local anaesthetic epidural infusions in early infancy.

A number of recent trials have reported effective and safe use of a newly introduced ropivacaine local anaesthetic in infants and children. In a double-blind multicentre study involving 245 children age 1–10 years, a single injection of 1 ml/kg of ropivacaine 0.2% produced similar onset time of approximately 10 minutes and equivalent effective postoperative analgesia of approximately 4.5 hours compared to 1 ml/kg of bupivacaine 0.25%. There was no measurable motor weakness with either local anaesthetic (Ivani et al. 2005). A second study compared postoperative analgesia and degree of motor block in a randomized double-blind study of a single injection of caudal 1 ml/kg of ropivacaine 0.25% or bupivacaine 0.25% in 80 children aged 2–5 years and demonstrated a significantly shorter duration (5 ± 4 hours) of motor block in the ropivacaine compared to the bupivacaine group (Da Conceicao et al. 1999). As expected, concentrations of ropivacaine higher than 0.2% produced greater motor weakness

(Da Conceicao and Coelho 1998, Da Conceicao et al. 1999). Interestingly, a higher concentration of ropivacaine of 0.375% did not appear to increase the duration of analgesia (5 ± 3 hours) but produced significantly less motor weakness compared to a similar concentration and volume (1 ml/kg) of caudal bupivacaine (Da Conceicao and Coelho 1998). The time to peak plasma concentration is significantly longer and plasma concentrations significantly higher with ropivacaine compared to similar concentration and volume of bupivacaine 0.2% (1 ml/kg) in children over the age of 2 years (Ala-Kokko et al. 2000). A lower concentration of ropivacaine 0.1% alone provides significantly less effective and shorter median duration of caudal analgesia compared to 0.2% (1.7 vs. 4.5 hours respectively) (Luz et al. 2000).

Few studies have investigated epidural levobupivacaine (equipotent to racemic bupivacaine) efficacy and safety in infants below the age of 6 months. A randomized observer-blinded comparison of three concentrations of levobupivacaine (0.125%, 0.2%, 0.25%) administered at a dose of 1 ml/kg for caudal block in 60 children aged 1–7 years demonstrated a clear dose–response effect of postoperative analgesia (time to the first analgesic rescue) and motor block (Ivani et al. 2003). Although there were no significant differences in the intraoperative analgesia between the

Table 11.2 Continuous caudal epidural anaesthesia in awake infants (Henderson et al. 1993, Peutrell and Hughes 1993, 1994)

Postconceptual age at the time of surgery	Local anaesthetic concentration and dose	Sensory segment level	Surgical duration in minutes	Advantages and disadvantages
40 ± 4 weeks	2-chloroprocaine 3% 84 ± 30 mg/kg/h*	T4–T2	95 ± 35	A prospective trial Longest anaesthetic duration was 170 min Effective in all 10 infants No plasma toxicity detected No complications
41 ± 2.5 weeks	Bupivacaine 0.25% and 0.375% 2.8 ± 0.7 mg/kg*	Not specified	Not specified In some infants > 95	A prospective trial Effective in 8 out of 9 infants One infant required supplementation Dose requirement was lower compared to a single-dose technique in Table 11.1 No complications
41.2 ± 7 weeks**	Bupivacaine 2.8 mg/kg (range 2.5–3.7 mg/kg)†	Not determined	40 ± 18 (range 20–80)	A retrospective trial Effective in 9 out 9 infants Complications. One premature infant developed transient self-limiting apnoea. A second premature infant with bronchopulmonary dysplasia developed transient apnoea and desaturation

* = cumulative dose
** = Combined subarachnoid-caudal epidural anaesthesia.
† = Initial dose of subarachnoid bupivacaine 0.5% was 0.87 ± 0.2 mg/kg, 20 minutes later it was followed by bupivacaine infusion and top up doses as needed.
(Modified from Regional Anesthesia and Analgesia 1998)

three concentrations, the 0.125% concentration produced significantly shorter postoperative duration of analgesia (median 60 minutes) and least motor block. The postoperative analgesia and motor block did not significantly differ between the other two concentrations of 0.25% and 0.2% of levobupivacaine. Yet the 0.2% concentration was considered to be the clinically useful concentration because of the longer median duration of analgesia of 118 minutes (range 60–660 minutes) with moderate weakness in 20% of the children. Another randomized controlled trial of 99 children aged 0.5–10 years compared the analgesic effects of similar concentrations of 0.25% caudal levobupivacaine to bupivacaine and ropivacaine. The results showed no difference in the surgical analgesic onset time (mean 8 ± 4 minutes) between the three groups. Bupivacaine produced significantly greater postoperative analgesia (2.5 ± 0.6 hours) and more intense residual motor block within the first hour of emerging from anaesthesia but no difference was noted between the three groups at 3 hours after administration of the local anaesthetic (Locatelli et al. 2005).

Adjuvant analgesics

Application of clonidine in adult anaesthesia and analgesia is well established (Sveticic et al. 2004). In children, clonidine is increasingly used by enteral and systemic routes for diagnostic and therapeutic purposes and in the past decade the application has been extended to perioperative management of anxiety, sympathetic arousal, emesis and to prolong analgesia (Nishina et al. 1999). In recent years, the analgesic property of clonidine has been expanded to epidural and intrathecal application in infants and children (Nishina et al. 1999, Rochette et al. 2004).

Table 11.3 Recommended local anaesthetics for continuous epidural infusion in young children based on elimination half-lives (Morgan et al. 1978, Ecoffey et al. 1985, Mazoit et al. 1988, Kost-Byerly et al. 1993, Luz et al. 1996, Hansen et al. 2000, Lonnqvist et al. 2000, McCann et al. 2001, Chalkiadis et al. 2004)

Local anaesthetic	Mean elimination half-lives (hours)			Maximum continuous infusion rates*
	Neonates	Infants (1-6 months)	Children ≥1 year	
Bupivacaine or levobupivacaine	8.1	7.7		Term neonates: ≤0.2 mg/kg/h 1–3 months: 0.25 mg/kg/h Infants >6 months: 0.4 mg/kg/h
Lidocaine	3.2	NA**		Term infants: 1 mg/kg/h Plasma levels should be monitored
Ropivacaine	6.7***	4.5 (0–12 months)***	3.2 ± 8 4.9 (range 3–6.7 h)	Term neonates: ≤0.2 mg/kg/h 1–3 months: 0.25 mg/kg/h ≥3 months: 0.4 mg/kg/h
Ropivacaine plus clonidine				Children ≥1 year: ropivacaine 0.08% plus clonidine 0.08–0.12 µg/kg/h

*Based on term infants and infusion duration of 48 hours. Lower doses are recommended in premature infants.
**NA = not available
***Clearance is slow in the first 0–3 months and increases by threefold after 6 months of age
(Modified from Regional Anesthesia and Analgesia 1998)

Clonidine exerts its analgesic action by activation of pre- and postsynaptic alpha-2-adrenergic subtype receptors at the dorsal horn grey matter neurons that results in inhibition of release of nociceptive neurotransmitters (Kamibayashi and Maze 2000). Epidural administration of clonidine produces dose-dependent sedation that correlates with the systemic absorption and blood concentrations (Ivani et al. 1998b). Clonidine is probably a safer alternative to opioids as an adjunct to neuroaxial local anaesthetics because, unlike opioids, at analgesic dose range it does not cause respiratory depression, motor blockade, pruritus or urinary retention. These advantages of clonidine prompted its application in paediatric regional anaesthesia and a number of investigators have documented the effectiveness and safety of a single injection and continuous infusion of epidural clonidine as an adjunct to bupivacaine and ropivacaine in children aged one year and older (Nishina et al. 1999, Ivani et al. 2000, De Negri et al 2001).

Clonidine alone is ineffective unless it is used in large doses that may also produce excessive sedation and haemodynamic instability, hypotension and bradycardia. Addition of 2 µg/kg of clonidine to variable doses of caudal-epidural local anaesthetics in children aged 1–10 years suggests enhancement of efficacy and prolongation of analgesic duration to a mean of 6–9.8 (median 3.7–6) hours but the optimal dose remains undetermined (Cook et al. 1995, Ivani

et al. 1996, Motsch et al. 1997, Constant et al. 1998, Dupeyrat et al. 1998, Klimscha et al. 1998, Luz et al. 1999).

Controlled trials of a single injection of caudal-epidural clonidine in children over the age of 1 year show a wide variation in analgesic duration and sedation due to variable systemic absorption of clonidine and differences in study designs. In general, caudal blocks with clonidine when combined with bupivacaine or ropivacaine appear to provide analgesia lasting 50–100% as long as with local anaesthetics alone (Klimscha et al. 1998, Ivani et al. 2000, Hansen et al. 2004). Comparison of a single dose of clonidine 1–5 µg/kg combined with bupivacaine, mepivacaine or ropivacaine to local anaesthetics alone in children over the age of 1 year demonstrated; (1) similar intensity and significantly longer duration with better quality of analgesia, (2) significant, but clinically insignificant, reduction in mean arterial blood pressure and heart rate with higher dose, 5 µg/kg, (3) no motor weakness or respiratory depression but significantly greater transient sedation, and (4) pharmacological profile similar to that reported in adults (Ivani et al. 1998a).

To date, very few safety data are available in infants below the age of 1 year. The potential risk of clonidine-induced life-threatening respiratory depression was recently highlighted in three case reports of term and former premature infants who received single-dose injections of caudal clonidine at 1.25, 1.8 and 2 µg/kg with lidocaine and/or bupivacaine (Breschan et al. 1999, Bouchut et al. 2001a, Fellmann et al. 2002). Although the respiratory depression may not entirely be attributed to clonidine alone, it probably contributed considerably to the untoward respiratory events. It is, therefore, prudent not to expose infants who are high risk for respiratory depression and those under the age of 1 year to epidural clonidine until safety data are available.

In view of a relatively short duration of a single dose of caudal clonidine, supplementation of smaller doses of clonidine to continuous epidural local anaesthetic infusion can provide prolonged postoperative pain relief and may reduce the sedative and possibly the respiratory depressant effects of clonidine (De Negri et al. 2001). An observer-blinded controlled trial of continuous infusion of epidural clonidine demonstrated a clear dose–response effect of 0.04, 0.08 and 0.12 µg/kg/h. Clonidine doses of 0.08–0.12 µg/kg/h enhanced the analgesic effect of a low and ineffective concentration of epidural ropivacaine (0.08%) when used alone. These are regarded optimal adjunct doses for children aged 1–4 years following hypospadias correction (De Negri et al. 2001).

Thoracic extrapleural paravertebral analgesia

As discussed previously, the advancement of caudal and lumbar-to-thoracic epidural catheters in infants and children has a high incidence of failure rate and requires radiological or other means of confirmation for proper placement. The efficacy and safety of thoracic epidural local anaesthetic and/or opioid in newborns and infants have not yet been fully investigated. Recently, thoracic extrapleural paravertebral catheter placement is described as a safer option to thoracic epidural catheter placement in neonates after unilateral thoracotomy and an effective means to provide postoperative analgesia with an infusion of bupivacaine 0.25%, at a rate range of 0.2–0.5 ml/kg/h for 48 hours (Karmakar et al. 1996, Cheung et al. 1997).

The placement of epidural catheters in the extrapleural paravertebral space is performed prior to the closure of a thoracotomy incision and is effective for unilateral intercostal and sympathetic nerve block. It is technically easier and probably safer than advancing epidural catheters to the thoracic epidural space from caudal or lumbar routes. While this technique is less likely to cause neurological injury compared to epidural catheter placement and has a high success rate of 86–90%, the systemic absorption of bupivacaine is much higher than from the epidural space due to high vascularity and so the potential for systemic toxicity may be higher (Karmakar et al. 1996). With the advent of less toxic local anaesthetics such as ropivacaine and levobupivacaine the safety of this technique could be improved.

PERIPHERAL NERVE BLOCKS

Although there are fewer indications for primary use of peripheral nerve blocks in infants undergoing procedures, the increasing demand for adequate and reliable postoperative pain relief has reignited the enthusiasm for use of these techniques in infants. Caution has to be exercised regarding dosage and the total volume of local anaesthetic solution administered. There are no conclusive studies that have determined the exact dose of local anaesthetic solution needed to provide an adequate peripheral nerve block in infants and children. Nevertheless we will attempt to provide the reader of this chapter with a dose based on safety and the potential avoidance of adverse reactions to local anaesthesia used in infants.

The most common peripheral nerve blocks used in infants are listed in Table 11.4.

Head and neck blocks

These are common nerve blocks used in one of the authors' institutions (SS) for most neonatal neurosurgical procedures. The advantage of using peripheral nerve block is the absence of pain with the potential avoidance of opioids during placement of Omaya reservoirs in neonates, particularly low-birth-weight premature infants, who have significant cardiovascular instability (Suresh and Bellig 2004).

Table 11.4 Peripheral nerve blocks in infants

Head and neck
Supraorbital, supratrochlear
Occipital
Superficial cervical plexus
Infraorbital
Lower extremity
Femoral
Lateral femoral cutaneous
Trunk
Intercostal
Penile
Ilioinguinal
Rectus sheath

Supraorbital/supratrochlear nerve block

The first division of the trigeminal nerve, the ophthalmic division, exits from the supraorbital foramen as it exits the roof of the orbit. It supplies the sensory innervation to the anterior portion of the scalp, anterior to the coronal suture. The supratrochlear nerve exits from the supratrochlear foramen and supplies the mid-portion of the forehead. This nerve is a purely sensory nerve. The most common use for this nerve block is for controlling pain from frontal ventriculo-peritoneal shunts, Omaya reservoir placement and frontal dermoid excision.

The block is performed by palpating the supraorbital area. The supraorbital foramen is usually located at about the mid-point of the pupil. After aseptic preparation of the supraorbital area, a 30-G needle is inserted subcutaneously. After aspiration, 0.5 ml of local anaesthetic solution is injected. To block the supratrochlear nerve, the needle is directed towards the midline at the supratrochlear margin and 0.5 ml of local anaesthetic is injected. Pressure is applied to the area and gentle massage of the area is performed to prevent haematoma formation.

Complications include haematoma and intravascular placement.

Greater occipital nerve block

The occipital nerve is a branch of the cervical root C2. It has a paramedian course inferior to the occipital protuberance and then crosses the occipital artery to run a lateral course providing the sensory supply to the occiput and the scalp over the vertex and a muscular branch to the semispinalis capitis. This block is useful to alleviate pain from posterior fossa craniotomy and posterior shunt revisions (Suresh and Bellig 2004).

The block is performed by identification of the occipital protuberance, the midline and palpation of occipital artery pulsation. The occipital nerve is located immediately medial to the occipital artery. A subcutaneous dose of local anaesthetic solution is injected after careful aspiration.

Potential complications include inadvertent intravascular injection and potential for traumatic neuralgia.

Infraorbital nerve block

The infraorbital nerve is the terminal cutaneous nerve of the maxillary division of the trigeminal nerve that supplies the upper lip, choana and the maxillary antrum. This is a purely sensory nerve and anaesthetizing the nerve is useful to control pain from cleft lip repair (Prabhu et al. 1999) and choanal surgery.

There are two approaches to the maxillary division of the trigeminal nerve. The infraorbital foramen is located about 2 cm from the midline of the face (Crista Galii) on the floor of the orbital rim. The extraoral route entails placing the needle directly into the infraorbital foramen using an external route through the maxilla. We prefer an intraoral sub-sulcal approach for infraorbital nerve block to avoid direct nerve injury (Fig. 11.2). The upper lip is everted. A 27-G needle is introduced using a sub-sulcal route and passed cephalad towards the infraorbital foramen. A volume of 0.5 ml of local anaesthetic is injected on each side. This provides excellent analgesia for patients undergoing upper lip procedures. Possible complications are haematoma and accidental intravascular injection.

Superficial cervical plexus block

The superficial cervical plexus is derived from the roots of the C2–C4 nerve roots. The superficial cervical plexus becomes superficial at about the middle of the sternocleidomastoid muscle and wraps around the belly of the sternocleidomastoid muscle and sends out four branches: the lesser occipital nerve that supplies the posterior auricular area; the great auricular nerve that supplies the mastoid area and the pinna; the transverse cervical nerve that supplies the anterior portion of the neck and; the supraclavicular nerve that supplies the anterior portion of the shoulder. This block can be used in conjunction with a supraorbital or an occipital nerve for temporo-parietal blockade of the scalp.

The block is accomplished by outlining the posterior border of the sternocleidomastoid. A 27-G needle is then passed at the middle of the posterior border of the sternocleidomastoid muscle in a cephalad fashion. The injection of local anaesthetic solution is in a subcutaneous plane after careful aspiration to rule out intravascular placement. Usually 0.5 ml to 1 ml of local anaesthetic solution is injected for pain relief.

Trunk blocks

Intercostal nerve block

This block is useful for providing analgesia for thoracotomy and upper abdominal procedures as well as for rib fractures and chest tube pain relief. It is particularly useful for chest tube placement in neonates. Although the commonly used regional technique in neonates is local infiltration of the chest wall for pain relief, the use of intercostal nerve blocks may offer longer and more effective pain relief (Bricker et al. 1989, Fernandez and Rees 1994, Anand et al. 2005). They may be used in an operating room setting or in an emergency setting in the neonatal intensive care unit. The pharmacokinetic profile of bupivacaine

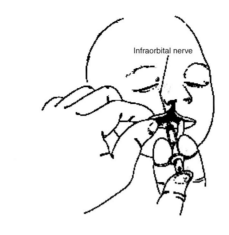

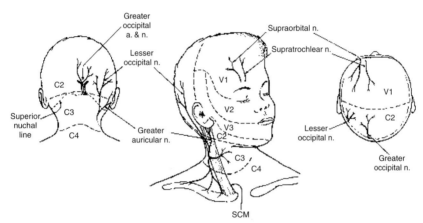

Figure 11.2 Infraorbital nerve block in an infant: intraoral approach. (Reproduced from Polaner et al. 2000 with permission from Elsevier.)

used for intercostal nerve blocks has been studied in neonates and infants 0–6 months and it was found that a dose not exceeding 1.5 mg/kg is not associated with systemic toxicity (Bricker et al. 1989).

The intercostal nerves are derived from the ventral rami of the first through the 12th thoracic nerves (Gray 1985). Each intercostal nerve has four branches; (1) a gray communicantes; (2) posterior cutaneous branch supplying the skin over the paravertebral area; (3) a lateral cutaneous branch supplying the subcutaneous area inferiorly and posteriorly; (4) a cutaneous branch supplying the midline of the chest and the abdomen.

The intercostal nerve is best approached in the mid-axillary line; it affords the easiest approach and has fewer complications associated with the block. The lower border of the rib is identified. The anterior axillary line is marked. The skin is penetrated and the needle is advanced until the needle encounters the lower border of the rib. At this point, the skin is gently moved down caudally and the needle is 'walked off' the inferior edge of the rib. The needle is advanced a few millimetres until a 'pop' is felt as the needle enters the space between the internal and medial intercostal space and, after careful aspiration to rule out intravascular placement, 2–5 ml of local anaesthetic solution is injected. This will allow the needle to enter the neurovascular bundle thereby providing adequate analgesia. Our experience with this technique has dramatically reduced the incidence of pneumothorax.

The most feared complications are accidental intravascular injection and pneumothorax. Local anaesthetic solutions have a greater propensity for toxic levels when used for intercostal blocks than in any other peripheral or central neuraxial blockade. Hence it is prudent to limit the total dose of local anaesthetic solution used in the intercostal space.

Ilioinguinal nerve block

For most hernia surgery in infants and neonates, caudal epidural analgesia is the block of choice. However, if there is a relative contraindication to a caudal block due to the presence of a sacral dimple, or if the infant is obese and the caudal space is not easily identifiable, an ilioinguinal nerve block is utilized (Gibson et al. 1995, Robinson et al. 2005).

The ilioinguinal and iliohypogastric nerves originate from the T12 (subcostal nerve) and L1 (ilioinguinal, iliohypogastric) nerve roots of the lumbar plexus (Gray 1985). These nerves pierce the internal oblique aponeurosis 2–3 cm medial to the anterior superior iliac spine. It travels between the internal oblique and the external oblique aponeurosis where it accompanies the spermatic cord and is part of the neurovascular bundle to the genital area.

The nerve block is carried out by drawing a line between the umbilicus and anterior superior iliac spine and the line is divided into three sections. The needle is inserted at the junction of the lateral third and the medial two-thirds. The needle is advanced towards the inguinal canal and advanced in until a pop is felt; local anaesthetic solution is injected after aspiration to rule out intravascular injection. Alternatively, an ilioinguinal nerve block can be performed through the surgical incision by having the surgeon flood the site of surgery with 10 ml of local anaesthetic solution. Another approach is to fan local anaesthetic solution medial to and below the anterior superior iliac spine.

Although ilioinguinal nerve block is relatively safe, perforation of the bowel wall can occur if the needle is advanced too deep inappropriately.

Rectus sheath block

The rectus sheath block was first described in 1899 for surgery performed around the umbilical area. It is gaining popularity particularly in children for umbilical area surgery.

The umbilical area is innervated by the 10th thoraco-abdominal intercostal nerve bilaterally. Each nerve then passes behind the costal cartilage and between the transversus abdominis muscle and the internal oblique muscle. The nerve runs between the sheath and the posterior wall of the rectus abdominis muscle and ends as the anterior cutaneous branch supplying the skin of the umbilical area.

The aim of this block is to deposit local anaesthetic solution between the muscle and the posterior aspect of the sheath. The technique has been well described by Ferguson et al. (1996). A 23-G needle is inserted above or below the umbilicus 0.5 cm medial to the linea semilunaris in a perpendicular plane. After the belly of the muscle is entered, the needle is further advanced until the posterior aspect of the rectus sheath is appreciated with a scratching sensation as the needle is moved again with a back and forth motion. Once the sheath is encountered, it is pierced and local anaesthetic solution is deposited posterior to the sheath. The usual depth of needle entry is about 0.5–1 cm. After aspiration, 2–3 ml of local anaesthetic solution is injected on either side. If resistance is felt to injection, the needle is advanced deeper since it may be in the body of the muscle.

A lateral approach may not allow appreciation of the passage of the needle through the various layers; a superficial injection after passage through the anterior rectus sheath may not allow spread of local anaesthetic due to the presence of tendinous bands. Intravascular injection, particularly if a large volume is injected directly into the rectus muscle, is a potential hazard and hence the volume of local anaesthetic solution injected has to be limited.

Penile nerve block

Although newborn circumcision remains medically controversial, it is the most widely performed operation worldwide for a variety of reasons, including medical, religious and cultural motivations. There is a growing body of prospective placebo-controlled, randomized trials to suggest that local and regional anaesthesia effectively relieves pain and attenuates the physiological (increased heart and respiratory rates, increased blood pressure, decreased haemoglobin oxygen saturation and increased transcutaneous carbon dioxide tension), behavioural (crying intensity, irritability, sleep and feeding disturbance), and endocrine (rise in plasma cortisol and beta-endorphin) responses to neonatal circumcision. Although the physiological and endocrine responses to the surgical trauma are transient, lasting 0.5–1.5 hours, the behavioural distress may last 24 hours to 3 weeks (Williamson and Williamson 1983, Dixon et al. 1984, Maxwell et al. 1987, Stang et al. 1988). These findings may have greater implications in sick and premature infants in whom the stress response is likely to last longer and have a greater magnitude than term infants (Anand et al. 1985, 1987). Furthermore, a recent study showed that infants circumcised without anaesthesia or analgesia during the neonatal period have increased pain responses during routine vaccinations 4–6 months after the circumcision compared to infants circumcised after pretreatment of the surgical site with EMLA cream. The investigators postulated that untreated circumcision pain can produce long-lasting alteration in the developing nervous system, a state of latent central neural sensitization, that amplifies subsequent nociceptive input (Taddio et al. 1997a). Nevertheless, many physicians still perform circumcision without the benefit of analgesia or use ineffective analgesia (Guide for the Care and Use of Laboratory Animals 1985, Howard et al. 1998). This practice is unwarranted due to the overwhelming evidence that even premature newborns are capable of experiencing pain and that the regulatory and ethical guidelines prohibit even minor surgical procedures on research animals without the use of anaesthesia (Guide for the Care and Use of Laboratory Animals 1985). Based on knowledge gained in the field of fetal and neonatal neurobiology and the evidence presented by numerous randomized controlled analgesic trials on the safety of local and regional analgesics for neonatal circumcision, the major professional and accrediting paediatric organizations have mandated analgesia and anaesthesia to be incorporated as the standard of care for infant circumcision (American Academy of Pediatrics 2000).

The most effective methods of providing anaesthesia for circumcision are dorsal penile nerve block (DPNB) and 'ring block'. The ring block is performed by circumferential infiltration of local anaesthetics in the subcutaneous layer of the penile mid-shaft. The DPNB consists of infiltration of a local anaesthetic deep to Buck's fascia at two dorsolateral locations of the base of the penile shaft where the dorsal penile nerves and vessels enter. Although both blocks are simple low-risk procedures in skilled hands, there is reluctance among practitioners to perform these blocks probably due to lack of appropriate training in performing nerve blocks and undue concerns over the potential serious local and systemic complications (Howard et al. 1998). A survey of 491 neonates who had undergone DPNB for circumcision by trained paediatricians reported a very low incidence of adverse events. The only complications noted were bruising at the site of injection in 54 (11%) and one infant developed a frank haematoma (0.2%); all of which resolved within 2 weeks without long-term sequelae (Snellman and Stang 1995).

Numerous studies have described the safety and effectiveness of DPNB relative to no analgesia for circumcision (Holve et al. 1983, Williamson and Williamson 1983, Dixon et al. 1984, Maxwell et al. 1987, Stang et al. 1988, Masciello 1990, Taddio et al. 1997a, b). Comparison of DPNB with topical anaesthesia EMLA cream and ring block in a randomized placebo-controlled trial demonstrated significantly greater analgesia with ring block throughout all stages of the circumcision compared to DPNB and 90-minute application of EMLA cream; the latter two anaesthetics were less effective particularly during foreskin preparation and incision (Lander et al. 1997). Similar findings were reported in another randomized controlled trial that compared local anaesthetic skin infiltration just proximal to the foreskin to DPNB. Local anaesthetic infiltration provided greater efficacy of attenuating pain-associated behaviour, physiological changes and plasma cortisol rise compared to DPNB (Masciello 1990). Nonetheless, skin infiltration in itself could be a more painful procedure than DPNB as it requires multiple injections.

Although the effectiveness of these techniques to blunt the physiological, behavioural and endocrine responses to neonatal circumcision is variable, and none are capable of entirely abolishing all the markers of the stress response, the ring block appears to be the most appealing because it is technically easy to perform, effective, requires minimal training or expertise, and is less time-consuming than other techniques (Masciello 1990, Lander et al. 1997, Hardwick-Smith et al. 1998).

In view of the imperfections of all the available anaesthetic techniques, other measures, such as the use of enteral acetaminophen, oral sucrose, a pacifier and maternal consolation (Blass and Hoffmeyer 1991, Marchette et al. 1991) should be considered in combination with the penile analgesic techniques to enhance comfort and reduce distress.

Lower extremity blocks

The lumbar and sacral plexuses supply the lower extremity. The lumbar plexus is contained in the psoas compartment and consists of a small portion of T12 and lumbar nerves L1–L4. The femoral nerve, lateral femoral cutaneous nerve and the obturator nerves are branches of the lumbar plexus that supply most of the thigh and the upper extremity. The lower leg is innervated by the sacral plexus, which is derived from the anterior rami of L4, L5, S1, S2 and S3. This plexus gives rise to the sciatic nerve which is the largest nerve in the body.

Femoral nerve block

This is the most commonly performed peripheral nerve block in children. It is used extensively for providing pain relief following femoral fractures (Grossbard and Love 1979, Ronchi et al. 1989, Johnson 1994, Tobias 1994). Although a femoral nerve block can be performed without the aid of a nerve stimulator, use of nerve stimulation improves the success rate. The femoral nerve is located at the level of the crease at the groin, lateral to the pulsation of the femoral artery. Topical landmarks are used to identify the location of the nerve prior to utilizing a sheathed needle.

The femoral pulse is located and a surface mapping electrode is placed lateral to the pulsation of the artery; a good quadriceps contraction is indicative of the correct location of the needle. Once the entry site is marked, a sheathed needle is advanced with the nerve stimulator initially set at 1 mA and gradually reduced to 0.4 mA. It is important to continue to obtain quadriceps muscle contractions at 0.4–0.5 mA indicating appropriate closeness to the nerve. After negative aspiration for blood the local anaesthetic solution is injected at volumes of 0.2–0.3 ml/kg.

Inadvertent intravascular injection can be prevented by carefully aspirating for blood prior to injection. It is advisable to inject small aliquots of local anaesthetic to avoid accidental intravascular injection (Sethna and McGowan 2005).

Lateral femoral cutaneous nerve block

The lateral femoral cutaneous nerve is derived from the L3 and L4 segments of the lumbar plexus. It is a purely sensory nerve that passes superficially along the lateral border of the iliac crest as it exits into the fascia iliaca compartment to supply the lateral aspect of the thigh. It is useful for providing analgesia for surgery on the lateral aspect of the thigh including muscle biopsies and harvesting donor skin graft (Maccani et al. 1995). It is a relatively easy block to perform with very few side effects and hence is easily applicable in neonates and infants.

The anterior superior iliac spine is identified and a point 1.5 inches below and medial to the anterior superior iliac spine is identified. After careful aseptic preparation of the area, a blunt needle is introduced into the marked site. An initial 'pop' is felt as the needle enters the skin and the fascia lata; a second 'pop' is felt as the needle enters the fascia iliaca compartment. Once the needle is lodged in this space, loss of resistance can be easily felt as the local anaesthetic solution is injected. A total volume of 0.2–0.3 ml/kg is injected.

TOPICAL LOCAL ANAESTHETICS

Several investigators have examined the efficacy of 5% EMLA® cream (eutectic mixture of lidocaine and prilocaine cream) in infants and children for a variety of superficial cutaneous and invasive medical procedures such as blood drawing, lumbar puncture, bladder tap, vaccination and superficial cutaneous surgery. It poorly permeates the glabrous skin and thus produces weak topical analgesia for a heel lancing procedure (Taddio et al. 1998). A major concern with the use of EMLA cream in newborns and infants is prilocaine toxicity. Prilocaine's metabolite, orto-toluidine, can oxidize a significant amount of haemoglobin to methaemoglobin. Neonates and premature infants are at increased risk for prilocaine toxicity due to reduced activity of the enzyme NADH-dependent methaemoglobin reductase. Other possible risk factors for systemic toxicity are presence of anaemia, sepsis, metabolic acidosis, hypoxaemia, G-6-PD deficiency, and the concomitant administration of sulfonamides, acetaminophen, phenytoin, phenobarbital, nitroglycerin, nitroprusside, benzocaine and other methaemoglobin-inducing agents (Jakobson and Nilsson 1985, Nilsson et al. 1990).

The effectiveness of EMLA cream is determined by the dose, size of skin area over which it is applied and duration of application (Table 11.5). There may be racial differences in the absorption of EMLA cream, and therefore differences in the effectiveness. The skin permeability is lower in African-American adult subjects due to increased thickness of the stratum corneum and the dose requirement for EMLA may be higher (Hymes and Spraker 1986).

Local skin reactions associated with EMLA cream are primarily related to the prilocaine component. Initial blanching is presumably caused by vasoconstriction at lower doses and redness is due to vasodilatation at higher concentrations. Transient purpuric lesions have been described in areas of repeated

Table 11.5 Maximum recommended dose and application area based on application to normal intact skin and normal renal and hepatic function (Taddio et al. 1995, Taddio et al. 1997a, EMLA full prescription. In: Astra USA, Inc., Westborough, MA 01581–4500)

Age	Body weight	Maximum total dose of EMLA	Maximum application area
30–37 weeks gestational age*	Mean 1.9 kg	0.5 g	Unspecified
= 37 weeks gestational age	= 2.5 kg	1 g	Unspecified
1 to 3 months	< 5 kg	1 g	10 cm^2
4 to 12 months	5 to 10 kg	2 g	20 cm^2

* A preliminary study in a small sample size

applications within the first 4 days of life in premature infants (Gourrier et al 1996).

Use of EMLA in premature infants

Application of a single dose of EMLA cream 0.5 g for 60 minutes per day on normal intact skin of premature infants older than 30 gestational weeks appears to be safe and effective. The blood methaemoglobin concentrations obtained at 4, 8 and 12 hours post-application were not significantly different from baseline. These infants did not have any additional risk factors that predispose to methaemoglobinaemia (Taddio et al. 1995). Uncontrolled trials suggest repeated application of EMLA cream in term and premature infants during the first week of life can result in high blood methaemoglobin concentration and while no clinical evidence of methaemoglobin toxicity was observed, caution is advised (Gourrier et al. 1995, 1996).

Use of EMLA in neonatal circumcision

The safety and efficacy of EMLA cream analgesia for control of circumcision pain in full-term neonates has been investigated in prospective placebo-controlled randomized trials (Benini et al. 1993, Taddio et al. 1995, Taddio et al. 1997b). The largest of these trials included 68 neonates; 38 received EMLA cream and 30 received placebo (Taddio et al. 1997b). The circumcision was effectively performed 60–80 minutes after application of EMLA cream. To ensure even spread of the cream over the penile skin one-third of a total dose of 1 ml (1 g) was applied to the lower abdomen and the penis was extended upward and gently pressed against the abdomen. The remainder of the dose was applied to a transparent occlusive dressing that was placed over the penis and secured against the abdomen. No adverse effects were observed clinically. Plasma lidocaine and prilocaine were detectable in 61% and 55% of the infants respectively. Neither drug was detectable at 18 hours after the EMLA cream application. The prilocaine metabolite O-toluidine was undetectable in all infants. The apparent safety of a similar dose of EMLA cream (1 g) has been confirmed in a smaller series of full-term infants undergoing circumcision. Blood methaemoglobin concentration increased in these infants but did not exceed the upper limit of the normal range (Law et al. 1996).

Although EMLA cream effectively decreases the pain associated with neonatal circumcision as assessed by decreased facial activity, the duration of crying and heart rate increases, it is less effective than dorsal penile nerve block and ring block with local anaesthetic (Lander et al. 1997). Despite the safety, efficacy and simplicity of EMLA cream application, it has not received widespread use due to fear of methaemoglobinaemia in newborns (Couper 2000). Recently, a 4% tetracaine gel (not available in the USA) was introduced as a safer substitute to 5% EMLA cream and the preliminary studies show that 4% tetracaine gel is as efficacious as 5% EMLA cream for veni-puncture in infants and children (Choy et al. 1999, Carceles et al. 2002). Several randomized controlled trials in moderately premature and term neonates found tetracaine gel to be safe and effective for venous puncture and cannulation (Jain and Rutter 2000, Moore 2001). As with EMLA cream, it requires occlusive dressing but the onset time of analgesia is relatively faster than EMLA; 30–45 minutes. Transient erythema is the most common adverse effect and it is contraindicated in the presence of hypersensitivity to ester local anaesthetics (O'Brien et al. 2005).

In summary, regional and topical anaesthetic techniques are appropriate and effective for most infants and young children undergoing invasive procedures. Simple and safe techniques, such as the use of EMLA cream and tetracaine gel, are available to all practitioners who care for children, while more complex techniques should only be performed by trained operators and anaesthesiologists with specialty training in paediatrics. Although knowledge of the advantages, limitations, technical issues and the relative risk/benefit balance with various regional techniques are evolving in the paediatric population, the clinical application of regional anaesthetic techniques in infants and young children is rapidly growing.

Controlled trials of regional anaesthesia techniques in newborns and young infants are scant and are difficult to perform compared to older children because of difficulties with pain assessment, grading of sensory and motor block, and limitation of the amount of blood samples necessary for local anaesthetic assay. Nevertheless, such trials in infants are necessary to fully characterize the techniques' safety and efficacy and whether they are likely to be more beneficial in a particular age group and in specific conditions. Hopefully, investigators will continue to evaluate these techniques in infants and children with controlled and randomized trials to further define efficacy and safety and support their use (O'Brien et al. 2005).

REFERENCES

Abajian JC, Mellish RW, Browne AF, et al. (1984). Spinal anesthesia for surgery in the high-risk infant. Anesth Analg 63: 359–362.

Afshan G, Khan FA. (1996). Total spinal anaesthesia following caudal block with bupivacaine and buprenorphine. Paediatr Anaesth 6: 239–242.

Agarwal R, Gutlove DP, Lockhart CH. (1992). Seizures occurring in pediatric patients receiving continuous infusion of bupivacaine. Anesth Analg 75: 284–286.

Ala-Kokko TI, Partanen A, Karinen J, et al. (2000). Pharmacokinetics of 0.2% ropivacaine and 0.2% bupivacaine following caudal blocks in children. Acta Anaesthesiol Scand 44: 1099–1102.

American Academy of Pediatrics. (2000). Prevention and management of pain and stress in the neonate. Pediatrics 105: 454–461.

Anand KJS, Hickey PR. (1992). Halothane-morphine compared with high-dose sufentanil for anesthesia and postoperative analgesia in neonatal cardiac surgery. New Engl J Med 326: 1–9.

Anand KJS, Brown MJ, Causon RC, et al. (1985). Can the human neonate mount an endocrine and metabolic response to surgery? J Pediatr Surg 20: 41–48.

Anand KJS, Sippell WG, Aynsley-Green A. (1987). Randomised trial of fentanyl anaesthesia in preterm babies undergoing surgery: effects on the stress response. Lancet 1: 62–66.

Anand KJS, Johnston CC, Oberlander TF, et al. (2005). Analgesia and local anesthesia during invasive procedures in the neonate. Clin Ther 27: 844–876.

Bardsley H, Gristwood R, Baker H, et al. (1998). A comparison of the cardiovascular effects of levobupivacaine and rac-bupivacaine following intravenous administration to healthy volunteers. Br J Clin Pharmacol 46: 245–249.

Benini F, Johnston CC, Faucher D, et al. (1993). Topical anesthesia during circumcision in newborn infants [published erratum appears in JAMA 1994 Jan 26;271(4):274]. JAMA 270: 850–853.

Blanco D, Llamazares J, Rincon R, et al. (1996). Thoracic epidural anesthesia via the lumbar approach in infants and children. Anesthesiology 84: 1312–1316.

Blass EM, Hoffmeyer LB. (1991). Sucrose as an analgesic for newborn infants. Pediatrics 87: 215–218.

Bosenberg AT. (1998). Epidural analgesia for major neonatal surgery. Paediatr Anaesth 8: 479–483.

Bosenberg AT, Bland BA, Schulte SO, et al. (1988). Thoracic epidural anesthesia via caudal route in infants. Anesthesiology 69: 265–269.

Bosenberg AT, Hadley GP, Wiersma R. (1992). Oesophageal atresia: caudo-thoracic epidural anaesthesia reduces the need for post-operative ventilatory support. Pediatr Surg Int 7: 289–291.

Bosenberg AT, Thomas J, Cronje L, et al. (2005). Pharmacokinetics and efficacy of ropivacaine for continuous epidural infusion in neonates and infants. Paediatr Anaesth 15: 739–749.

Bouchut JC, Dubois R, Foussat C, et al. (2001a). Evaluation of caudal anaesthesia performed in conscious ex-premature infants for inguinal herniotomies. Paediatr Anaesth 11: 55–58.

Bouchut JC, Dubois R, Godard J. (2001b). Clonidine in preterm-infant caudal anesthesia may be responsible for postoperative apnea. Reg Anesth Pain Med 26: 83–85.

Breschan C, Krumpholz R, Likar R, et al. (1999). Can a dose of 2microg.kg(-1) caudal clonidine cause respiratory depression in neonates? Paediatr Anaesth 9: 81–83.

Bricker SR, Telford RJ, Booker PD. (1989). Pharmacokinetics of bupivacaine following intraoperative intercostal nerve block in neonates and in infants aged less than 6 months. Anesthesiology 70: 942–947.

Carceles MD, Alonso JM, Garcia-Munoz M, et al. (2002). Amethocaine-lidocaine cream, a new topical formulation for preventing venopuncture-induced pain in children. Reg Anesth Pain Med 27: 289–295.

Chalkiadis GA, Eyres RL, Cranswick N, et al. (2004). Pharmacokinetics of levobupivacaine 0.25% following caudal administration in children under 2 years of age. Br J Anaesth 92: 218–222.

Chawathe MS, Jones RM, Gildersleve CD, et al. (2003). Detection of epidural catheters with ultrasound in children. Paediatr Anaesth 13: 681–684.

Cheung SL, Booker PD, Franks R, et al. (1997). Serum concentrations of bupivacaine during prolonged continuous paravertebral infusion in young infants. Br J Anaesth 79: 9–13.

Choy L, Collier J, Watson AR. (1999). Comparison of lignocaine-prilocaine cream and amethocaine gel for local analgesia before venepuncture in children. Acta Paediatr 88: 961–964.

Constant I, Gall O, Gouyet L, et al. (1998). Addition of clonidine or fentanyl to local anaesthetics prolongs the duration of surgical analgesia after single shot caudal block in children. Br J Anaesth 80: 294–298.

Cook B, Grubb DJ, Aldridge LA, et al. (1995). Comparison of the effects of adrenaline, clonidine and ketamine on the duration of caudal analgesia produced by bupivacaine in children. Br J Anaesth 75: 698–701.

Cote CJ, Zaslavsky A, Downes JJ, et al. (1995). Postoperative apnea in former preterm infants after inguinal herniorrhaphy. A combined analysis. Anesthesiology 82: 809–822.

Couper RT. (2000). Methaemo-globinaemia secondary to topical lignocaine/prilocaine in a circumcised neonate. J Paediatr Child Health 36: 406–407.

Craven PD, Badawi N, Henderson-Smart DJ, et al. (2003). Regional (spinal, epidural, caudal) versus general anaesthesia in preterm infants undergoing inguinal herniorrhaphy in early infancy. Cochrane Database Syst Rev: CD003669.

Da Conceicao MJ, Coelho L. (1998). Caudal anaesthesia with 0.375% ropivacaine or 0.375% bupivacaine in paediatric patients. Br J Anaesth 80: 507–508.

Da Conceicao MJ, Coelho L, Khalil M. (1999). Ropivacaine 0.25% compared with bupivacaine 0.25% by the caudal route. Paediatr Anaesth 9: 229–233.

de Beer DA, Thomas ML. (2003). Caudal additives in children–solutions or problems? Br J Anaesth 90: 487–498.

De Negri P, Ivani G, Visconti C, et al. (2001). The dose–response relationship for clonidine added to a postoperative continuous epidural infusion of ropivacaine in children. Anesth Analg 93: 71–76.

Desparmet JF. (1990). Total spinal anesthesia after caudal anesthesia in an infant. Anesth Analg 70: 665–667.

Dixon S, Snyder J, Holve R, et al. (1984). Behavioral effects of circumcision with and without anesthesia. J Develop Behav Ped 5: 246–250.

Dohi S, Naito H, Takahashi T. (1979). Age-related changes in blood pressure and duration of motor block in spinal anesthesia. Anesthesiology 50: 319–323.

Dupeyrat A, Goujard E, Muret J, et al. (1998). Transcutaneous CO2 tension effects of clonidine in paediatric caudal analgesia. Paediatr Anaesth 8: 145–148.

Ecoffey C, Desparmet J, Maury M, et al. (1985). Bupivacaine in children: pharmacokinetics following caudal anesthesia. Anesthesiology 63: 447–448.

Eisenach JC, Yaksh TL. (2003). Epidural ketamine in healthy children–what's the point? Anesth Analg 96: 626; author reply 626–627.

Eisenach JC, James FM 3rd, Gordh T Jr, et al. (1998). New epidural drugs: primum non nocere. Anesth Analg 87: 1211–1212.

Emmanuel ER. (1994). Post-sacral extradural catheter abscess in a child. Br J Anaesth 73: 548–549.

Fellmann C, Gerber AC, Weiss M. (2002). Apnoea in a former preterm infant after caudal bupivacaine with clonidine for inguinal herniorrhaphy. Paediatr Anaesth 12: 637–640.

Ferguson S, Thomas V, Lewis I. (1996). The rectus sheath block in paediatric anaesthesia: new indications for an old technique? Paediatr Anaesth 6: 463–466.

Fernandez CV, Rees EP. (1994). Pain management in Canadian level 3 neonatal intensive care units. CMAJ 150: 499–504.

Frawley G, Ragg P, Hack H. (2000). Plasma concentrations of bupivacaine after combined spinal epidural anaesthesia in infants and neonates. Paediatr Anaesth 10: 619–625.

Fried E, Bailey A, Valley R. (1994). Electrocardiographic and hemodynamic changes associated with unintentional intravascular injection of bupivacaine with epinephrine in infants. Anesthesiology 79: 394–398.

Frumiento C, Abajian JC, Vane DW. (2000). Spinal anesthesia for preterm infants undergoing inguinal hernia repair. Arch Surg 135: 445–451.

Giaufre E, Conte-Devolx B, Morisson-Lacombe G, et al. (1985). Caudal epidural anesthesia in children. Study of endocrine changes. Presse Medicale 14: 201–203.

Giaufre E, Dalens B, Gombert A. (1996). Epidemiology and morbidity of regional anesthesia in children: A one-year prospective survey of the French-language society of pediatric anesthesiologists. Anesth Analg 83: 904–912.

Gibson PJ, Britton J, Hall DM, et al.

(1995). Lumbosacral skin markers and identification of occult spinal dysraphism in neonates. Acta Paediatr 84: 208–209.

Goobie SM, Montgomery CJ, Basu R, et al. (2003). Confirmation of direct epidural catheter placement using nerve stimulation in pediatric anesthesia. Anesth Analg 97: 984–988.

Gourrier E, Karoubi P, el Hanache A, et al. (1995). Use of EMLA cream in premature and full-term newborn infants. Study of efficacy and tolerance. Arch Pediatr 2: 1041–1046.

Gourrier E, Karoubi P, el Hanache A, et al. (1996). Use of EMLA cream in a department of neonatology. Pain 68: 431–434.

Gray H. (1985). Anatomy of the human body: Gray's anatomy. Williams & Wilkins, Baltimore.

Grossbard GD, Love BR. (1979). Femoral nerve block: a simple and safe method of instant analgesia for femoral shaft fractures in children. Aust NZ J Surg 49: 592–594.

Grunau RV, Whitfield MF, Petrie JH. (1994). Pain sensitivity and temperament in extremely low-birth-weight premature toddlers and preterm and full-term controls. Pain 58: 341–346.

Guide for the Care and Use of Laboratory Animals. (1985). Publication (NIH) 8523. US Department of Health and Human Services.

Guinard J-P, Borboen M. (1993). Probable venous air embolism during caudal anesthesia in a child. Anesth Analg 76: 1134–1135.

Gunter JB. (2000). Thoracic epidural anesthesia via the modified Taylor approach in infants. Reg Anesth Pain Med 25: 561–565.

Gunter JB, Eng C. (1992). Thoracic epidural anesthesia via the caudal approach in children. Anesthesiology 76: 935–938.

Gunter JB, Watcha MF, Forestner JE, et al. (1991). Caudal epidural anesthesia in conscious premature and high-risk infants. J Pediatr Surg 26: 9–14.

Guyer B, Strobino DM, Ventura SJ, et al. (1995). Annual summary of vital statistics–1994. Pediatrics 96: 1029–1039.

Habre W, Bergesio R, Johnson C, et al. (2000). Pharmacokinetics of ropivacaine following caudal analgesia in children. Paediatr Anaesth 10: 143–147.

Hansen TG, Ilett KF, Lim SI, et al. (2000). Pharmacokinetics and clinical efficacy of long-term epidural ropivacaine

infusion in children. Br J Anaesth 85: 347–353.

Hansen TG, Henneberg SW, Walther-Larsen S, et al. (2004). Caudal bupivacaine supplemented with caudal or intravenous clonidine in children undergoing hypospadias repair: a double-blind study. Br J Anaesth 92: 223–227.

Hardwick-Smith S, Mastrobattista JM, Wallace PA, et al. (1998). Ring block for neonatal circumcision. Obstet Gynecol 91: 930–934.

Harnik EV, Hoy GR, Potolicchio S, et al. (1986). Spinal anesthesia in premature infants recovering from respiratory distress syndrome. Anesthesiology 64: 95–99.

Hassan SZ. (1977). Caudal anesthesia in infants. Anesth Analg 56: 686–689.

Henderson K, Sethna NF, Berde CB. (1993). Continuous caudal anesthesia for inguinal hernia repair in former preterm infants. J Clin Anesth 5: 129–133.

Holve RL, Bromberger PJ, Groveman HD, et al. (1983). Regional anesthesia during newborn circumcision. Effect on infant pain response. Clin Ped 22: 813–818.

Howard CR, Howard FM, Garfunkel LC, et al. (1998). Neonatal circumcision and pain relief: current training practices. Pediatrics 101: 423–428.

Hymes JA, Spraker MK. (1986). Racial difference in the effectiveness of a topically applied mixture of local anesthetics. Regional Anesthesia 11: 11–13.

Ivani G, Mattioli G, Rega M, et al. (1996). Clonidine-mepivacaine mixture vs plain mepivacaine in paediatric surgery. Paediatr Anaesth 6: 111–114.

Ivani G, Bergendahl HT, Lampugnani E, et al. (1998a). Plasma levels of clonidine following epidural bolus injection in children. Acta Anaesthesiol Scand 42: 306–311.

Ivani G, Lampugnani E, Torre M, et al. (1998b). Comparison of ropivacaine with bupivacaine for paediatric caudal block. Br J Anaesth 81: 247–248.

Ivani G, De Negri P, Conio A, et al. (2000). Ropivacaine-clonidine combination for caudal blockade in children. Acta Anaesthesiol Scand 44: 446–449.

Ivani G, De Negri P, Lonnqvist PA, et al. (2003). A comparison of three different concentrations of levobupivacaine for caudal block in children. Anesth Analg 97: 368–371.

Ivani G, De Negri P, Lonnqvist PA, et al. (2005). Caudal anesthesia for minor pediatric surgery: a prospective randomized comparison of ropivacaine 0.2% vs levobupivacaine 0.2%. Paediatr Anaesth 15: 491–494.

Jain A, Rutter N. (2000). Does topical amethocaine gel reduce the pain of venepuncture in newborn infants? A randomised double blind controlled trial. Arch Dis Child Fetal Neonatal Ed 83: F207–210.

Jakobson B, Nilsson A. (1985). Methemoglobinemia associated with prilocaine-lidocaine cream and trimetoprim sulphametonazole. A case report. Acta Anesth Scand 29: 453–455.

Johnson CM. (1994). Continuous femoral nerve blockade for analgesia in children with femoral fractures. Anaesth Intens Care 22: 281–283.

Kamibayashi T, Maze M. (2000). Clinical uses of alpha2-adrenergic agonists. Anesthesiology 93: 1345–1349.

Karmakar MK, Booker PD, Franks R, et al. (1996). Continuous extrapleural paravertebral infusion of bupivacaine for post-thoracotomy analgesia in young infants. Br J Anaesth 76: 811–815.

Klimscha W, Chiari A, Michalek-Sauberer A, et al. (1998). The efficacy and safety of a clonidine/bupivacaine combination in caudal blockade for pediatric hernia repair. Anesth Analg 86: 54–61.

Knudsen K, Beckman Suurkula M, Blomberg S, et al. (1997). Central nervous and cardiovascular effects of i.v. infusions of ropivacaine, bupivacaine and placebo in volunteers. Br J Anaesth 78: 507–514.

Kost-Byerly S, Greenberg RS, Billett CA, et al. (1993). Continuous lidocaine epidural analgesia in neonates. Anesthesiology 81: A1343.

Kost-Byerly S, Tobin JR, Greenberg RS, et al. (1998). Bacterial colonization and infection rate of continuous epidural catheters in children. Anesth Analg 86: 712–716.

Krane EJ, Haberkern CM, Jacobson LE. (1995). Postoperative apnea, bradycardia, and oxygen desaturation in formerly premature infants: prospective comparison of spinal and general anesthesia. Anesth Analg 80: 7–13.

Kurth CD, Spitzer AR, Broennle AM, et al. (1987). Postoperative apnea in preterm infants. Anesthesiology 66: 483–488.

Lander J, Brady-Fryer B, Metcalfe JB, et al. (1997). Comparison of ring block, dorsal penile nerve block, and topical anesthesia for neonatal circumcision: a randomized controlled trial. JAMA 278: 2157–2162.

Larousse E, Asehnoune K, Dartayet B, et al. (2002). The hemodynamic effects of pediatric caudal anesthesia assessed by esophageal Doppler. Anesth Analg 94: 1165–1168.

Larsson BA, Lundeberg S, Olsson GL. (1997). Epidural abscess in a one-year-old boy after continuous epidural analgesia. Anesth Analg 84: 1245–1247.

Law RM, Halpern S, Martins RF, et al. (1996). Measurement of methemoglobin after EMLA analgesia for newborn circumcision. Biol Neonate 70: 213–217.

Lerman J, Strong A, LeDez KM, et al. (1989). Effects of age on the serum concentration of alpha-acid glycoprotein and the binding of lidocaine in pediatric patients. Clin Pharmacol Ther 46: 219–224.

Liu LM, Cote CJ, Goudsouzian NG, et al. (1983). Life-threatening apnea in infants recovering from anesthesia. Anesthesiology 59: 506–510.

Locatelli B, Ingelmo P, Sonzogni V, et al. (2005). Randomized, double-blind, phase III, controlled trial comparing levobupivacaine 0.25%, ropivacaine 0.25% and bupivacaine 0.25% by the caudal route in children. Br J Anaesth 94: 366–371.

Lonnqvist PA, Westrin P, Larsson BA, et al. (2000). Ropivacaine pharmacokinetics after caudal block in 1-8 year old children. Br J Anaesth 85: 506–511.

Luz G, Innerhofer P, Bachmann B, et al. (1996). Bupivacaine plasma concentrations during continuous epidural anesthesia in infants and children. Anesth Analg 82: 231–234.

Luz G, Innerhofer P, Oswald E, et al. (1999). Comparison of clonidine 1 microgram kg^{-1} with morphine 30 micrograms kg^{-1} for post-operative caudal analgesia in children. Eur J Anaesthesiol 16: 42–46.

Luz G, Innerhofer P, Haussler B, et al. (2000). Comparison of ropivacaine 0.1% and 0.2% with bupivacaine 0.2% for single-shot caudal anaesthesia in children. Paediatr Anaesth 10: 499–504.

Maccani RM, Wedel DJ, Melton A, et al. (1995). Femoral and lateral femoral cutaneous nerve block for muscle biopsies in children. Paediatr Anaesth 5: 223–227.

Malviya S, Swartz J, Lerman J. (1993). Are all preterm infants younger than 60 weeks postconceptual age at risk for postanesthetic apnea? Anesthesiology 78: 1076–1081.

Marchette L, Main R, Redick E, et al. (1991). Pain reduction interventions during noenatal circumcision. Nurs Res 40: 241–244.

Masciello AL. (1990). Anesthesia for neonatal circumcision: local anesthesia is better than dorsal penile nerve block. Obstet Gynecol 75: 834–838.

Maxwell LG, Yaster M, Wetzel RC, et al. (1987). Penile nerve block for newborn circumcision. Obstet Gynecol 70: 415–419.

Mazoit JX, Denson DD, Samii K. (1988). Pharmacokinetics of bupivacaine following caudal anesthesia in infants. Anesthesiology 68: 387–391.

McCann ME, Sethna NF, Mazoit JX, et al. (2001). The pharmacokinetics of epidural ropivacaine in infants and young children. Anesth Analg 93: 893–897.

McCloskey JJ, Haun SE, Deshpande JK. (1992). Bupivacaine toxicity secondary to continuous caudal epidural infusion in children. Anesth Analg 75: 287–290.

McNeely JK, Farber NE, Rusy LM, et al. (1997a). Epidural analgesia improves outcome following pediatric fundoplication. A retrospective analysis. Reg Anesth 22: 16–23.

McNeely JK, Trentadue NC, Rusy LM, et al. (1997b). Culture of bacteria from lumbar and caudal epidural catheters used for postoperative analgesia in children. Reg Anesth 22: 428–431.

Meunier JF, Norwood P, Dartayet B, et al. (1997). Skin abscess with lumbar epidural catheterization in infants: is it dangerous? Report of two cases. Anesth Analg 84:1248–1249.

Moore J. (2001). No more tears: a randomized controlled double-blind trial of Amethocaine gel vs. placebo in the management of procedural pain in neonates. J Adv Nurs 34: 475–482.

Morgan D, McQuillan D, Thomas J. (1978). Pharmacokinetics and metabolism of the anilide local anaesthetics in neonates. II Etidocaine. Europ J Clin Pharmacol 13: 365–371.

Motsch J, Bottiger BW, Bach A, et al. (1997). Caudal clonidine and bupivacaine for combined epidural and general anaesthesia in children. Acta Anaesthesiol Scand 41: 877–883.

Murat I, Walker J, Esteve C, et al. (1988). Effect of lumbar epidural anaesthesia on plasma cortisol levels in children. Can J Anaesth 35: 20–24.

Nilsson A, Engberg G, Henneberg S, et al. (1990). Inverse relationship between age-dependent erythrocyte activity of methaemoglobin reductase and prilocaine-induced methaemoglobinaemia during infancy. Br J Anaes 64: 72–76.

Nishina K, Mikawa K, Shiga M, et al. (1999). Clonidine in paediatric anaesthesia. Paediatr Anaesth 9: 187–202.

Oberlander TF, Berde CB, Lam KH, et al. (1995). Infants tolerate spinal anesthesia with minimal overall autonomic changes: analysis of heart rate variability in former premature infants undergoing hernia repair. Anesth Analg 80: 20–27.

O'Brien L, Taddio A, Lyszkiewicz DA, et al. (2005).A critical review of the topical local anesthetic amethocaine (Ametop) for pediatric pain. Paediatr Drugs 7: 41–54.

Pascucci RC, Hershenson MB, Sethna NF, et al. (1990). Chest wall motion of infants during spinal anesthesia. J Appl Physiol 68: 2087–2091.

Payen D, Ecoffey C, Carli P, et al. (1987). Pulsed Doppler ascending aortic, carotid, brachial, and femoral artery blood flows during caudal anesthesia in infants. Anesthesiology 67: 681–685.

Peutrell JM, Hughes DG. (1993). Epidural anaesthesia through caudal catheters for inguinal herniotomies in awake ex-premature babies. Anaesthesia 48: 128–131.

Peutrell JM, Hughes DG. (1994). Combined spinal and epidural anaesthesia for inguinal hernia repair in babies. Paediatr Anaesth 4: 221–227.

Polaner D, Suresh S, Cote CJ. (2000). A practice of anesthesia for infants and children. In: Cote CJ, Todres ID, Ryan JF, Goudsouzian NG (eds), Pediatric regional anesthesia, pp. 636–675. WB Saunders, Philadelphia.

Porter FL, Grunau RE, Anand KJS. (1999). Long-term effects of pain in infants. J Dev Behav Pediatr 20: 253–261.

Prabhu KP, Wig J, Grewal S. (1999). Bilateral infraorbital nerve block is superior to peri-incisional infiltration for analgesia after repair of cleft lip. Scand J Plast Reconstr Surg Hand Surg 33: 83–87.

Rapp HJ, Grau T. (2004). Ultrasound imaging in pediatric regional anesthesia. Can J Anaesth 51: 277–278.

Rapp HJ, Molnar V, Austin S, et al. (2004). Ropivacaine in neonates and infants: a population pharmacokinetic evaluation following single caudal block. Paediatr Anaesth 14: 724–732.

Robinson AJ, Russell S, Rimmer S. (2005). The value of ultrasonic examination of the lumbar spine in infants with specific reference to cutaneous markers of occult spinal dysraphism. Clin Radiol 60: 72–77.

Rochette A, Raux O, Troncin R, et al. (2004). Clonidine prolongs spinal anesthesia in newborns: a prospective dose-ranging study. Anesth Analg 98: 56–59.

Ronchi L, Rosenbaum D, Athouel A, et al. (1989). Femoral nerve blockade in children using bupivacaine. Anesthesiology 70: 622–624.

Rose JB. (2003). Spinal cord injury in a child after single-shot epidural anesthesia. Anesth Analg 96: 3–6.

Santos AC, DeArmas PI. (2001). Systemic toxicity of levobupivacaine, bupivacaine, and ropivacaine during continuous intravenous infusion to nonpregnant and pregnant ewes. Anesthesiology 95: 1256–1264.

Schwartz N, Eisenkraft JB. (1993). Probable venous air embolism during epidural placement in an infant. Anesth Analg 76: 1136–1138.

Sethna NF, Berde CB. (1993). Venous air embolism during identification of the epidural space in children. Anesth Analg 76: 925–927.

Sethna NF, Berde CB. (2002). Pediatric regional anesthesia. In: Gregory GA (ed.) Pediatric anesthesia, fourth edition, pp. 267–316. Churchill Livingstone, New York.

Sethna NF, McGowan FX Jr. (2005). Do results from studies of a simulated epidural test dose improve our ability to detect unintentional epidural vascular puncture in children? Paediatr Anaesth 15: 711–715.

Somri M, Gaitini L, Vaida S, et al. (1998). Postoperative outcome in high-risk infants undergoing herniorrhaphy: comparison between spinal and general anaesthesia. Anaesthesia 53: 762–766.

Snellman LW, Stang HJ. (1995). Prospective evaluation of complications of dorsal penile nerve block for neonatal circumcision. Pediatrics 95: 705–708.

Spear RM, Deshpande JK, Maxwell LG. (1988). Caudal anesthesia in the awake, high-risk infant. Anesthesiology 69: 407–409.

Stang HJ, Gunnar MR, Snellman L, et al. (1988). Local anesthesia for neonatal circumcision. Effects on distress and cortisol response. JAMA 259: 1507–1511.

Steward DJ. (1982). Preterm infants are more prone to complications following minor surgery than are term infants. Anesthesiology 56: 304–306.

Strafford MA, Wilder RT, Berde CB. (1995). The risk of infection from epidural analgesia in children: a review of 1620 cases. Anesth Analg 80: 234–238.

Suresh S, Bellig G. (2004). Regional anesthesia in a very low-birth-weight neonate for a neurosurgical procedure. Reg Anesth Pain Med 29: 58–59.

Suresh S, Barcelona SL, Young NM, et al. (2002). Postoperative pain relief in children undergoing tympanomastoid surgery: is a regional block better than opioids? Anesth Analg 94: 859–862, table of contents.

Sveticic G, Gentilini A, Eichenberger U, et al. (2004). Combinations of bupivacaine, fentanyl, and clonidine for lumbar epidural postoperative analgesia: a novel optimization procedure. Anesthesiology 101: 1381–1393.

Taddio A, Shennan AT, Stevens B, et al. (1995). Safety of lidocaine-prilocaine cream in the treatment of preterm neonates. J Pediatr 127: 1002–1005.

Taddio A, Katz J, Ilersich AL, et al. (1997a). Effect of neonatal circumcision on pain response during subsequent routine vaccination. Lancet 349: 599–603.

Taddio A, Stevens B, Craig K, et al. (1997b). Efficacy and safety of lidocaine-prilocaine cream for pain during circumcision. N Eng J Med 336: 1197–1201.

Taddio A, Ohlsson A, Einarson TR, et al. (1998). A systematic review of lidocaine-prilocaine cream (EMLA) in the treatment of acute pain in neonates. Pediatrics 101: E1.

Tamai H, Sawamura S, Kanamori Y, et al. (2004). Thoracic epidural catheter insertion using the caudal approach assisted with an electrical nerve stimulator in young children. Reg Anesth Pain Med 29: 92–95.

Tanaka M, Nitta R, Nishikawa T. (2001). Increased T-wave amplitude after accidental intravascular injection of lidocaine plus bupivacaine without epinephrine in sevoflurane-anesthetized child. Anesth Analg 92: 915–917.

Tobias JD. (1994). Continuous femoral nerve block to provide analgesia following femur fracture in a paediatric ICU population. Anaesth Intens Care 22: 616–618.

Touloukian RJ, Wugmeister M, Pickett LK, et al. (1971). Caudal anesthesia for neonatal anoperineal and rectal operations. Anesth Analg 50: 565–568.

Tsui BC, Gupta S, Finucane B. (1998). Confirmation of epidural catheter placement using nerve stimulation. Can J Anaesth 45: 640–644.

Tsui BC, Seal R, Koller J, et al. (2001). Thoracic epidural analgesia via the caudal approach in pediatric patients undergoing fundoplication using nerve stimulation guidance. Anesth Analg 93: 1152–1155.

Tsui BC, Wagner AM, Cunningham K, et al. (2005). Threshold current of an insulated needle in the intrathecal space in pediatric patients. Anesth Analg 100: 662–665.

Tucker GT. (1986). Pharmacokinetics of local anaesthetic agents. Br J Anesth 58: 717–731.

van Niekerk J, Bax-Vermeire BM, Geurts JW, et al. (1990). Epidurography in premature infants. Anaesthesia 45: 722–725.

Ved SA, Pinosky M, Nicodemus H. (1993). Ventricular tachycardia and brief cardiovascular collapse in two infants after caudal anesthesia using a bupivacaine-epinephrine solution. Anesthesiology 79: 1121–1123.

Welborn LG, Hannallah RS, Fink R, et al. (1989). High-dose caffeine suppresses postoperative apnea in former preterm infants. Anesthesiology 71: 347–349.

Welborn LG, Rice LJ, Hannallah RS, et al. (1990). Postoperative apnea in former preterm infants: prospective comparison of spinal and general anesthesia. Anesthesiology 72: 838–842.

Welborn LG, Hannallah RS, Luban NL, et al. (1991). Anemia and post-operative apnea in former preterm infants. Anesthesiology 74: 1003–1006.

William JM, Stoddart PA, Williams SA, et al. (2001). Post-operative recovery after inguinal herniotomy in ex-premature infants: comparison between sevoflurane and spinal anaesthesia. Br J Anaesth 86: 366–371.

Williamson PS, Williamson ML. (1983). Physiologic stress reduction by a local anesthetic during newborn circumcision. Pediatrics 71: 36–40.

Wilson GA, Brown JL, Crabbe DG, et al. (2001). Is epidural analgesia associated with an improved outcome following open Nissen fundoplication? Paediatr Anaesth 11: 65–70.

Wolf AR, Hughes D, Hobbs AJ, et al. (1991). Combined morphine-bupivacaine caudals for reconstructive penile surgery in children: systemic absorption of morphine and postoperative analgesia. Anaesth Intens Care 19: 17–21.

Wolf AR, Eyres RL, Laussen PC, et al. (1993). Effect of extradural analgesia on stress responses to abdominal surgery in infants. Br J Anaesth 70: 654–660.

Wolf AR, Doyle E, Thomas E. (1998). Modifying infant stress responses to major surgery: spinal vs extradural vs opioid analgesia. Paediatr Anaesth 8: 305–311.

Wulf H, Peters C, Behnke H. (2000). The pharmacokinetics of caudal ropivacaine 0.2% in children. A study of infants aged less than 1 year and toddlers aged 1–5 years undergoing inguinal hernia repair. Anaesthesia 55: 757–760.

CHAPTER 12

The social and environmental context of pain in neonates

C Celeste Johnston
Marilyn Aita
Marsha Campbell-Yeo
Lenora J Duhn
Margot A Latimer
Kathryn J McNaughton

INTRODUCTION

The context in which pain occurs influences its perception and experience. This idea has been recognized in the literature since Beecher's now widely quoted observation that wounded soldiers who realized that their injuries were extensive enough to send them home from the battlefield did not appear to be distressed by pain from significant tissue damage (Beecher 1956). That observation, as well as numerous other situations in which people seemingly do not feel pain in certain social contexts despite significant tissue damage, helped Melzack conceptualize the importance of descending pathways from higher brain centres in the modulation of pain (Melzack and Wall 1996, Melzack 1999).

Context can be broadly defined to include the physical setting, such as light and sound, or the psychosocial setting, such as who is present, is the setting familiar or strange and is the pain expected or not. In children, for example, there is a large literature on parental presence during painful events (Broome and Endsley 1989, Piira et al. 2005). In a recent systematic review that reported on 28 studies investigating the effect of parental presence during medical procedures, in spite of mixed results, with more rigourous studies showing no effect for the child, it was concluded that having parents present during painful events is beneficial, at least for parents (Broome and Endsley 1989, Piira et al. 2006). There is the possibility that indicators of benefit were not sensitive to the intervention in these studies and that a child demonstrating distress could reflect a comfort level in expressing emotion. In a recent study on adults suffering from fibromyalgia it was found that in the presence of a loved one, not only did patients report less pain when stimulated at pressure points, but there was a concomitant decrease in somatosensory brain activity (Montoya et al. 2004).

There is less known about the context in which infants experience pain, although there is now more interest in this topic. They are the most vulnerable to repeated and prolonged exposure to pain without benefit of analgesia (McLaughlin et al. 1993, Anand and Selankio 1996, Johnston et al. 1997a). For preterm neonates the transition from the womb to the outside world, a stressful event for all newborns, comes at a time when they are developmentally less prepared to cope with that transition than healthy full-term neonates (Als 1982, Als et al. 1988).

PRIOR EXPERIENCE WITH PAIN

Animal model studies have shown that repeated exposure to pain early in life leads to hypersensitization later (Fitzgerald and Shortland 1988, Anand et al. 1999, Narsinghani and Anand 2000, Howard et al. 2001, Johnston et al. 2002). Taddio has reported both memory for pain in newborns as demonstrated by anticipatory reactivity (Taddio et al. 2002) and increased sensitivity in response to subsequent painful stimuli (Taddio et al. 1997). In contrast, preterm neonates who have been exposed to pain without analgesia appear to have decreased responsiveness (Johnston and Stevens 1996, Grunau et al. 2001). In one study it was reported that the more recent the last invasive procedure the less likely the preterm infant would be to respond behaviourally (Johnston et al. 1999). Thus it would seem that the context of how much pain the infant has experienced will affect their response. In another study of very low-birth-weight infants, Grunau reported that after approximately 20 invasive procedures, the infant's response was diminished. In a recent study in which there was a 24-hour period between heel lances, infants between 32–36 weeks gestational age showed greater physiological response in the second session regardless of the intervention, which had been randomly assigned. In addition, in a study conducted by Holsti et al. (2005), preterm neonates undergoing heel lance prior to clustering care demonstrated heightened facial, body and heart rate responses during the presumably non-painful care interventions, such as bathing and diaper change. These study results suggest that exposure of preterm neonates to non-painful or painful neonatal intensive care unit (NICU) stimuli may initially increase responsiveness even to presumably non-painful stimuli but eventually the infant is unable to mount a robust response, possibly due to exhaustion.

THE NEURO-BEHAVIOURAL STATE

The neuro-behavioural state (Prechtl 1974) the infant is in at the time of a painful event can be considered as context. Grunau first reported that full-term neonates who were in a quiet state at the time of a painful event showed less response (Grunau and Craig 1990, Grunau 1991). Stevens and others (Stevens and Johnston 1994, Stevens et al. 1994) corroborated this observation and explicitly considered state to be the infant-related context in which pain occurs (Stevens et al. 1996).

There are various behavioural strategies that have been tested either to improve quiet state which might in turn decrease pain response as well as strategies that have been tested in the context of procedural pain. These strategies, described below, include physical interventions such as positioning, rocking, or touch, maternal and other family members being present, environmental light and noise, and finally, the socio-professional context of the NICU itself.

TOUCH, POSITION, VESTIBULAR ACTION

Touch and massage can have a soothing effect that results in promotion of growth (Field 2002a, 2002b), but in ill or compromised infants, it may have a destabilizing effect (Scafidi et al. 1993). The way in which the touch is performed will affect the response. In one study it was reported that handling an infant just prior to a painful event resulted in greater physiological instability in response to that painful event (Porter et al. 1991). The type of handling in that study was in preparation for the impending lumbar puncture, whereas touch given gently is more appropriate. Firmly holding an infant in midline position, referred to as facilitative tucking, resulted in a more rapid recovery from heel lance (Corff et al. 1995). However, positioning in the prone position while nested, without touch, was not found to have an effect on pain responses (Stevens et al. 1999, Grunau et al. 2004), although prone positioning and nesting promotes physiological stability and a quiet behavioural state (Campos 1989, Als et al. 1994). Similarly, rocking water beds were shown to promote quiet state, physiological stability and reduce irritability, but was unsuccessful when tested for procedural pain reduction (Johnston et al. 1997b). It could be concluded that simply the act of promoting quiet state and physiological stability may not be sufficient to blunt pain. In the rocking study that had shown effectiveness (Campos 1989), the infants were full-term, were in an upright position, and were held by their mothers. The notion that mothers may be the key for comfort has led to studies with promising results.

SIGNIFICANT OTHERS: MOTHER

Mothers across species have instinctively comforted their young as a means of survival of the species. Only recently have the complex neurochemical relationships been studied which has allowed us to understand the basic mechanisms underlying the maternal comforting process. Interestingly, from the perspective of pain, the opioid system is an important one in early maternal–infant interactions (Panksepp et al. 1994, Nelson and Panksepp 1998). Also, oxytocin, which not only is circulating within lactating mothers but also spills into breast milk, is known to promote bonding and regulation, and is also implicated in pain modulation via endogenous opiate release (Carter et al. 1992, Lund et al. 2002). Essentially, maternal contact releases opiates.

There have been some recent studies that have exploited the idea that maternal contact would decrease pain. Kangaroo care, or skin-to-skin care, is gaining acceptance as a standard of care in NICUs throughout the world (Engler et al. 2002). It was first developed as a method of home care for low-birth-weight infants in Bogota, Columbia by Rey and Martinez in 1979 as an alternative to incubator care (Whitelaw and Sleath 1985). During kangaroo care a diaper-clad infant is held upright, at an angle of approximately 60°, between the mother's breasts, providing maximal skin-to-skin contact between baby and mother.

Several studies have shown kangaroo care to have positive effects upon autonomic behaviour and state (Acolet et al. 1989, deLeeuw et al. 1991, Bier et al. 1995, Mooncey et al. 1997, Ludington-Hoe et al. 2000, Chwo et al. 2002, Feldman et al. 2002, Feldman and Eidelman 2003). A recent Cochrane review on kangaroo care for lactation success, maternal–infant behaviour and infant physiology, although not pain response, (Anderson et al. 2005) concluded that it was useful in promoting breastfeeding and decreasing crying.

There have been two reported studies on the efficacy of kangaroo care for procedural pain, one on full-term neonates (Gray et al. 2000) and the other with preterm neonates 32–36 weeks gestational age (Johnston et al. 2003). Thirty full-term neonates undergoing heel lance for routine testing for phenylketonuria were randomly assigned to kangaroo care or being swaddled in an incubator. Differences in amount of crying and facial grimacing were less than half as frequent in the kangaroo care group and heart rate was significantly lower (Gray et al. 2000). In the study on preterm neonates ($n = 74$) a cross-over design was used comparing kangaroo care and incubator conditions on pain response. The scores on the composite pain measure for procedural pain, the PIPP (Stevens et al. 1996), were lower for the kangaroo care group and the facial grimacing was reduced by 30% (Johnston et al. 2003).

Amniotic fluid and breastmilk, especially colostrum and foremilk, share the same chemical profile peculiar to each lactating woman (Varendi et al. 1996, Porter and Winberg 1999) and infants will migrate towards the unwashed breast compared to the washed breast of their mother (Varendi and Porter 2001).

Breastfeeding as an analgesic has been tested on full-term neonates. Gray and colleagues (Gray et al. 2002) studied 30 full-term breast-fed neonates during heel lance for routine blood testing in a randomized control trial. Crying and grimacing were almost extinguished (90% difference) and heart rate significantly reduced in the breastfeeding situation. In a similar study, but using venepuncture instead of heel lance as the procedure to obtain blood, Carbajal and colleagues (2003) also found significant reduction in the breastfeeding condition along with the glucose and pacifier condition on both the Douleur Aigue Neonatal (DAN) (Carbajal et al. 1997) and the PIPP scales (Stevens et al. 1996). There was a non-significant trend for the pain scores in the breastfeeding condition to be lower on the DAN than glucose with pacifier.

Although studies showed breastfeeding as analgesia to be effective, it seems to have been the holding of the infant that was effective in those studies (Gormally et al. 2001). In that study, 85 full-term neonates were randomly assigned to holding plus sucrose, holding with water, not held with sucrose and the control group received water and were not held during routine heel lance. Holding alone or holding with sucrose had lower facial expressions of pain than sucrose while not being held. There have been no studies of aromatherapy, specifically breast milk for pain. Breast milk given by syringe was not shown to be analgesic in two studies (Ors et al. 1999, Bilgen et al. 2001) but was in a third (Upadhyay et al. 2004), leaving open the question of its olfactory potential for comfort.

Infants may learn certain characteristics about their mother while still in utero. For example, infants prefer their own mother's voice to other female voices (DeCasper and Fifer 1980, DeCasper and Spence 1986, DeCasper et al. 1994), demonstrating evidence of auditory memory. This notion was tested in a cross-over design in which the mother's voice was played in the experimental condition but no sound was played in the control condition during routine heel lance. There was no effect of the mother's voice on the pain response, suggesting that auditory stimulation may not be sufficient as an analgesic.

There is enough evidence to support the effect of maternal interventions involving direct physical contact with the infant to believe that it is effective in providing comfort to neonates during an acute painful event. The question arising from the studies on maternal comfort is whether or not another caring person would have a similar effect, or does it need to be someone for whom the infant has some memory.

SIGNIFICANT OTHERS: FATHER

The literature regarding care of the neonate and infant has focused in large part on maternal involvement, to the exclusion of paternal contributions. Yet socio-economic changes and evolving societal perceptions and expectations of fathers' role (Coleman et al. 2004, St. John et al. 2005) have inspired greater consideration of the importance of the role of fathers and the impact of 'fathering' on the family system. In so doing, a growing body of evidence profiles the importance of fathers' contributions to childcare, in particular to healthy child development and a secure infant–paternal relationship. These findings offer new directions for paternal role involvement as it relates to innovative pain management strategies for neonates and infants.

While in Kampala, Uganda in 1954–1955, Ainsworth's (1967) longitudinal research of 28 babies during their first 15 months of life detailed some of the earliest findings on the power of paternal influence and involvement in infant development and attachment. Her writings speak of the child's attachment to his/her mother but acknowledge, in addition, a special quality in the father's interaction with his infant that seemed apart from the mother's, and for some infants the father represented the preferred attachment figure despite limited interactions. The elusive quality in the father's interaction, queried as 'tenderness or intense delight', had profound effects on some of the infants wherein they are described as having a preference to seek out their fathers over all others, even when tired or ill. Interestingly quality of interaction has been identified as an important predictor for secure infant–father attachment in other investigations (Cox et al. 1992). As well, Brazelton (1992) notes a pattern of paternal preference that many newborn infants demonstrate by turning their heads to their father's voice as opposed to the voice of a stranger.

More recent studies provide information on the impact of the infant–father connection. In a longitudinal study by Levy-Shiff et al. (1990) the impact of fathers' hospital visits with their preterm infants was explored with data collection occurring during the hospital stay, at discharge, at 8 months of age, and at 18 months of age. The frequency of visits was associated with infant weight gain during hospitalization as well as higher scores on behavioural and social-development aspects of later infant development during the first 18 months.

Yogman and colleagues (1995) also report an equally powerful image of the infant–father relationship. In their longitudinal study, 985 low-birth-weight preterm infants were followed from birth to age 3 years. One of the findings from this study was an association within the Afro-American ethnic subgroup between higher father involvement with their infant and improved cognitive outcome, suggesting that paternal involvement plays a unique role in a child's cognitive development.

The practice of kangaroo care has provided an enhanced opportunity for parents of preterm infants to become more involved in the care of their infant, and as Dodd (2005) notes it facilitates parents' recognition and understanding of their infants' cues allowing them to respond as needed. Most investigations of kangaroo care have studied the role of the mother, however three studies in particular examined the father's role in providing kangaroo care. The first, a descriptive study by Ludington-Hoe and colleagues (1992) of 11 healthy preterm infants, examined their cardiorespiratory, thermal and state behaviour responses to 2 hours of paternal kangaroo care within the first 17 hours of birth. They concluded that fathers were able to keep their infants sufficiently warm, and offer that fathers may be an under-used source of warmth and comfort for these infants.

Christensson (1996) found a similar result in studying 44 healthy, full-term elective caesarean section-delivered infants when exploring skin and body temperature and metabolic adaptation in infants randomized to either an incubator, a cot, or skin-to-skin with their father during the first 2 hours after birth. The mean axillary temperature increase was significantly greater in the skin-to-skin cared-for infants compared to those infants who were cared for in a cot, while no significant difference was seen with the incubator group. Catecholamine levels were normal and not different between the groups, but blood glucose increase was significant only in the skin-to-skin group, suggestive of possible conservation of energy. Additionally it was noted that at 24 hours after birth the temperature was significantly higher in the skin-to-skin group than in the incubator group.

Bauer et al. (1996) investigated the effects of maternal and paternal kangaroo care on 11 preterm infants with gestational ages ranging from 28 to 31 weeks, birth weight of 560 to 1390 grams, and postnatal ages of 8 to 48 days. The variables that were analyzed included oxygen consumption, carbon dioxide production, energy expenditure, skin and rectal temperature, heart and respiratory rates, arterial saturation, and behavioural states. Only skin temperature increased significantly during both maternal and paternal kangaroo care, while the remaining variables did not change during either type of care.

Collectively these outcomes provide beginning evidence that early paternal involvement in the care of their healthy or compromised infant is necessary, meaningful and even critical. What has not been explored is the full contribution that fathers can make through their involvement in the care of their sick or preterm infant, specifically in the area of providing comfort against pain. Since it has been shown that paternal involvement can be successful in helping infants maintain body regulatory behaviours such as temperature maintenance, as well as the powerful role of paternal attachment, it is possible that fathers could provide comfort to neonates as effectively as mothers. Initial research projects could be conducted to compare paternal presence to no one, paternal presence to a non-family member, and paternal presence to maternal presence.

SIGNIFICANT OTHERS: SIBLINGS

Some neonates are born with a relationship with a sibling or siblings. This is the case with multiple births. The incidence of twin and higher-order multiple (HOM) births is continuing to rise in both the United States and Canada to approximately 2.5% of live births (Millar et al. 1992). A rise in births to older mothers, increased fertility treatments and interventions augmenting conception have been reported as the main reasons for this increase (Millar et al. 1992, Wilcox et al. 1996). Twins and higher-order multiples are at higher risk of prematurity (Newman and Ellings 1995), intrauterine growth restriction, retinopathy of prematurity, intraventricular haemorrhage and bronchopulmonary dysplasia (Millar et al. 1992). Approximately 50% of twins and 90% of triplets are born prematurely (before 37 weeks gestation). At birth, twins are separated as individual health needs are met. Thus they face the harsh, often painful environment of the NICU alone, without their sibling(s) with whom they have spent the last several months feeling and hearing. It has been demonstrated that maternal contact may have a blunting effect on infant pain response and may facilitate physiologic stability (recovery) following painful procedures (Johnston et al. 2003). Is it then possible that the contact or presence of a sibling who has shared the same uterine space since conception would have a similar comforting effect?

Gottfried et al. (1994) examined the attachment relationship in infant twins at 18–34 months (median age 21 months) and found that when separated from their mothers, twin infants showed minimal distress, measured as amount and type of crying, if their twin remained present. Separation from both their twin and mother created a high level of distress. Furthermore, when reunited with their mothers, twin dyads that had not been separated were able to quickly restore normal social behaviours. In those infants separated from their mother and twin, both the separated and the non-separated twin remained distressed during reunion and both solicited physical contact and comfort from their mother.

Twins spend their entire lives before birth in close quarters, growing and developing in the presence of another fetus. Twin siblings have been observed on ultrasound as early as 14 weeks sucking on their sibling's face and fingers and appearing to be touching and exploring their sibling's face, activity which has been interpreted as preparation for self-soothing and comfort measures (Klaus and Klaus 1998). Mothers of twins have reported that their babies appeared to have similar periods of activity and sleep while in utero (Gallagher et al. 1992). Studies have consistently demonstrated that twins, when monitored by non-stress tests (NSTs), exhibit a remarkably high incidence (~58%) of coincident fetal heart rate (FHR) acceleration. FHR accelerations appeared to be independent of gestational age, growth patterns or placental type. Synchronous FHR accelerations remained constant with increasing gestational age (27–42 weeks) (Devoe and Azor 1981, Sherer et al. 1990). In a later study examining FHR accelerations, fetal movements and behaviour patterns, twins were found to have synchronous behaviour (sleep or awake patterns) 94.7% of the time (Gallagher et al. 1992). Twins appeared to have some form of 'interfetal communication'. This bond may provide a basis for sibling comforting and improved physiologic stability (recovery) following painful procedures if placed in contact with each other. In older children, the presence of a sibling as a co-therapist, during central venous port-access in children with acute lymphoplastic leukaemia, had a positive effect. Physical resistance was eliminated and anxiety responses were reduced (Barrera 2000).

Als (1986) hypothesized that infants actively communicate how they perceive and cope with their environment in her Synactive Theory of Development which Nyquist and Lutes (1998) used to provide an explanatory model for understanding how co-bedding may assist preterm twins in coping with the extrauterine environment. Co-bedding is a developmental care practice in which twins and higher-order multiples are cared for in one incubator versus being separated and cared for individually in separate incubators. Suggestions for co-bedding are based on the premise that extrauterine adaptation of twin neonates is enhanced by continued physical contact with the other twin, rather than the sudden deprivation of such stimuli (Als 1986, Nyquist and Lutes 1998, Fowler et al. 2003). Swaddling multiples in the same blanket provides them with the opportunity to co-regulate. Hayward (2003) described co-bedding as a natural extension of the socialization process that allows twins to adjust the extrauterine environment by co-regulating their body temperatures, sleep/wake cycles, infant state and initiating co-soothing measures. Extensive research on infant cues and state modulation provides evidence of the newborn infant's ability to not only respond to his/her external environment, but also to initiate communication through the use of cues (Sumner and Spietz 1996, Klaus and Klaus 1998). Studies on the psychological and social effects of co-sleeping reveal positive consequences on child development (McKenna and Mosko 1994, McKenna 1997, Lewis and Janda 1998). Co-bedding is theorized to enhance twin co-regulation, improve respiratory status, decrease oxygen requirements, increase weight gain, facilitate mutuality in their circadian rhythms and sleep/awake patterns (Nyquist and Lutes 1998, Lutes and Altimier 2001, Fowler et al. 2003, Hayward 2003). Anecdotal evidence and case reports have described the comforting aspects of co-bedding. When placed together, twins appear to touch and soothe one another (Lutes 1996, DellaPorta et al. 1998, Gannon 1999). When mothers of twins being co-bedded were interviewed, they reported that their infants appeared to be more restless and irritable when separated and 'complained' more when nurses took blood samples and performed other medical procedures (Nyquist and Lutes 1998). Despite the mounting evidence of the benefits of maternal contact related to infant pain response, scien-tific studies examining the effect of the continued presence of a sibling(s) have not yet been done. If twins have established a physiological responsivity to each other prenatally, a psychobiological model may help us to theoretically understand the potential for siblings to comfort one another.

The increased incidence of multiple gestation births and admission of these fragile babies to neonatal units raises questions regarding the differences in care of HOMs versus singletons. If sibling contact while co-bedding is determined to have a positive effect then changes in current neonatal care practices to include co-bedding for twins may be an inexpensive, non-invasive method to help twins and higher-order multiples maintain physiologic stability and decrease long-term psychological impacts of procedural pain in this high-risk population.

CONTEXT AS THE PHYSICAL ENVIRONMENT: LIGHT AND SOUND

The previous sections have considered the infant's own context (state) or social context, that is, presence of family members. However, context also includes the physical environment of the NICU to be considered. For more than three decades, light and noise have been identified as important sources of environmental stress that preterm and high-risk neonates are exposed to in the NICU (Als 1982, 1986, Lotas 1992, Glass 1999, Goldson 1999, Perlman 2001, Warren 2002, Holditch-Davis et al. 2003). These physical factors have been reported to create physiological instability in preterm neonates (Shiroiwa et al. 1986, Blackburn and Patteson 1991, Zahr and Balian 1995, Graven 2000). However, less is known about the effect of light and noise in the NICU environment on the experience of pain in preterm neonates. Yet, theoretical hypotheses (Anand and Scalzo 2000) suggest that non-painful sensory stimulation in the environment may heighten pain response in preterm infants, further supporting the importance of limiting their exposure to NICU light and noise.

Researchers' and clinicians' attentiveness towards NICU environmental light and noise arises mainly from the *Synactive Theory of Development* elaborated by Heidelise Als in 1982. Als proposed that sensory stimulation induced by NICU noise and light can influence preterm neonates' brain development. Input to the auditory and visual sensory systems is particularly noteworthy given that input to these systems is muted or absent in the intrauterine environment. In addition, White-Traut et al. (1994) suggested that there is a strong probability of visual and auditory over-stimulation in premature neonates since vision and hearing are the last two senses to develop in utero and the exposure to light and noise is nearly incessant in the NICU environment. The preterm neonates' brain is believed to be functional in transmitting and integrating visual, auditory and tactile sensory stimuli (Anand and Scalzo 2000). As such, when the central nervous system has integrated environmental stressors such as noise and light, the autonomic nervous system then reflects the stress response of physiological and behavioural responses (Johnson et al. 1992).

Light and noise have been reported to produce physiological responses in preterm neonates. Infants exposed to continuous lighting over 24 hours in the NICU have shown increased mean heart rate and motor activity levels during the evening/night time hours compared to the ones exposed to cycled lighting (Blackburn and Patteson 1991). Similarly, Shiroiwa et al. (1986) reported that when the eyes of 10 preterm neonates were not shielded during the night they had a higher mean and variation in respiratory rate as well as longer-lasting movements. Noises in the NICU also decrease infants' oxygen saturation and clinically increase infants' heart and respiratory rates (Zahr and Balian 1995). After a comprehensive review of the literature, Graven (2000) concluded that sudden intense noises disturb the physiological stability of preterm neonates. These stimuli cause depletion of energy resources that would otherwise be used to promote growth and development as well as subsystems' organization (Sammons and Lewis 1985, Blackburn 1998). In the context of pain, the exposure of premature neonates to NICU light and noise would use energy that would no longer be available to deal with a painful procedure.

Reducing exposure to NICU light and noise levels is advocated by pain experts as an appropriate environmental strategy to prevent and manage pain in preterm neonates (Franck and Lawhon 1998, Stevens et al. 2000). Anand and the International Evidence-Based Group for Neonatal Pain (2001) also recommend using environmental strategies to reduce stress in preterm neonates and manage pain. Additionally, Stevens et al. (2000) profiled the need for researchers to investigate the effect of reduced overall noxious stimuli in the NICU environment on pain response of preterm infants. Interestingly, some experienced pain researchers have acknowledged the importance of controlling for light and noise in their studies evaluating pain response. For example, Johnston and Stevens (1996) reported in their study that prior pain exposures increased pain response in preterm neonates, and recognized that light and noise, although not assessed in the study, might have influenced the premature infants' pain responses. Despite the lack of empirical evidence to confirm the beneficial effect of reducing light and noise on pain response in preterm neonates, theoretical knowledge provides a promising direction for pain research, specifically to evaluate the effect of interventions that increase the physiological stability of preterm infants. For example, reduced illumination such as day and night cycling (Blackburn and Patteson 1991), and shielding preterm infants' eyes (Shiroiwa et al. 1986), as well as reduction of noises by infants wearing earmuffs (Zahr and de Traversay 1995) and placing acoustical foam pieces inside the incubators (Johnson 2001) have all been reported as interventions being physiologically beneficial for premature neonates. Therefore, testing the effect of these interventions on the pain response of preterm neonates, either separately or combined, would significantly contribute to the body of knowledge for the pain management of these infants.

THE CONTEXT OF THE NICU: HOSPITAL WORK ENVIRONMENT

The environment in which neonates are cared for is complex. Environmental factors may influence how infants perceive pain and how staff deliver pain care. While we do not know at this point in time how the work environment directly affects pain management, we do know that it affects staff performance in other areas of care. Nurses and doctors who have, and are able to use, pain assessment and management knowledge in their work environment are likely to prevent pain and discomfort in neonates. Efforts to increase pain knowledge uptake and use to enhance pain care could be directed more comprehensively at the work environment.

There is evidence that staff 'know' that infants and children experience pain. Franck and Miaskowski (1997) reported that nurses and physicians believed infants could feel as much pain as adults, however adequate pain relief was not provided for procedures such as circumcision and chest tube insertion. Neonatal nurses in Reyes' study (2003) scored high on pain assessment knowledge but chart reviews revealed that knowledge did not translate to practice of pain relief (Reyes 2003). Similar discrepancies were reported between knowledge and practice by Jacob and Puntillo (1999). Other researchers have reported an increase in knowledge as a result of interventions to change practice but question whether the changes have been sustained (Dahlman et al. 1999, Howell et al. 2000). Work environment factors such as access to professional development, interdisciplinary collaboration, leadership, adequate staffing and skill mix are emerging as vital components potentially increasing knowledge use for better care outcomes.

The top four sources of nurse practice knowledge are identified as; personal nursing experience, patient/clinical experiences, nurse–physician discussions and in-services (Estabrooks et al. 2004). Knowledge transfer researchers have demonstrated a relationship between attendance at conferences/in-services and innovation adoption (Coyle and Sokop 1990, Estabrooks 1999). Specifically in the area of pain research, Johnston et al. (2004) found a positive correlation between pain knowledge and pain course/workshop attendance while Dufault and Sullivan (2000) reported significantly lower pain intensity by patients cared for by nurses and physicians who attended pain in-services. Access to interdisciplinary opportunities where both nurses and physicians share and learn effective pain care strategies together are a fundamental component of the work environment. These would include weekly pain rounds involving presentation of patient case studies where pain is the central care issue. Informal presentations by all disciplines and attendance at pain and paediatric conferences where staff could present potentially better practices tested on their units could be highly useful.

Opportunities to learn are just as important as the chances to use the knowledge at work. Information exchange between nurses and physicians is a crucial process for knowledge use resulting in better pain care. Given the fact that a major source of nurses' knowledge is derived from clinical experience and discussions with physicians, interventions facilitating open sharing of pain practice knowledge are reasonable. Any informal and formal opportunities that facilitate nurse–physician discussions could potentially increase the translation of pain care strategies across disciplines creating work climates that sustain more widespread unit changes. There is strong evidence demonstrating the impact on patient outcomes when good nurse–physician collaboration exists. Pain care will likely be potentiated when high pain knowledge is paired with high interdisciplinary collaboration.

Collaboration has been defined as 'nurses and physicians cooperatively working together, sharing responsibilities for solving problems and making decisions to formulate and carry out plans for patient care' (Baggs and Schmidt 1988, p. 145). Significant positive correlations between nurses' perceptions of nurse–doctor collaboration and satisfaction with decision-making have been reported (Dechario-Marino et al. 2001, Krairiksh and Anthony 2001). Krairiksh and Anthony indicated that only nurse–physician collaboration positively contributed to greater participation in decision-making directly influencing care outcomes. Recently, Estabrooks et al. (2005) reported that after adjusting for patient co-morbidities and age, the presence of better nurse–physician relationships was one of the top four predictors of lower 30-day mortality rates. This finding is consistent with previous research reporting lower mortality rates and fewer re-admissions to the ICU associated with better nurse–doctor communication (Knaus et al. 1986, Baggs et al. 1992, Aiken et al. 1994, Miller et al. 2001). Furthermore, good doctor–nurse relations have been associated with patient reports of better pain care (Wild and Mitchell 2000), higher incidence of medication administration enhancing patient functional mobility (Schmidt and Svarstad 2002), and reducing pain post surgery (Willson 2000). Specific interventions enhancing nurse–physician pain care collaboration would include a routine time during the shift for nurses to share their assessment of infant pain, and opportunities to discuss the co-ordination of management strategies for upcoming painful procedures agreed upon between nurses and physicians.

Leaders/managers can create the organizational processes necessary to sustain collaborative strategies and enhance knowledge uptake that is important for practice. McClelland found that organizational climate explained 36% of the variance of one group's success over another. Senior business executive leadership styles impacted 70% of the climate as experienced by those reporting to the leader (Lepelley 2002). For nurses, Wilson and Laschinger (1994) discovered that nurses' views on access to power and opportunity in their own jobs depended on their perceptions of their managers' powerfulness. Physicians and nurse leaders/administrators are in a unique position to influence pain outcomes. These leaders can actively support staff attendance at professional development opportunities, implement pain care accreditation guidelines, establish unit routines, engage healthcare professionals in relevant discussions about care, and effectively use resources such as equipment and staff to influence better care in busy workplaces.

There has been an overall increase in work intensity and complexity in downsized organizations (O'Brien-Pallas et al. 2001) and credible research links organizational structures, staffing levels and patient outcomes (Aiken et al. 1994, 2002, McGillis-Hall and Doran 2001). Workload has been defined as a balance between job demands with sufficient resources such as adequate staffing and time available to plan and perform work (Koehoorn et al. 2003). Infant mortality rate was reported to increase by 50% with higher nurse workloads on full versus half-capacity units (Tucker 2002). Workload was measured by occupancy rates and nurse-to-infant ratio. In other neonatal research, odds of mortality adjusted for initial risk and infant dependency scores (nurse workload) were improved by 82% when an infant–staff ratio greater than 1.71 occurred (Callaghan et al. 2003). The Agency for Healthcare Research and Quality report on working conditions and patient safety found that lower nurse–patient ratios in neonatal intensive care were associated with more complex errors such as poor prioritization of clinical tasks and failure to perform diagnostic assessments resulting in adverse outcomes. Lee et al. (2003) reported higher mortality rates among infants admitted to intensive care units on nights. Nurse–patient ratios were not predictive of higher mortality rates, however nurses' level of experience and specific descriptions of nurse–patient ratios including acuity across units were not examined. The night shift is not the most desirable shift to work and likely to be staffed by the least-experienced nurses with the lowest seniority.

Scheduling nurses with appropriate levels of expertise to care for infants 24/7 is as important as securing an adequate complement of nurses. While staff factors such as age and education are not considered modifiable variables, hiring and scheduling decisions made by leaders are. O'Brien-Pallas et al. (2004) reported experienced, full-time baccalaureate staff provided a higher quality of pain care to adult patients, while Tibby et al. (2004) demonstrated that factors associated with decreased adverse patient events in a paediatric intensive care unit included the presence of a senior nurse in charge, a high proportion of the shift filled by permanent staff and/or senior nurses. A sample of patient-related adverse events included drug-related errors, intravenous/arterial line extravasations requiring restarts (additional tissue-damaging procedures) and needle stick injuries to patients. An adequate number of nurses with relevant professional attributes matched to care needs working in a supportive work environment enhances the likelihood of optimum pain care while decreasing adverse painful events.

Anecdotal and research evidence of work factors indicating use of best practices for pain care knowledge include: standing medication orders for analgesics to be given based on nurses' pain assessment; availability of validated and appropriate pain scales; official places to document pain scores and assessments on medical records regularly consulted by all disciplines (Faries et al. 1991, Reyes 2003); availability of equipment like patient-controlled analgesia (PCA) infusion pumps, and accessibility and proximity of analgesics to the bedside.

In fact, unit design may be a factor underlying effective pain care delivery. With less time to provide more intensive care, nurses and physicians are challenged to find ways to share knowledge more effectively. The 'time' to travel from the bedside to the medication room for analgesics, or to find someone to assist and hold the baby for painful procedures is limited. Units with open designs and easier visual contact with others may facilitate more collaborative pain practices as nurses may consult nurse and physician colleagues more readily if they can see them. Nurses may be more apt to ask for assistance with a procedure or for an analgesic order if they can see that someone is available to assist them. Infants cared for by staff working in units designed to facilitate

knowledge exchange may experience better management for painful procedures. Less-experienced nurses requiring more intense mentoring opportunities may be challenged to effectively manage procedures in the newly designed private 'pod'-like care settings created to reduce ambient factors and support better infection control principles.

Creating collaborative and well-designed workplaces where knowledgeable staff have time to conduct developmentally appropriate pain assessments and opportunities to act on and share this knowledge either in face-to-face discussions or through documentation will be environments conducive to 'better' pain care practices. Discussions and documentation provide the feedback loop building trust among caregivers while creating a natural knowledge translation strategy across shifts and between professionals.

CONCLUSION

The context in which the neonate experiences pain is multidimensional and complex. How environmental and contextual factors affect pain perception and response in neonates is only beginning to be explored and data are scanty. There are data that support the real presence of the mother, as opposed to her photograph. Paternal and sibling presence have been shown to promote physiological stability and a quiet state, so these are avenues to explore in terms of their effect on pain experienced by neonates. Physical aspects of the context such as reduction of light and noise have been shown to promote physiological stability and thus may also decrease pain response, but research is needed to test this possibility. Finally, the complex work environment of the NICU affects staff performance, which will affect pain management, but the direct link between work environment and pain experience in the neonate has not specifically been studied. The early information that we do have suggests that the contextual environment in which pain is experienced does influence response in neonates, including critically ill preterm neonates, as it does in older persons. It is an area worthy of further exploration and possible manipulation for the benefit of neonates, especially those undergoing multiple painful events.

REFERENCES

Acolet D, Sleath K, Whitelaw A. (1989). Oxygenation, heart rate, and temperature in very low birthweight infants during skin-to-sin contact with their mothers. Acta Paediatr 78: 189–193.

Aiken LH, Smith HL, Lake ET. (1994). Lower medicare mortality among a set of hospitals known for good nursing care. Med Care 2: 771–787.

Aiken LH, Clarke S, Sloane DM, et al. (2002). Hospital nurse staffing and

patient mortality, nurse burnout, and job satisfaction. JAMA 288: 1987–1993.

Ainsworth MDS. (1967). Infancy in Uganda: infant care and the growth of love. The Johns Hopkins Press, Baltimore, Maryland.

Als H. (1982). Towards a synactive theory of development: Promise for the assessment of infant individuality. Infant Ment Health J 3: 229–243.

Als H. (1986). A synactive model of neonatal behavioral organization: Framework for the assessment of neurobehavioral development in the premature infant and for support of infants and parents in the neonatal intensive care environment. Phys Occup Ther Pediatr 6: 3–53.

Als H, Duffy FH, McAnulty G. (1988). Behavioural differences between preterm and full-term newborns as measured with the APIB system scores: I. Infant Behav Develop 11: 305–318.

Als H, Lawhon G, Duffy FH, et al. (1994). Individualized developmental care for the very low birth weight preterm infant: Medical and neurofunctional effects. JAMA 272: 853–858.

Anand KJS, International Evidence-Based Group for Neonatal Pain. (2001). Consensus statement for the prevention and management of pain in the newborn. Arch Pediatr Adolesc Med 155: 173–180.

Anand KJS, Scalzo FM. (2000). Can adverse neonatal experiences alter brain development and subsequent behavior? Biol Neonate 77: 69–82.

Anand KJS, Selankio JD. (1996). SOPAIN Study Group. Routine analgesia practices in 109 neonatal intensive care units (NICU's). Pediatr Res 39: 192A.

Anand KJS, Coskun V, Thrivikraman KV, et al. (1999). Long-term behavioral effects of repetitive pain in neonatal rat pups. Physiol Behav 66: 627–637.

Anderson GC, Moore E, Hepworth J, et al. (2005). Early skin-to-skin contact for mothers and their healthy newborn infants. Cochrane Database Syst Rev: CD003519

Baggs JG, Schmidt MH. (1988). Collaboration between nurses, physicians. Image 20: 145–149.

Baggs JG, Phelps CE, Johnson JE. (1992). The association between inter-disciplinary collaboration and patient outcomes in a medical intensive care unit. Heart Lung 21: 18–24.

Barrera M. (2000). Brief clinical report: procedural pain and anxiety management with mother and sibling as co-therapists. J Pediatr Psychol 25: 117–121.

Bauer J, Sontheimer D, Fischer C, et al. (1996). Metabolic rate and energy balance in very low birth weight infants during kangaroo holding by their mothers and fathers. J Pediatr 129: 608–611.

Beecher HK. (1956). Relationship of significance of wound to pain experienced. JAMA 161: 1609–1613.

Bier JAB, Ferguson A, Liebling JA, et al. (1995). Skin-to-skin contact improves physiologic stress of breastfed low birthweight infants. Pediatr Res 37: 103A.

Bilgen H, Ozek E, Cebeci D, et al. (2001). Comparison of sucrose, expressed breast milk, and breast-feeding on the neonatal response to heel prick. J Pain 2: 301–305.

Blackburn S. (1998). Environmental impact of the NICU on developmental outcomes. J Pediatr Nurs 13: 279–289.

Blackburn S, Patteson D. (1991). Effects of cycled light on activity state and cardiorespiratory function in preterm infants. J Perinat Neonatal Nurs 4: 47–54.

Brazelton TB. (1992). Touchpoints: your child's emotional and behavioral development. Addison-Wesley, Reading, MA.

Broome ME, Endsley RC. (1989). Maternal presence, childrearing practices, and children's response to an injection. Res Nurs Health 12: 229–235.

Callaghan LA, Cartwright DW, O'Rourke P, et al. (2003). Infant to staff ratios and risk of mortality in very low birthweight infants. Arch Dis Child Fetal Neonatal Ed 88: F94–97.

Campos RG. (1989). Soothing pain elicited distress in infants with swaddling and pacifiers. Child Dev 60: 781–792.

Carbajal R, Paupe A, Hoenn E, et al. (1997). [APN: evaluation behavioral scale of acute pain in newborn infants]. [French]. Arch Pediatr 4: 623–628.

Carbajal R, Veerapen S, Couderc S, et al. (2003). Analgesic effect of breast feeding in term neonates: randomized controlled trial. BMJ 326: 313.

Carter CS, Williams JR, Witt DM, et al. (1992). Oxytocin and social bonding. Ann NY Acad Sci 652: 204–211.

Christensson K. (1996). Fathers can effectively achieve heat conservation in healthy newborn infants. Acta Paediatr 85: 1354–1360.

Chwo MJ, Anderson GC, Good M, et al. (2002). A randomized controlled trial of early kangaroo care for preterm infants: Effects on temperature, weight, behavior, and acuity. J Nurs Res 10: 129–142.

Coleman W, Garfield C, the Committee on Psychosocial Aspects of Child and Family Health. (2004). Fathers and pediatricians: Enhancing men's roles in the care and development of their children. Pediatrics 113: 1406–1411.

Corff KE, Seideman R, Venkataraman PS, et al. (1995). Facilitated tucking: A nonpharmacologic comfort measure for pain in preterm neonates. J Obstet Gynecol Neonatal Nurs 24: 143–147.

Cox MJ, Owen MT, Henderson VK, et al. (1992). Prediction of infant–father and infant–mother attachment. Dev Psychol 28: 474–483.

Coyle LA, Sokop AG. (1990). Innovation adoption behavior among nurses. Nurs Res 39: 176–180.

Dahlman GB, Dykes AK, Elander G. (1999). Patients' evaluation of pain and nurses' management of analgesics after surgery. J Adv Nurs 30: 866–874.

DeCasper AJ, Fifer WP. (1980). Of human bonding: Newborns prefer their mothers voices. Science 208: 1174–1176.

DeCasper AJ, Spence MJ. (1986). Prenatal maternal speech influences newborn's perception of speech sounds. Infant Behav Develop 9: 133–150.

DeCasper AJ, Lecanuet JP, Busnel MC, et al. (1994). Fetal reactions to recurrent maternal speech. Infant Behav Develop 17: 159–164.

Dechario-Marino AE, Jordan-Marsh M, Traiger G, et al. (2001). Nurse/physician collaboration: Action research and the lessons learned. J Nurs Adm 31: 232.

deLeeuw R, Colin EM, Dunnebier EA, et al. (1991). Physiologic effects of kangaroo care in very small preterm infants. Biol Neonate 59: 149–155.

DellaPorta K, Aforismo D, Butler-O'Hara M. (1998). Co-bedding of twins in the neonatal intensive care unit. Pediatr Nurs 24: 529–531.

Devoe LD, Azor H. (1981). Simultaneous nonstress fetal heart rate testing in twin pregnancy. Obstet Gynecol 58: 450–455.

Dodd V. (2005). Implications of Kangaroo Care for growth and development in preterm infants. J Obstet Gynecol Neonatal Nurs 34: 218–232.

Dufault MA, Sullivan M. (2000). A collaborative research utilization approach to evaluate the effects of pain management standards on patient outcomes. J Prof Nurs 16: 240–250.

Engler AJ, Ludington-Hoe SM, Cusson RM, et al. (2002). Kangaroo care: National survey of practice, knowledge, barriers, and perceptions. MCN Am J Matern Child Nurs 27: 146–153.

Estabrooks CA. (1999). Modelling the individual determinants of research utilization. West J Nurs Res 21: 758–772.

Estabrooks CA, Scott-Findlay S, Rutakumwa W, et al. (2004). The determinants of research utilization in acute care: Pain management in adult and pediatric settings. Faculty of Nursing, University of Alberta, Edmonton, AB.

Estabrooks CA, Midodzi W, Cummings G, et al. (2005). The impact of hospital nursing characteristics on 30-day mortality. Nurs Res 54: 74–84.

Faries JE, Mills DS, Goldsmith KW, et al. (1991). Systematic pain records and their impact on pain control. A pilot study. Cancer Nurs 14: 306–313.

Feldman R, Eidelman AI. (2003). Skin-to-skin contact (Kangaroo Care) accelerates autonomic and neurobehavioural maturation in preterm infants. Dev Med Child Neurol 45: 274–281.

Feldman R, Weller A, Sirota L, et al. (2002). Skin-to-skin contact (kangaroo care) promotes self-regulation in premature infants: Sleep-wake cyclicity, arousal modulation, and sustained exploration. Dev Psychol 38: 194–207.

Field T. (2002a). Massage therapy. [Review]. Med Clin North Am 86: 163–171.

Field T. (2002b). Preterm infant massage therapy studies: an American approach. [Review]. Semin Neonatol 7: 487–494.

Fitzgerald M, Shortland P. (1988). The effect of neonatal peripheral nerve section on the somadendritic growth of sensory projection cells in the rat spinal cord. Brain Res 470: 129–136.

Fowler Byers J, Yovaish W, Lowman LB, et al. (2003). Co-bedding versus single-bedding premature multiple-gestation infants in incubators. J Obstet Gynecol Neonatal Nurs 32: 340–347.

Franck LS, Lawhon G. (1998). Environmental and behavioural strategies to prevent and manage neonatal pain. Semin Perinatol 22: 434–443.

Franck LS, Miaskowski C. (1997). Measurement of neonatal responses to painful stimuli: A research review. J Pain Symptom Manage 14: 343–378.

Gallagher MW, Costigan K, Johnson TRB. (1992). Fetal heart rate accelerations, fetal movement, and fetal behavior patterns in twin gestations. Am J Obstet Gynecol 167: 1140–1144.

Gannon J. (1999). So happy together. Neonatal Network 18: 39–40.

Glass P. (1999). The vulnerable neonate and the neonatal intensive care environment. In: Avery GB, Fletcher MA, MacDonald MG (eds). Neonatology: pathophysiology and management of the newborn (5th edn), pp. 91–108. Lippincott Williams and Wilkins, New York.

Goldson E. (1999). The environment of the neonatal intensive care unit. In: Goldson E (ed.) Nurturing the premature infant: developmental interventions in the neonatal intensive care nursery, pp. 4–17. Oxford University Press, New York.

Gormally S, Barr RG, Wertheim L, et al. (2001). Contact and nutrient caregiving effects on newborn infant pain responses. Dev Med Child Neurol 43: 28–38.

Gottfried NW, Seay BM, Leake E. (1994). Attachment relationships in infant twins: The effect of co-twin presence during separation from mother. J Genet Psychol 155: 273–282.

Graven SN. (2000). Sound and the developing infant in the NICU: Conclusions and recommendations for care. J Perinatol 20: S88–S93.

Gray L, Watt L, Blass EM. (2000). Skin-to-skin contact is analgesic in healthy newborns. Pediatrics 105: e14.

Gray L, Miller LW, Philipp BL, et al. (2002). Breastfeeding is analgesic in healthy newborns. Pediatrics 109: 590–593.

Grunau R. (1991). Neonatal responses to invasive procedures. Nurs Times 87: 53–54.

Grunau R, Craig KD. (1990). Facial activity as a measure of neonatal pain expression. In: Tyler DC, Krane EJ (eds). Advances in pain therapy and research, Vol 15. Pediatric pain, pp. 147–156. Raven Press, New York.

Grunau R, Oberlander TF, Whitfield MF, et al. (2001). Demographic and therapeutic determinants of pain reactivity in very low birth weight neonates at 32 weeks' postconceptional age. Pediatrics 107: 105–112.

Grunau RE, Linhares MB, Holsti L, et al. (2004). Does prone or supine position influence pain responses in preterm infants at 32 weeks gestational age? Clin J Pain 76–82.

Hayward KM. (2003). Co-bedding of twins: A natural extension of the socialization process. MCN Am J Matern Child Nurs 28: 260–263.

Holditch-Davis D, Blackburn ST, Vandenberg K. (2003). Newborn and infant neurobehavioral development. In: Kenner C, Lott JW (eds).

Comprehensive neonatal nursing: a physiologic perspective (3rd edn), pp. 236–284. W. B. Saunders, Montreal.

Holsti L, Grunau RE, Oberlander TF, et al. (2005). Prior pain induces heightened motor responses during clustered care in preterm infants in the NICU. Early Hum Dev 81: 293–302.

Howard RF, Hatch DJ, Cole TJ, et al. (2001). Inflammatory pain and hypersensitivity are selectively reversed by epidural bupivacaine and are developmentally regulated. Anesthesiology 95: 421–427.

Howell D, Butler L, Vincent L, et al. (2000). Influencing nurses' knowledge, attitudes, and practice in cancer pain management. Cancer Nurs 23: 55–63.

Jacob E, Puntillo KA. (1999). A survey of nursing practice in the assessment and management of pain in children. J Pediatr Nurs 25: 278–286.

Johnson AN. (2001). Neonatal response to control of noise inside the incubator. Pediatr Nurs 27: 600–605.

Johnson EO, Kamilaris TC, Chrousos GP, et al. (1992). Mechanisms of stress: A dynamic overview of hormonal and behavioral homeostasis. Neurosci Biobehav Rev 16: 115–130.

Johnston CC, Stevens BJ. (1996). Experience in a neonatal intensive care unit affects pain response. Pediatrics 98: 925–930.

Johnston CC, Collinge JM, Henderson S, et al. (1997a). A cross sectional survey of pain and analgesia in Canadian neonatal intensive care units. Clin J Pain 13: 1–5.

Johnston CC, Stremler RL, Stevens BJ, et al. (1997b). Effectiveness of oral sucrose and simulated rocking on pain response in preterm neonates. Pain 72: 193–199.

Johnston CC, Stevens BJ, Franck LS, et al. (1999). Factors explaining lack of response to heel stick in preterm newborns. J Obstet Gynecol Neonatal Nurs 28: 587–594.

Johnston CC, Walker CD, Boyer K. (2002). Animal models of long-term consequences of early exposure to repetitive pain. Clin Perinatol 29: 395–414.

Johnston CC, Stevens B, Pinelli J, et al. (2003). Kangaroo care is effective in diminishing pain response in preterm neonates. Arch Pediatr Adolesc Med 157: 1084–1088.

Johnston CC, Gagnon A, Ritchie JA, et al. (2004). Coaching one-to-one for pain practices of pediatric nurses. Unpublished data.

Klaus MH, Klaus PH. (1998). Your amazing newborn. Perseus Books, Massachusetts.

Knaus W, Draper EA, Wagner DP, et al. (1986). An evaluation of outcome from intensive care in major medical centers. Ann Intern Med 104: 410–418.

Koehoorn M, Ratner PA, Shamian J. (2003). Feasibility of using existing Statistics Canada surveys to describe the health and work of nurses. Can J Nurs Leadersh 16: 94–106.

Krairiksh M, Anthony M. (2001). Benefits and outcomes of staff nurses participation in decisionmaking. J Nurs Adm 31:16–23.

Lee SK, Lee DS, Andrews WL, et al. and Canadian National Neonatal Network. (2003). Higher mortality rates among inborn infants admitted to neonatal intensive care units at night. J Pediatr 11: 592–596.

Lepelley D. (2002). Exploring the adaptability of leadership styles in senior business executives: Life narratives and self discovery of factors contributing to adaptability. Dissertation Abstracts International Section A. Humanities Social Sci 62(12A): 4245.

Levy-Shiff R, Hoffman MA, Mogilner S, et al. (1990). Fathers' hospital visits to their preterm infants as a predictor of father–infant relationship and infant development. Pediatrics 86: 289–293.

Lewis RJ, Janda H. (1998). The relationship between adult sexual adjustment and childhood experience regarding exposure to nudity, sleeping in the parental bed, and parental attitudes toward sexuality. Arch Sex Behav 17: 349–362.

Lotas MJ. (1992). Effects of light and sound in the neonatal intensive care unit environment on the low-birth-weight infant. NAACOG Clin Issues 3: 34–44.

Ludington-Hoe SM, Hashemi MS, Argote LA, et al. (1992). Selected physiologic measures and behavior during paternal skin contact with Colombian preterm infants. J Dev Physiol 18: 223–232.

Ludington-Hoe SM, Nguyen N, Swinth JY, et al. (2000). Kangaroo care compared to incubators in maintaining body warmth in preterm infants. Biol Res Nurs 2: 60–73.

Lund I, Yu LC, Uvnas-Moberg K, et al. (2002). Repeated massage-like stimulation induces long-term effects on nociception: contribution of oxytocinergic mechanisms. Eur J Neurosci 16: 330–338.

Lutes L. (1996). Bedding twins/multiples together. Neonatal Network 15: 61–62.

McGillis Hall L, Doran D. (2001). A study of the impact of nursing staff mix models and organizational change on patient, system and nurse outcomes. Online. Available: http://chsrf.ca/final_research/ogc/mcgillis_e.php.

McKenna JJ. (1997). Co-sleeping (bed sharing) among infants and toddlers. J Dev Behav Pediatr 18: 4089–4100.

McKenna J, Mosko S. (1994). Sleep and arousal, synchrony and independence among mothers and infants sleeping apart and together (same bed): An experiment in evolutionary medicine. Acta Paediatr Suppl 397: 94–102.

McLaughlin CR, Hull JG, Edwards WH, et al. (1993). Neonatal pain: a comprehensive survey of attitudes and practices. J Pain Symptom Manage 8: 7–16.

Melzack R. (1999). From the gate to the neuromatrix. [Review]. Pain Suppl 6: S121–126.

Melzack R, Wall PD. (1996). The challenge of pain, 2nd edn. Basic Books, Inc., New York.

Millar WJ, Wadhera S, Nimrod C. (1992). Multiple births: trends and patterns in Canada, 1974–1990. Health Report 4: 223–250.

Miller PA. (2001). Nurse–physician collaboration in an intensive care unit. Am J Crit Care 10: 341–350.

Montoya P, Larbig W, Braun C, et al. (2004). Influence of social support and emotional context on pain processing and magnetic brain responses in fibromyalgia. Arthritis Rheum 50: 4035–4044.

Mooncey S, Giannakoulopoulos X, Glover V, et al. (1997). The effect of mother–infant skin-to-skin contact on plasma cortisol and betaendorphin concentrations in preterm newborns. Infant Behav Develop 20: 553–557.

Narsinghani U, Anand KJS. (2000). Developmental neurobiology of pain in neonatal rats. Lab Anim 29: 27–39.

Nelson EE, Panksepp J. (1998). Brain substrates of infant-mother attachment: contributions of opioids, oxytocin, and norepinephrine. [Review]. Neurosci Biobehav Rev 22: 437–452.

Newman RB, Ellings JM. (1995). Antepartum management of the multiple gestation: the case for specialized care. Semin Perinatol 19: 387–403.

Nyquist KH, Lutes LM. (1998). Co-bedding twins: A developmentally supportive care strategy. J Obstet Gynecol Neonatal Nurs 27: 450–456.

O'Brien-Pallas L, Thomson D, Alksnis C, et al. (2001). The economic impact of nurse staffing decisions: Time to turn down another road? Hosp Q 4: 42–50.

O'Brien-Pallas L, Thomson D, McGillis Hall L, et al. (2004). Evidence-based standards for measuring nurse staffing and performance. Online. Available: http://www.chsrf.ca/final_research/ogc/o'brien_e.php.

Ors R, Ozek E, Baysoy G, et al. (1999). Comparison of sucrose and human milk on pain response in newborns. Eur J Pediatr 158: 63–66.

Panksepp J, Nelson E, Siviy S. (1994). Brain opioids and mother–infant social motivation. [Review]. Acta Paediatr Suppl 397: 40–46.

Perlman JM. (2001). Neurobehavioral deficits in premature graduates of intensive care: Potential medical and neonatal environmental risk factors. Pediatrics 108: 1339–1348.

Piira T, Sugiura T, Champion GD, et al. (2005). The role of parental presence in the context of children's medical procedures: A systematic review. Child Care Health Dev 31: 233–243.

Piira T, Hayes B, Goodenough B, et al. (2006). Effects of attentional direction, age, and coping style on cold-pressor pain in children. Behav Res Ther 44: 835–848.

Porter FL, Miller JP, Cole FS, et al. (1991). A controlled clinical trial of local anesthesia for lumbar punctures in newborns. Pediatrics 88: 663–669.

Porter RH, Winberg J. (1999). Unique salience of maternal breast odors for newborn infants. [Review]. Neuro Biobehav Rev 23: 439–449.

Prechtl HFR. (1974). The behavioral states of the newborn infant: a review. Brain Res 76: 185–212.

Reyes S. (2003). Nursing assessment of infant pain. J Perinat Neonatal Nurs 17: 291–303.

Sammons WAH, Lewis JM. (1985). Premature babies: A different beginning. Mosby, Toronto.

Scafidi FA, Field T, Schanberg SM. (1993). Factors that predict which preterm infants benefit most from massage therapy. J Dev Behav Pediatr 176–180.

Schmidt IK, Svarstad BL. (2002). Nurse–physician communication and quality of drug use in Swedish nursing homes. Soc Sci Med 54: 1767–1777.

Sherer DM, Nawrocki MN, Peco NE, et al. (1990). The occurrence of simultaneous fetal heart rate accelerations in twins during nonstress testing. Obstet Gynecol 76: 817–821.

Shiroiwa Y, Kamiya Y, Uchibori S, et al. (1986). Activity, cardiac and respiratory responses of blindfold preterm infants in a neonatal intensive care unit. Early Hum Dev 14: 259–265.

Stevens BJ, Johnston CC. (1994). Physiological responses of premature infants to a painful stimulus. Nurs Res 43: 226–231.

Stevens BJ, Johnston CC, Horton L. (1994). Factors that influence the behavioral pain responses of premature infants. Pain 59: 101–109.

Stevens B, Johnston C, Petryshen P, et al. (1996). Premature Infant Pain Profile: development and initial validation. Clin J Pain 12: 13–22.

Stevens BJ, Johnston C, Franck L, et al. (1999). The efficacy of developmentally sensitive interventions and sucrose for relieving procedural pain in very low birth weight neonates. Nurs Res 98: 35–43.

Stevens B, Gibbins S, Franck LS. (2000). Treatment of pain in the neonatal intensive care unit. Pediatr Clin North Am 47: 633–650.

St John W, Cameron C, McVeigh C. (2005). Meeting the challenge of new fatherhood during the early weeks. J Obstet Gynecol Neonatal Nurs 34: 180–189.

Sumner G, Spietz A. (1996). NCAST: caregiver/parent–child interaction teaching manual. NCAST Publications, University of Washington, School of Nursing, Seattle.

Taddio A, Katz J, Ilersich AL, et al. (1997). Effect of neonatal circumcision on pain response during subsequent routine vaccination. Lancet 349: 599–603.

Taddio A, Shah V, Gilbert-MacLeod C, et al. (2002). Conditioning and hyperalgesia in newborns exposed to repeated heel lances. JAMA 288: 857–861.

Tibby SM, Correa-West J, Durward A, et al. (2004). Adverse events in a pediatric intensive care unit: Relationship to workload, skill mix and staff supervision. Intensive Care Med 30: 1160–1166. Online. Available: http:// www.springerlink.com.

Tucker J. (2002). UK Neonatal Staffing Study Group. Patient volume, staffing, and workload in relation to risk adjusted outcomes in a random stratified sample of UK neonatal intensive care units: A prospective evaluation. Lancet 12: 99–107.

Upadhyay A, Aggarwal R, Narayan S, et al. (2004). Analgesic effect of expressed breast milk in procedural pain in term neonates: A randomized, placebo-controlled, double-blind trial. Acta Paediatr 93: 518–522.

Varendi H, Porter RH. (2001). Breast odour as the only maternal stimulus elicits crawling towards the odour source. Acta Paediatr 90: 372–375.

Varendi H, Porter RH, Winberg J. (1996). Attractiveness of amniotic fluid odor: evidence of prenatal olfactory learning? Acta Paediatr 85: 1223–1227.

Warren I. (2002). Facilitating infant adaptation: The nursery environment. Semin Neonatol 7: 459–467.

Whitelaw A, Sleath K. (1985). Myth of the marsupial mother: Home care of the very low birth weight babies in Bogota, Colombia. Lancet I: 1208.

White-Traut RC, Nelson MN, Burns K, et al. (1994). Environmental influences on the developing premature infant: Theoretical issues and applications to practice. J Obstet Gynecol Neonatal Nurs 23: 393–401.

Wilcox LS, Kiely JL, Melvin CL, et al. (1996). Assisted reproductive technologies: Estimates of their contribution to multiple births and newborn hospital days in the United States. Fertil Steril 5: 361–366.

Wild LR, Mitchell PH. (2000). Quality pain management outcomes: The power of place. Outcomes Manage Nurs Pract 4: 136.

Willson H. (2000). Factors affecting the administration of analgesia to patients following repair of fractured hip. J Adv Nurs 31: 1145–1154.

Wilson B, Laschinger H. (1994). Staff nurse perception of job empowerment and organizational commitment. J Nurs Adm 24: 39–47.

Yogman M, Kindlon D, Earls F. (1995). Father involvement and cognitive/ behavioral outcomes of preterm infants. J Am Acad Child Adolesc Psychiatry 34: 58–66.

Zahr LK, Balian S. (1995). Responses of premature infants to routine nursing interventions and noise in the NICU. Nurs Res 44: 179–185.

Zahr LK, de Traversay J. (1995). Premature infant responses to noise reduction by earmuffs: Effects on behavioral and physiologic measures. J Perinatol 15: 448–455.

13 Pain and the human fetus

Vivette Glover
Nicholas M Fisk

INTRODUCTION

The subject of fetal pain remains very controversial. This controversy exists, in part, due to our lack of knowledge; we still do not know when the fetus starts to feel pain or when it starts to become conscious (Glover and Fisk 1996). By conscious, we mean aware or sentient, not the more complex type of consciousness, such as consciousness of self, or thinking in words, which must develop much later. The subject is particularly difficult because the understanding of the physical basis of conscious awareness in the human adult is still limited. However, with an adult we can ask them what they feel and whether it hurts; with the fetus, as with animals, and indeed the neonate, we have to make an educated guess. There may not be a single moment when consciousness, or the potential to experience pain, is turned on; it may come on gradually like a dimmer switch (Greenfield 1995). It is also most unlikely that the pain in the fetus is the same as in the adult. For example, it is improbable that the fetus would be able to anticipate distress.

Current discussions emphasize that, for conscious experience in the human adult, there needs to be activity of a large network of neurons involving both the thalamus and the cerebral cortex (Crick 1994). Conscious experience is associated with the activation and inactivation of populations of neurons that are widely distributed in the thalamocortical system. The activity in the cortex may well be important for the specific content of a particular experience and lesions of specific cortical regions are closely linked to loss of specific aspects, such as colour perception. The driving force of the activations of the thalamic–cortical connections comes from lower in the brainstem, in the reticular activating system, which is located in the evolutionary older part of the brain (Edelman and Tononi 2000). Lesions in this system, but not in others, cause a loss of consciousness. However positron emission tomography (PET) scanning and other imaging studies have shown that every conscious task is associated with the activation or deactivation of large parts of the brain. Unconsciousness either in sleep or deep anaesthesia is associated with a profound depression of neural activity in both the thalamus and the cortex. Waking consciousness is associated with low-level irregular activity in the electroencephalogram (EEG) ranging from 12–70 Hz (Seth et al. 2005). However sufficient conditions for consciousness are hard to establish. Edelman and colleagues have discussed evidence for consciousness in different animal species and concluded that birds may well be conscious and it is even possible that the octopus is conscious (Edelman et al. 2005, Seth et al. 2005). Both birds and octopi have brains as different from an adult human as a mid-trimester fetus. Therefore, these arguments suggest that, for conscious experience, we cannot be sure that it is necessary to have a functional cerebral cortex similar to that in the human adult.

For the fetus to feel pain, there must be functional connections between the peripheral nociceptive receptors and the sites in the brain necessary for conscious experience of pain. There is considerable evidence, from PET scan studies in adults, that when pain is experienced as unpleasant, there is activation of a thalamic pathway which projects to areas of the cortex including the anterior insula, the anterior cingulate and the prefrontal cortex (Apkarian et al. 2005, Fink 2005, Kulkarni et al. 2005, Lorenz and Casey 2005). When these pathways are functional it is likely that the fetus or baby will feel pain. At earlier stages, we have to make an informed guess.

We can suggest the type of evidence that may give us a better understanding of whether and when the fetus may start to feel pain. We need to know when potentially relevant pathways in the brain become established anatomically, and when they become functional in the human fetus. We can obtain some clues from studies in animals, but cannot be sure how applicable they are to the human situation, as fetal development occurs at different rates in different species. We can also examine hormonal and physiological responses, and use other evidence such as the development of different patterns of behaviour in the human fetus. These aspects are discussed below and in more detail in Chapter 2.

DEVELOPMENT OF FETAL NERVOUS SYSTEM

The nervous system of the human fetus develops gradually throughout gestation, with the anatomical pathways and synapses forming first in the periphery and spinal cord and then moving upwards into the brain. In the brain the lower structures are connected first and then anatomical pathways are formed towards the thalamus, the subplate zone (a region specific to the fetus which lies underneath the cortex) and finally the cerebral cortex (Fig. 13.1).

The first essential requirement for nociception is the presence of sensory receptors, which start to develop in the perioral area at around 7 weeks gestational age (GA) (Fitzgerald 1994) (Table 13.1). (Gestational ages are given as postmenstrual.) Sensory receptors then

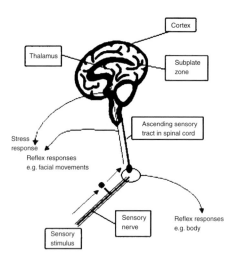

Figure 13.1 Fetal sensory pathways

develop in the rest of the face, and in the palmar surfaces of the hands and soles of the feet from 11 weeks. By 20 weeks GA, they are present throughout the skin and mucosal surfaces. In the first trimester stimulation of sensory receptors can result in local reflex movements involving the spinal cord but not the brain. Thus the fact that a fetus of 12 weeks will move away if touched is most unlikely to be associated with any conscious experience. As neurodevelopment continues these reflex pathways connect with the brainstem, and sensory stimulation can cause other responses such as increases in heart rate and blood pressure.

Development of the brain and spinal cord begins when the neural tube forms from neuroectoderm. Neural crest cells migrate out laterally to form peripheral nerves from 4 weeks, with the first synapses between them forming a week later (Okado et al. 1979). Synapses within the spinal cord develop from 8 weeks GA (Konstantinidou et al. 1995). In general, motor synapses develop before the equivalent sensory ones; the first spinal reflexes are present from 8 weeks. Between 8 and 18 weeks GA is the time of maximal neuronal development in the brain, with approximately 200 000 new neurons laid down every minute (Rabinowicz et al. 1996). The first neurons develop in the ventricular zone (an epithelial layer) along with glia. These glia adopt a radial arrangement, along which the newly formed neurons migrate out in waves to form the neocortex. Neurons are first laid out in the deeper layers and then in the superficial layers. After neural proliferation, synaptogenesis occurs, first in peripheral structures and then more centrally. From around 20 weeks GA, this process is at least partly dependent on sensory stimulation. Initially, many more neurons are laid down than are functionally

Table 13.1 Gestational ages at which fetal behaviours, sensory responses and stress responses appear

GA weeks	Movement or behaviour	Sensory responses	Stress responses
7	Just discernible movement		
8	Startle General movement	Moves if touched on lips	
9–10	Hiccup, isolated arm, leg or head movement, isolated head rotation		
10	Fetal breathing movements, arm twitch, leg twitch, hand–face contact, stretch, rotation of fetus		
11	Jaw movement, yawn		
12	Finger movement, sucking and swallowing	Moves if touched on face	
13	Clonic movement of arm or leg	Kinaesthetic response. The fetus's hand makes contact with its mouth, and the fetus may be observed sucking its thumb	
14	Rooting	Moves if touched on body	
16	Eye movements		Brain sparing redistribution of blood flow
18			Norepinephrine and endorphin response
20		Motor response to sound	Cortisol response
26		Motor response to external light stimulus	
28		Heart rate response to sound	

necessary. This leads to a large percentage of these redundant neurons undergoing apoptosis prior to birth, with estimates varying from 30 to 70% (Rabinowicz et al. 1996). During the second half of gestation, the folding of the cortex becomes much more complex and the brain increases considerably in weight.

The cerebral cortex starts to form at 10 weeks, although at this stage it is isolated from the rest of the brain (Marin-Padilla 1983). Cortical development involves the structural differentiation and maturation of cortical neurons, fibres, glia and blood vessels, and these processes start only at about 17 weeks GA with layers VI and V, but continue until long after birth. From 15 weeks GA, histological studies have shown that the cortex is underlain by the subplate zone (Kostovic and Judas 1998). Synapses appear within the cortical plate from mid-gestation. The subplate zone expands considerably between 17 and 20 weeks, while from about 17 weeks, there is a shifting

population of connections from the thalamus to this region (Kostovic and Rakic 1990, Kostovic et al. 1992, 1993, 2002, Kostovic and Judas 1998, Altman and Bayer 2002, Kostovic and Judas 2002). Thalamic fibres have been shown to penetrate the cortical plate from 24 to 28 weeks GA (Kostovic and Judas 2002).

Assuming that activity in the cerebral cortex or subplate zone is necessary for consciousness, then for the fetus to be conscious of an external stimulus, these regions need to be connected with incoming nervous activity. Most incoming pathways, including nociceptive ones, are routed through the thalamus and, as stated above, start to penetrate the subplate zone from about 17 weeks GA. However no human studies have examined the development of thalamo-cortical circuits specifically associated with pain perception. It must also be emphasized that the few histological studies that have been carried out on the development of thalamocortical pathways in the human fetal brain are based on small numbers, with often only one fetal brain studied at a specific GA. Much more evidence will be needed to determine when the potentially relevant anatomical pathways become established.

Based on the current anatomical evidence, it seems probable that the necessary pathways for pain perception are present from 26 weeks GA, and may be present in rudimentary form from 20 weeks GA. Before 17 weeks GA, the required pathways do not appear to be present.

It is possible that the older fetus actually perceives pain as being more severe than in the adult. Descending inhibition is the process whereby the sensation of pain transmitted in the ascending spinal neurons is dampened via inhibitory descending serotonin neurons in the dorsal horn of the spinal cord. In the rat, descending inhibition has been found not to be functionally effective until the tenth postnatal day (Fitzgerald and Koltzenburg 1986), corresponding in neurological maturity to 27–28 weeks of human gestation.

DEVELOPMENT OF FUNCTIONAL ACTIVITY IN THE FETAL BRAIN

Physiological evidence concerning the function of these pathways is even more limited than their anatomical development. There is evidence for a primitive EEG from 19 to 20 weeks. Sustained EEGs are obtainable from preterm infants of 23 weeks gestation. Studies of evoked responses in preterm infants show that both visual and somatosensory potentials can be elicited from 24 weeks and are well developed by 27 weeks (Klimach and Cook 1988). Clinical observations with preterm babies suggest that the nociceptive system is functional at 24–26 weeks. The flexor reflex, a measure of nociceptive function in the central nervous system, also is present in preterm infants tested from 26 weeks (Fitzgerald 1993). Thus the nociceptive system does appear to be active by 24–26 weeks, but when exactly it starts to function prior to this is not known.

Fetal responses to stress

Human fetal endocrine responses to stress have been demonstrated from 18 weeks gestation. Our group first demonstrated increases in fetal plasma concentrations of cortisol and β-endorphin in response to needling of the intrahepatic vein (IHV) for intra-uterine transfusion (Giannakoulopoulos et al. 1994). The magnitude of these stress responses correlated with the duration of the procedure. The median increase was 590% in cortisol and 183% in β-endorphin. Fetuses receiving the same procedure of transfusion,

but via the non-innervated placental cord insertion, failed to show these hormonal responses. In a larger series, our group confirmed this rise in β-endorphin during intrahepatic transfusion, and showed that it occurred from at least 18 weeks gestation onwards independent of both gestation and the maternal response (Gitau et al. 2001a). The fetal cortisol response, again independent of the mother's, was observed from 20 weeks gestation, but increased with gestational age. A similar but faster response is seen in fetal plasma norepinephrine levels to IHV needling. This, too, is observed in fetuses from at least 18 weeks, and is independent of the maternal response (Giannakoulopoulos et al. 1999).

Adults respond to the stress of cold, hypoxia or significant haemorrhage by a sympathetically controlled redistribution of blood flow to maximize blood flow to the body's more vital organs, the brain, the heart and the adrenal glands, at the expense of the peripheral circulation. These changes have been demonstrated in the fetus in animal studies, in response to reduced uterine blood flow, hypoxaemia and haemorrhage. Using Doppler ultrasound, human fetal studies have confirmed similar circulatory changes in response to the chronic stress of growth restriction, whereas studies of the response to acute stress are limited to the investigation of fetuses undergoing clinically indicated invasive procedures as acute stressors. Human intrauterine needling studies that involve transgression of the fetal trunk have shown that brain sparing, as assessed by colour Doppler ultrasound, affects the human fetus from at least 16 weeks gestation, with a decrease in the pulsatility index of the middle cerebral artery, indicative of increased blood flow to the brain (Teixeira et al. 1999) and an increase in pulsatility index of the femoral artery (Smith et al. 2003). Thus, from these studies, one can conclude that (a) the human blood flow redistribution response to an invasive stimulus is functional from at least 16 weeks GA, (b) the hypothalamic–pituitary–adrenal axis is functionally mature enough to produce a β-endorphin response by 18 weeks GA, and a cortisol response from 20 weeks gestation, and (c) the sympathetic system with the release of norepinephrine is functional from at least 18 weeks GA.

Stress responses and blood flow redistribution do not show that the fetus is feeling pain. Production and release of stress hormones such as cortisol can be mediated by the hypothalamus, without involvement of the cortex or other higher brain regions involved in sentience. Although stress hormones are increased when an individual suffers pain, many other situations that are not painful, such as exercise, also increase levels. However, if the stress hormone levels did not rise, it would be less likely that the fetus was having pain. Stress responses may also be used to give some sort of index, though imperfect, of the degree of tissue injury caused, and thus can be used as surrogate markers to determine the effects of analgesia or anaesthesia.

Fetal behaviour and responses to sensory stimuli

The ontogeny of fetal nociception is informed by studies of the onset of fetal behaviour (Roodenburg et al. 1991) and fetal responses to sensory stimuli. These responses can be measured by stimulating the fetus in various ways and observing its behaviour by ultrasound or by measuring heart rate. The available evidence indicates that all the senses adults have are, to some degree, functional in the fetus, although they become detectable at different stages of fetal life.

Touch is the first sense of the fetus to develop. At 8 weeks gestation, the fetus moves if touched on the lips (Hooker 1952). Tactile sensitivity then spreads to the cheeks, the forehead and the palms, followed by the upper arms. By 14 weeks gestation, most of the body, excluding the back and top of the head, is responsive to touch. The fetus receives tactile stimulation from contact with the walls of the uterus. It might also stimulate itself; for example, the fetus touches its own face from about 13 weeks gestation (de Vries et al. 1985).

The fetal response to sound is the most studied of its sensory modalities, because of the relative ease with which auditory stimuli can be presented to the fetus (Lecanuet et al. 2000). In the normal course of pregnancy, sound from the mother's internal organs, such as her heart beat and borborygmi (rumbling sounds heard in the uterus), and from the external environment, such as voices and music, form a natural part of the fetus's environment. Experimental auditory stimuli elicit motor responses from 20–24 weeks gestation, and increases in heart rate from 28 weeks gestation. The fetus begins hearing in the low-frequency part (250 Hz, 500 Hz) of the adult hearing range (20–20 000 Hz) and its range of hearing extends as the fetus matures (Hepper and Shahidullah 1994). The response of the fetus is influenced by the type of sound presented, its frequency, intensity, duration and the fetus's behavioural state (Hepper and Shahidullah 1994, Kisilevsky et al. 2004). For example, louder intensities elicit a rapid startle response, whereas lower-intensity sounds may elicit an orienting reaction similar to that seen in the newborn. Towards the end of pregnancy the fetus is able to discriminate between speakers, languages and even individual speech sounds (Lecanuet et al. 1987).

From early gestation the fetus is immersed in an ever-changing environment of potential smells and tastes. Substances from the maternal diet are transmitted to the fetus through the maternal blood stream. In early pregnancy they can also diffuse into the amniotic fluid and be swallowed by the fetus. In animal models at least, there is good evidence that the fetus can both detect and remember chemosensory information across birth (Schaal and Orgeur 1992).

The sense of kinaesthesia refers to the position of the various parts of the body in relation to one another. It is the sense we use, for example, to direct our arm, hand and fingers to pick up a cup. From about 13 weeks gestation, the fetus's hand makes contact with its mouth, and the fetus may be observed sucking its thumb (Hepper et al. 1991).

In summary, with the exception of vision, all of the fetus's senses will be stimulated at least to some degree naturally during the course of pregnancy. Moreover, the fetus has the ability to detect these stimuli from as early as 8 weeks, in the case of touch, and 20 weeks in the case of sound. However these responses, especially those of movement to touch, can just involve a reflex arc through the spinal cord, and may not indicate anything about the involvement of higher centres.

FETAL SURGERY AND ANALGESIA

There are several intrauterine procedures where it may now be appropriate to consider pain relief or anaesthesia for the fetus (Myers et al. 2002). These include open surgery, ultrasound-guided and endoscopic therapeutic procedures and some terminations (Glover and Fisk 1996, 1999). A large number of invasive techniques for prenatal diagnosis and treatment of the fetus have been developed. Most of the simpler procedures involve needling the placenta, amniotic fluid or umbilical cord without piercing the fetus. However, fetal tissue biopsy, body cavity or cyst aspiration, and blood sampling from the intra-hepatic vein for prenatal diagnosis are clearly potentially painful. Longer procedures such as feto–amniotic shunt insertion for bladder obstruction or hydrothoraces, cardiac balloon valvotomy for outlet valve obstruction (Tulzer et al. 2002) and fetal blood transfusion are now regularly performed in the second and third trimesters. Open fetal surgical techniques to repair major anomalies such as cystic adenomatoid malformation and sacrococcygeal teratoma are also occasionally used (Harrison et al. 1993). Open proce-dures involve fetal thoracotomy, abdominal incisions and resections, and such proce-dures are certainly potentially painful. The main indication for open surgery, diaphragmatic hernia, is now more usually approached endoscopically, but will still involve laryngoscopy and intratracheal deposition of a fetal balloon (McNiece and Dierdorf 2004). Other endoscopic procedures, such as fetal cystoscopy, involve fetal puncture, and considerable manipulation (Welsh et al. 2003) and are thus presumably similarly painful.

The subject of anaesthesia for fetal surgery has been reviewed by Myers and her co-workers (Myers et al. 2002, Myers 2005), and will not be discussed in detail here. The anaesthetist has to consider maternal, uteroplacental and fetal factors. Giving analgesia directly to the fetus without open surgery poses a considerable challenge. A variety of fetal routes can be used; intra-amniotic, intramuscular or intravenous. Each involves an additional invasive procedure with the small risk of fetal loss or delivery. Transplacental administration via the mother may be appropriate in some cases, although general anaesthesia is increasingly avoided in modern obstetric practice; it is also necessary to show that a dose which is safe and effective for the mother, is also effective for the fetus. It has been demonstrated by cord sampling, at the time of caesarean section, that on average under 50% of a maternal dose of fentanyl reaches the fetus, and that there is considerable individual variation (Desprats et al. 1991). Uptake of inhaled anaesthetics occurs more slowly in the fetus than the mother (Myers et al. 2002).

There has been little research addressing the delivery and efficacy of analgesia and anaesthesia in the human fetus. In infancy, opioids have been widely used for analgesia, for both minor and major procedures. They have been shown to reduce stress responses and postoperative mortality and morbidity. Fentanyl (a selective μ receptor agonist) is often used in preterm neonates; doses of 3 μg/kg, administered at the start of minor surgical procedures, appear to be effective in reducing postoperative pain without causing respiratory depression (Attia et al. 1986). Doses of 10 μg/kg of fentanyl provide anaesthesia and ablate operative stress responses (Anand et al. 1987). For analgesia to be effective, it is essential that the necessary receptors are present. The fact that there are abundant μ opioid receptors in the fetal brain and spinal cord from as early as 20 weeks gestation (Magnan and Tiberi 1989, Ray and Wadhwa 1999) makes opioids a good option for fetal analgesia. Clearance is predominantly by hepatic metabolism. In general the half-life of drugs administered intravascularly to the fetus is shorter than when the same drug is used in the neonate. This shorter half-life probably reflects placental binding and metabolism, the increased volume of distribution provided by the placental circulation together with

transplacental transfer into the maternal circulation. The usual practice, therefore, is to administer larger doses per kilogram of estimated fetal weight, typically by an empiric 25%, than would be used in the preterm neonate.

Our research group has investigated the use of fentanyl for pain relief in the fetus. We recruited women undergoing clinically indicated intrauterine transfusions between 20 and 35 weeks. Before commencing transfusion through the intrahepatic vein, a bolus of fentanyl was administered directly to the fetus. The effect of fentanyl on fetal plasma levels of cortisol and β-endorphin after transfusion, as well as on the middle cerebral artery pulsatility index, were determined. A pilot experiment showed that a bolus of 3 μg/kg had little effect. However a bolus of 10 μg/kg significantly reduced the increase in β-endorphin, and prevented any change in the pulsatility index. There was a 50% reduction in cortisol levels also, but this did not achieve statistical significance (Fisk et al. 2001). This study provided the first evidence that direct fetal analgesia reduces stress responses to invasive procedures in utero. However, much research is still needed. Higher doses of fentanyl may be more effective, but need to be used with caution. Fetuses may manifest cardiovascular response to analgesic drugs; our group recently demonstrated that the late-gestation ovine fetus shows changes in fetal heart rate and carotid blood flow with decreased pH and PO_2 after high-dose intravenous fentanyl administration (Smith et al. 2004). Sedgwick et al. have recently confirmed this finding in sheep and also suggest that caution is needed with higher-dose fentanyl (100–500 μg/g) until further studies are conducted (Sedgwick et al. 2005).

Late therapeutic abortion is also an intervention for which it is appropriate to consider the reduction of potential fetal pain, if conducted after 20 weeks and if surgical dismemberment is involved. In Britain, most surgical terminations take place under general anaesthesia, which is believed to affect the fetus, though evidence for this is sparse.

The experience of the baby during childbirth is a subject that is not widely considered. Assisted deliveries in particular can be very stressful for the infant, as shown by high cord cortisol levels (Gitau et al. 2001b).

Given that there is now general agreement that the nociceptive system is in place and functional by 40 weeks gestation, the huge extrinsic pressures from maternal tissues and expulsive forces, and the evidence of their direct effect on the fetus in terms of soft tissue and skull deformation at birth, the lack of consideration of the infant's presumably painful experience is quite puzzling. Some argue that it is unlikely that the baby feels pain because the childbirth procedure is a natural process. However the mother's experiences are also natural and can be very painful, and pain relief during labour is a major maternal issue.

LONG-TERM PROGRAMMING ISSUES

When considering the effects of pain on the developing fetus, and the possible benefits of analgesia, we must bear in mind not just the humanitarian need to alleviate the distress of pain from surgery or other interventions, but also whether being subjected to pain or stress during early development causes permanent alterations. This concept is known as programming, defined by Barker as 'the process whereby a stimulus or insult at a critical, sensitive period of development has permanent effects on structure, physiology and metabolism' (Barker 2000).

There is now a large literature documenting this phenomenon in response to perinatal stress. Animal studies, mainly in rats but also in monkeys, have shown that prenatal stress can cause long-term changes in the hypothalamic–pituitary–adrenal axis. These changes include permanent reductions in the numbers of hippocampal glucocorticoid receptors in the offspring of antenatally stressed animals (Henry et al. 1994). This attenuates the negative feedback response, resulting in increased basal and stress-induced cortisol or corticosterone levels. In humans, it has been shown that children of mothers who have experienced prenatal stress or anxiety, have long-term behavioural changes, including attention deficit/hyperactivity disorder and increased anxiety (O'Connor et al. 2002, 2003). They also have raised cortisol levels (O'Connor et al. 2005).

In rats, specific programming attributed to early pain has been demonstrated. Injection of the irritant Freund's adjuvant into a paw on the first postnatal day causes permanent increases in density and excitability in the ipsilateral afferent nerves from that region that persist into adulthood (Ruda et al. 2000). This phenomenon was not observed if the injection of irritant was delayed until day 14 postnatally. Neonatally, skin wounds were associated with increased sprouting of local sensory nerves, resulting in a permanent area of hyperinnervation, with skin innervation density in the wound area increasing threefold. This effect was greatest if done on the first neonatal day and decreased with age (Reynolds and Fitzgerald 1995). Human babies are born at a later stage of neurological development than the rat, so that neonatal rats are in some ways developmentally analogous to the late-gestation human fetus.

Data in humans concerning the long-term effects of perinatal pain are comparatively sparse. Taddio and colleagues demonstrated that boys circumcised in the first 4–5 days of the neonatal period had higher behavioural scores and cried longer in response to their vaccination injection at 4–6 months of age. This response was partially attenuated with the use of local anaesthetic cream at the time of circumcision (Taddio et al. 1995, 1997). Our own studies have demonstrated a significant correlation between stress at the time of birth, shown by infant cord blood cortisol levels, and the cortisol response to vaccination at 2 months (Taylor et al. 2000, Miller et al. 2005). A detailed discussion of the long-term consequences of pain in human neonates and animal models can be found in Chapters 4 and 5 respectively.

Jacobson and Bygdeman have suggested that the long-term effects of birth stress might last into adulthood. In a retrospective case control study of 242 Swedish adults who committed suicide, they found using multivariate analysis, that the risk of suicide by violent means was more than fourfold higher in men who had had a traumatic birth. If opiate analgesia had been administered at birth, presumably minimizing discomfort to both mother and baby, this may have reduced the relative risk (Jacobson and Bygdeman 1998). In a case sibling control study of opiate addicts, this group also found that maternal use of multiple opiate doses in labour was associated with opiate addiction of the offspring in later life (Jacobson et al. 1990). These studies raise the possibility of long-term sequelae from obstetric interventions, traumatic delivery and drugs administered during both pregnancy and labour. Robust studies are now needed to determine more about possible long-term effects of both early stress and pain, and the risk/benefit of drugs used to minimize these effects.

CONCLUSIONS

Lee et al. (2005) have recently stated that the capacity 'for conscious perception of pain can arise only after thalamocortical pathways begin to function, which may occur in the third trimester around 29–30 weeks' gestational age'. As discussed above, given the limitations of our current knowledge, this is unduly definite. Pain perception in the fetus may not use the same pathways as in the human adult, just as other species, such as the octopus, may not (Edelman et al. 2005). Many fetal structures are different from those in the adult, and may function in a different way. We do not know that, in the fetus, thalamocortical pathways are essential for any perception of pain; connections from the thalamus to the subplate zone may be sufficient. If Lee et al.'s reasoning were correct, it would imply that the majority of premature babies in intensive care do not feel pain either. This may be so, but is not consistent with clinical assessment or the judgements of most neonatal health professionals who prefer to treat their patients as though they do experience pain.

We suggest that the current evidence, although still limited, makes it quite likely that the fetus can feel pain from 26 weeks, and very unlikely before 17 weeks. It is possible that some sensory experience of pain may start by about 20 weeks.

The possibility of fetal pain should be considered in relation to fetal interventions, terminations in the second half of gestation, and possibly also for traumatic births. However, we still need to know much more about the most appropriate drugs to use, in what dose to use them, and how to deliver them. These issues are important, not only because of immediate suffering, but also because of increasing evidence for the long-term effects of early experience.

REFERENCES

Altman J, Bayer SA. (2002). Regional differences in the stratified transitional field and the honeycomb matrix of the developing human cerebral cortex. J Neurocytol 31: 613–632.

Anand KJS, Sippell WG, Aynsley-Green A. (1987). Randomised trial of fentanyl anesthesia in preterm babies undergoing surgery: effects on the stress response. Lancet 1: 62–66.

Apkarian AV, Bushnell MC, Treede RD, et al. (2005). Human brain mechanisms of pain perception and regulation in health and disease. Eur J Pain 9: 463–484.

Attia J, Ecoffey C, Sandouk P, et al. (1986). Epidural morphine in children: pharmacokinetics and CO_2 sensitivity. Anesthesiology 65: 590–594.

Barker DJ. (2000). In utero programming of cardiovascular disease. Theriogenology 53: 555–574.

Crick F. (1994). The astonishing hypothesis. Touchstone Books, Simon and Schuster Ltd, London.

de Vries JI, Visser GH, Prechtl HF. (1985). The emergence of fetal behavior. II. Quantitative aspects. Early Hum Dev 12: 99–120.

Desprats R, Dumas JC, Giroux M, et al. (1991). Maternal and umbilical cord concentrations of fentanyl after epidural analgesia for caesarean section. Eur J Obstet Gynecol Reprod Biol 42: 89–94.

Edelman DB, Baars BJ, Seth AK. (2005). Identifying hallmarks of consciousness in non-mammalian species. Conscious Cogn 14: 169–187.

Edelman GE, Tononi G. (2000). A universe of consciousness. Basic Books, New York.

Fink WA Jr. (2005). The pathophysiology of acute pain. Emerg Med Clin North Am 23: 277–284.

Fisk NM, Gitau R, Teixeira JM, et al. (2001). Effect of direct fetal opioid analgesia on fetal hormonal and hemodynamic stress response to intrauterine needling. Anesthesiology 95: 828–835.

Fitzgerald M. (1993). Development of pain pathways and mechanisms. In: Anand KJS, McGrath PJ (eds) Pain research and clinical management Vol 5. Pain in neonates, pp 19–38. Elsevier, New York.

Fitzgerald M. (1994). Neurobiology of fetal and neonatal pain. In Wall P, Melzack ER (eds) Textbook of pain. Churchill Livingstone, Edinburgh.

Fitzgerald M, Koltzenburg M. (1986). The functional development of descending inhibitory pathways in the dorsolateral funiculus of the newborn rat spinal cord. Brain Res 389: 261–270.

Giannakoulopoulos X, Sepulveda W, Kourtis P, et al. (1994). Fetal plasma cortisol and b-endorphin response to intrauterine needling. Lancet 344: 77–81.

Giannakoulopoulos X, Teixeira J, Fisk N, et al. (1999). Human fetal and maternal noradrenaline responses to invasive procedures. Pediatr Res 45: 494–499.

Gitau R, Fisk NM, Teixeira JM, et al. (2001a). Fetal hypothalamic-pituitary-adrenal stress responses to invasive procedures are independent of maternal responses. J Clin Endocrinol Metab 86: 104–109.

Gitau R, Menson E, Pickles V, et al. (2001b). Umbilical cortisol levels as an indicator of the fetal stress response to assisted vaginal delivery. Eur J Obstet Gynecol Reprod Biol 98: 14–17.

Glover V, Fisk N. (1996). Do fetuses feel pain? We don't know; better to err on the safe side from mid-gestation. BMJ 313: 796.

Glover V, Fisk N. (1999). Fetal pain: implications for research and practice. Br J Obstet Gynaecol 106: 881–886.

Greenfield SA. (1995). Journeys to the centres of the mind. Towards a science of consciousness. W.H.Freeman and Company. New York.

Harrison MR, Adzick NS, Flake AW, et al. (1993). Correction of congenital diaphragmatic hernia in utero: VI. Hard-earned lessons. J Pediatr Surg 28: 1411–1417; discussion 1417–1418.

Henry C, Kabbaj M, Simon H, et al. (1994). Prenatal stress increases the hypothalamo-pituitary-adrenal axis response in young and adult rats. J Neuroendocrinol 6: 341–345.

Hepper PG, Shahidullah BS. (1994). Development of fetal hearing. Arch Dis Child 71: F81–87.

Hepper PG, Shahidullah S, White R. (1991). Handedness in the human fetus. Neuropsychologia 29: 1107–1111.

Hooker D. (1952). The prenatal origin of behavior. University of Kansas Press, Kansas.

Jacobson B, Bygdeman M. (1998). Obstetric care and proneness of offspring to suicide as adults: case-control study. BMJ 317: 1346–1349.

Jacobson B, Nyberg K, Gronbladh L, et al. (1990). Opiate addiction in adult offspring through possible imprinting after obstetric treatment. BMJ 301: 1067–1070.

Kisilevsky S, Hains SM, Jacquet AY, et al. (2004). Maturation of fetal responses to music. Dev Sci 7: 550–559.

Klimach VJ, Cook RWI. (1988). Maturation of the neonatal somatosensory evoked response in preterm infants. Develop Med Child Neurol 30: 208–214.

Konstantinidou AD, Silos-Santiago I, Flaris N, et al. (1995). Development of the primary afferent projection in human spinal cord. J Comp Neurol 354: 11–12.

Kostovic I, Judas M. (1998). Transient patterns of organization of the human fetal brain. Croat Med J 39: 107–114.

Kostovic I, Judas M. (2002). Correlation between the sequential ingrowth of afferents and transient patterns of cortical lamination in preterm infants. Anat Rec 267: 1–6.

Kostovic I, Rakic P. (1990). Developmental history of the transient subplate zone in the visual and somatosensory cortex of the macaque monkey and human brain. J Comp Neurol 297: 441–470.

Kostovic I, Knezevic S, Wisniewski HM, et al. (1992). Neurodevelopment, aging and cognition. Birkhauser, Boston.

Kostovic I, Petanjek Z, Judas M. (1993). Early areal differentiation of the human cerebral cortex: entorhinal area. Hippocampus 3: 447–458.

Kostovic I, Judas M, Rados M, et al. (2002). Laminar organization of the human fetal cerebrum revealed by histochemical markers and magnetic resonance imaging. Cereb Cortex 12: 536–544.

Kulkarni B, Bentley DE, Elliott R, et al. (2005). Attention to pain localization and unpleasantness discriminates the functions of the medial and lateral pain systems. Eur J Neurosci 21: 3133–3142.

Lecanuet JP, Granier-Deferre C, DeCasper AJ, et al. (1987). [Fetal perception and discrimination of speech stimuli; demonstration by cardiac reactivity; preliminary results]. C R Acad Sci III 305: 161–164.

Lecanuet JP, Graniere-Deferre C, Jacquet AY, et al. (2000). Fetal discrimination of low-pitched musical notes. Dev Psychobiol 36: 29–39.

Lee SJ, Ralston HJP, Drey EA, et al. (2005). Fetal pain. A systematic multidisciplinary review of the evidence. JAMA 294: 947–954.

Lorenz J, Casey KL. (2005). Imaging of acute versus pathological pain in humans. Eur J Pain 9: 163–165.

Magnan J, Tiberi M. (1989). Evidence for the presence of mu- and kappa- but not of delta-opioid sites in the human fetal brain. Brain Res Dev Brain Res 45: 275–281.

Marin-Padilla M. (1983). Structural organisation of the human cerebral cortex prior to the appearance of the cortical plate. Anat Embryol 168: 21–40.

McNiece WL, Dierdorf SF. (2004). The pediatric airway. Semin Pediatr Surg 13: 152–165.

Miller NM, Fisk NM, Modi N, et al. (2005). Stress responses at birth: determinants of cord arterial cortisol and links with cortisol response in infancy. BJOG 112: 921–926.

Myers L. (2005). Anesthesia for fetal intervention and surgery: BC Decker Inc., New York.

Myers LB, Cohen D, Galinkin J, et al. (2002). Anesthesia for fetal surgery. Paediatr Anesth 12: 569–578.

O'Connor TG, Heron J, Golding J, et al. (2002). Maternal antenatal anxiety and children's behavioral/emotional problems at 4 years. Report from the Avon Longitudinal Study of Parents and Children. Br J Psychiatry 180: 502–508.

O'Connor TG, Heron J, Golding J, et al. (2003). Maternal antenatal anxiety and behavioral/emotional problems in children: a test of a programming hypothesis. J Child Psychol Psychiatry 44: 1025–1036.

O'Connor TG, Ben-Shlomo Y, Heron J, et al. (2005). Prenatal anxiety predicts individual differences in cortisol in pre-adolescent children. Biol Psychiatry 58: 211–217.

Okado N, Kakimi S, Kojima T. (1979). Synaptogenesis in the cervical cord of the human embryo: sequence of synapse formation in a spinal reflex pathway. J Comp Neurol 184: 491–518.

Rabinowicz T, de Courten-Myers GM, Petetot JM, et al. (1996). Human cortex development: estimates of neuronal numbers indicate major loss late during gestation. J Neuropathol Exp Neurol 55: 320–328.

Ray SB, Wadhwa S. (1999). Mu opioid receptors in developing human spinal cord. J Anat 195: 11–18.

Reynolds ML, Fitzgerald M. (1995). Long-term sensory hyperinnervation following neonatal skin wounds. J Comp Neurol 358: 487–498.

Roodenburg PJ, Wladimiroff JW, van Es A, et al. (1991). Classification and quantitative aspects of fetal movements during the second half of normal pregnancy. Early Hum Dev 25: 19–35.

Ruda MA, Ling QD, Hohmann AG, et al. (2000). Altered nociceptive neuronal circuits after neonatal peripheral inflammation. Science 289: 628–631.

Schaal B, Orgeur P. (1992). Olfaction in utero: can the rodent model be generalized? Q J Exp Psychol B 44: 245–278.

Sedgwick JA, Schenbeck JL, Eghtesady P. (2005). Harmful effects of fentanyl on the fetus and placenta? Am J Obstet Gynecol 193: 303–304; author reply 304.

Seth AK, Baars BJ, Edelman DB. (2005). Criteria for consciousness in humans and other mammals. Conscious Cogn 14: 119–139.

Smith RP, Glover V, Fisk NM. (2003). Acute increase in femoral artery resistance in response to direct physical stimuli in the human fetus. BJOG 110: 916–921.

Smith RP, Miller SL, Igosheva N, et al. (2004). Cardiovascular and endocrine responses to cutaneous electrical stimulation after fentanyl in the ovine fetus. Am J Obstet Gynecol 190: 836–842.

Taddio A, Goldbach M, Ipp M, et al. (1995). Effect of neonatal circumcision on pain responses during vaccination in boys. Lancet 345: 291–292.

Taddio A, Katz J, Ilersich AL, et al. (1997). Effect of neonatal circumcision on pain response during subsequent routine examination. Lancet 349: 599–603.

Taylor A, Fisk NM, Glover V. (2000). Mode of delivery and subsequent stress response. Lancet 355: 120.

Teixeira JM, Glover V, Fisk NM. (1999). Acute cerebral redistribution in response to invasive procedures in the human fetus. Am J Obstet Gynecol 181: 1018–1025.

Tulzer G, Arzt W, Franklin RC, et al. (2002). Fetal pulmonary valvuloplasty for critical pulmonary stenosis or atresia with intact septum. Lancet 360: 1567–1568.

Welsh A, Agarwal S, Kumar S, et al. (2003). Fetal cystoscopy in the management of fetal obstructive uropathy: experience in a single European centre. Prenat Diagn 23: 1033–1041.

Visceral pain in infancy

Elie D Al-Chaer
Paul E Hyman

OVERVIEW OF ABDOMINAL PAIN IN INFANCY

Abdominal pain falls into three categories: visceral pain, parietal pain and referred pain (Leung and Sigalet 2003). Visceral pain is caused by disorders of the stomach, kidney, gallbladder, urinary bladder, intestines, pancreas, spleen and liver. Such pain, often associated with nausea, is caused in hollow viscera by distension from obstruction by atresia, stenosis, tumour, ischaemia, inflammation or muscle spasm. In solid viscera, pain is caused by distension of the capsule from extramedullary haematopoiesis, venous congestion or tumour. Also, pain may be caused by traction on the mesentery. Pain and nausea result from activation of sensory afferent nerves. Because visceral pain fibres are bilateral and enter the spinal cord at multiple levels, visceral pain usually is dull, poorly localized, and felt in the midline. In the adult, severe abdominal pain can be associated with benign conditions such as gas or the cramping of viral gastroenteritis, while relatively mild pain (or no pain) may be present with severe and life-threatening conditions such as cancer of the colon or early appendicitis. In otherwise healthy people, solid organs are least sensitive, whereas the serosal membranes of hollow organs are most sensitive to acute pain (Giamberardino and Vecchiet 1995). On the other hand, mildly painful or even innocuous stimuli such as gas or passage of fecal material can be exquisitely painful (hyperalgesia/allodynia) when acting on inflamed or otherwise chronically affected tissue (e.g. irritable bowel syndrome).

Children under the age of seven are poor at localizing pain, and often are unable to discriminate between physical and emotional distress. Therefore a range of causes needs to be considered. Causes are age-related, e.g. necrotizing enterocolitis mostly occurs in preterm neonates, intussusception is most common between 4 and 24 months, but rare beyond that except in children with cystic fibrosis or polyps. Acute abdominal pain in children is frequently accompanied by vomiting, but this does not necessarily indicate obstruction or upper gastrointestinal pathology. Chronic abdominal pain may be caused by organic pathology or neuropathic origin.

Parietal pain arises from noxious stimulation of the parietal peritoneum caused by ischaemia, inflammation or stretching. Parietal pain usually is sharp, intense, discrete, and well localized, and coughing or movement can aggravate it. In the adult, this pain is transmitted through myelinated afferent fibres to specific dorsal root ganglia on the same side and at the same dermatomal level as the origin of the pain. In infants, these fibres may still be in the process of myelination.

Referred pain has many of the characteristics of parietal pain, but the originating stimulus may be a diseased visceral organ, and the pain is felt in remote areas supplied by the same dermatome as the diseased organ. It results from shared central pathways.

Age is a key factor in evaluating pain; the incidence and symptoms of different conditions vary over the paediatric age spectrum. This chapter provides a comprehensive basic and clinical overview of the mechanisms and approach to the evaluation of the neonate and infant with abdominal pain.

ANATOMY OF THE ENTERIC NERVOUS SYSTEM

Peripheral pathways

Knowledge of the innervation of the neonatal or paediatric viscera derives mostly from comparisons with the adult visceral innervation. Innervation of visceral organs consists of two types of neurons; intrinsic neurons (the enteric nervous system (ENS) proper) and extrinsic neurons with cell bodies outside the viscera. This chapter will focus on extrinsic primary afferents because they tend to be more involved in visceral sensory processing and relay to the central nervous system.

Unlike somatic tissue, the viscera are innervated by two sets of primary afferent fibres that project to distinct regions of the central nervous system (CNS). Innervation of the gastrointestinal (GI) tract from the oesophagus through the transverse colon is provided by vagal afferent fibres originating in the nodose ganglia and projecting centrally to the nucleus of the solitary tract. Pelvic nerve afferent fibres, originating in the sacral (human; lumbosacral in rat) dorsal root ganglia, innervate the remaining lower bowel and project centrally to the sacral spinal cord. The entire GI tract is also innervated by afferent fibres in the splanchnic nerves projecting to the T5–L2 segments of the spinal cord. For example, colonic afferent fibres project in both the pelvic and the splanchnic nerves (Berkley et al. 1993, Traub et al. 1999).

In contrast to somatic afferent fibres, visceral afferents have no end organs or morphological specialization. Endings of vagal and spinal sensory neurons terminate within the muscle, mucosal epithelia and ganglia of the ENS (Berthoud et al. 1995). Spinal afferents terminate also in the serosa and mesenteric attachments and form a dense network around mesenteric blood vessels and their intramural tributaries. Vagal afferent endings in the mucosa are in close association with the lamina propria, adjacent to the mucosal epithelium, where they monitor the chemical nature of luminal contents either following their passage across the epithelium or via input from epithelial enteroendocrine cells. Nutrients cross the epithelium to reach the afferent nerve terminals in the lamina propria. In addition, luminal nutrients release messenger molecules (e.g. cholecystokinin and 5-HT) from mucosal enteroendocrine cells. These molecules activate afferent terminals that lie in close proximity to the lamina propria (Kirkup et al. 2001).

Spinal afferents are subdivided into splanchnic and pelvic afferents. They follow the path of sympathetic and parasympathetic efferents that project to the gut wall. Somatic afferents that innervate the striated musculature of the pelvic floor project to the sacral spinal cord via the pudendal nerve. Axons of spinal afferents are almost exclusively thinly myelinated A-delta and unmyelinated C-fibres; they exhibit chemosensitivity, thermosensitivity and/or mechanosensitivity. There are two physiological classes of nociceptive viscerosensory receptors: (1) low-threshold afferents respond to physiological distension but continue to encode levels of distension that cause pain in humans or pain behaviour in animals; and (2) high-threshold afferents respond to noxious distension (Sengupta and Gebhart 1994). Experimental data suggest that the viscera also contain spinal nociceptive afferent fibres that are normally considered 'silent' and are sensitized by inflammation. Silent nociceptors do not respond at all in the normal intestine but become responsive to distension when the intestine is injured or inflamed (McMahon and Koltzenberg 1994). This receptor behaviour illustrates how mechanosensitivity is not fixed either in terms of the threshold for sensory activation or the relationship between stimulus and response. Injury and inflammation decrease the threshold and increase the magnitude of the response for a given stimulus, a phenomenon known as peripheral sensitization (Cervero and Laird 2003). The distribution of these fibres also varies among organs. High-threshold receptors exclusively innervate organs from which pain is the only conscious sensation (i.e. ureter, kidney, lungs, heart), but are relatively few in organs that provide innocuous and noxious sensations (e.g. colon, stomach, bladder).

Spinal afferents have multiple receptive fields extending over a relatively wide area. Those in the serosa and mesenteric attachments respond to distortion of the viscera during distension and contraction. Other endings detect changes in the submucosal chemical milieu following injury, ischaemia or infection and may play a role in generating hypersensitivity. Intramural spinal afferent fibres have collateral branches that innervate blood vessels and enteric ganglia. These contain and release neurotransmitters during local axon reflexes that influence GI blood flow, motility and secretory reflexes (Maggi and Meli 1988). Spinal afferents en route to the spinal cord also give off collaterals that innervate prevertebral sympathetic ganglia neurons. The same sensory information is thereby transmitted to information-processing circuits in the spinal cord, ENS and prevertebral ganglia. The main transmitters are calcitonin gene-related peptide (CGRP) and substance P – both peptides that are implicated in the induction of neurogenic inflammation.

Sensory transduction depends upon the modulation of ion channels and/or receptors on the sensory nerve terminal (Kirkup et al. 2001). Mechanosensitivity may arise indirectly following the release of chemical mediators such as adenosine triphosphate (ATP) that, in turn, act on purinergic receptors located on afferent nerve terminals. Alternatively, there may be direct activation via mechanosensitive ion channels in these afferent nerve terminals. Mechanical deformation of the nerve ending opens or closes ion channels, depolarizing the terminal to threshold and causing action potential firing.

Peripheral sensitization

Sensitizing mediators are released by platelets, leukocytes, lymphocytes, macrophages, mast cells, glia, fibroblasts, blood vessels, muscle and epithelial cells and neurons. Several mediators can be released from a single cell to either act directly on the sensory nerve terminal or indirectly by stimulating the release of agents from other cells in a series of cascades.

Chemical mediators, including biogenic amines, purines, prostanoids, proteases and cytokines act on receptors expressed upon any one sensory ending (Bueno et al. 2000, Kirkup et al. 2001). Three processes are involved in the actions of these substances on visceral afferent nerves. First, the terminals are depolarized by direct activation of receptors coupled to the opening of ion channels present on nerve terminals, and impulses are initiated. Second, sensitization develops and results in hyperexcitability to both chemical and mechanical modalities. Sensitization may involve post-synaptic receptor signal transduction that includes G-protein coupled alterations in second messenger systems which in turn lead to phosphorylation of membrane receptors and ion channels that control excitability of the afferent endings. Third, ion channels and receptors expressed

by the afferent nerve could alter the sensitivity of the afferent terminals by genetic changes in the phenotype of mediators, for example a change in the ligand-binding characteristics or coupling efficiency of newly expressed receptors. Neurotrophins, in particular nerve growth factor (NGF) and glial-derived neurotropic factor (GDNF), influence different populations of visceral afferents and play an important role in adaptive responses to nerve injury and inflammation (McMahon 2004).

Peripheral sensitization can occur rapidly and be short-lived, because the changes taking place at sensory nerve terminals are dependent on release of one or more algesic mediators. However, in sustained tissue injury or inflammatory states, changes in gene expression prolong peripheral sensitization. These changes include alterations in genes that determine the amount and pattern of neurotransmitters released from the sensory nerve terminals in the spinal cord and the brain, thereby altering CNS processing of sensory information. Peripheral sensitization integrated with central sensitization is a factor determining nociception.

Central pathways

Upon entering the dorsal horn, visceral afferents terminate in spinal cord laminae I, II, V and X (Ness and Gebhart 1990). Visceral afferents constitute 10% of afferent inflow into the spinal cord. This is a relatively small number when considering the large surface area of some organs. Both anatomical and electrophysiological studies have demonstrated viscerosomatic convergence in both the dorsal horn and supraspinal centres (Ness and Gebhart 1990, Al-Chaer et al. 1996a, 1996b, 1997a, 1998). There is also evidence of viscerovisceral convergence onto these second-order neurons. Examples include the convergence of pelvic visceral inputs such as colon/rectum, bladder, uterine cervix and vagina (Ness and Gebhart 1990, Berkley et al. 1993). Along with the low density of visceral nociceptors and the functional divergence of visceral input within the central nervous system, viscerovisceral convergence in the spinal cord may explain poorly localized visceral pain.

Visceral information carried by the pelvic nerve converges onto spinal neurons in the lumbosacral segments of the cord and those carried by the splanchnic nerves on thoracolumbar segments (see Traub 2000). Centrally, ascending pathways involved in the transmission of visceral nociceptive information include the spinothalamic tract (STT), spinohypothalamic tract, spinosolitary tract, spinoreticular tract, spino-parabrachial tract and others (Al-Chaer et al. 1999). In addition, a number of recent studies have pointed to a possible role of the dorsal column (DC) in viscerosensory processing, opening the door for a new role of the DC in visceral pain (for reviews see Al-Chaer et al. 1998, Willis et al. 1999).

One difference between the DC and the STT is that the DC axons ascend ipsilaterally near the midline before converging onto the DC nuclei (nucleus gracilis and nucleus cuneatus). From there, internal arcuate fibres transmit nociceptive input to the contralateral ventroposterolateral (VPL) nucleus of the thalamus. Experimental data from different groups (Al-Chaer et al. 1996a, 1996b, 1998, 1999, Ness 2000) have identified the DC as being more important in visceral nociceptive transmission than the STT and spinoreticular tracts. In monkeys, colorectal distension stimulates the firing of viscero-sensitive VPL thalamic neurons. After a DC lesion at T10 level, the responses are reduced despite ongoing stimulation. A similar lesion of the STT at T10 does not achieve the same effect (Al-Chaer et al. 1998). The DC also has a role in signalling epigastric nociception (see Willis et al. 1999). The DC, however, is not simply a conduit of viscerosensory information onto supraspinal centres, but may also facilitate visceral input upon other sensory channels originating in the spinal cord and the rekindling of spinal neuronal sensitization of visceral origin. A lesion of the DC suppressed spinal neuronal responses to colorectal distension (CRD) and reduced spinal neuronal sensitization in Al-Chaer's model of chronic visceral pain (Saab et al. 2004). It remains to be determined whether similar pathways subserve visceral pain in infants.

Central sensitization

Central sensitization is the neural mechanism underlying secondary hyperalgesia – increased pain sensitivity in regions distant to the site of injury or inflammation. Central sensitization arises because altered transmitter mechanisms in the spinal cord lead to decreased threshold, increased responsiveness and an expansion of spinal neuronal receptive fields (Al-Chaer et al. 1997b). Central sensitization could contribute to visceral hypersensitivity in functional or idiopathic visceral disorders. Changes in synaptic transmission may persist beyond the initial injury or inflammation (Al-Chaer et al. 2000, Ma et al. 2002). Non-methyl-D-aspartate (NMDA) receptors and neurokinin receptors mediate visceral pain. Transient distension of the ureter evokes a pressor response that is inhibited by NMDA receptor antagonists (Olivar and Laird 1999). Likewise, NMDA receptor antagonists attenuate primary afferent (McRoberts et al. 2001) and spinal neuron responses to acute noxious and innocuous colorectal stimuli (Zhai and Traub 1999, Ji and Traub 2001). The contribution of NMDA receptors to the signalling of innocuous colonic stimuli leads to speculation that excessive activity at these receptors in the absence of inflammation could produce central sensitization leading to visceral hyperalgesia (Ji and Traub 2001). NK-1 receptors and NK-3 receptors partially mediate spinal responses to colonic distension. However, the particular receptor involved in the signal transduction depends upon the mechanism for producing inflammation. NK-1 receptors signal neurogenic inflammation but not non-neurogenic inflammation (Laird et al. 2000). Likewise, a different mediator works through NK-3 and/or NMDA receptors (Coutinho et al. 1996, Kamp et al. 2001). Because most visceral afferents contain substance P, the natural ligand at the NK-1 receptor, a role for NK-1 receptors would be expected (Kawasaki et al. 2000).

For a detailed discussion of supraspinal processing of pain, see Chapter 3.

DEVELOPMENTAL CHANGES IN VISCERAL AFFERENT SIGNALLING

Sensory neurons go through a number of processes during development that include programmed cell death and functional differentiation. Excess neurons are generated during development of the vertebrate peripheral nervous system (PNS), and numbers are reduced to the required complement during a phase of programmed cell death that occurs shortly after the neurons innervate their targets. For most neurons in the PNS, this process is regulated by members of the neurotrophin family of growth factors that includes NGF, brain-derived neurotrophic factor (BDNF), neurotrophin 3 (NT3) and neurotrophin 4 (NT4) (Hohn et al. 1990, Maisonpierre et al. 1990, Rosenthal et al. 1990, Huang and Reichardt 2001, Kirstein and Farinas 2002). The mechanisms by which PNS neurons begin their differentiation are to a certain extent dependent upon the organs they innervate. However, within the first hours of extrauterine life, there are many rapid physiologic changes that take place and explain how a few hours and a few meals may, for example, alter gastric neuromuscular function. One possible factor is the surge and ebb of stress hormones during and after delivery. Accommodation to luminal distension may be diminished in the first hours of life because of the dominance of sympathetic tone over parasympathetic tone (see Zangen et al. 2001).

VISCERAL PAIN IN NEONATES AND INFANTS

Understanding sensory processing in preverbal children presents a challenge to human neuroscience.

Consequently, pain in infants may be an under-recognized and undertreated symptom, including pain arising from recurrent or chronic conditions (Cummings et al. 1996, Porter and Anand 1998). This under-recognition and undertreatment of pain is a problem because the incidence of chronic conditions is high, and visceral involvement makes them more life-threatening than those arising from somatic pain (Giamberardino 2000). In adults, visceral pain is often poorly localized and hard to quantify (Giamberardino 2000), so when it arises in infants, in whom quantification of pain is already difficult, it becomes particularly hard to define. In recent studies, measuring the abdominal skin reflex (ASR) was used to monitor the development of referred visceral hypersensitivity in infants diagnosed prenatally with unilateral hydronephrosis (Andrews et al. 2002).

Acute visceral pain

Causes
Acute visceral pain may be caused by stretching of the viscus, stretching of the peritoneum, or by tissue destruction and inflammation. For a list of causes by age, see Table 14.1.

Clinical presentation
The neonate or infant with an acute abdomen appears distressed: crying, grimacing, knees to chest, breathing rapidly, twisting from side to side. Touching the abdomen causes increasing distress, and attempts to withdraw. There may be vomiting, retching or diarrhoea. The abdomen may be distended and firm. Heart rate, respirations and pulse pressure are increased.

Chronic abdominal pain

Causes
Chronic abdominal pain in infants may be organic, functional or developmental in origin. Presentation, particularly with non-organic pain, is more frequent in children 5 years and over. Under that age the pain is more likely to have an organic basis. For a list of causes by age, see Table 14.2.

Clinical presentation
The clinical presentation of chronic abdominal pain varies with the condition causing the pain. The most common cause for chronic abdominal pain in infancy is functional constipation.

Functional constipation Functional constipation occurs in otherwise well infants at the time of weaning from breast milk to infant formula. Stools become firm with the transition to formula. If a child experiences pain in the anal sphincter while passing a large hard bowel movement, the child becomes conditioned to avoid defecation. The anticipation of pain with defecation causes infants to contract the pelvic floor, and stool does not pass. High-amplitude propagating colonic contractions (HAPCs) move colon contents from the proximal colon to the rectum over a minute or two after each meal in infants (Di Lorenzo

Table 14.1 Common causes of acute visceral pain

Infant	Toddler	Older
Bowel obstruction	Intussusception	In addition to the causes for infants and toddlers:
Sepsis and peritonitis	Gastroenteritis	Ovarian pathology
Gastroenteritis	Appendicitis	Pregnancy complication
Acute intervertebral discitis	Bowel perforation	Acute ulcerative colitis
	Intestinal perforation	Crohn's disease
	Renal pathology	Typhlitis
	Abdominal mass	Sickling crisis
	Mesenteric adenitis	
	Perforated Meckel's diverticulum	
	Inflammatory bowel disease	
	Haemolytic uraemic syndrome	
	Henoch–Schonlein purpura	
	Acute spinal infection	

Source: Medcyclopedia™, Leung and Sigalet 2003.

Table 14.2 Common causes of recurrent abdominal pain in children

Infant	Toddler	Older
Constipation	Constipation	In addition to the causes for infants and toddlers:
Malabsorption syndrome	Malabsorption syndrome	Inflammatory bowel disease
Renal pathology: hydronephrosis, urinary tract anomalies	Cystic fibrosis	Gastro-oesophageal reflux, gastritis, gastric or duodenal ulcer
	Meckel's diverticulum	Ovarian pathology
	Transient intussusception	Recurrent appendicitis
	Mesenteric adenitis (usually recurrent pain)	Psychosomatic
	Postoperative, recurrent, or partial obstruction Renal pathology: pyelonephritis, urinary tract infection, cystitis, urinary calculi	Rare liver, gallbladder, pancreatic disease, worms and infestations, pseudo-obstruction, connective tissue diseases

Source: Medcyclopedia™.

et al. 1995). When a healthy child senses the start of an HAPC, the child relaxes the pelvic floor and increases intra-abdominal pressure, facilitating a bowel movement. In contrast, children with painful defecation or fear of defecation are unable to relax the pelvic floor. The HAPC pushes against an obstructed anal sphincter with pressures of 80 mmHg and more (Hamid et al. 1998), well above the threshold for rectal pain (Mertz et al. 1995).

Treatment for functional constipation includes: (1) education and effective reassurance for the family and (2) assuring painless defecation for the child. Most clinicians do not alter diet; diet changes alone are ineffective for assuring painless defecation. Most clinicians prescribe polyethylene glycol (PEG) every day, mixed in water or another transparent beverage (Youssef et al. 2002). PEG is an inert particle too large to cross the mucosa. It keeps water in the stool by osmotic force. PEG is titrated to a daily dose that makes stool the same consistency as oatmeal or applesauce. Milk of magnesia and mineral oil also assure painless defecation, but PEG is often the most palatable preparation.

Protein intolerance-associated enteritis and colitis Enteritis or colitis associated with protein intolerance occurs in about one in 50 neonates. It often presents with diarrhoea or constipation and failure-to-thrive. The inflammation secondary to an abnormal mucosal immune response alters intestinal motility and sensitizes pain receptors, causing pain to occur with normal luminal distension and wall contractions. The infant may refuse to eat, regurgitate or cry after meals. Crying due to pain from protein sensitivity may be distinguished from infant colic (intractable fussing without failure-to-thrive) by the 'Rule of Ones'. In infant colic, crying is the one and only symptom (see Chapter 7). In protein intolerance there are other symptoms and signs. Laboratory studies may show occult blood and white blood cells in the stool of infants with protein intolerance. Stool pH may be low, and there may be evidence of malabsorption when the small bowel is involved.

Treatment for protein intolerance requires removal of the offending antigen(s) from the diet. Paediatricians who care for patients with mild symptoms tend to switch from cow's milk to soy protein formula. However, there is a 30% chance that the infant with cow's milk intolerance may have sensitivity to soy milk. Paediatric gastroenterologists who care for patients with more severe symptoms order a predigested protein formula.

Dyspepsia Dyspepsia is defined as pain or other discomfort in the upper abdomen (Rasquin-Weber et al. 1999). Traditional definitions of dyspepsia include the caveat that the child must be capable of providing an accurate pain history. Apart from poor appetite or other transient conditions, however, there are only two reasons why infants refuse to eat: (1) it hurts to eat, and (2) they fear it will hurt to eat. Infants and toddlers with repeated perinatal visceral pain experiences suffer from oral aversion syndrome or food refusal that is likely due to dyspepsia. Other potential causes of chronic food refusal due to gastrointestinal pain include oesophagitis, diffuse oesophageal spasm and achalasia.

Infants with the highest incidence of feeding problems are those with chronic disease and developmental delay (Burklow et al. 1998). Preterm infants after prolonged endotracheal intubation, infants with bronchopulmonary dysplasia, or surgery to correct congenital cyanotic heart disease are frequently affected by dyspepsia or oral aversion syndrome. These children may regurgitate recently ingested food to relieve their discomfort, therefore, Nissen fundoplication may be performed in an attempt to avoid calorie loss and other complications of gastro-oesophageal reflux disease (GERD). After fundoplication they refuse to eat, sometimes retching when tube fed. Fundoplication may increase pain sensitivity in the gastric fundus by inducing hyperalgesia or by reducing receptive relaxation and the effective gastric volume.

Treatment for infants with dyspepsia varies in complexity, depending on the severity of the symptoms, growth and development of the child and wishes of the family.

Reducing the volume in each feeding may reduce intragastric pressure, but the number of feedings or caloric density must increase to provide enough calories for growth. Continuous drip feedings will distend the stomach less than bolus feedings. Continuous drip post-pyloric feedings distend the stomach least. Post-pyloric feeding for 6 weeks or more seems to improve symptoms of food refusal when oral feedings are reintroduced (Hyman, unpublished data).

For intractable conditions, medication for chronic neuropathic pain may be useful. Tricyclics (e.g. amitriptyline, imipramine) and anticonvulsants (e.g. gabapentin) can be used in children 6 months of age or older. If the child has sleep problems, amitriptyline, with its sedating properties, may be titrated up until the child and parents enjoy a restful night of sleep. If the child is constipated, imipramine may be preferable to amitriptyline. Doses for these two drugs are identical. The initial dose range is 0.2–0.3 mg/kg/day given an hour or two before bedtime. The dose is increased by 0.2–0.3 mg/kg/day weekly, until the desired endpoint is reached (e.g. increased voluntary oral intake or sleep through the night), up to a maximum dose of 1 mg/kg/day. The cardiac arrhythmias occasionally seen with 10–20-fold higher doses for depression are unlikely with these low doses. Although sleepiness is the rule, hyperactivity may occur with tricyclics in about one in 30 children. Gabapentin may be preferred in children with a history of seizures or those who get undesirable side effects from a tricyclic. Gabapentin may be added

to a tricyclic to achieve an additive response. An optimal dose is 50 mg twice daily for infants and 100 mg twice daily for toddlers (Hyman, unpublished data).

The histamine-1 and serotonin-1 receptor antagonist cyproheptidine improves appetite in about a third of these patients. Perhaps it works centrally or perhaps by enhancing gastric receptive relaxation to a meal. Cyproheptidine is safe but effective in only a minority of patients. Tolerance to the appetite-stimulating effect of cyproheptidine develops after 3–4 weeks.

Often, a multidisciplinary approach speeds recovery. It helps to avoid all unnecessary pain experiences and stressful situations. Immunizations may be delayed until the visceral hypervigilence subsides. Birthday parties at the end of the first year may be quiet affairs limited to a few familiar faces. Reassurance and routine reduces arousal. If the infant enjoys massage or music, those sensory experiences may reduce pain and hyperarousal.

Nausea Acute nausea in infants occurs most commonly during acute gastroenteritis. Infants turn pale, sweaty, look vacant and quiet, and may vomit or retch. Other causes of acute nausea include recovery from inhalant anaesthesia and cancer chemotherapy.

Chronic nausea may accompany emotional distress. Chronic nausea may be due to functional dyspepsia, and so may present in infancy as food refusal (Richards and Andrews 2004). Episodes of intense unremitting nausea accompanied by vomiting lasting hours to days with intervening baseline periods lasting weeks to months occur in the cyclic vomiting syndrome (Rasquin-Weber et al. 1999).

LONG-TERM EFFECTS OF NEONATAL PAIN EXPERIENCES

Emotional stress and traumatic events during childhood increase the risk of social (e.g. school failure, victimization, anti-social behaviour), neuropsychiatric (e.g. post-traumatic stress disorder, conduct disorders) and other medical problems (e.g. heart disease, gastrointestinal disorders and chronic pain symptoms) (Perry 1994, Graham et al. 1999).

Perinatal brain plasticity, while important for normal development and necessary for learning, may increase the vulnerability to early adverse experiences, thus leading to abnormal development and atypical behaviours. During the neonatal period, the developing nervous system is highly plastic, overproduction of synapses is widespread, and only used synapses are maintained. Neonatal 'use-dependence' affects the brain wiring of the maturing adult and its consequences are apparent in the somatosensory systems, where normal stimulation during an early sensitive period is required for normal neuronal development (Hughes and Carr 1978).

Early adverse experiences often contribute to adaptive or maladaptive functions of the nervous system, and possibly to the development of chronic pain disorders occurring in the absence of identifiable structural problems, hence the cognomen functional pains (e.g. fibromyalgia, functional abdominal pain, etc.). Models of early-life incidents, such as repetitive pain, inflammation, sepsis, or maternal separation in rodents and other species have noted multiple alterations in the adult brain, correlated with specific behavioural phenotypes depending on the timing and nature of the insult (see Chapter 5).

To study the effect of neonatal peripheral irritation on developmental structural and functional outcomes in adults, newborn rat pups were exposed to nociceptive or inflammatory visceral treatments and followed through adulthood. Exposing newborn rat pups to painful colorectal distension – a painful, reproducible experimental form of physical abuse – or to colon inflammation during pre-adolescence, caused long-term visceral and somatic hypersensitivity long after the initial injury had resolved (Al-Chaer et al. 2000). This hypersensitivity was associated with central and peripheral neural sensitization (Lin and Al-Chaer 2003) and changes in pain-processing pathways (Park and Al-Chaer 2002). For example, changes in the role of the DC in the processing of visceral pain were documented in adult rats exposed to neonatal visceral pain compared to controls. In addition, there was a shift in the role of the thalamus and descending pathways between rats with neonatal colon pain and controls (Saab et al. 2004). Thalamic stimulation in the ventrobasal complex (VBC) caused inhibition of nociceptive neuronal responses in the dorsal horn under normal conditions; however, in adult rats exposed to neonatal colon pain, thalamic stimulation had a facilitatory effect. In addition to these neuronal changes, alterations in exploratory activity and faecal output were seen in adult rats with neonatal colon pain; symptoms commonly seen in patients with IBS. These observations were made in male and female rats. The hypersensitivity and changes in exploratory activity were aggravated by stress (Hinze et al. 2002).

In general, voluntary exploratory behaviour of animals in a new environment may be used as a measure of discomfort that may be associated with ongoing pain (Palecek et al. 2002), distress and anxiety (Griebel et al. 1998), socio-sexual behaviour (Gonzales et al. 1996), adaptation to or fear of leaving a familiar place, otherwise known as agoraphobia.

Neonatal rats exposed to somatic pain or the stress of maternal separation as adults exhibited increased input and segmental changes in nociceptive primary afferent axons, spinal neural circuits as well as altered responses to sensory stimulation (Ruda et al. 2000, Lidow et al. 2001, Coutinho et al. 2002), proving that there is a long-lasting impact of postnatal events on the neural processing of sensory information. This impact includes changes in afferent pathways, hyperexcitability or sensitization of receptive neurons, and possibly a shift in dynamics of sensory channels and descending controls, which in turn determines the adult visceral sensitivity and predisposes to chronic visceral pain. (For a complete description of animal models of neonatal pain, see Chapter 5.)

Similar observations were made clinically. Exposure to painful stimuli in the early postnatal period can alter the physiological and behavioural profile of the adult and predispose to chronic pain disorders. Drossman et al. (1990) documented a high level of early (pre-adolescent) sexual and physical abuse among female patients with functional GI disorders. In one study, 47.1% of IBS patients reported childhood sexual abuse (Blanchard and Scharff 2002). In a prospective cohort matched case-control study, using siblings as controls, gastric suction at birth was associated with an increased prevalence of functional intestinal disorders in later life possibly linked to the development of long-term visceral hypersensitivity and cognitive hypervigilance (Anand et al. 2004). In a retrospective assessment, children who had gastric suction at birth were 2.99 times more likely to be admitted to hospital for abdominal pain than children who were not intubated at birth. Thus, consideration of the long-term consequences of early neonatal pain is important for a complete understanding of use-dependent plasticity in sensation and other functional outcomes.

REFERENCES

Al Chaer ED, Lawand NB, Westlund KN, et al. (1996a). Visceral nociceptive input into the ventral posterolateral nucleus of the thalamus: a new function for the dorsal column pathway. J Neurophysiol 76: 2661–2674.

Al Chaer ED, Lawand NB, Westlund KN, et al. (1996b). Pelvic visceral input into the nucleus gracilis is largely mediated by the postsynaptic dorsal column pathway. J Neurophysiol 76: 2675–2690.

Al Chaer ED, Westlund KN, Willis WD. (1997a). Nucleus gracilis: an integrator for visceral and somatic information. J Neurophysiol 78: 521–527.

Al Chaer ED, Westlund KN, Willis WD. (1997b). Sensitization of postsynaptic dorsal column neuronal responses by colon inflammation. Neuroreport 8: 3267–3273.

Al Chaer ED, Feng Y, Willis WD. (1998). A role for the dorsal column in nociceptive visceral input into the thalamus of primates. J Neurophysiol 79: 3143–3150.

Al Chaer ED, Feng Y, Willis WD. (1999). Comparative study of viscerosomatic input onto postsynaptic dorsal column and spinothalamic tract neurons in the primate. J Neurophysiol 82: 1876–1882.

Al Chaer ED, Kawasaki M, Pasricha PJ. (2000). A new model of chronic visceral hypersensitivity in adult rats induced by colon irritation during postnatal development. Gastroenterology 119: 1276–1285.

Anand KJS, Runeson B, Jacobson B. (2004). Gastric suction at birth associated with long-term risk for functional intestinal disorders in later life. J Pediatr 144: 449–454.

Andrews KA, Desaib D, Dhillonb HK, et al. (2002). Abdominal sensitivity in the first year of life: comparison of infants with and without prenatally diagnosed unilateral hydronephrosis. Pain 100: 35–46.

Berkley KJ, Hubscher CH, Wall PD. (1993). Neuronal responses to stimulation of the cervix, uterus, colon, and skin in the rat spinal cord. J Neurophysiol 69: 545–556.

Berthoud HR, Kressel M, Raybould HE, et al. (1995). Vagal sensors in the rat duodenal mucosa: distribution and structure as revealed by in vivo DiI-tracing. Anat Embryol (Berl) 191: 203–212.

Blanchard EB, Scharff L. (2002). Psychosocial aspects of assessment and treatment of irritable bowel syndrome in adults and recurrent abdominal pain in children. J Consult Clin Psychol 70: 725–738.

Bueno L, Fioramontin J, Garcia-Villar R. (2000). Pathobiology of visceral pain: molecular mechanisms and therapeutic implications. III. Visceral afferent pathways: a source of new therapeutic targets for abdominal pain. Am J Physiol Gastrointest Liver Physiol 278: G670–G676.

Burklow KA, Phelps AN, Schultz JR, et al. (1998). Classifying complex pediatric feeding disorders. J Pediatr Gastroenterol Nutr 27: 143–147.

Cervero F, Laird JM. (2003). Role of ion channels in mechanisms controlling gastrointestinal pain pathways. Curr Opin Pharmacol 3: 608–612.

Coutinho SV, Meller ST, Gebhart GF. (1996). Intracolonic zymosan produces visceral hyperalgesia in the rat that is mediated by spinal NMDA and non-NMDA receptors. Brain Res 736: 7–15.

Coutinho SV, Plotsky PM, Sablad M, et al. (2002). Neonatal maternal separation alters stress-induced responses to viscerosomatic nociceptive stimuli in rat. Am J Physiol 282: G307–316.

Cummings EA, Reid GJ, Finley GA, et al. (1996). Prevalence and source of pain in pediatric inpatients. Pain 68: 25–31.

Di Lorenzo C, Flores A, Hyman PE. (1995). Age-related changes in colon motility. J Pediatr 127: 593–597.

Drossman DA, Leserman J, Nachman G, et al. (1990). Sexual and physical abuse in women with functional or organic gastrointestinal disorders. Ann Intern Med 113: 828–833.

Giamberardino MA. (2000). Visceral hyperalgesia. In: Devor M, Rowbotham MC, Wiesenfeld-Hallin Z (eds) Proceedings of the 9th World Congress on Pain, pp. 523–550. IASP Press, Seattle, WA.

Giamberardino MA, Vecchiet L. (1995). Visceral pain, referred hyperalgesia and outcome: new concepts. Eur J Anaesth 12 (suppl. 10): 61–66.

Gonzalez MI, Albonetti E, Siddiqui A, et al. (1996). Neonatal organizational effects of the 5-HT2 and 5-HT1A subsystems on adult behavior in the rat. Pharm Biochem Behavior 54: 195–203.

Graham YP, Heim C, Goodman SH, et al. (1999). The effects of neonatal stress on brain development: implications for psychopathology. Dev Psychopathol 11: 545–565.

Griebel G, Perrault G, Sanger DJ. (1998). Limited anxiolytic-like effects of non-benzodiazepine hypnotics in rodents. J Psychopharm 12: 356–365.

Hamid SA, Di Lorenzo C, Reddy SN, et al. (1998). Bisacodyl and high amplitude propagating colonic contractions in children. J Pediatr Gastroenterol Nutr 27: 398–402.

Hinze CL, Lin C, Al-Chaer ED. (2002). Estrous cycle and stress related variations of open field activity in adult female rats with neonatal colon irritation (CI). Program No. 155.14. 2002 Abstract Viewer/Itinerary Planner. Society for Neuroscience, Washington, DC. CD-ROM.

Hohn A, Leibrock J, Bailey K, et al. (1990). Identification and characterization of a novel member of the nerve growth factor/brain-derived neurotrophic factor family. Nature 344: 339–341.

Huang EJ, Reichardt LF. (2001). Neurotrophins: roles in neuronal development and function. Annu Rev Neurosci 24: 677–736.

Hughes A, Carr V. (1978). The interaction of periphery and center in the development of dorsal root ganglia. In: Jacobsen M (ed.) Handbook of sensory physiology: IX Development of sensory systems, pp. 85–114. Springer-Verlag, New York.

Ji Y, Traub RJ. (2001). Spinal NMDA receptors contribute to neuronal processing of acute noxious and nonnoxious colorectal stimulation in the rat. J Neurophysiol 86: 1783–1791.

Kawasaki M, Pasricha PJ, Al-Chaer ED. (2000). Blockade of NK1 receptors in the spinal cord reduces the hyper-sensitivity associated with colorectal distension in an animal model of the irritable bowel syndrome. Gastroenterology 118: A841.

Kamp EH, Beck DR, Gebhart GF. (2001). Combinations of neurokinin receptor antagonists reduce visceral hyperalgesia. J Pharmacol Exp Ther 299: 105–113.

Kirkup AJ, Brunsden AM, Grundy D. (2001). Receptors and transmission in the brain–gut axis: potential for novel therapies. I. Receptors on visceral afferents. Am J Physiol 280: G787–794.

Kirstein M, Farinas I. (2002). Sensing life: regulation of sensory neuron survival by neurotrophins. Cell Mol Life Sci 59: 1787–1802.

Laird JM, Olivar T, Roza C, et al. (2000). Deficits in visceral pain and hyperalgesia of mice with a disruption of the tachykinin NK1 receptor gene. Neuroscience 98: 345–352.

Leung AK, Sigalet DL. (2003). Acute abdominal pain in children. Am Fam Physician 67: 2321–2326.

Lidow MS, Song ZM, Ren K. (2001). Long-term effects of short-lasting early local inflammatory insult. NeuroReport 12: 399–403.

Lin C, Al-Chaer ED. (2003). Long-term sensitization of primary afferents in adult rats exposed to neonatal colon pain. Brain Res 971: 73–82.

Ma H, Park Y, Al-Chaer ED. (2002). Functional outcomes of neonatal colon pain measured in adult rats. J Pain 3 (Suppl 1): 27.

Maggi CA, Meli A. (1988). The sensory-efferent function of capsaicin-sensitive sensory neurons. Gen Pharmacol 19: 1–43.

Maisonpierre PC, Belluscio L, Friedman B, et al. (1990). NT-3, BDNF, and NGF in the developing rat nervous system: parallel as well as reciprocal patterns of expression. Neuron 5: 501–509.

McMahon SB. (2004). Sensitisation of gastrointestinal tract afferents. Gut 53 (Suppl 2): 13–15.

McMahon SB, Koltzenberg M. (1994). Silent afferents and visceral pain. In: Pharmacological approaches to the treatment of chronic pain: new concepts and critical issues. Progress in pain research and management, Vol 1, pp. 11–30. IASP Press, Seattle, Washington.

McRoberts JA, Coutinho SV, Marvizon JC, et al. (2001). Role of peripheral N-methyl-D-aspartate (NMDA) receptors in visceral nociception in rats. Gastroenterology 120: 1737–1748.

Medcyclopedia. http://www.amershamhealth.com/medcyclopaedia/medical/index.asp.

Mertz H, Naliboff B, Munakata J, et al. (1995). Altered rectal perception is a biomarker in irritable bowel syndrome. Gastroenterology 109: 40–52.

Ness TJ. (2000). Evidence for ascending visceral nociceptive information in the dorsal midline and lateral spinal cord. Pain 87: 83–88.

Ness TJ, Gebhart GF. (1990). Visceral pain: a review of experimental studies. Pain 41: 167–234.

Olivar T, Laird JM. (1999). Differential effects of N-methyl-D-aspartate receptor blockade on nociceptive somatic and visceral reflexes. Pain 79: 67–73.

Palecek J, Paleckova V, Willis WD. (2002). The roles of pathways in the spinal cord lateral and dorsal funiculi in signaling nociceptive somatic and visceral stimuli in rats. Pain 96: 297–307.

Perry BD. (1994). Neurobiological sequelae of childhood trauma: post traumatic stress disorders in children. In: Murburg M (ed.) Catecholamine function in post traumatic stress disorder: emerging concepts, pp. 253–276. American Psychiatric Press, Washington, DC.

Porter FL, Anand K. (1998). Epidemiology of pain in neonates. Res Clin Forum 20: 9–18.

Rasquin-Weber A, Hyman PE, Cucchiara S, et al. (1999). Childhood functional gastrointestinal disorders. Gut 45 (suppl. II): II60–II68.

Richards CA, Andrews PL. (2004). Food refusal: a sign of nausea? J Pediatr Gastroenterol Nutr 38: 227–228.

Rosenthal A, Goeddel DV, Nguyen T, et al. (1990). Primary structure and biological activity of a novel human neurotrophic factor. Neuron 4: 767–773.

Ruda MA, Ling QD, Hohmann AG, et al. (2000). Altered nociceptive neuronal circuits after neonatal peripheral inflammation. Science 289: 628–631.

Saab CY, Arai Y-CP, Al-Chaer ED. (2004). Modulation of visceral nociceptive processing in the lumbar spinal cord following thalamic stimulation or inactivation and after dorsal column lesion in rats with neonatal colon irritation. Brain Res 1008: 186–192.

Sengupta JN, Gebhart GF. (1994). Characterization of mechanosensitive pelvic nerve afferent fibers innervating the colon of the rat. J Neurophysiol 71: 2046–2060.

Traub RJ. (2000). Evidence for thoracolumbar spinal cord processing of inflammatory, but not acute colonic pain. Neuroreport 11: 2113–2116.

Traub RJ, Hutchcroft K, Gebhart GF. (1999). The peptide content of colonic afferents decreases following colonic inflammation. Peptides 20: 267–273.

Willis WD, Al-Chaer ED, Quast MJ, et al. (1999). A visceral pain pathway in the dorsal column of the spinal cord. In: The Neurobiology of Pain. Proceedings of the National Academy of Sciences (USA). The National Academy of Science, Washington, D.C., 96 (14): 7675–7679.

Youssef NN, Peters JM, Henderson W, et al. (2002). Dose response of PEG 3350 for the treatment of childhood fecal impaction. J Pediatr 141: 410–414.

Zangen S, Di Lorenzo C, Zangen T, et al. (2001). Rapid maturation of gastric relaxation in newborn infants. Pediatr Res 50: 629–632.

Zhai QZ, Traub RJ. (1999). The NMDA receptor antagonist MK-801 attenuates c-Fos expression in the lumbosacral spinal cord following repetitive noxious and non-noxious colorectal distention. Pain 83: 321–329.

Ethical issues in the treatment of neonatal and infant pain

John Lantos
William Meadow

INTRODUCTION

The treatment of pain in neonates and infants is a topic that raises passions. Newborn and young babies are among the most helpless and vulnerable of citizens. They deserve care and protection. Neonatal intensive care is an idealistic attempt to treat each newborn life as of inestimable value. It has been one of the most phenomenally successful medical developments of the last century. However, it has also been ethically controversial. Some of the ethical controversies associated with neonatal intensive care focus on the implications of saving babies with debilitating chronic conditions. Some would argue that in certain circumstances, it seems preferable to forego life-sustaining treatment and, instead, to let nature take its course.

Another set of controversies associated with neonatal intensive care focus on the painful nature of many of the interventions and the lack of attention to prevention and analgesic treatment for those painful procedures. As in many areas of biomedical ethics, the dilemma is with us because the choices before us are not clear. If there was a simple, risk-free intervention that would ameliorate pain during neonatal intensive care, most healthcare professionals would likely adopt it immediately. The problem is that most interventions are of uncertain efficacy and all are associated with both costs and risks. Furthermore, pain relief is a difficult goal to precisely quantify so it is not always clear whether the risks and costs are associated with commensurate benefits.

HISTORICAL APPROACHES TO THE ETHICS OF PAIN TREATMENT

The two previous editions of this textbook had excellent chapters on the ethical issues associated with the treatment of pain in infants and children. Interestingly, they took very different approaches to the problem.

In the first edition, Nance Cunningham examined 'the belief system and culture in which the existence of infant pain has been doubted or denied, in which infant pain has been discounted, and in which changes in practice may very well be resisted'.

Cunningham presented a series of commonly held beliefs about pain or pain treatment, and then argued against them. For example, one common belief is that because pain is a subjective experience, it cannot be measured.

She argued against the belief that pain is subjective by showing that not only does everybody experience pain but that we are able to recognize the pain of others by recognizing distinctive signals and gestures. Furthermore, she noted, it is rational to assume that others who are like us feel the same things that we do. We can then use these beliefs as the basis for the use of analgesia and anaesthesia in a wide variety of clinical circumstances. Cunningham argued that such use of our knowledge of others' pain to develop ways to relieve pain fulfils one of the central moral functions of medicine.

She then talked about some beliefs about infants' pain. In particular, she sought to obliterate the belief, then widespread, that because infants may not be able to remember pain, it therefore 'doesn't count' in the way that it would 'count' for an adult. She also sought to show that the treatment of pain in neonates was not inherently more dangerous than in adults. Against these beliefs, she cited both moral principles and empirical data indicating that neonates have the same physiologic responses to painful stimuli as do adults, and that painful experiences leave infants with long-term sequalae, suggesting that they have a bodily memory, if not conscious memory, of pain. She acknowledged the need for studies to find safe and effective means of treating pain and that such studies would not be impossible to do.

Her conclusions were that standards of care for neonates that allow inadequate attention to pain are the results of '1) a series of well-accepted, unexamined, bad arguments and 2) a willingness by caregivers themselves to allow major differences between beliefs and moral rules inside the medical context, on the one hand, and beliefs and moral rules outside the medical context, on the other hand.' Her chapter is an attempt to convince individuals to reexamine the contradictions in their own beliefs. Once they do, she believes, they will realize that it is time to 're-examine and discard where appropriate those beliefs and arguments that have left them in a kind of moral darkness and some of their infant charges in what must have been an existential darkness'.

In the second edition, Walco and Cassidy took a somewhat different approach to exploring ethical issues in infants. They began with an ethical challenge to caregivers: 'Since pain seems harmful to patients, and caregivers are categorically committed to preventing harm to their patients, not using all available means of relieving pain must be justified'.

They then discussed three common justifications that are used for the undertreatment of pain. One is that the pain is not that bad. A second is that the burdens of relieving pain are greater than the burdens of unrelieved pain. Finally, some caregivers think that unrelieved pain is necessary to produce something better.

Against the first belief, they offered scientific data showing that infants have the neural capability to experience pain and, therefore, we have every reason to believe that the subjective experience of pain is every bit as severe for the infant as the subjective experience of pain for an adult. They also cited data from studies of physiological and behavioural responses to painful stimuli showing that the sympathetic nervous system and the endocrine system both have measurable responses to painful stimuli. Furthermore, infants behave in ways that suggest that they experience pain and that the pain can be relieved.

Walco and Cassidy acknowledged that the burdens associated with some methods for treating pain are real and thus require a balancing of the burdens of the pain itself against the burdens of such treatments. In this discussion, they specifically note the need to use painful procedures, such as an intramuscular injection, to deliver pain medication as well as the risks of complications, such as respiratory depression from the use of opioids that arise from some pain therapy. They suggested, however, that the response to these challenges should not be to withhold analgesic medications but, instead, to figure out less painful ways to deliver them and better approaches to monitoring infants to prevent harmful consequences. They concluded that 'the administration of analgesic medication depends on an analysis of relative benefits and risks… Any comparative justification for withholding pain relief must be rigorously controlled by a careful analysis of all the risks and benefits and the disciplined use of empirical data, not speculation or undocumented lore'.

Finally, they talked about situations in which unrelieved pain may be necessary for good medical treatment. As an example, they described the situation in which a patient suffers from abdominal pain. In this situation, they say, it is important for the physician to be able to elicit and reproduce the pain to diagnose the problem. Pain relief, in this situation, may lead to misdiagnosis and a worse outcome for the patient. They claimed, however, that such situations, though real, are rare, and should not be used to justify undertreatment of pain in situations where such counterbalancing benefits are not present.

Cunningham's discussion was more passionate and exhortatory. Walco and Cassidy were more measured. Both come to relatively similar conclusions – that the treatment of pain is a moral imperative and that the reasons commonly given by professionals for not treating pain are often inadequate.

RECENT DEVELOPMENTS

Since these previous editions of the textbook were published, there have been a number of interesting developments and challenges in the field of neonatal and infant pain treatment. These developments allow for new understandings of the ethical dilemmas associated with the treatment of neonatal pain.

Following up on the calls of many practitioners for enhanced research rigour in relation to the treatment of neonatal pain, a number of studies were carried out. The design of these studies highlighted some of the ethical controversies associated with clinical research in neonatology and the difficulties of pain research in neonates.

A single-centre, randomized controlled trial compared the clinical efficacy and side effects of fentanyl or morphine analgesia in ventilated newborn infants. Among 163 infants allocated to receive fentanyl or morphine infusions for 24–48 hours after birth, the analgesic effects were similar in both groups, but side effects were less frequent in the fentanyl group (23% vs. 47%, P < 0.01) (Saarenmaa et al. 1999). In the design of this trial, the authors asserted that it would have been unethical to use a placebo control group. In a commentary on the article, Kennedy and Tyson argued for placebo-controlled trials. They wrote:

> *Narcotics can be considered a proven and ethically mandatory therapy for infants receiving mechanical ventilation only if the value has been established in one or more masked randomized trials with sufficient numbers of infants to assess all important potential benefits and hazards… Administration of narcotics or sedatives in neonates receiving mechanical ventilation should not be considered obligatory and should be undertaken with skepticism and recognition that there are significant side effects and perhaps major, as yet unidentified, hazards.*
>
> *Kennedy and Tyson 1999*

Placebo-controlled trials are ethically appropriate when there is no evidence-based standard treatment. When there is such a treatment, it would be unethical to randomize research subjects to a no-treatment placebo control. At the time of this study, there did not seem to be a standard treatment for ventilated neonates. Therefore, placebo controls were ethically acceptable.

Other issues in study design were associated with the power and generalizability of particular studies. Some of the earliest placebo-controlled trials yielded promising results. Anand et al. (1999) randomized ventilated infants to morphine, midazolam or placebo.

They found 'Two neonates in the placebo group and 1 neonate in the midazolam group died; no deaths occurred in the morphine group. Poor neurologic outcomes occurred in 24% of neonates in the placebo group, 32% in the midazolam group, and 4% in the morphine group (likelihood ratio χ^2 = 7.04, P = .03). Secondary clinical outcomes and neurobehavioral outcomes at 36 weeks' postconceptional age were similar in the 3 groups. Responses elicited by endotracheal tube suction (Premature Infant Pain Profile scores) were significantly reduced during the morphine (P < .001) and midazolam (P = .002) infusions compared with the placebo group'. However, the number of patients in this study was small although it was a multi-centre study. Therefore, it could be concluded that the study was underpowered to answer the research question and that results needed to be viewed with extreme caution. However, the study did provide important pilot data on the safety of midazolam in this population, which ultimately precluded inclusion of this treatment in future studies.

Other studies did not yield similar results. For example, Simons et al. (2003) randomized ventilated infants in two level II neonatal intensive care units (NICUs) in the Netherlands to morphine or placebo. They reported that 'The analgesic effect did not differ between the morphine and placebo groups, judging from the following median (interquartile range) pain scores: Premature Infant Pain Profile, 10.1 (8.2–11.6) vs. 10.0 (8.2–12.0) (P = .94); Neonatal Infant Pain Scale, 4.8 (3.7–6.0) vs. 4.8 (3.2–6.0) (P = .58); and visual analog scale, 2.8 (2.0–3.9) vs. 2.6 (1.8–4.3) (P = .14), respectively. Routine morphine infusion decreased the incidence of IVH (23% vs. 40%, P = 0.04) but did not influence poor neurologic outcome (10% vs. 16%, P = 0.66)'. They concluded that the 'Lack of a measurable analgesic effect and absence of a beneficial effect on poor neurologic outcome do not support the routine use of morphine infusions as a standard of care in preterm newborns who have received ventilatory support'.

The multicentre, randomized Neurologic Outcomes and Pre-emptive Analgesia in Neonates (NEOPAIN) trial was much larger than any previous study (Anand et al. 2004). Nearly 900 ventilated infants from 16 centres were randomized to either morphine infusions or placebo control groups. Although the primary neurological outcomes were similar in the two randomized groups (Anand et al. 2004), the side effect of respiratory depression, occurred more frequently in the morphine infusion group (Bhandari et al. 2005). Other side effects, such as hypotension appeared to be related to the infant's condition or severity of illness at birth, rather than the use of morphine versus placebo infusions (Hall et al. 2005). Specifically, for the respiratory outcomes:

Infants in the morphine group required ventilator therapy significantly longer, compared with the placebo group (median [interquartile range]: 7 days [4–20 days] vs. 6 days [3–19 days])… After adjustment for birth weight, Clinical Risk Index for Babies scores, maternal chorioamnionitis, RDS requiring surfactant, and patent ductus arteriosus in a logistic regression model, the use of additional analgesia with morphine was associated independently with increased air leaks and longer durations of high-frequency ventilation, nasal continuous positive airway pressure, and oxygen therapy.

Bhandari et al. 2005

Despite these differences, the NEOPAIN randomized trial was designed to examine a composite primary outcome including intraventricular haemorrhage, periventricular leukomalacia, or death. The placebo and morphine groups had similar rates of the composite outcome (105/408 [26%] vs. 115/419 [27%]), neonatal death (47/449 [11%] vs. 58/449 [13%]), severe IVH (46/429 [11%] vs. 55/411 [13%]), and PVL (34/367 [9%] vs. 27/367 [7%]). For neonates who were not given open-label morphine, rates of the composite outcome (53/225 [24%] vs. 27/179 [15%], p = 0.0338) and severe IVH (19/219 [9%] vs. 6/189 [3%], p = 0.0209) were higher in the morphine group than the placebo group. Placebo-group neonates receiving open-label morphine had worse rates of the composite outcome than those not receiving open-label morphine (78/228 [34%] vs. 27/179 [15%], p < 0.0001). Morphine-group neonates receiving open-label morphine were more likely to develop severe IVH (36/190 [19%] vs. 19/219 [9%], p = 0.0024)' (Anand et al. 2004).

The investigators concluded that morphine did not improve short-term outcomes in ventilated infants. However, morphine did seem to be effective in relieving pain. In a systematic review, investigators from the Cochrane Database wrote,

Thirteen studies on 1505 infants were included. Infants given opioids showed reduced premature infant pain profile (PIPP) scores compared to the control group (weighted mean difference –1.71; 95% confidence interval –3.18 to –0.24).

Bellu et al. 2005

Prior to the availability of these data, some clinicians had concluded that, in spite of the risks, morphine infusions should be used for ventilated neonates. For example, based on empirical data available before these randomized trials, Taddio proposed that:

Opioids have been demonstrated to blunt the physiologic effects of pain and may prevent some of the clinical consequences of unmanaged pain. There are sufficient data to recommend the clinical use of opioid analgesics for the treatment of pain in the neonate.

Taddio 2002

CAN PAIN BE WORSE THAN DEATH?

The opposing opinions about the interpretation of study results suggests that different people weigh the value of different outcomes according to their own ideas about which outcomes count the most. A thought experiment might highlight this. Let us imagine that the results of the NEOPAIN study were strongly in favour of using morphine, such that infants in the morphine group had shorter courses of ventilation, fewer side effects and lower rates of IVH than those in the placebo group. Investigators might have justifiably concluded that morphine was clearly indicated and morally imperative as treatment for such babies. Given the equivocal results, however, the investigators did not conclude that morphine is clearly contraindicated or morally problematic. Instead, they concluded that more research was necessary and that it should be used with caution. The meaning of results can only be arrived at after both rigorous statistical analysis and an ethical balancing of the value of pain relief compared to value of survival.

One can quantify thresholds for such analyses. Suppose, for example, the pain associated with mechanical ventilation for preterm infants could be relieved by a drug that increased mortality rates by 1%. Would it be worth it to have a slightly higher mortality rate and less pain, or a slightly lower mortality rate and more pain? In most clinical situations involving adults, patients are willing to take some gamble on the risk of mortality in order to achieve better pain relief. Surgical procedures, for example, could be done with only neuromuscular blockade rather than general anaesthesia and would likely be safer. However, most people prefer the pain relief associated with general anaesthesia, even though it may be associated with slightly higher risks of side effects and morbidity.

EXTRAPOLATING FROM ADULT INTENSIVE CARE UNITS TO NEONATAL INTENSIVE CARE UNITS

One possible way to determine whether the risks of analgesia outweigh the benefits would be to use a form of substituted judgement. By this technique, we might ask what competent adults who face the burdens and suffering of ICU care generally choose. That issue is complicated because it is often not the adults who are choosing options for themselves.

Regardless of how these choices are arrived at, it seems clear that, in most cases, the choice is to provide analgesia and sedation for ventilated adults. The rationale for this seems to be both to relieve the acute experience of pain and also to try to minimize any memory of the NICU. Some of the studies specifically note that patients vividly recollect their painful experiences in the intensive care unit (Puntillo 1990). Some have noted psychological problems akin to post-traumatic stress disorder that persist long after their medical recovery (Cuthbertson et al. 2004).

The short-term and long-term symptoms of pain and suffering in the adult ICU are so dreaded that most intensivists will treat every intubated adult patient for pain. One recent editorial described the situation thus, 'Because the environment in the intensive care unit is so stressful, intensive intravenous sedation has evolved from adjunct therapy to a central component of critical care. Initially administered as continuous infusions to promote comfort in patients receiving mechanical ventilation, various combinations of narcotics, benzodiazepines, major tranquilizers, and anesthetic agents are now given almost routinely for numerous indications. Physicians prescribe these drugs in stupor-producing doses for intubated patients to induce amnesia, prevent patients from removing their endotracheal tubes, decrease oxygen consumption, and promote synchronous breathing with mechanical ventilators. It is now common in a busy intensive care unit to find that most, if not all, patients receiving mechanical ventilation are in a drug-induced state of suspended animation' (Heffner 2000).

Interestingly, while there are many surveys documenting the use of analgesia and sedation, there are few reports of the side effects. Instead, these drugs are seen as essential. If the side effects would not be a reason to withhold treatment, then, for some, there is little reason to study them. This cavalier attitude leads to some predictable problems. Heffner notes, 'Despite the widespread use of high-dose, continuous infusions of sedatives in the intensive care unit, there is little evidence that such sedation improves patients' outcomes... Moreover, practical and validated scoring systems to allow accurate adjustment of the doses of sedatives given to patients receiving mechanical ventilation do not exist'. He highlights some of the gaps in knowledge, '... most of our knowledge of the pharmacokinetics of sedative drugs derives from short-term studies in normal subjects. Critical illnesses

and drug interactions alter the volumes of distribution, availability, and elimination of drugs, essentially converting "short-acting" sedatives to drugs with long-term effects. There have been few rigorous studies of the comparative usefulness of various sedative drugs administered in the intensive care unit. Appropriate administration of these drugs is further complicated by the poor understanding of their pharmacokinetics and therapeutic properties on the part of many caregivers in the intensive care unit' (Heffner 2000).

It seems somewhat ironic that such issues seem to be getting studied more rigorously in neonates than they have been in adults. The willingness of intensivists in adult ICUs to use sedatives and analgesics in the absence of practice guidelines, evidence of efficacy, and in the presence of known risks suggests that, in the adult units, the moral balance between the risks of pain relief and the benefits tips slightly differently than it does in the NICU. In neonates, many see pain relief as a goal that is only worth pursuing if it can be achieved without any trade-offs in survival or in other worthwhile goals. In adult ICUs, by contrast, pain relief is seen as primary, and the side effects of analgesia are seen as tolerable. Based upon this, my guess would be that, in adult ICUs, it would be considered morally intolerable to do the sort of placebo-controlled trials that have been carried out in NICUs.

THE CENTRAL ETHICAL ISSUE: HOW MUCH RISK OF MORTALITY IS PAIN CONTROL WORTH?

In both groups, children and adults, the central ethical issue in pain control is the question of balancing the risks against the benefits. The problem, in neonates, is that it is harder to quantify the benefits because patients cannot tell us how much pain they are experiencing. In addition, neonates need to be on mechanical ventilation for longer periods of time than do most adults in medical ICUs. This could make the risks of sedation or analgesia even higher.

The recognition that pain relief in neonates will not come without a price brings us full-circle in our considerations about pain treatment in newborns. Twenty or thirty years ago, many reasonable people denied that newborns could feel pain. In the intervening decades, this view has been discredited. In its place, new scientific studies have allowed us to quantify both the efficacy and the risks of pain relief in newborns. The data from these studies, though, presents a new sort of moral dilemma for practitioners and parents alike. How do we decide when pain is worse than death?

In the Netherlands, this issue is addressed more explicitly than it is in other countries. In a recent paper reviewing actual practices in Dutch NICUs, van der Heide and colleagues noted, 'A distinction between intentionally ending life and providing adequate terminal care by alleviating pain or other symptoms, which is important in moral and judicial terms, is probably not easily made for some of these patients' (van der Heide et al. 2000).

A shift in attitudes toward newborn pain has been incorporated into practice by Dutch physicians. In a recent essay in the *New England Journal of Medicine*, two Dutch neonatalogists, Verbagan and Sauer (2005) wrote, 'Suffering is a subjective feeling that cannot be measured objectively, whether in adults or in infants. But we accept that adults can indicate when their suffering is unbearable. Infants cannot express their feelings through speech, but they do so through different types of crying, movements, and reactions to feeding. Pain scales for newborns, based on changes in vital signs (blood pressure, heart rate, and breathing pattern) and observed behavior, may be used to determine the degree of discomfort and pain. Experienced caregivers and parents are able to evaluate the degree of suffering in a newborn, as well as the degree of relief afforded by medication or other measures'.

This statement, unobjectionable in itself, was used as a justification for the Groningen protocol, a protocol designed to identify infants whose suffering was so intractable that they were considered by their paediatricians to be candidates for euthanasia. The Dutch practice of infant euthanasia highlights what appears to be the logical extreme of one algorithm for balancing the harm associated with pain against the limits of analgesia.

CONCLUSION

The ethical issues associated with the treatment of neonatal pain have gotten harder, rather than easier, as a result of the scientific studies of various approaches to the treatment of such pain. Put simply, treatments that work well enough to relieve pain seem to worsen other outcomes. We know from both surgical experience and from experiences in adult ICUs that we can control pain. However, to do so in the NICU would likely require higher doses of opioids than most doctors feel comfortable administering. Such doses would likely lead to adequate pain relief, but might also lead to higher mortality rates. The judgement about the ethics of such treatment must turn on assessments of three factors – pain relief, effect of treatment on mortality, and the effect of treatment on long-term morbidity. The complexity of these assessments can be illustrated by thought experiments that seek to determine appropriate thresholds for each of these variables.

Imagine, for example, that continuous high-dose morphine or fentanyl infusions can completely control pain but with an increased mortality rate of 2%, and a decrease in IVH of 5%. Would it be worth it? What if it led to higher mortality as well as higher incidence of IVH? Who should make the decision – doctors or parents? What if doctors disagree?

Until a safe and effective analgesic comes along, it seems that decisions about pain control in the NICU will turn on people's responses to multifactorial equations of risks and benefits such as these. Until then, the ethical issues associated with such treatments will likely become more complicated rather than simpler.

REFERENCES

Anand KJS, McIntosh N, Lagercrantz H, et al. (1999). Analgesia and sedation in preterm neonates who require ventilatory support: results from the NOPAIN trial. Arch Pediatr Adolesc Med 153: 331–338.

Anand KJS, Hall RW, Desai N, et al. (2004). NEOPAIN Trial Investigators Group. Effects of morphine analgesia in ventilated preterm neonates: Primary outcomes from the NEOPAIN randomised trial. Lancet 363: 1673–1682.

Bellu R, de Waal KA, Zanini R. (2005). Opioids for neonates receiving mechanical ventilation. Cochrane Database Syst Rev, CD004212.

Bhandari V, Bergqvist LL, Kronsberg SS, et al. (2005). NEOPAIN Trial Investigators Group. Morphine administration and short-term pulmonary outcomes among ventilated preterm infants. Pediatrics 116: 352–359.

Cuthbertson BH, Hull A, Strachan M, et al (2004). Post-traumatic stress disorder after critical illness requiring general intensive care. Intensive Care Med 30: 450–455.

Hall RW, Kronsberg SS, Barton BA, et al. (2005). Morphine, hypotension and adverse outcomes in preterm neonates: Who's to blame? Pediatrics 115: 1351–1359.

Heffner JE. (2000). A wake up call in the ICU. N Engl J Med 342: 1520–1522.

Kennedy KA, Tyson JE. (1999). Narcotic analgesia for ventilated newborns: are placebo-controlled trials ethical and necessary? J Pediatr 134: 127–129.

Puntillo KA. (1990). Pain experiences of intensive care unit patients. Heart Lung 19: 526–533.

Saarenmaa E, Huttunen P, Leppaluoto J, et al. (1999). Advantages of fentanyl over morphine in analgesia for ventilated newborn infants after birth: A randomized trial. J Pediatr 134: 144–150.

Simons SH, van Dijk M, van Lingen RA, et al. (2003). Routine morphine infusion in preterm newborns who received ventilatory support: a randomized controlled trial. JAMA 290: 2419–2427.

Taddio A. (2002). Opioid analgesia for infants in the neonatal intensive care unit. Clin Perinatol 29: 493–509.

van der Heide A, van der Maas PJ, van der Wal G, et al. (2000). Using potentially life-shortening drugs in neonates and infants. Crit Care Med 28: 2595–2599.

Verbagen E, Sauer PJJ. (2005). The Groningen protocol – euthanasia in severely ill newborns. N Eng J Med 352: 959–962.

Neonatal and infant pain in a social context

Patrick J McGrath
Anita M Unruh

INTRODUCTION

To be fully understood, neonatal and infant pain must be placed in a larger social context. All health issues arise in a social context and are resolved or not resolved in a context. We have a tendency to ignore the role of social context and believe that factors such as advances in science or personal beliefs are much more important. Because we are all immersed in our social context, the effects of social context always appear to be the normal or natural way. In this chapter, we will highlight some examples of how the social context is critical for understanding and ameliorating infant and neonatal pain.

Social context refers to the web of meaning, expectations, shared beliefs, attitudes, values and norms of behaviour that form the non-physical infrastructure of all organizations and institutions. Sometimes referred to as 'culture', it emerges from that which is shared amongst those in an organization. The idea of social context can be applied to almost any grouping. This would include a specific unit in a hospital, such as 'the social context of the neonatal intensive care unit at the Health Centre' to a set of units as 'the social context of family physicians' offices in the Netherlands' or a religious, political or ethnic group such as 'people in the United States who vote for the Democrats and attend the Episcopalian Church regularly'. Different individuals in a given physical space will experience different social contexts or cultures. For example, a parent whose child is in the neonatal intensive care unit (NICU) will not experience the same social context as the neonatologist who is caring for the child. There will be elements of the culture that are shared but there will also be distinct differences.

Different social contexts will prompt different behaviours. So, for example, neonatologists in NICUs that differ in terms of the expectation that pain will be treated, will engage in different pain management strategies. Individual differences will be nested within these social contexts.

This chapter discusses the most relevant issues related to social context. There is very limited research on infant and neonatal pain and social context. This chapter is an attempt to prompt interest of clinicians and researchers in how social context influences all aspects of infant and neonatal pain rather than a definitive treatment of all social context issues in neonatal and infant pain.

NICU: A STRANGE SOCIAL CONTEXT

Most parents are both joyous and a bit stressed by the birth of a child. The situation of parents of babies in the NICU is strange, frightening and stressful. Babies admitted to the NICU are at risk. Parents worry about the health and survival of their baby. The physical environment from the layperson's point of view is unreal. Babies are installed in incubators surrounded by high-tech equipment with nurses and doctors almost constantly around them.

A significant issue for parents of babies in the NICU is that the expected parental role of caring for their baby is dramatically altered. They no longer have the primary responsibility for caregiving and protection of their infant. Gale et al. (2004) examined parents' views of their experiences observing and coping with their infant's clinical course, infant pain experiences, and the parenting experience during and after their stay in the NICU.

Two themes emerged: infant pain as a source of parental stress and relief of parental stress due to the relief of infant pain. Parents were distressed by their inability to protect their babies from pain and to comfort their babies when they had pain. Some parents experienced a mismatch between their own perceptions of the pain experienced by their babies and the perception of staff. Many parents were frustrated by the barriers to them caring for their babies, including the baby's severity of illness, their jealousy of nurses' greater competencies and just not knowing how to help their baby.

Parents were upset by the distress of their baby and the tissue damage from procedures. Finally, they felt unprepared for the pain their babies were having. They felt they lacked information about procedures that caused pain and the management of infant pain.

Parents found that support from the NICU staff and from visiting nurses after discharge was important in relieving their distress. Participating in care in the NICU reduced parental distress. The Internet was a source of information and support from other parents was helpful. Written information provided by the unit developmental specialists was also helpful.

Although many parents of babies in the NICU are stressed and worried, few develop clinical anxiety or depression and most cope quite well with this difficult time (Carter et al. 2005).

DEMOCRATIZATION OF HEALTH KNOWLEDGE

At one time, access to scientific knowledge in health was limited to physicians and a very small coterie of non-physicians who had the skills to read it. However,

in the last 25 years this has dramatically changed. The lay public is becoming more aware of healthcare issues and practices because of the broad coverage of medical issues in the press and on the Internet. Parents of infants and neonates are becoming more sophisticated in their knowledge and more demanding that infant and neonatal pain be considered.

A social standard widely held in our society is the right to protection from unnecessary harm inflicted by others. Pain is clearly an important form of harm. This standard is particularly important for those who are unable to protect themselves. This expectation or value becomes obvious in our laws about child abuse and neglect. Almost all jurisdictions have enacted and enforce laws that make the harming of children, or, in certain circumstances, the failure to prevent harm to children, a criminal matter. As a society, we believe that infants should be protected from harm including pain. Healthcare professionals share this general social expectation and have both a legal and ethical obligation to protect their patients from harm. Parents see protection of their children from unnecessary pain as their responsibility as well.

In the medical context, parents delegate this responsibility to healthcare professionals in the trust that professionals will do everything they can to prevent their children from suffering pain. Paradoxically, much of the pain suffered by neonates in the medical context is due to medical care, albeit it is pain for the purpose of diagnosis and treatment. But pain from surgery and pain from procedures are iatrogenic. Pain is an unintended and unwanted side effect. The trust that parents have given to healthcare providers to prevent pain is violated if doctors and nurses do not use the best scientific evidence available to assess the infant's pain and then, based on this assessment, provide safe and effective pain relief. The only justification to permit the violation involved in hurting an infant is if the procedure is necessary for the health of the infant and if pain management or prevention were impossible or dangerous.

The expectation that efforts should be made to protect infants from pain have not changed. Parents have always expected that health professionals would do everything they could to prevent pain. What has changed is that parents now have information about neonatal pain and are able to challenge what health professionals are doing.

The most striking example of how parental knowledge has been used to challenge typical clinical practice is that of Jeffrey Lawson. In 1985, a 1-pound, 11-ounce neonate, Jeffrey Lawson, was operated on to correct a patent ductus arteriosus. His mother had heard of the failure to anaesthetize infants during surgery from a popular report of research. She spoke to her son's neonatologist and was reassured by him that her baby would be anaesthetized (Harrison 1987). The infant died a month after surgery. When his mother, Jill Lawson, later reviewed her child's medical chart, she found that at no point during the surgical procedure had her son been given anaesthesia. Her discovery led to an unrelenting struggle to confront the practice of lack of anaesthesia in neonatal surgery.

Jeffrey had holes cut on both sides of his neck, another cut in his right chest, an incision from his breastbone around to his backbone, his ribs pried apart, and an extra artery near his heart tied off. This was topped off with another hole cut in his left side for a chest tube. This operation lasted hours. Jeffrey was awake through it all. The anesthesiologist paralyzed him with Pavulon, a curare drug that left him unable to move, but totally conscious. When I questioned the anesthesiologist later about her use of Pavulon, she said Jeffrey was too sick to tolerate powerful anesthetics. Anyway, she said, it had never been demonstrated to her that premature babies feel pain.

Lawson 1986, p. 125

Ms. Lawson's confrontation of current neonatal practice was strongly resisted by many in the medical establishment. She was patronized and discouraged from pursuing redress. But some physicians were outraged. Scanlon, her son's neonatologist who had reassured Ms. Lawson that her son would be having anaesthesia described neonatal surgery with only muscle relaxant and minimal anaesthesia as based on 'ignorance, hubris and barbarism' (Scanlon 1987, p. 82). It was not until August 1986, when The Washington Post published her account that the resistance to examining neonatal pain practice in the NICUs of the United States began to change (Harrison 1987). The individual action of Jill Lawson, when it reached the public press, generated collective pressure. Other parents (see for example, Rovner 1986, in the San Francisco Chronicle; Fischer 1987, in Redbook; Stern 1987, in the Oakland Tribune) also supported her efforts. Criticism from parents such as Ms. Lawson changed neonatal pain practices in a variety of settings, beginning in the hospital where her son was operated on, the Children's Hospital National Medical Center in Washington, DC (Fletcher 1987).

Ms. Lawson's efforts may have begun with reasoned appeals to change anaesthetic practice. But she made her son's situation the focus of an impassioned and, at times, bitter crusade. The language she used was not that of scientific discourse and the attacks were often personal, pointed and, perhaps unfair, from the point of view of those who were their targets. But a mother reacting to the suffering of her child has every reason to be passionate. The passion and the vehemence of her efforts certainly contributed to them being taken up by the popular press. Her work has made a major contribution to the re-examination of neonatal pain. We doubt that a calm, reasoned, dispassionate discourse would have been as effective. The singular contribution of Jeffrey Lawson's experience and his mother's efforts to changing pain management has been recognized by the American Pain Society developing an award in his name to recognize advocacy in paediatric pain. Making her the first recipient of this award recognized the incredible efforts of Jill Lawson.

Parents also lobby in a more private way with health professionals for recognition and treatment of pain in their own infants and neonates. Harrison (1987) and Butler (1988) suggested that parents consider the following options to ensure adequate pain management of their newborn. First, infant pain and NICU procedures can be discussed prior to birth with the obstetrician and paediatrician when a premature delivery is a possibility. Parents can choose not to have optional surgery, such as circumcision, for their baby. When babies are hospitalized, parents should discuss with the physician and nurses how pain in neonates is assessed and managed and what medication and comfort measures will be given. Parents should seek a second opinion when conflict arises. Anaesthesia should be discussed with both the surgeon and the anaesthesiologist prior to surgery. Risks of anaesthesia and analgesics, risks of alternatives to them and additional methods of providing comfort may be discussed with the physician and nurses. Parents may also choose to sign a limited consent form specifying consent only for anaesthetized surgery. However, many physicians may not accept a limited consent because it impinges on their professional responsibility to follow what they think is most appropriate. Similarly, parents can ask for pain management when their infants are receiving procedures such as immunization.

Physicians, nurses and other allied health professionals are also in a position to lobby for changes in neonatal pain practice within their own institutions and associations. This can be a difficult endeavour when professionals perceive that they themselves do not have the power or authority to change practices.

SOME PAIN INFLICTED ON INFANTS AND NEONATES IS SOCIALLY APPROVED

Certain painful practices have widespread social approval. Taking blood for diagnostic tests and giving injections are socially approved. Health professionals and parents alike typically view these practices as justified because they are medically necessary. This acceptance of needles as a necessity is part of our modern culture. We seldom examine activities that are widely socially approved within our own society.

Blood tests are only ethically justified when they are done for a good reason that has real potential benefit for the infant or neonate. It is not ethical to subject a neonate or infant to painful procedures simply because the procedure is scheduled. If there is not a clinical judgement of the need for a blood test, it is hard to see how it can be ethical. It is not good enough that many blood draws are for the benefit of specific infants. A general social approval of doing needle procedures 'because they are needed' is insufficient as a justification for subjecting specific children to specific incidents of unnecessary pain. Is every one of the hundreds of needle procedures that the average neonate in intensive care receives needed? Is there any way, with a little planning, of eliminating some of the blood draws by not doing some and by using the same blood draw for more than one test? The general social approval should be replaced by careful consideration of the necessity of each individual needle procedure.

A second example of culturally sanctioned infliction of pain on neonates and infants is routine non-therapeutic male circumcision. Male circumcision is a particularly interesting illustration of a culturally sanctioned painful procedure in infants because within the culture it is seen as normal but outside the culture it is very difficult to understand. Circumcision appears to have two major sociocultural roots. Religious circumcision has been common in Middle Eastern areas for centuries and continues today in our own society in some religious groups such as Judaism.

The second cultural root of circumcision relates to routine, non-religious circumcision and appears to have arisen out of the anti-masturbation hysteria of the late 19th century (e.g. Stall 1897). Circumcision was thought to discourage masturbation and assist through this mechanism or other unspecified mechanisms in the prevention of many diseases such as insanity, alcoholism, epilepsy, asthma, gout, rheumatism, curvature of the spine and headache, paralysis, malnutrition, night terrors, clubfoot, eczema, convulsions and mental retardation, promiscuity, syphilis and cancer. Recently, the justification for circumcision switched from prevention of sexual excesses to hygiene, especially the prevention of urinary tract infections.

The interpretation of the world evidence for a medical benefit of circumcision and recommendation

shows a sociocultural pattern. A recent meta-analysis from Australia (Singh-Grewal et al. 2005) found the improvement of risk of urinary tract infection to be present but insignificant for normal infants. An American commentator vehemently disagreed and endorsed the medical benefit of circumcision (Schoen 2005).

The rate of circumcision varies considerably by country and even by area of the same country. In the United States, except in the Western states, most males are still circumcised (National Centre for Health Statistics, accessed December 18, 2005, American Academy of Pediatrics 1999). Canadians have lower rates but it is not uncommon and in the UK circumcision is now rare.

Although social context is seldom cited in discussions of scientific evidence because scientists assume that they are immune to these influences, most commentators agree that parents make decisions about circumcision because of social considerations, especially whether the infant's father is circumcised.

It is not the purpose of this chapter to argue that social factors are the only factors in the decision to circumcise or to give needles but merely to emphasize that the understanding of needles or circumcision is more complete if social factors are considered.

INFANT AND NEONATAL PAIN HAS NOT BENEFITED MUCH FROM (OR BEEN HARMED BY) INDUSTRY INTEREST

Health issues such as infant and neonatal pain are typically seen as primarily influenced by scientific knowledge of a specialized group of professionals and scientists. There may be differing views in science and practice but these issues are seen as simply professional rather than social issues. It is no accident that major attention and resources are devoted to some health issues and other issues languish. The reasons for this are at least as much due to social influences as because of health burden or need.

For example, health problems that have patented drugs, especially recently patented drugs, as their solution is promoted by pharmaceutical companies funding research, by marketing to physicians, by so-called public education campaigns and by direct consumer marketing. Although the health benefits of these efforts have been severely criticized (Mansfield et al. 2005), these health issues become part of the public discourse, have resources devoted to them and are likely to be treated.

Let us look at some ways that having a drug company wanting to promote a product helps move the agenda of a problem forward. In terms of the patented drug market, the critical feature is obtaining an indication for use from the appropriate governmental agency (the Federal Drug Administration (FDA) in the United States). When a pharmaceutical is being developed for a market by a major pharmaceutical company, clinical trials must be developed by the company with consultation from scientists and professionals, clinical trials will be conducted in dozens of health centres, professional meetings will be funded to present the results of the trials, special issues of journals may be funded to ensure a venue for discussion, and scientists and professionals will be employed as speakers and consultants. The profile of a health problem will be enhanced in the professional and scientific arena.

Very few companies seek approval for drugs for neonatal and infant pain because the market is not large enough to justify the cost of the application for an indication. In spite of efforts by governments to interest companies in paediatric indications for drugs, it is often not financially advantageous for pharmaceutical companies to seek and obtain paediatric indications.

This lack of participation by pharmaceutical companies impacts on many aspects of infant and neonatal pain. For example, it is more difficult to maintain a research lab if there are no drug company studies to keep staff employed. Attendance at scientific and professional meetings and obtaining support to have speakers is more challenging without the support of industry. Funding of educational material and educational meetings for practitioners is more difficult if there is no major pharmaceutical company support.

Once the appropriate regulatory agency approves a drug for an indication, an army of drug company representatives is unleashed on the medical subspeciality most likely to prescribe the drug. The relationships of doctors to drug companies are complex as doctors need drugs to appropriately treat patients and companies sell products only if doctors prescribe it. However, the wooing of doctors is so aggressive that both physician organizations (e.g. Canadian Medical Association 2001) and organizations of pharmaceutical companies (e.g. Pharmaceutical and Research Manufacturers of America 2002) have found it necessary to develop ethical codes for relationships between physicians and industry. These ethical codes seek to restrict undue influence that pharmaceutical companies may have on what doctors prescribe.

Because analgesics for infants and neonates do not have a large market potential, few companies seek regulatory approval for their drugs. Many drugs used in infant and neonatal pain are generic drugs or drugs nearing the end of patent protection. As a result,

investigators are not drawn to the area, their research labs are not supported and there are fewer resources to bring infant and neonatal pain to the forefront. On the other hand, the lack of commercial incentive helps reduce industry-driven drug use.

SOCIAL CONTEXT INFLUENCES CHANGES IN PAIN MANAGEMENT

The past 20 years have seen significant change in behaviour of healthcare professionals in assessing and managing pain in neonates. However, these advances are not primarily attributable to technological discoveries or the development of new pharmacologic agents. The basic armamentarium of pain management in the neonate has not dramatically changed in this time, although research studies demonstrating the effectiveness and safety of pharmacological and non-pharmacological treatments have increased dramatically. More notably, there has been a clear shift in specific beliefs, attitudes and behaviour about neonatal pain. The changes in beliefs and attitudes and the influence on behaviour are well illustrated by a survey of paediatric anaesthetists in the United Kingdom and the Republic of Ireland that was completed in 1988 (Purcell-Jones et al. 1988) and then repeated in 1995 (De Lima et al. 1996). One of the first questions asked was whether perception of pain occurred in newborn infants less than a week old, neonates aged 1 week to 1 month, infants aged 1–3 months, infants aged 3–12 months and infants of less than 60 weeks' postconceptual age. In 1988, 13% thought newborns and 7% thought infants did not feel pain and 23% were undecided. By 1995, there was almost universal agreement that all groups perceived pain. This change in attitudes and beliefs was accompanied by changes in the behaviours of health professionals. The change in the prescribing of systemic opioids for babies of different ages is detailed in Figure 16.1. As the figure indicates, the use of systemic opioids increased at all ages, over the 7-year span. However, this increase was most dramatic in the newborns. Similarly, the rate of use of regional analgesia showed very sharp increases over time (see Fig. 16.2). Again, the increase was most evident in the youngest age groups but was very significant at all ages. The use of local anaesthetics and acetaminophen for minor surgery was also increased in 1995 as compared to 1988. These data reflect what anaesthetists say they do and, although one would expect that they are related to actual behaviour, there are likely to be some self-serving biases. Moreover, these data were gathered from paediatric anaesthesiologists and likely do not reflect the practice of those not in this

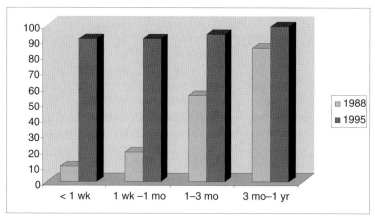

Figure 16.1 Percentage of UK anaesthetists reporting that they always or usually used systemic opioids in babies of different ages following major surgery (data from De Lima et al. 1996).

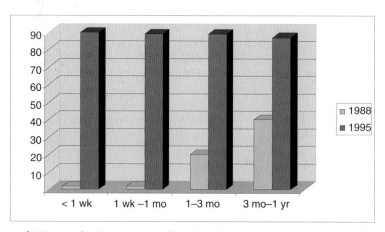

Figure 16.2 Percentage of UK anaesthetists reporting that they always or usually used regional analgesia in babies of different ages following major surgery (data from De Lima et al. 1996).

subspecialty. In the last 10 years this trend appears to have continued but the studies have not been done to firmly document this.

A Canadian study completed over a decade ago (Johnston et al. 1997) had 14 NICUs report from the medical records of their patients on pain management for 1 week. They found good analgesic coverage for postoperative pain but pain from procedures was less well managed. There were 2134 invasive procedures performed on 239 infants. Medication was given specifically for invasive procedures on 17 occasions. One hundred and twenty-nine invasive procedures were carried out while the infant was receiving analgesia for other reasons (e.g. surgery). The procedures for which analgesia was used at least 50% of the time were insertion of peripheral arterial line, urinary bladder catheterization and chest tube insertion.

Porter and colleagues (1997) focused on procedures in a survey of 374 clinicians (nurses and physicians) working in 11 Level II and four Level III nurseries in a large metropolitan area in the United States. Most physicians (59%) and nurses (64%) believed that infants can feel the same amount of pain as adults. About 27% believed that infants feel more pain and only 10% considered that infants feel less pain than adults. Clinicians rated the following nine procedures as at least moderately painful: endotracheal intubation, insertion of chest tube, circumcision, arterial or venous cutdown, lumbar puncture, intramuscular injection, insertion of peripheral intravenous line, heel stick and insertion of a radial or tibial arterial catheter. Three procedures, insertion of gavage tube, tracheal suctioning and insertion of umbilical catheter were seen as somewhat painful. Circumcision and insertion of chest tubes were considered the most painful procedures. Pharmacological agents were not thought to be used frequently even for the most painful procedures. Physicians thought that pharmacotherapy was used more often than did nurses. Com-fort measures were also not believed to be used commonly, although comfort measures were seen to be used more often than pharmacological agents. Both nurses and physicians felt that pharmacological and comfort measures should be used more frequently for the management of pain from procedures.

More recent studies in the Netherlands (Simons et al. 2003), in France (Debillon et al. 2002) and in Italy (Lago et al. 2005) have shown that only minor progress has been made in providing routine pain relief in NICUs. The number of needle sticks given and protection from pain in NICU babies has not dramatically changed. Some of this lack of progress is due to the current limits of science but much is because of local social context that does not see that it is necessary to protect neonates and infants from medical pain. Evidence for this comes from the wide variation in management of procedures where there is scientific and professional agreement on analgesic management. For example, Lago et al. (2005) found low rates but wide variation in the use of analgesia for endotracheal intubation even though an International Consensus statement stated that intubation without analgesia and sedation should be restricted to life-threatening situations when no intravenous access is available (Anand et al. 2001). The descriptive design of these studies precludes definitive statements about causal relationships between social context and pain management practices but does suggest that social context is important.

Controversy over what is appropriate management of neonatal pain has, and will continue to have, an impact on healthcare professionals who are caught between the current practices in their own unit, the comfort of their neonatal patients, the concerns of parents, and the debate in the scientific and professional literature and the popular press. The debate has shifted over the past decade. By the turn of the 21st century, we accept that neonates have pain and, in most centres, standard practice dictates that infants and neonates should, in most circumstances, receive analgesia for surgery. However, there is widespread agreement amongst idea leaders in the health professions that there is an urgent need for more aggressive pain management for painful procedures using both pharmacology and comfort measures as the practice of pain management for invasive procedures lags far behind other types of pain management, including postoperative pain. Part of the reason for this lag is the absence of unequivocal scientific information about effective management of procedure-related pain. However, the lack of knowledge is not as incomplete as practice would indicate. For example,

there are effective pharmacologic methods to control pain from the most painful procedures such as circumcision and chest tube insertion but they are not widely used. An extensive discussion of treatment of procedure-related pain can be found in appropriate chapters using both traditional and novel approaches.

Another area where there is little research is in the examination of pain in significantly cognitively impaired neonates and infants. Although there is an emerging interest in pain in cognitively impaired children (Guisiano et al. 1995, McGrath et al. 1998) there has been very little research on infants or neonates with cognitive impairment (Breau et al. 2004). They may be at particular risk for pain because of the nature and complexity of their medical conditions.

HOW HAS CHANGE OCCURRED?

Although neonatal pain management has changed, and continues to change, change has also been resisted. What has triggered change? Why did it take so long for us to be concerned about neonatal pain? Why does change in practice still lag behind what we know is possible from research? One can examine these questions from several different perspectives. In this section, we will briefly discuss how research scientists believe change occurs, how theorists knowledgeable about research utilization and innovation diffusion view change and our own perception of how change has occurred in neonatal pain. We will also examine some of the barriers that are evident in changing neonatal pain practices and speculate about how change is likely to occur in the future.

Scientists seem to believe that change will occur once they have results supporting the best strategy. For example, scientists assume that if a better way to manage pain from a procedure is developed, everyone will welcome and adopt this new way.

We have evidence that this belief is clearly wrong as, in spite of ample evidence of how the pain from some painful procedures such as circumcision can be decreased, these strategies are often not used. Our naive beliefs and assumptions about the use of research as a basis for changing practice fail to recognize that change is a multidimensional process that requires social influence as well as scientific evidence.

Changing practice is not a simple matter of applying what we know (research) to what we do (practice). In an extensive review of the literature, Scott-Findlay and Estabrooks (2006) concluded that research utilization is influenced by individual determinants, organizational determinants, the local context (e.g. the hospital unit) and the attributes of the innovation (e.g. the characteristics of the research and the clinical context).

None of these categories of determinants have been well studied, although more work has been done on individual determinants than on the others. Of nearly two dozen individual variables that have been identified, only three exerted statistically significant effects in terms of research utilization, attitudes towards research, in-services attended and belief suspension (Estabrooks 1997).

Theoretical models about how innovation occurs have also been developed. Rogers' (1995) work suggests that both the local context and innovation attributes are important. Estabrooks (1999a, 1999b) reported that a conceptual structure of research utilization, first described by social scientists and later introduced into nursing, asserts that research is used in different ways; instrumentally (procedurally), conceptually and persuasively (to influence decision makers). However, well-designed studies have not been possible on the process of research utilization, as (a) the descriptive work on the three main categories of determinants (individual, organizational and innovation) has been poorly developed and (b) studies that have included design interventions from research outside of nursing have not been able to demonstrate significant effects, because the interventions they have selected have been drawn from other work contexts that are not reflective of the nature and structure of the work of nursing in hospitals.

Hester and colleagues (1998) have applied Rogers' (1995) model of adoption of new practices to the case of pain measurement in children. They note that five attributes of any innovation influence the rate of adoption. These five attributes are:

1. relative advantage, the degree to which an innovation is seen as being better than what it supercedes;
2. compatibility, the degree that the innovation is seen as consistent with the values, past experiences and the needs of those who would adopt the innovation;
3. complexity, the degree that an innovation is seen as difficult to understand and use;
4. trialability, the degree that an innovation can be tried out on a limited basis;
5. observability, the degree to which the results of innovation are visible to others.

The vector of change in health practice is not entirely understood. Nurses report that they use knowledge gained through personal experience and interactions with co-workers and with individual patients rather than journal articles or textbooks (Estabrooks et al. 2005). According to a recent review of meta-analyses,

physician behaviour appears to be changed most effectively by interactive techniques (audit/feedback, academic detailing/outreach, and reminders) whereas clinical practice guidelines and opinion leaders are less effective. Lectures and distributing printed information have little or no beneficial effect in changing what physicians do (Bloom 2005). It may be that different professions use different approaches to knowledge transfer but sufficient research has not been done to determine that this is so.

Models of research utilization and innovation diffusion have not been sufficiently applied to neonatal pain but could assist in addressing the problem of research application to practice for individuals, institutions, professional organizations and policy makers.

Scattered scientific reports and reviews have appeared for years suggesting that full-term and premature neonates feel pain and should be treated for pain (e.g. Raju et al. 1980, Waugh and Johnson 1984). Even the ancient Greeks believed that infants were capable of pain sensation. In fact, Plato (about 400 BC) thought that, for infants, all feeling was essentially painful (Keele 1962). In 1656, the physician, Felix Wurtz questioned:

If a new skin in old people be tender, what is it you think in a newborn Babe? Doth a small thing pain you so much on a finger, how painful is it then to a Child, which is tormented all the body over, which hath but tender grown flesh? If such a perfect Child is tormented so soon, what shall we think of a Child, which stayed not in the womb its full time? Surely it is twice worse with him.

Quoted in Rurah (1925), pp. 204–205

In spite of the long history of scattered scientific reports, the randomized controlled trials conducted in the University of Oxford (UK) during the early 1980s were instrumental in popularizing the issue of pain in the neonate. Although these research studies were important in themselves, they were misinterpreted and sensationalized by the lay press, thus generating a public controversy that brought the issue of neonatal pain to national prominence in the UK. The authors of these studies, Anand and Aynsley-Green, set out to characterize and measure the physiological stress responses of neonates undergoing surgery. Their initial data, showing markedly accentuated hormonal responses in neonates, presented totally unexpected patterns (Anand and Aynsley-Green 1985). In trying to explain these findings, they discovered the prevalence of minimal anaesthesia used for the surgical correction of patent ductus arteriosus (Anand and

Aynsley-Green 1985). Of the 1157 neonates reported in published studies, only 23% were given analgesia (in small doses), whereas 77% received minimal (muscle relaxant with nitrous oxide) or no anaesthesia (muscle relaxant and oxygen). This practice was commonly known as the 'Liverpool technique', and it was employed as the standard anaesthetic technique in many hospitals around the world, including the John Radcliffe Hospital in Oxford.

Following this review, these researchers developed a pilot study to examine the stress responses of preterm neonates undergoing surgical ligation of a patent ductus. This study demonstrated that all preterm babies mounted massive hormonal and metabolic stress responses to the operative procedure (Anand and Aynsley-Green 1985). Finally, the research team devised randomized controlled trials to conclusively determine whether or not deep anaesthesia could blunt neonatal stress responses. This research group consulted methodological experts to ensure that the studies were scientifically sound and an independent ethics committee subjected all studies to careful ethical review. These clinical trials basically showed that potent anaesthesia substantially blunted the neonatal stress responses, and may have contributed to a better clinical outcome as compared to the neonates receiving minimal anaesthesia. This work was briefly mentioned in an editorial in the *British Medical Journal* (Richards 1985) and, when presented at the annual meeting of the British Paediatric Association in April 1986, it received the Michael Blacow Award as the best paper. The first report of these randomized clinical trials was published in January 1987 in *The Lancet* (Anand et al. 1987). The study was carefully scrutinized by the medical profession and reported in the press but did not receive a great deal of public notice. However, in June 1987, the Daily Mail, a London UK tabloid, featured this research in an article titled 'Pain-killer shock in babies' operations and questioned the ethics of the research. When Professor Aynsley-Green contacted the journalist to correct this misinformation, he was once again attacked in the Daily Mail under the headline: 'This test is a crying shame'. Thereafter, this controversy died down until 14 Members of the British Parliament, who belonged to the All-Party Parliamentary Pro-Life Group, issued a press release under the heading 'Inhumane baby operations slammed'.

This press release came at the same time that Anand was presenting additional data from full term neonates at the Fifth World Congress on Pain, sponsored by the International Association for the Study of Pain in August 1987 and planning the first edition of this book. The press release accused these investigators of barbarous experimentation and demanded an investigation by the General Medical Council Disciplinary Committee for misconduct and medical negligence. The uproar was immediate and widespread. Initially, the focus of press reports was on the accusations of the Members of Parliament.

However, quickly there was a rush of distinguished researchers and clinicians who pointed out that the studies were eminently ethical and, in fact, would lead to better care of babies. The control group had received what was standard practice, a practice that was unequivocally challenged by this research. Over the next few months several editorials in leading medical journals recounted the controversy and supported the ethical basis of these studies. Although the initial attacks by the Daily Mail and the All-party Parliamentary Pro-life Group were followed by a public apology, they had garnered a great deal of publicity for this research.

In this situation, as in the Lawson case, public controversy appeared to be effective in bringing about change. Unfortunately, public pressure is a very crude instrument for influencing change.

Public pressure may not distinguish between well-validated scientific findings and wild speculation. If public pressure is effective in changing practice without adequate research, harmful analgesic practices could become standard practice. As Eugene Braunwald (cited in Silverman 1985) has emphasized, the premature dissemination of a new medical technique, before evaluation by carefully designed clinical trials, is like the proverbial genie escaped from the bottle. It is impossible to undo the confusion resulting from unrestrained therapeutic exuberance.

Institutional change does not occur rapidly and the spotlight of the media on neonatal pain is inconsistent and notoriously short. Those intending to influence policies might consider attempting media coverage of neonatal pain but should be cautious as one cannot control the media or the reaction of one's colleagues to media coverage.

Change in neonatal pain management has occurred within the larger social matrix. Continued change may benefit from a larger social systems view that considers the social factors that influence policies and behaviour in the NICU.

HOW COULD MEDICAL PEOPLE IGNORE PAIN IN INFANTS AND NEONATES?

One might well wonder how intelligent, dedicated and decent individuals who care deeply for their patients could continue to ignore pain in infants or neonates that they are caring for. Parents of infants and laypersons generally believe that the relief of pain and suffering is a primary end point of medical care. Unfortunately, as Cassell (1982) notes, this goal is often not shared by physicians. With infants and neonates, there may be particular forces that encourage ignoring pain.

'It took me a few days to stop thinking of them as people, as human beings, and to revert to seeing them primarily as receivers of treatment' (the comment of a Neonatology Fellow on returning to service in the NICU after an absence of several months). Two potent factors that may permit ignoring of infant and neonatal pain are denial and desensitization. In order to function effectively in the NICU and to perform invasive procedures on neonates without analgesia or with limited pain relief, physicians and nurses may rely on denial. Denial may consist of blunting of emotions or rationalizing the validity of the procedures that are being performed without any pain relief or with inadequate pain relief. Such denial or rationalization occurs for a variety of emotive and cognitive reasons.

The first reason is that, in the past, medical and allied health training had tended to give little attention to paediatric pain management. This situation has dramatically changed. For example, pediatric pain research presented at the Pediatric Academic Societies Annual meetings (the principal American venue for paediatric research) quadrupled from fewer than ten abstracts in 1988 to more than 40 in 1993 (Schechter 1997). Similarly, Rana (1987) reviewed the leading English language textbooks of paediatrics and found that there was virtually no information on pain (less than one page out of 12 000 pages). Today, every major paediatric text has full chapters on pain and pain management and pain is discussed throughout the texts. Similarly, the production of published papers in paediatric pain has risen dramatically (Guardiola and Banos 1993, Schechter 1997). Although we have no documentation as to the change in neonatal pain literature, the changes in the paediatric field, in general, have included changes in the neonatal literature.

Although education has improved and awareness of neonatal pain has increased, denial may still play a role. Infant responses to pain may be explained away as reflexive or random movement. Denial in professionals, who hold to this point of view, is primarily a cognitive reaction since neonatal pain perception is not believed to be possible. Denial also becomes emotive when professionals are confronted with their own suspicion and increasing evidence that their hypotheses about neonatal pain are erroneous. To acknowledge that one has caused pain to infants even though one's practice has been accepted medical

practice and has arisen from the highest of motives, is a difficult task.

A second difficulty in medicine is the understandable preoccupation with survival, in some cases to the exclusion of all else (Fletcher 1987). Pain treatment may be considered of secondary importance, especially if methods of pain relief are believed to be potentially harmful to the patient. These views are harder to maintain as the evidence for safety of analgesia improves.

Even 20 years ago, in spite of the prevailing view that neonatal pain was of little consequence, many healthcare professionals were concerned with neonatal pain. As Fletcher (1987) emphasized, neonatal pain perception was not denied by all:

Certainly not by those of us at the bedside of critically ill infants, who see them flinch from procedures, startle in response to loud noises, and turn from bright lights and various other forms of stimulation. Not by those who have heard infants' anguished cries and seen their vigorous withdrawals from painful stimuli. Not by those who have observed their increasing heart and respiratory rates and profuse sweating in response to heel sticks or circumcision.

Fletcher 1987, p. 1347

A professional who has come to know a neonate intimately has more chance to learn how to differentiate between neonatal pain behaviour and behaviour related to other needs. However, they may be tempted to attribute behavioural distress to the absence of a parent or disruptions in routine rather than to painful stimuli.

Third, there are also social factors about neonates themselves and about work in a NICU, which may limit the extent that professionals will become personally familiar with their patients. Neonates who are surrounded by complex medical equipment, essential to maintaining life, do not have the same cuddly appeal that one anticipates on seeing a newborn. The very premature baby also has very thin limbs, underdeveloped facial features, little visible bodily hair and high-pitched, irritating cries. In addition, the neonate may have been born with an apparent disability and/or congenital anomalies. The problem of appearing, in some sense, less like the expected healthy newborn is compounded by the neurological and physiological immaturity of neonates as compared to older infants.

Fourth, reduced social reciprocity between the health professional and the neonate may also lead to less intimacy between the health professional and the neonate. Healthy neonates enjoy eye contact, vocalizing and physical interaction with their parents and their professional caregivers.

The responsiveness of the neonate encourages increased attention and nurturing behaviour on the part of parents and healthcare professionals. However, an ill neonate has very little capability to engage in social exchanges, thereby reducing the likelihood that a health caregiver will initiate social attention. Moreover, reduction in handling of sick neonates because of the potential distress that may come from handling may limit the opportunities for social interaction. As discussed in Chapter 22, this may have an important effect on the parent–child attachment.

Fifth, the demands of caring for ill neonates will limit the time that is available for observation and social contact. Moreover, in the busy, highly stressful context of the NICU environment, the importance of and the time for social contact may not be recognized.

Sixth, social reciprocity between neonate and health professional is also hindered by the very real life and death struggle that exists for many neonates, especially the very preterm infant. Professionals may reserve their attachment to a neonate whose state can alter rapidly between life and death. There may be considerable anxiety over the expected quality of life that would result if the baby lives. Limited social reciprocity and detachment between neonate and health professional leads to a greater ability to distance oneself from the neonate, to be less observant of pain-related behaviours and to consciously or subconsciously deny that the neonate is capable of feeling or expressing pain.

Finally, the highly technical environment of the NICU itself allows for dehumanization in the same way that other ICU environments are characterized by bright lights without periods of darkness, excessive auditory stimulation and heightened levels of activity with frequent medical crises. Complex and highly technical solutions to problems can easily be seen as the only solutions in the NICU environment (Butler 1986, Fletcher 1987).

Desensitization has negative consequences for the neonate, the parents and the parent–professional relationship, and for professionals themselves. The most serious consequence of desensitization is that symptoms of pain behaviour and the sequelae of pain are undetected, minimized, or denied and changes in neonatal pain management are resisted. These scenarios result in unnecessary suffering for neonates with further possible health trauma as a result of physiological distress and the potential for long-term sensitization to pain.

Most parents approach a sick neonate naively expecting the infant to be as responsive to pain as an older baby. Parents have a strong emotional investment in wanting to love, nurture and protect this new baby and will be especially observant of behaviours in the neonate which may be indicative of pain. Parents will assume that their neonates are anaesthetized for surgical procedures and that they are given pain relief for invasive procedures. If neonates do not receive adequate analgesia, parents may feel they have failed in protecting their child (Harrison 1986, Lawson 1986, Stern 1987).

It has long been known that parents of babies in the NICU are highly stressed (Miles et al. 1993). Sources of parental distress include the physical environment (bright lights, noisy equipment and smells), seeing their babies hooked up to equipment and the loss of their expected, and in particular the parental caregiving and protective, roles that they were anticipating to fulfil (Franck et al. 2005a).

If parents also observe that professionals are not perceptive to symptoms of pain behaviour in their baby or that they do not provide adequate pain relief, hostility, a sense of failure or, ironically, acceptance of professional denial of neonatal pain may occur. Increased public awareness of controversy in neonatal pain (e.g. Fischer 1987, Stern 1987) may exacerbate the friction between parents and professionals. Such early, negative, experiences between parents and healthcare professionals may have deleterious effects on future health care for the child and the family.

Franck and colleagues (2005b) conducted a study of nine neonatal units (196 parents) in the United Kingdom and two neonatal units in the United States (61 parents). Parents thought that their babies had experienced moderate to severe pain that was considerably greater than they had expected. Only 4% of parents reported receiving written information about infant pain but 58% said that they had been told about pain. Few parents said they had been told about how to determine if their baby was in pain but about half were told ways to comfort their infant. The methods that were suggested (and the percentage receiving each suggestion) were: positioning (41%); pacifier (25%); patting or rocking (21%); swaddling (21%); feeding (15%); music or toys (5%) and other methods (14%). Across all units in both countries, parents were stressed by the extent of their infant's pain and the lack of ability to care for their babies.

Unfortunately, for some parents, the resultant feelings of guilt that, as parents, they were unable to protect their child from unnecessary pain might be very stressful and may lead to over-sensitization and hostility towards health professionals.

Health professionals who are convinced by the scientific evidence and their clinical experience in a NICU that neonates do feel pain, but who are unable to provide relief because they either do not have the authority to do so or they believe they cannot challenge or change current practices of their unit, may feel increasingly helpless, depressed and disillusioned about neonatal care. In addition, those who recognize pain are presented with another problem. Although there are good strategies of pain management for some procedures, there remains significant scientific uncertainty about how to control pain from some of the most common procedures in neonates (e.g. heel sticks). The inability to provide adequate pain relief may cause internal conflict or arouse feelings of guilt or hopelessness.

Changes in pain management per se have worked in concert with widespread efforts to change the environment of NICUs. The most comprehensive approach is that developed by Als and her collaborators (e.g. Als et al. 1986). More efforts are being made to decrease noxious stimuli in the neonatal environment by decreasing light intensity and auditory stimulation, by providing more opportunity for uninterrupted sleep, by comforting infants using positioning and swaddling. A more detailed discussion of behavioural and environmental approaches to pain management can be found in Chapter 12.

STANDARDS OF CARE IN NEONATAL PAIN ARE CHANGING

Institutions in their general standards and professional associations in their ethical standards seldom detail exact procedures that should be followed in specific situations but rather expect a standard of care that should be provided. Detailed protocols in many different forms are in place in some institutions for specific aspects of neonatal pain. In addition, professional associations or other organizations have developed more specific practice guidelines. Practice guidelines and institutional protocols are intended to guide behaviour but are phrased to allow professional judgement. Along with research articles, professional articles and material in widely used textbooks, these documents combine with actual practice to set a standard of care. Although often invoked in a non-legal context, standard of care has been most widely discussed in the legal literature, especially in the negligence literature. The non-legal notion of standard of care is very similar to the concepts involved in civil negligence with one important difference. Institutional and professional standards may be designed to provide both a minimum acceptable level but also to present goals to be attained. Standards of care in

negligence law are minimum standards. An important question is 'What is the standard of care against which a specific physician or nurse dealing with a specific infant should be ethically and legally judged?' Clearly, it is not good enough for a physician or nurse just to do his or her best if it is below what is an acceptable standard of care. On the other hand, the law and ethical guidelines do not insist that care must be the best possible care, just reasonably good care.

Standard of care has received many interpretations. Historically, the standard of care of rural doctors was lower than that of urban doctors. This locality rule was designed to protect rural doctors in a time when isolation prevented those outside the major centres from keeping up with medical advances. Sharpe (1987) has outlined four levels of standard of care. These levels are: (1) common practice in the immediate locality of the professional accused of negligence; (2) common practice in similar locations; (3) common practice in relation to the medical resources available to the health professional; (4) national minimum standard of a reasonable and prudent practitioner.

Sharpe (1987) suggests that both American and Canadian courts have tended to use the third level to determine standard of care in negligence. This standard is also likely to be true of professional ethical bodies. The third level requires the appropriate use of consultation and referral to a major medical centre if one is available. Due to the rapid dispersal of medical knowledge and the ready access to consultation and referral, it is no longer accepted that standards of care should vary across most geographic areas. A person practicing in a NICU in one setting would generally not be held to a different, lower, standard of care than someone practicing in another NICU. However, they might be legitimately practicing at a lower level than the most advanced unit.

Standards of care develop both from the top down, in the form of statements by professional bodies but also bottom up, in the form of common practice by prudent practitioners. Documenting top down guidelines is much easier than determining what is common practice.

The concept of standard of care does not necessarily mean that the average standard of care is acceptable if that average is deficient. The standard of care that the courts or ethical boards would expect is that of a reasonable and prudent professional. In rapidly changing areas such as neonatal pain, the reasonable and prudent professional, one might argue, should not rely on past practice or standard texts that may be out of date. Furthermore, it is always open to a court or ethical board to raise the standard of care if they feel it is appropriate. We know of no legal or ethics cases on this topic. However, standards of care are helpful in prompting behaviour outside of the legal and ethical domains.

Statements and guidelines of professional or governmental agencies play an important role in determining what a reasonable physician or nurse should do and consequently, what the standard of care is. However, only the most naïve would believe that these top down approaches automatically cause changes in practice.

Many policy and consensus documents have influenced what the standard of care in neonatal pain should be. We will review several of the most influential. The first was the joint statement of the American Academy of Pediatrics (1987) and the American Society of Anesthesiologists (1987). This statement includes the following opinion:

local or systemic pharmacologic agents are now available to permit relatively safe administration of anesthesia or analgesia to neonates undergoing surgical procedures, and that such administration is indicated according to the usual guidelines for the administration of anesthesia to high-risk, potentially unstable patients [any decision to withhold an algesia or anesthesia] should be based on the same medical criteria used for older patients. The decision should not be based solely on the child's age or perceived degree of cortical maturity.

American Society of Anesthesiologists 1987, p. 12

The second document was the Clinical Practice Guideline for Acute Pain Management published by the US Agency for Health Care Policy and Research (Acute Pain Management Guideline Panel 1992). This guideline discusses the measurement, strategies for treatment and institutional responsibility for pain management. The importance of this document for neonatal pain lies in the unequivocal endorsement of the need for neonatal pain management by a blue ribbon panel, who studied and reviewed the research literature at the request of the US Department of Health and Human Services. These documents provided official sanction for the necessity of pain management in neonates and have had an important influence on practice.

Both of these early documents put the prevention and amelioration of infant and neonatal pain on the clinical and research agenda. As previously noted, policy documents and consensus statements do not change practice by themselves but they provided a justification for change.

One of the most significant landmarks in the efforts to obtain better pain care in healthcare institutions was the issuing and subsequent implementation of pain assessment and management standards by the Joint Commission on Accreditation of Healthcare Organizations (JCAHO). The standards were developed in close collaboration with the American Pain Society. JCAHO accredits healthcare organizations in the United States. Inclusion of pain standards in accreditation was landmark because it signalled that the healthcare establishment recognized that pain was an important issue in health care. Healthcare institutions take accreditation very seriously as their reputation and financial health depend on maintaining accreditation.

Accreditation standards differ from clinical guidelines. Most importantly, accreditation standards are not directed to clinicians dealing with individual patients but are directed to organizations and the administrators. Accreditation standards require institutional change and are used in judgement of the adequacy of an organization rather than guidance in clinical cases.

The JCAHO accreditation standards in pain (JCAHO 2003) are based on the need to recognize the right of patients to appropriate assessment and management of pain. The standards require screening all patients for pain and recording the results, ensuring staff knowledge and competence in pain measurement and ensuring that policies and procedures support pain management and that monitoring of pain management is incorporated into performance activities of the health organization.

The JCAHO standards are for all patients and thus include pain in infants and neonates. The standards do not provide any specific directions for infants or neonates. It is not clear how much accreditation standards have improved pain management as primarily anecdotal reports are all that are available (Gallagher 2003).

Two consensus documents have recently focused on pain in neonates and infants. The joint statement by the American Academy of Pediatrics and the Canadian Paediatric Society (2000) endorsed the need to measure pain in the neonate using appropriate measures and to provide safe and effective pharmacological, behavioural or environmental interventions to prevent and treat neonatal pain and stress. The joint statement has been very influential because it specifically focused on neonates and infants and was from the pre-eminent organizations in infant health. The credibility of the sponsoring organizations is of the highest order across all areas of infant and neonatal health. The guidance is clear and endorses the latest research on pain in the neonate. For example, the long-term negative impact of pain, the need to avoid unnecessary pain, the need to use drugs that are not approved for use in neonates, the validity of pain measures in neonates and the need for staff education are all discussed.

A more recent consensus document (Anand et al. 2001) sponsored by an educational grant from a drug company, was headed by Anand and included a very wide variety of specialists from many different countries. The document was more detailed and inclusive than previous documents. A list of eight general principles provides the basis for a change in the entire social context of pain. For example, after stating that pain occurs frequently in neonates and is often unrecognized and untreated, the basic principles note that many different behavioural, environmental and pharmacological treatments are effective. Finally, individual health professionals and units are tasked with the responsibility to assess, prevent and manage pain and to develop and implement protocols and guidelines for neonatal pain.

Anand et al. (2001) document 25 common painful procedures done in the NICU and outline four published neonatal pain measures. Recommended doses for analgesics for neonates are detailed. The authors outline 13 specific procedures and general strategies for reducing and managing pain and discuss adverse events associated with analgesics.

This consensus document does not attempt to replace clinical judgement but the expertise and breadth of the authors and the detailed prescriptive recommendations establishes a new standard of care for pain in the NICU.

The standards of care for infant and neonatal pain have become well established and now provide a clear basis for research-based care. The ways that guidelines, consensus statements and accreditation documents influence care are difficult to determine. However, they provide an important part of the structure upon which change in neonatal and infant pain has been built.

CONCLUSIONS

Social context influences many aspects of infant and neonatal pain and pain management. Neonatal pain occurs in contexts that are influenced by social factors. Although there has been little research on the influence of social context of neonatal pain perception, work with infants would suggest that there may even be social influences on pain perception in neonates. Changes in the practice of pain management have clearly occurred over the last 25 years. Changes appear to be due to both scientific research and to socio-political lobbying, primarily by parents. Although the standard of care for neonatal pain has risen dramatically in the past 15 years, much remains to be done. Procedural pain appears to be a continuing issue and pain in the cognitively handicapped neonate has not been widely addressed.

ACKNOWLEDGEMENTS

Patrick McGrath is supported by a Canada Research Chair in paediatric pain. His research on pain in neonates and infants is supported by the Canadian Institutes of Health Research. Anita Unruh's research is supported by the Social Sciences and Humanities Research Council.

REFERENCES

Acute Pain Management Guideline Panel. (1992). Management of postoperative and procedural pain in infants, children, and adolescents: Clinical Practice Guideline. United States Department of Health and Human Services, Public Health Service.

Als H, Lawhon G, Brown E, et al. (1986). Individualized behavioral and environmental care for the very low birth weight preterm infant at high risk for bronchopulmonary dysplasia: Neonatal intensive care unit and developmental outcome. Pediatrics 78: 1123–1132.

American Academy of Pediatrics. (1987). Neonatal anesthesia. Pediatrics 80: 446

American Academy of Pediatrics, Task Force On Circumcision. (1999).

Circumcision policy statement. Pediatrics 103: 686–693.

American Academy of Pediatrics and Canadian Paediatric Society. (2000). Prevention and management of pain and stress in the neonate. A joint statement. Pediatr Child Health 5: 31–38.

American Society of Anesthesiologists. (1987). Neonatal anesthesia. ASA Newsletter 51: 12.

Anand KJS, Aynsley-Green A. (1985). Metabolic and endocrine effects of surgical ligation of patent ductus arteriosus in the human preterm neonate: are there implications for further improvement of postoperative outcome? Mod Prob Pediatr 23: 143–157.

Anand KJS, Sippell WG, Aynsley-Green A. (1987). Randomized trial of fentanyl

anesthesia in preterm babies undergoing surgery: Effects on the stress response. Lancet January: 243–247.

Anand KJS and the International Evidence-based Group for Neonatal Pain. (2001). Consensus statement for the prevention and management of pain in the newborn. Arch Pediatr Adolesc Med 155: 173–180.

Bloom BS. (2005). Effects of continuing medical education on improving physician clinical care and patient health: a review of systematic reviews. Int J Technol Assess Health Care 21: 380–385.

Breau LM, Camfield CS, McGrath PJ, et al. (2004). Risk factors for pain in children with severe cognitive impairments. Develop Med Child Neurol 46: 364–371.

Butler NC. (1986). The NICU culture

versus the hospice culture: Can they mix? Neonatal Netw 5: 35–42.

Butler NC. (1988). More on neonatal pain. Perinatal Press 11: 19–21.

Canadian Medical Association. (Update 2001). Physicians and the pharmaceutical industry. CMA Policy. Online. Available: http://policybase.cma.ca/PolicyPDF/PD01-10.pdf

Carter JD, Mulder RT, Bartram AF, et al. (2005). Infants in a neonatal intensive care unit: parental response. Arch Dis Child Fetal Neonatal Ed 90: F109–F113.

Cassell EJ. (1982). The nature of suffering and the goals of medicine. New Engl J Med 306: 639–645.

Debillon T, Bureau V, Savagner C, et al. (2002). Pain management in French neonatal intensive care units. Acta Paediatr 91: 822–826.

De Lima J, Lloyd-Thomas AR, Howard RF, et al. (1996). Infant and neonatal pain: Anaesthetists' perceptions and prescribing patterns. BMJ 313: 787.

Estabrooks CA. (1997). Research utilization in nursing: An examination of formal structure and influencing factors. Unpublished doctoral dissertation, Faculty of Nursing, University of Alberta, Edmonton, Alberta.

Estabrooks CA. (1999a). The conceptual structure of research utilization. Res Nurs Health 22: 203–216.

Estabrooks CA. (1999b). Modeling the individual determinants of research utilization. West J Nurs Res 21: 758–772.

Estabrooks CA, Chong H, Brigidear K, et al. (2005). Profiling Canadian nurses' preferred knowledge sources for clinical practice. Can J Nurs Res 37: 118–140.

Fischer A. (1987). Babies in pain. Redbook October: 124–125, 184–186.

Fletcher AB. (1987). Pain in the neonate. N Engl J Med 317: 1347–1348.

Franck LS, Cox S, Allen A, et al. (2005a). Measuring neonatal intensive care unit-related parental stress. J Adv Nurs 49: 608–615.

Franck LS, Allen A, Cox S, et al. (2005b). Parents' views about infant pain in neonatal intensive care. Clin J Pain 21: 133–139.

Gale G, Franck LS, Kools S, et al. (2004). Parents' perceptions of their infant's pain experience in the NICU. Int J Nurs Stud 41: 51–58.

Gallagher RM. (2003). Physician variability in pain management: are the JCAHO standards enough? Pain Med 4: 1–3.

Guardiola E, Banos J. (1993). Is there an increasing interest in pediatric pain? Analysis of the biomedical articles published in the 1980s. 1. Pain Symptom Man 8: 449–450.

Guisiano B, Jimeno MT, Collignon P, et al. (1995). Utilization of a neural network in the elaboration of an evaluation scale for pain in cerebral palsy. Meth Inf Med 34: 498–502.

Harrison H. (1986). Letter to the editor. Birth 13: 124.

Harrison H. (1987). Pain relief for premature infants. Twins 10-1(1): 53.

Hester NO, Foster RL, Jordan Marsh M, et al. (1998). Putting pain measurement into clinical practice. In: Finley GA, McGrath PJ (eds). Measurement of pain in infants and children, pp. 179–198. IASP Press, Seattle.

JCAHO (Joint Commission on Accreditation of Healthcare Organizations). (2003). Improving the quality of pain management through measurement and action. Online. Available: http://www.JCAHO.org accessed December 29, 2005.

Johnston CC, Collinge JM, Henderson SJ, et al. (1997). A cross-sectional survey of pain and pharmacological analgesia in Canadian neonatal intensive care units. Clin J Pain 13: 308–312.

Keele KD. (1962). Some historical concepts of pain. In: Keele CA, Smith R (eds) Proceedings of the International Symposium held under the auspices of the University Federation for Animal Welfare, Middlesex Hospital, London, pp. 12–27.

Lago P, Guadagni A, Merazzi D, et al. (2005). Pain management in the neonatal intensive care unit: a national survey in Italy. Paediatr Anaesth 15: 925–931.

Lawson JR. (1986). Letter to the editor. Birth 13: 124–125.

McGrath PJ, Rosmus C, Camfield C, et al. (1998). Behaviours care givers use to determine pain in non-verbal, cognitively impaired individuals. Dev Med Child Neurol 40: 340–343.

Mansfield PR, Mintzes B, Richards D, et al. (2005). Direct to consumer advertising. BMJ 330: 5–6.

Miles MS, Funk SG, Carlson J. (1993). Parent stressor scale: Neonatal intensive care. Nurs Res 42: 148–152.

National Centre for Health Statistics, National Hospital Discharge and Ambulatory Surgery Data. Online. Available: http://www.cdc.gov/nchs/about/major/hdasd/nhds.htm. Accessed December 18, 2005.

Pharmaceutical and Research Manufacturers of America. (2002). PhRMA code on interactions with healthcare professionals. Online. Available: http://www.phrma.org/files/PhRMA%20Code.pdf.

Porter EL, Wolf CM, Gold J, et al. (1997). Pain and pain management in newborn infants: a survey of physicians and nurses. Pediatrics 100: 626–632.

Purcell-Jones G, Dormon E, Sumner E. (1988). Pediatric anaesthetists perceptions of neonatal and infant pain. Pain 33: 181–187.

Raju TNK, Vidyasagar D, Torres C, et al. (1980). Intracranial pressure during intubation and anesthesia in infants. Pediatrics 96: 860–862.

Rana SR. (1987). Pain – A subject ignored. Pediatrics 79: 309–310.

Richards T. (1985). Can a fetus feel pain? Br Med J 291: 1220–1221.

Rogers EM. (1995). Lessons for guidelines from the diffusion of innovations. 1. Quality Impr 21: 324–328, 366–368.

Rovner S. (1986). Surgery on premises done without pain killers. San Francisco Chronicle August 26: 15, 17.

Ruhrah J. (1925). Pediatrics of the past. Paul B. Hoeber, New York.

Scanlon JW. (1987). The stress of unanesthetized surgery. Perinatal Press 10: 82.

Schechter NL. (1997). The status of pediatric pain control. Child Adolesc Psychiat Clin North Am 6: 687–702.

Schoen EJ. (2005). Circumcision for preventing urinary tract infections in boys. North American view. Arch Dis Child 90: 772–773.

Scott-Findlay S, Estabrooks C. (2006). Knowledge translation and pain management. In: Finley GA, McGrath PJ, Chambers CT (eds) Bringing pain relief to children. Humana Press, Totowa, NJ.

Sharpe G. (1987). The law and medicine in Canada, 2nd edn. Butterworth, Toronto.

Silverman WA. (1985). Human experimentation: a guided step into the unknown. Oxford University Press, Oxford.

Simons SHP, van Dijk M, Anand KJS, et al. (2003). Do we still hurt newborn babies? A prospective study of procedural pain and analgesia in neonates. Arch Pediatr Adolesc Med 157: 1058–1064.

Singh-Grewal D, Macdessi J, Craig J. (2005). Circumcision for the prevention of urinary tract infection in boys: a systematic review of randomised trials and observational studies. Arch Dis Child 90: 853–858.

Stall S. (1987). What a young boy ought to know. Vir Publishing, Philadelphia, PA.

Stern S. (1987). Shielding infants from surgical pain. The Tribune, Oakland, CA. Feb 5, CI, C2.

Waugh R, Johnson GG. (1984). Current considerations in neonatal anesthesia. Can Anaesth Soc J 31: 700–709.

17

Evidence-based practice as a means for clinical decision making

Arne Ohlsson
Vibhuti Shah

INTRODUCTION

This chapter provides an introduction on understanding how the clinical decision-making process for neonatal and infant pain management can be informed by applying the concepts of evidence-based medicine/practice, randomized controlled trials, systematic reviews and clinical practice guidelines. A brief history of how evidence regarding neonatal pain evolved is provided. The decision-making process is illustrated using a synopsis approach (evidence based on reviews and individual studies) to the clinical question 'Do local anaesthetics reduce pain associated with venepuncture in neonates/infants?'

EVIDENCE-BASED MEDICINE/PRACTICE

The term 'evidence-based medicine' (EBM) was introduced by Guyatt (Guyatt 1991). He stated: 'For the clinician, evidence-based medicine requires skills of literature retrieval, critical appraisal, and information synthesis. It also requires judgment of the applicability of the evidence to the patient at hand and systematic approaches to make decisions when direct evidence is not available'. EBM was later described as the 'conscientious, explicit, and judicious use of current best evidence in making decisions about the care of individual patients' (Sackett et al. 1996). It is not 'cookbook' medicine but requires the integration of individual clinical expertise and the best external evidence (Sackett et al. 1996). The essential steps in the emerging science of EBM (Greenhalgh 1997) include:

- Converting informational needs into answerable questions.
- Collecting, with maximum efficiency, the best evidence to answer these questions, which may come from the clinical examination, the diagnostic laboratory, the published literature or other sources.
- Appraising the evidence critically to assess validity (i.e. closeness to truth), reliability (i.e. reproducibility) and utility (i.e. applicability) in clinical practice.
- Implementing the results of this appraisal in clinical practice.
- Evaluating performance.

EBM requires that the healthcare professional critically appraises the best available research papers at the appropriate time and, if indicated, alters his/her behaviour (and, what might be more difficult, alters the behaviour of other people) in light of relevant evidence (Greenhalgh 1997). The concepts of EBM apply to all healthcare providers; therefore, given that pain management is a transdisciplinary team approach to patient care, we will use the term evidence-based practice (EBP) throughout this chapter.

RANDOMIZED CONTROLLED TRIALS AND SYSTEMATIC REVIEWS

Randomized controlled trials (RCTs) and systematic reviews of RCTs form a sound foundation to develop EBP guidelines and guide further research (Ohlsson 1994, 1996, Cook et al. 1997, Mulrow et al. 1997). The idea of the controlled trial to assess the effectiveness of an intervention goes back to biblical times (Daniel, The Holy Bible). However, the methodology of the RCT as used today was introduced by Bradford-Hill in a trial of streptomycin in pulmonary tuberculosis over half a century ago (MRC Streptomycin in Tuberculosis Trials Committee 1948). The idea of critical appraisal of available information is not new. James Lind's (1953) 'Treatise of the scurvy (in three parts)', published in 1753 contains 'An inquiry into the Nature, Causes and Cure, of that Disease together with a Critical and Chronological View of what has been published on the subject'. One hundred and fifty years later, the James Lind Library was established in the UK by Chalmers, the founder of the Cochrane Collaboration (Chalmers 2005). The James Lind Library website (http://www.jameslindlibrary.org) is dedicated to patients and professionals whose involvement in clinical research has contributed evidence about the effects of treatments in health care.

THE COCHRANE COLLABORATION

When the practicing healthcare professional asks a question regarding the effectiveness of a certain intervention for a clinical condition, she/he is often overwhelmed by the amount of available information. In 1972, Cochrane published his seminal work 'Effectiveness and efficiency; random reflections on health services' (Cochrane 1972). He stressed the lack of an adequate knowledge base for much of the care provided and made a strong case for the evaluation of new and existing forms of care in controlled trials. He later proposed a need to review research evidence systematically. Cochrane stated: 'It is surely a great criticism of our profession that we have not organized a critical summary, by specialty or subspecialty adapted periodically of all relevant randomized controlled trials' (Cochrane 1979). Mulrow (1987) identified the lack of scientific methods to identify,

assess and synthesize information in medical review articles. These ideas and observations led to the creation by Chalmers of the Oxford Database of Perinatal Trials, innovative textbooks based on systematic reviews (Chalmers et al 1989, Sinclair and Bracken 1992) and the first Cochrane Centre in Oxford, England in 1992 (Ohlsson 1996).

The Cochrane Collaboration aims to help individuals make well-informed decisions about health care by preparing, maintaining and promoting the accessibility of systematic reviews of the effects of healthcare interventions (The Cochrane Library 2005). The Cochrane Library is an electronic publication that publishes quarterly the results of systematic reviews in all areas/fields of health care. The Cochrane Library is a valuable source for identifying RCTs. There are currently (as of September, 2005) 454 449 entries to RCTs in The Cochrane Library compared to 218 355 in February, 1999 (The Cochrane Library 1999). Of these citations, 18 316 RCTs involve neonates or infants; identified using the search terms 'Infant' OR 'Newborn'. The Cochrane Collaboration has developed methods to systematically review and synthesize the evidence from RCTs using meta-analytic techniques (The Cochrane Library 2005). This technique allows for an increase in statistical power and more precise estimates of the effect size. Cochrane systematic reviews tend to have greater methodological rigour and are more frequently updated than systematic reviews published in non-electronic format (Jadad et al. 1998). However, in a comparison of the quality of Cochrane reviews and systematic reviews published in paper-based journals, Shea et al. (2002) found that Cochrane reviews were better at reporting some items and paper-based reviews were better at others. The overall quality was found to be low but the authors reported that the Cochrane Collaboration had taken steps to improve the quality of its reviews, through more thorough prepublication refereeing, developments in the training and support offered to reviewers, and in the system for post-publication peer review.

The evidence from Cochrane Systematic Reviews should be interpreted in conjunction with other available evidence outside of RCTs. Policy and decision makers need to interpret evidence in the context of the needs, resources and priorities in the local setting, be it a specific health region or an individual neonatal/perinatal/paediatric unit. Systematic review, like any other research method, is open to critique (Feinstein 1995, Crombie and McQuay 1998, Gardosi 1998). However, critics agree that a systematic approach to the review of a healthcare-related topic is a major advance over the narrative review by one or several experts in the field that previously was the norm.

Guidelines on reading systematic reviews and interpreting the results of discordant reviews are readily available (Oxman and Guyatt 1998, Akobeng 2005) on the Critical Appraisal Skills Programme web site: http://www.phru.nhs.uk/ casp/casp.htm. The advantage of an electronic publication like The Cochrane Library is that critique can be incorporated in subsequent editions (updated quarterly) and errors can be addressed and corrected shortly after being detected. The systematic review is a powerful tool for teaching current evidence regarding healthcare interventions (Badgett et al. 1997). There is evidence that neonatologists use systematic reviews and modify their practice accordingly (Jordens et al. 1998).

The Cochrane Library (2005) currently lists six systematic reviews regarding pain management in the neonate/infant (Table 17.1), three references to reviews published in paper-based journals (included in the Database of Abstracts of Reviews of Effects (DARE)) but no reference to Health Technology Assessments. Of the six reviews related to neonatal/ infant pain, two conclude that there is insufficient data to draw conclusions and make recommendations for practice (Bellù et al. 2005, Craven et al. 2005). This conclusion is not surprising as a survey of reviewers' conclusions found that more evidence was needed in 90 of the113 Cochrane Neonatal Reviews published at that time (Sinclair et al. 2003). Two somewhat overlapping reviews on pain related to circumcision (Brady-Fryer et al. 2005, Taddio and Ohlsson 2005) give clear recommendations as do reviews on the use of sucrose (Stevens et al. 2005) and on venepuncture versus heel lance (Shah and Ohlsson 2005) (Table 17.1). Both of these reviews (first published in 1998 and 1999 respectively) were updated twice when new information became available; this updating is a

valuable and important feature of The Cochrane Library.

A BRIEF HISTORY OF THE EVOLVING EVIDENCE THAT NEONATES/INFANTS EXPERIENCE PAIN

Evidence that newborn infants experience pain was documented as early as 1518 when Jörgen Ratgeb painted Jesus' circumcision (Luke, The Holy Bible, Ohlsson et al. 2000). In this picture, it is evident that the two male grown-up bystanders show the facial expressions of pain, clearly expressing empathy with the boy and perhaps remembering their own painful experiences? An old man comforts Jesus and a young man holds a chalice likely containing sweet wine as means of managing Jesus' pain (Fig. 17.1a). The crying Jesus shows the same facial expressions that were later depicted in an etching of the same event by Rembrandt in 1630 (Schwartz 1977) (Fig. 17.1b). Darwin (1872) also commissioned photographs and described the facial, vocal and bodily expressions of pain in infants (Figure 17.1c). He wrote:

- 'Infants, when suffering even slight pain, moderate hunger, or discomfort, utter violent and prolonged screams.
- Whilst thus screaming their eyes are firmly closed, so that the skin around them is wrinkled, and the forehead contracted into a frown.
- The mouth is widely opened with the lips retracted in a peculiar manner, which causes it to assume a squarish form; the gums or teeth being more or less exposed.'

Similar observations form the basis for several validated neonatal pain scales today.

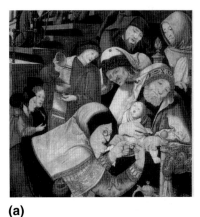
(a)

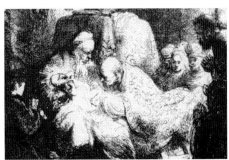
(b)

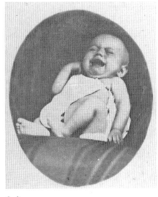
(c)

Figure 17.1 (a) Circumcision. Altar in Herrenberg, Germany by J. Ratgeb, 1518/1519. (b) Circumcision. Etching by Rembrandt 1630. (c) Photo of crying child. Commissioned by Darwin 1872.

Table 17.1 Systematic reviews on pain in neonates and/or infants in The Cochrane Library, Issue 3, 2005

Authors, year of 1st publication and updates if any	Title	Number of trials/patients included	Implications for practice*	Implications for research*	Conclusions*
Taddio et al. 1999	Lidocaine-prilocaine cream for analgesia during circumcision in newborn boys	3/139	Routine use of single dose EMLA for neonatal circumcision pain in settings where no analgesics are administered is recommended. EMLA is not recommended over other analgesic techniques with proven efficacy, such as regional nerve block with lidocaine	To determine the relative and combined efficacy of different analgesic techniques/dosage regimens for circumcision further research is recommended. To facilitate systematic review, investigators are encouraged to design research studies with similar outcomes, and report results consistently	EMLA reduces pain response during circumcision in newborn male infants. Other potentially more effective forms of analgesia for circumcision (such as dorsal penile nerve block (DPNB), ring block) should be subjected to systematic review
Bellù et al. 2005	Opioids for neonates receiving mechanical ventilation	13/1505	There is insufficient evidence to recommend routine use of opioids in mechanically ventilated newborns. Opioids should be used selectively, when indicated by clinical judgment and evaluation of pain indicators. If sedation is required, morphine is safer than midazolam	Only selective use of opioids in mechanically ventilated newborns is recommended. Future large, well-conducted studies should enroll only newborns who express indicators of pain (based on best available pain scores) when on mechanical ventilation. Medium/long term neuro-developmental consequences of opioid treatment have not been adequately addressed	There is insufficient evidence to recommend routine use of opioids in mechanically ventilated newborns. Opioids should be used selectively, when indicated by clinical judgment and evaluation of pain indicators. If sedation is required, morphine is safer than midazolam. Further research is needed

Table 17.1 Systematic reviews on pain in neonates and/or infants in The Cochrane Library, Issue 3, 2005—*cont'd*

Authors, year of 1st publication and updates if any	Title	Number of trials/patients included	Implications for practice*	Implications for research*	Conclusions*
Brady-Fryer et al. 2004	Pain relief for neonatal circumcision	35/1984	DPNB was the most effective for circumcision pain. EMLA was less effective. Both interventions were safe for use in newborns. No studied intervention completely eliminated the pain from circumcision	Future studies should compare two or more active interventions for pain relief. Although sucrose cannot be recommended for circumcision pain at this time, the effect of combining oral sucrose with other interventions should be pursued	DPNB was the most frequently studied intervention and was the most effective for circumcision pain. Compared to placebo, EMLA was also effective, but was not as effective as DPNB. Both interventions appear to be safe for use in newborns. No studied intervention completely eliminated pain from circumcision
Craven et al. 2003	Regional (spinal, epidural, caudal) versus general anaesthesia in preterm infants undergoing inguinal herniorrhaphy in early infancy	4/122	There is no convincing evidence to support the use of spinal anaesthesia in inguinal herniorrhaphy in ex-preterm infants. Spinal anaesthesia may reduce postoperative apnoea in infants not pretreated with respiratory depressants	Larger studies are needed to identify the risk benefit ratio of spinal anaesthesia versus general anaesthesia. Strict pre-study definitions of outcome measures are required and must be consistent between individual surgical centres	No reliable evidence concerning the effect of spinal as compared to general anaesthesia on the incidence of postoperative apnoea, bradycardia, or oxygen desaturation in ex-preterm infants undergoing herniorrhaphy exists. A large well designed randomised controlled trial is needed

Continued

Table 17.1 Systematic reviews on pain in neonates and/or infants in The Cochrane Library, Issue 3, 2005—*cont'd*

Authors, year of 1st publication and updates if any	Title	Number of trials/patients included	Implications for practice*	Implications for research*	Conclusions*
Stevens and Ohlsson 1998 Updated twice Last update 2004	Sucrose for analgesia in newborn infants undergoing painful procedures	21/1616	Sucrose reduces procedural pain from heel lance and venepuncture in neonates, with minimal to no side effects. The routine use of sucrose 0.012–0.12 g administered 2 min prior to single heel lance and venepuncture for pain relief in neonates is recommended. As pain scores were reduced by approximately 20%, other methods of pain relief should be considered for use in combination with sucrose administration to reduce or eliminate pain in this population	Repeated administrations of sucrose in neonates needs to be investigated. There is a need to evaluate the use of sucrose in combination with other behavioural and pharmacologic interventions for more invasive procedures and in neonates that are very low birth weight, unstable and/or ventilated. Replication of existing studies of high methodological quality and using identical validated outcomes would allow for combination of results in meta-analyses	Sucrose is safe and effective for reducing procedural pain from single painful events (heel lance, venepuncture). There was inconsistency in the effective dose of sucrose. An optimal dose for use in preterm and/or term infants could not be identified. The use of repeated doses of sucrose needs to be investigated. The use of sucrose in combination with other behavioural and pharmacologic interventions as well as in neonates who are of very low birth weight, unstable and/or ventilated needs to be addressed
Shah and Ohlsson 1999 Updated twice Last update 2004	Venepuncture versus heel lance for blood sampling in term neonates	3/357	Venepuncture, performed by a trained phlebotomist, appears to be the method of choice for blood sampling in term neonates	Further well-designed randomized controlled trials need to be conducted. The interventions should be compared in settings where several individuals perform the venepuncture and the heel lance	Venepuncture, performed by a skilled phlebotomist, appears to be the method of choice for blood sampling in term neonates. In future well designed randomized controlled trials the interventions should be compared in settings where several individuals perform the venepuncture and the heel lance

*The information under these three headings has been shortened by the authors of this chapter.

Over the centuries, there was little progress in the prevention and management of infant pain. We quote from a standard textbook of paediatric surgery (Swenson 1958):

- 'A skilled anaesthesiologist can provide such necessary conditions for the operation as proper relaxation of abdominal musculature which is an immense help to the surgeon.'

- 'Premature infants require no preoperative sedation.'

- 'Procaine 0.5% can be used satisfactorily for premature infants since pain perception seems to be less acute in them than in full-term infants.'

- 'Limiting the general anesthesia to those intervals of the operation which require the infant to be quiet and relaxed is less dangerous than maintaining a full general anesthesia for the whole procedure.'

In the early 1980s studies on the physiological, hormonal and behavioural responses to pain in neonates started to appear in the research literature. A decrease in transcutaneous PO_2 as a response to pain associated with circumcision (Rawlings et al. 1980), the hormonal responses to venepuncture (Fiselier et al. 1983) and increases in heart rate and crying as a reaction to heel lance were reported in the early 1980s (Owens and Todt 1984). Anand et al. (1985a, 1985b) studied the endocrine and metabolic stress responses to surgery in the neonate. These studies indicated that neonates/infants react to pain with physiologic and hormonal stress responses.

The first controlled trial of an intervention for pain in infants was probably by Palmer (1962), who in a double-blind controlled study involving 86 infants with teething pain found that an active gel (choline salicylate) was more effective than placebo. The major breakthrough for controlled trials studying neonatal/infant pain seems to have occurred in the early 1980s. The dorsal penile nerve block (DPNB) technique for neonatal circumcision was introduced by Kirya and Werthman (1978). In a controlled double-blind investigation by Holve et al. (1983), 15 infants received regional anaesthesia by DPNB by injection of lidocaine, eight underwent DPNB with saline and eight were circumcised without undergoing DPNB. DPNB with lidocaine was shown to significantly reduce the time spent crying and the mean increase in heart rate. The authors concluded 'Physicians who

circumcise newborns have good reason to employ the technique of DPNB with lidocaine to minimize infant pain and distress'. Harpin and Rutter (1983), in a RCT, demonstrated that a mechanical lancet was considerably less painful than manual heel lance. Blomquist et al. (1983) tested dicycloverin chloride solution as a remedy for infantile colic. Of these studies, only Harpin and Rutter (1983) used random allocation for assignment of infants to study groups.

AWARENESS AMONG PARENTS AND HEALTHCARE PROFESSIONALS THAT NEONATES/INFANTS EXPERIENCE PAIN

Owens (1984) suggested that our everyday usage of the term pain be applied to infants: 'Essentially this suggestion is that we infer that an infant has a subjective experience that is unpleasant when there is evidence of tissue damage and the infant responds with signs of distress, such as crying, increased heart rate, facial expression consistent with distress or other signs'. He advised that multidisciplinary research teams (physicians, nurses, psychologists, biologists and anthropologists) may develop the best research ideas. The inclusion of parents in perinatal research teams was proposed later (Ohlsson 1996).

By 1985 the public and healthcare professionals became more aware of the consequences of untreated neonatal pain. Scanlon wrote an editorial in Perinatal Press protesting the 'barbarism' of surgery without anaesthesia for newborn babies (Scanlon 1985). He had been alerted by a mother of a preterm baby boy, who was under his care and who developed a patent ductus arteriosus (PDA). Scanlon later referred the boy to another institution for operation of the PDA. The mother (Jill Lawson, see below) related that her son had been operated on without any anaesthesia – the only drug given was one causing muscular paralysis. Next year Jill Lawson and Helen Harrison, mothers of preterm infants who underwent surgery with muscle paralysis but no anaesthesia, wrote letters to the Editors of *Birth*. Jill Lawson's son Jeffery (Lawson 1986) was born preterm in February 1985 and underwent surgery for a PDA while paralyzed with Pavulon but not anaesthetized and he died a month later. Helen Harrison's baby boy Edward was shunted without anaesthesia for hydrocephalus, while paralyzed with curare (Harrison 1986). He survived with severe impairment. His mother noted later that 'he reacts to the simplest medical procedures or the mere sight of the hospital with violent trembling, profuse sweating, screaming, struggling, and vomiting'. Rovner (a journalist) published the Jeffery Lawson story in The Washington Post in August of 1986 (Rovner 1986). Lawson, Harrison and Scanlon became advocates for improved pain management in infancy.

Possibly in response to this debate, the Committee of Fetus and Newborn of the American Academy of Pediatrics published a one-page statement on neonatal anaesthesia in 1987 (American Academy of Pediatrics 1987) ascertaining that 'There is an increasing body of evidence that neonates, including those born preterm, demonstrate physiological responses to surgical procedures that are similar to those demonstrated by adults and that these responses can be lessened with anesthetic agents'. The decision to withhold anaesthetic agents should not be based solely on the infant's age or perceived degree of maturity.

In October 1999, Baños et al. (2001) performed a Medline search on articles on neonatal pain published from 1965 to 1999. They used a broad search strategy: 'pain' (MeSH terms) OR 'pain' (Title word) OR 'pain' (All fields), AND 'infant, newborn' (MeSH terms). The printout was reviewed to establish pertinence to the study's objective, which was to analyse articles on neonatal pain indexed in Medline from 1965 to 1999. Of 2490 references identified 545 were considered relevant to neonatal pain. Most papers were published in English. The first authors of 316 citations came (in descending order) from the US (38.6%), Canada (14.2%), the UK (13.3%) and other countries (33.9%). The main subjects of the articles were pain related to colic (20.4%), general neonatal pain issues (13.6%) and procedural pain (13.4%). Of the 545 articles identified, 70 (12.8%) were randomized clinical trials first appearing in the early 1980s. The authors concluded: 'Pain in neonates was a neglected subject of publication until the mid-1980s, and currently, only a few countries seem interested in this type of pain. This lack of interest may be related to the undertreatment of pain in the neonatal period'. There were very few articles published between 1965 and 1985 but a sharp rise occurred after 1985 (see Fig. 17.2). We repeated an identical Medline search from November 1999 to September 1st, 2005 and identified an additional 255 articles on neonatal/infant pain.

We suggest that it was consumers like Lawson and Harrison, supported by physicians like Anand and Scanlon, who exerted the greatest impact on making the general public and the healthcare professionals aware of neonatal pain. This awareness resulted in an increased interest in this topic after 1985 or at least a close temporal association is evident.

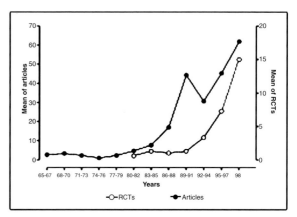

Figure 17.2 Temporal evolution of articles and randomized controlled trials (RCTs) on neonatal pain (1965 to 1998). The figure shows the mean number of articles and RCTs for every three consecutive years. The last point corresponds to 1998 and represents only the absolute number of papers in this year. Papers from 1999 are not represented because the indexing process of the database used was incomplete at the time the search was performed. (This information was originally published in Baños et al. (2001). Pain Research and Management 6(1): 45–50.)

THE NEED FOR EFFECTIVE PAIN MANAGEMENT IN NEONATES UNDERGOING PAINFUL/STRESSFUL PROCEDURES

Ample evidence has been presented that fetuses that are mature enough to survive outside of the womb with or without extensive life support have the anatomical, biochemical and physiological requisites in place to respond to painful stimuli (Anand and Hickey 1987, Perreault et al. 1997). Memories for early painful events may not be accessible to conscious recall, but are incorporated in the subconscious or procedural memory, coded by structural and functional changes within the pain system and other neuronal assemblies. In sharp contrast to previous views, a recent systematic review on fetal pain concluded that the 'evidence regarding the capacity for fetal pain is limited but indicates that fetal perception of pain is unlikely before the third trimester... the capacity for conscious perception of pain can arise only after thalamocortical pathways begin to function, which may occur in the third trimester around 29 to 30 weeks' gestational age, based on limited data available' (Lee et al. 2005). Based on the evidence that has been documented over the last decades regarding fetal and neonatal pain this systematic review is likely to result in a vivid debate among healthcare researchers, professionals and consumers. Issues associated with this debate are further described in Chapters 1 and 13.

Analgesics include acetaminophen, opioids, local anaesthetics and sweet-tasting substances. Comfort measures may also reduce stress and pain responses. All of these infant pain management strategies are described in detail in Chapters 9–12. Also, several extensive narrative reviews of the use of analgesics/anaesthetics including local anaesthetics in newborns have been published (Bell 1994, Bhatt-Mehta 1996, Bucher and Bucher-Schmid 1996). Systematic review techniques were first applied in the late 1990s to sucrose (Stevens et al. 1997, 2005), EMLA (Taddio et al. 1998, Taddio and Ohlsson 2005) and venepuncture vs. heel lance for blood sampling (Shah and Ohlsson 2005).

EVIDENCE-BASED NEONATAL PAIN GUIDELINES

Evidence-based guidelines regarding the prevention and management of neonatal pain have been published and have incorporated the findings of Cochrane reviews and systematic reviews published in paper-based journals in addition to other evidence (American Academy of Pediatrics and Canadian Paediatric Society 2000, Anand and International Evidence-Based Group for Neonatal Pain 2001, Larsson et al. 2002, Anand et al. 2005, Aranda et al. 2005). The uptake of these recommendations by healthcare providers remains low (Simons et al. 2003).

THE USE OF LOCAL ANAESTHETICS IN THE PREVENTION OF PAIN RELATED TO VASCULAR ACCESS IN NEONATES AND INFANTS

Guyatt has suggested a mnemonic '4S' for pre-processed EBM resources (Guyatt 2004):

- The individual *study*
- The *systematic review* of all the available studies on a given problem
- A *synopsis* of both individual studies and summaries, and
- *Systems* of information.

To illustrate how EBP can be applied to common interventions that are painful in neonates and infants, we chose the 'synopsis' approach suggested by Guyatt (2004) where we synthesized information from both systematic reviews and RCTs that were published following systematic reviews. We used the **PICO** (Population, Intervention, Comparison, Outcome) approach to frame our questions and to search the literature.

- P = Population (neonates/newborns and/or infants (≤ 1 year of age))

- I = Intervention (local anaesthetic agents (lidocaine, combination of lidocaine-prilocaine, amethocaine, liposomal lidocaine) in isolation or in combination with other analgesic agent, sweetening agent or behavioural/environmental procedures)
- C = Comparison (comparing one local anaesthetic agent vs. no intervention vs. another pain reducing intervention)
- O = Outcome (pain assessment according to a validated pain scale for neonates/infants, changes in behavioural, physiological and biochemical parameters).

Our main question was: In neonates/infants undergoing venepuncture/venous access, which local anaesthetic agent in isolation or in combination with other interventions compared to no intervention (placebo) or another intervention is effective and safe in reducing pain, as assessed by a validated outcome measure?

GENERAL SEARCH STRATEGY

Electronic databases including Medline (1966 – August 2005), EMBASE (1980 – August 2005), CINAHL (1982 – August 2005) and The Cochrane Library were searched using the following MeSH headings: [infant, newborn OR neonate]; AND [vascular access OR blood vessel catheterization OR vein catheterization OR central venous catheterization OR phlebotomy] AND [randomized controlled trial OR controlled clinical trial OR clinical trial OR random allocation] AND [local anaesthetic agent OR anaesthetic agent OR analgesic agent]. The search was expanded using the following terms/textwords: pain, pain assessment, venepuncture, long line, lidocaine, lidocaine-prilocaine cream, amethocaine and liposomal lidocaine. No language restrictions were applied. In addition, the databases were searched for reviews and guidelines. Abstracts and RCTs in which we could not extract information relevant to infants were excluded. The quality of identified trials was assessed independently by the two authors using the following criteria proposed by the Cochrane Neonatal Collaborative Review Group: blinding of randomization, blinding of intervention, blinding of outcome measure assessment and completeness of follow up. There are three potential answers to these questions: yes, no and cannot tell. There is no numerical weight assigned to the answers following these questions. Concealed allocation of study subjects to treatment and control groups is the most important design aspect of a randomized controlled study and can always be achieved even if the blinding of the interventions cannot be accomplished. A 'yes' answer to all four questions would indicate high study quality and that the results are likely to be valid. Data were abstracted onto data collection forms by one author and checked for accuracy by the second author and discrepancies were resolved by consensus. The statistical package RevMan 4.2.8 of the Cochrane Collaboration was used to combine data when at least two identified trials evaluated the same intervention, reported on the same outcome and were of sufficient quality (The Cochrane Library 2005).

SPECIFIC INTERVENTIONS

Using the synopsis approach we synthesized information from both systematic reviews and RCTs for different painful interventions.

Amethocaine gel vs. placebo for venepuncture, venous cannulation/peripheral insertion of central catheters (PICC)

One systematic review (O'Brien et al. 2005) and four studies evaluating the effectiveness of amethocaine gel

for venepuncture ($n = 2$), venous cannnulation ($n = 1$) and PICC insertion ($n = 1$) were identified. The quality of included trials was good (Table 17.2).

Jain and Rutter (2000) evaluated 40 infants of 27–41 (median 33) weeks gestation at 2–17 (median 7) days of age undergoing venepuncture. They were randomized to receive either 1.5 g of 4% (w/w) amethocaine gel or 1.5 g placebo on the dorsum of the hand. The gel was covered with Tegaderm and removed 60 min later. The infant was left to settle for 5 min and venepuncture was performed by one of several neonatal senior house officers with 3–24 months paediatric experience, or by a neonatal nurse practitioner using a 21-gauge needle. Pain response to needle insertion was assessed using a validated adaptation of the neonatal facial coding system (NFCS) and by the presence and duration of crying (Rushforth and Levene 1994). The infants were videotaped during the procedure. Independent assessors scored the presence or absence of eye squeeze, brow bulge, open mouth, deepened nasolabial folds, and cry for each second, starting 5 seconds before and ending

Table 17.2 Studies on venepuncture/venous cannulation/peripherally inserted central venous catheter

Trials	Interventions	Blinding of intervention	Blinding of follow-up	Complete outcome	Blinding of randomization measurement
Jain and Rutter 2000	Amethocaine gel vs. placebo	Yes	Yes	Yes	Yes
Long et al. 2003	Tetracaine patch vs. placebo	Yes	Yes	Yes	Yes
Moore and Stretton 2001	Amethocaine gel vs. placebo	Yes	Yes	Yes	Yes
Ballantyne et al. 2003	Tetracaine gel vs. placebo	Yes	Yes	Yes	Yes
Larsson et al. 1998	EMLA vs. placebo	Yes	Yes	Yes	Yes
Acharya et al. 1998	EMLA vs. placebo	Yes	Yes	Yes	Yes
Lindh et al. 2000	EMLA vs. placebo	Cannot tell	Yes	Yes	No
Gradin et al. 2002	EMLA vs. 30 % glucose	Yes	Yes	Yes	Yes
Abad et al. 2001	Four groups were compared: 2 ml of sucrose (24%) vs. EMLA alone vs. EMLA and sucrose (24%) vs. 2 ml of spring water (placebo)	Yes	Yes	Yes	Yes

5 seconds after needle insertion. A cumulative NFCS score of ≤10 in the first 5 seconds after needle insertion was considered to indicate no or minimal pain. The total length of crying in response to needle insertion (defined as a cry starting within 5 seconds of needle insertion and finishing with a gap of at least 30 seconds before any further cry) and the number of punctures required to obtain the sample were recorded. Of 40 subjects enrolled, one (amethocaine group) was excluded before the code was broken due to restlessness before the venepuncture. Demographic characteristics were similar between groups. Of the 19 amethocaine-treated infants, 16 (84%) showed little or no pain compared with six of 20 (30%) in the placebo group (P = 0.001). The median (interquartile range (IQR)) cumulative NFCS score over the 5 seconds after needle insertion was 3 (0–9) in the amethocaine group compared with 16 (8–18) in the placebo group (P = 0.001). Fifteen of 19 (79%) samples were collected at first attempt in the amethocaine group compared with 13 of 20 (65%) in the placebo group (non-significant (NS)). No adverse reactions were noted. The authors concluded that topical amethocaine provided effective pain relief during venepuncture in newborns.

Long et al. (2003) enrolled 34 (two withdrawn after randomization) infants with gestational age (GA) of 32–42 (median 36) weeks and postnatal age of 3–18 (median 6) days to receive a tetracaine-containing patch or placebo applied to the dorsum of the hand 30 min before venepuncture. Pain assessment was performed using a validated adaptation of the NFCS and the presence of cry. The infants were videotaped for 20 seconds before and after the procedure. The investigators used the same criteria as Jain and Rutter (2000) to define clinically effective anaesthesia (no or minimal pain). The baseline characteristics of the study infants were similar. The median cumulative NFCS scores during the 5 seconds immediately before the venepuncture were 0 in both groups. The median cumulative NFCS scores between the groups scored over the 5 seconds immediately following the venepuncture was 0 in the tetracaine group compared with 12.5 in the placebo group (P = 0.0002). Fourteen of 15 (93%) tetracine-treated neonates presented with little or no pain in response to the procedure compared with six of 17 (35%) in the placebo group (P = 0.01). No local skin reactions were noted in either group. The authors concluded that a tetracaine patch produced effective pain relief for venepuncture.

Moore and Stretton (2001) in a double-blind placebo-controlled RCT enrolled 40 infants of >32 weeks gestation to assess the effectiveness of amethocaine gel before cannulation. One duplicate publication of this trial was identified (Moore 2001). The appropriate gel (amount not provided in either paper) was administered and covered with Tegaderm for 30 min and baseline heart rate was recorded 30 min before its removal. The infant was then settled and cannulation performed by a physician. During the procedure, the doctor and a nurse observed responses in facial expression, cry and heart rate. A pain assessment tool was designed using the three variables and assigned a score from 0–3 (maximum score 9) for each parameter. An additional parameter, 'ease of cannulation' to indicate difficulty of intravenous access was incorporated. A good analgesic effect was demonstrated in the amethocaine group as there were significant differences (Mann-Whitney U test) in the mean (SD) pain scores between the groups (1.7 (1.45) vs. 5.7 (1.23) (P < 0.01)) favouring the amethocaine group. Moore concluded that amethocaine gel is an effective local anaesthetic for venepuncture.

Ballantyne et al. (2003) enrolled 49 infants (two infants with incomplete data were excluded from the original sample of 51) with GA from 27 to 41 (mean 33, SD 4.2) weeks and age at the time of insertion of catheter from 2 to 85 (mean 18, SD 22.5) days in a RCT to determine the efficacy of tetracaine gel for the treatment of pain associated with PICC line insertion. Thirty min before the procedure, infants randomized to the tetracaine gel group received 1 g of 4% (w/w) tetracaine gel and infants in the control group received 1 g of placebo cream. The cream was covered with an occlusive dressing. After the specified application time, the dressing was removed, and the drug was wiped off. Both groups received comforting measures of non-nutritive sucking and swaddling throughout the procedure. The same type of catheter was used in all infants and inserted by a group of five specially trained nurses. Pain responses were assessed using the Premature Infant Pain Profile (PIPP). Total scores of ≤6 indicate minimal or no pain and scores of ≥12 indicate moderate to severe pain (Stevens et al. 1996). Data were collected during the PICC procedure: application of the study medication, baseline (infant comfortably placed in either supine or lateral position and left undisturbed (1 min)), preparation (cleaning and draping of the site (1 to 5 min)), PICC (catheter insertion and application of dressing (3 min)) and recovery (infant was returned to the previous comfort position (1 min)). Even though the PICC procedure lasted from 3 to 8 min, the first 3 min were used to standardize the observation period across patients. Facial action was videotaped from baseline to recovery phase while physiologic indicators were recorded using a Hewlett-Packard monitor. No clinically significant differences in mean PIPP scores between the two groups across the PICC phases were noted, nor during the 3 min of the PICC insertion phase when analysed by GA group (<32 weeks and ≥32 weeks). The authors concluded that tetracaine gel was not effective for pain relief for PICC insertion.

The results for the outcome of pain excess of 'little or no pain' could be combined using meta-analysis from two studies (Jain and Rutter 2000, Long et al. 2003). The relative risk was 0.17 (95% confidence interval (CI) 0.07, 0.45), the risk difference (RD) was –0.56 (95% CI –0.37, –0.74). The number needed to treat (1/RD) to avoid one infant experience more than 'little or no pain' was 2 (95% CI 1–3). There was no between-study heterogeneity ($I^2 = 0$) for this outcome making the findings robust (Higgins et al. 2003).

In summary, available evidence indicates that the use of amethocaine gel or patch is effective in reducing pain from venepuncture/cannulation, but is ineffective in preventing pain associated with PICC insertion in infants. These conclusions agree with the recently published review by O'Brien et al. (2005).

Eutectic mixture of local anaesthetics (EMLA) vs. placebo

Taddio et al. (1998) included one study in abstract form (now published as a full paper) and one study that we could not verify as an RCT. Three RCTs were identified for inclusion in this review.

Larsson et al. (1998) randomized 120 neonates undergoing venepuncture to receive either EMLA or placebo. Five hundred mg of EMLA or placebo was placed on the dorsum of the hand and covered with Tegaderm for 60 min. After removal of Tegaderm and the test substance, the area was warmed for one min by placing the child's hand between the warm hands of the nurse. The skin was cleaned and the vein was penetrated with a needle measuring 0.9 × 40 mm. After skin puncture, the infants were left undisturbed for 60 s. Thereafter, if necessary, manipulation and additional skin punctures were made in order to obtain sufficient blood. One nurse performed all procedures while a second nurse spoke into audio-recording equipment and recorded the procedure. All infants were observed for 12 hours to ascertain the possibility of methaemoglobinaemia. Facial actions were videotaped and NFCS scores were analysed by two observers during the first 15 seconds after the skin was punctured (0–15 seconds) and again after a pause of 60 seconds, during the first 15 seconds when manipulation took place (60–75 seconds). Six facial actions were scored (total possible range 0–600). The audio-tape was reviewed to determine the latency to cry from skin puncture, duration of first cry and total time the infant cried during the procedure. Duration

of the procedure to obtain the required sample and number of skin punctures required were recorded. Five neonates were excluded in the EMLA group; two as they cried prior to skin puncture and three due to video-equipment failure. Four neonates were excluded in the placebo group; two as they cried prior to skin puncture, one due to video-equipment failure and one as consent was withdrawn. The median total NFCS score after skin puncture was 287 for the EMLA group vs. 374 for the placebo group (P = 0.016). The median total NFCS score during manipulation was not different between groups (288 vs. 407; P = 0.18). Infants in the EMLA group had shorter duration of the first cry than the placebo group (median 11 vs. 33 seconds; P < 0.05). The duration of the procedure was shorter in the placebo group (125 vs. 145 s; P = 0.01). The authors concluded that EMLA significantly reduced pain caused by venepuncture.

Acharya et al. (1998) in a double-blind placebo-controlled cross-over RCT enrolled 19 infants with a median and range GA of 31 (26–33) weeks, postnatal age of 21 (3–65) days and birth weight of 1.56 (0.92–2.25) kg. Infants randomly received EMLA or placebo on first venepuncture. The alternative cream was used on second venepuncture. Test substance (0.5 ml) was applied on the dorsum of the hand or foot and covered with Tegaderm for 60 min. After removal of the cream, the infant was allowed to settle for 10 min. The same doctor performed all venepunctures using a 21-gauge needle. The procedure was divided into three phases: pre-procedure (beginning of recording to needle insertion, lasting 2.5 min), procedure (from needle insertion to removal) and post-procedure phase (from needle removal to end of recordings, lasting 2.5 min). Heart rate and oxygen saturations were recorded every 30 seconds throughout while blood pressure was recorded twice during each phase. The infant's facial action and cry were video-recorded. Verbal cues were given by the doctor at the point of limb holding, needle insertion and removal. Thirty seconds of the tape before and after needle insertion were analysed by two authors on separate occasions and blinded to the study intervention. The duration of first cry (from onset to end of first cry (cessation of crying for 5 s)) and total duration of cry (from onset of first cry to cessation of all crying for 30 s) were analyzed. The difficulty to perform venepuncture and local changes at the site of cream application were recorded. Methaemoglobin concentrations were measured at 1 and 8 h after the application. There were no differences in physiological and behavioural responses between the groups. Methaemoglobin levels were increased at 8 h in the EMLA group with no evidence of clinical toxicity. The authors concluded that their findings did not support the routine use of EMLA for venepuncture in healthy preterm infants.

Lindh et al. (2000) evaluated the efficacy of EMLA on pain response to venepuncture in 60 3-day-old healthy (GA 37–42 weeks) newborns using frequency domain analysis of heart rate variability and incidence of crying compared to placebo. One g of EMLA or placebo was applied on the dorsum of the baby's left hand, covered with Tegaderm and removed after 60 min. Ten min after removal the hand was warmed with a water-filled glove for 2 min. Venepuncture was performed using a 20-gauge needle. The baby was breast-fed within 1 hour before the recording and one parent held the baby during the procedure. Heart rate recordings were divided into three different sequences (5 min baseline period, 2 min of warming the hand and venepuncture and 80 s of blood sampling). Three segments were selected for statistical analysis: from 60 to 140 seconds of the baseline, the last 80 seconds of the warming sequence and 80 seconds starting from the beginning of the venepuncture sequence. Mean heart rate and spectral analysis of heart rate variability were used to assess the pain response to venepuncture. Crying was taped and categorized as 'instant' if a cry occurred within 30 seconds after the venepuncture, 'delayed' if the baby started to cry 30–80 seconds after the skin puncture, and as 'silent' if no cry was present. The EMLA-treated group had a statistically significant lower mean (SD) heart rate when compared to the placebo group (130 (17) vs. 144 (20) (P = 0.03)); an increase in heart rate variability (4.31 (0.4) vs. 4.1 (0.35) (P = 0.05)); and low-frequency power (4.23 (0.44) vs. 4.0 (0.39) (P = 0.04)). Instant crying after venepuncture occurred in four babies in the EMLA and in nine in the placebo group (P = 0.212). Delayed crying was present in five cases in the EMLA and seven in the placebo group (P = 0.12) (NS). Based on the findings of mean heart rate and spectral analysis of heart rate variability the authors concluded that EMLA decreases the stress response during venepuncture in newborn infants.

The data from three trials identified for this review could not be combined because of differences in the reporting of the results. Two studies showed EMLA to be effective whereas a third did not.

Sweetening agent vs. EMLA

No systematic reviews and two RCTs were identified.

Gradin et al. (2002) enrolled 201 newborns with GA ≥36 weeks and postnatal age of >24 hours but <30 days. Infants were randomized to receive EMLA on the skin and oral placebo (sterile water) or glucose (30%) and placebo on the skin. EMLA (0.5 g) or

placebo was placed on the dorsum of the hand and covered with Tegaderm. Sixty min later Tegaderm and the test substance were removed. The infant was left undisturbed for 15 min to reduce any constriction of the vein and to recover from the stress associated with removal of the dressing. The infant was placed on a preheated nursing table and a pulse-oximeter was attached to record baseline heart rate and oxygen saturation. A 1 ml dose of 30% glucose or water was administered by syringe into the infant's mouth. The assistant nurse visualized the vein and cleaned the skin. A staff member or the parent stood by the infant's head and was encouraged to give the infant a pacifier or their own finger to suck on. After venepuncture (21-gauge needle) the infant was left undisturbed for 3 min. Pain response was measured by cry duration after the skin puncture and by PIPP. Changes in heart rate were measured on four occasions (before the test, as the highest value during the first 30 seconds of the test, immediately and 3 minutes after the blood sampling). Recordings were made of time since last feed, use of a pacifier, the presence of the parent gently holding the infant, the duration of blood sampling, any local effects of the cream, and the success of the procedure. Ninety-nine newborns received EMLA and 102 received glucose. Five infants were excluded: one in the EMLA and four in the glucose group (two infants were <36 weeks gestation, one infant received antibiotics, one developed seizures during the procedure, and parents withdrew consent for one infant). Baseline characteristics were similar between groups. The PIPP scores were significantly lower in the glucose compared to the EMLA group (mean (SD) 4.6 (3.3) vs. 5.7 (3.8) (P = 0.031)). Significantly fewer patients in the glucose group were scored as having pain (PIPP above 6): 19.3 % compared with 41.7% in the EMLA group (P = 0.0007). The duration of crying during the first 3 min was significantly shorter in the glucose (median 1 second, range 0–180) than in the EMLA group (median 18 seconds, range 0–176; P < 0.001). There were no significant differences in the increase in heart rate between the two groups. Sampling was successful in 74 in the EMLA and 77 in the glucose group. Successful completion of the procedure took 161 seconds in the EMLA and 169 seconds in the glucose group (NS). The authors concluded that glucose is effective in providing pain relief from venepuncture and seems to be better than EMLA.

In a RCT Abad et al. (2001) compared the efficacy of oral sucrose vs. EMLA cream for pain relief during venepuncture. Full-term neonates with GA between 37 and 42 weeks and a postnatal age of <4 days were eligible for inclusion. Before the venepuncture infants were randomized to one of four treatment groups: 2 ml of spring water (placebo), 2 ml of sucrose 24% (w/v), 1 g of EMLA and 1 g of EMLA plus 2 ml of sucrose 24% (w/v). The study protocol was completed in 55 of 64 scheduled venepunctures. Data from 51 neonates were obtained. Four neonates were tested on two occasions, separated by at least a 24-h period. For the second venepuncture, random allocation to a different treatment group and use of the other arm were additional criteria for inclusion. In the groups which received EMLA, the cream was applied 45–60 min before the procedure. Four min before venepuncture Tegaderm and cream were removed. Oral sucrose or placebo was administered 2 min prior to the procedure. Cry duration and changes in heart rate, respiratory rate and oxygen saturation were measured blindly at baseline, immediately post venepuncture, and 2 and 4 min afterwards. Venepuncture was performed by the same nurse using a 25-gauge needle. The baseline characteristics were similar for the four groups except that the GA of infants in the EMLA plus sucrose group was significantly lower compared to the water group (P = 0.01). The main effects observed were that the time spent crying and the immediate heart rate response to pain were significantly lower in the sucrose alone (P = 0.001) and EMLA plus sucrose (P = 0.008) groups. The concomitant use of EMLA did not increase further the analgesic efficacy of sucrose. The authors concluded that administration of 24% sucrose compared favourably with EMLA in decreasing pain response to venepuncture in newborns.

In summary, glucose and sucrose were more effective than EMLA.

CONCLUSIONS

As has been pointed out before in guidelines and individual systematic reviews, there is a need for consistent reporting of results from RCTs to be able to combine data using meta-analytic techniques. In this systematic review it was possible to combine data only for one outcome from two RCTs as pain was assessed using different outcome measures. Use of a few validated measures such as the NFCS or the PIPP would allow for more intervention trials to be included in the meta-analyses. Also, although there is good reason to report data as medians and ranges (data are often not normally distributed), there is a need to report data as mean and SD whenever possible to be able to combine data from several studies in meta-analyses and thus achieve more precise estimates of the effect size.

Based on our systematic review of the literature using a synopsis approach, available evidence indicates that the use of amethocaine gel or patch is effective in reducing pain from venepuncture/cannulation, but is ineffective in preventing pain associated with PICC insertion in infants. EMLA does decrease pain associated with venepuncture but sweet-tasting solutions (glucose or sucrose) appear to be more effective. The effectiveness of amethocaine vs. a sweet-tasting solution has not been tested. There is a definite need for additional systematic reviews of pain-relieving interventions for neonates and older infants. Only through careful examination of existing evidence will we be able to determine the best directions for decision making around individual strategies for relieving pain in infants and to identify areas for future intervention research.

ACKNOWLEDGEMENTS

We acknowledge with gratitude the help from Ms. Elizabeth Uleryk, Chief Librarian, the Hospital for Sick Children, in designing all literature searches for this chapter.

REFERENCES

Abad F, Díaz-Gómez NM, Domenech E, et al. (2001). Oral sucrose compares favourably with lidocaine-prilocaine cream for pain relief during venepuncture in neonates. Acta Paediatrica 90: 160–165.

Acharya AB, Bustani PC, Phillips JD, et al. (1998). Randomized controlled trial of eutectic mixture of local anaesthetics cream for venepuncture in healthy preterm infants. Arch Dis Child Fetal Neonatal Ed 78: F138–F142.

Akobeng AK. (2005). Understanding systematic reviews and meta-analysis. Arch Dis Child 90: 845–848.

American Academy of Pediatrics, Committee of Fetus and Newborn, Committee on Drugs, Section on Anesthesiology and Section on Surgery. (1987). Neonatal anesthesia. Pediatrics 80: 186.

American Academy of Pediatrics, Committee on Fetus and Newborn, Committee on Drugs, Section on Anesthesiology, Section on Surgery. Canadian Paediatric Society. Fetus and Newborn Committee. (2000). Prevention and management of pain and stress in the neonate. Pediatrics 105: 454–461.

Anand KJS, Hickey PR. (1987). Pain and its effects in the human neonate and fetus. N Engl J Med 317: 1321–1329.

Anand KJS, International Evidence-Based Group for Neonatal Pain. (2001). Consensus statement for the prevention and management of pain in the newborn. Arch Pediatr Adolesc Med 155: 173–180.

Anand KJS, Brown MJ, Causon RC, et al. (1985a). Can the neonate mount an endocrine and metabolic response to surgery? J Pediatr Surg 20: 41–48.

Anand KJS, Brown MJ, Bloom SR, et al. (1985b). Studies on the hormonal regulation of fuel metabolism in the human newborn infant undergoing anesthesia and surgery. Horm Res 22: 115–128.

Anand KJS, Johnston CC, Oberlander T, et al. (2005). Analgesia and local anesthesia during invasive procedures in the neonate. Clin Ther 27: 844–876.

Aranda JV, Carlo W, Hummel P, et al. (2005). Analgesia and sedation during mechanical ventilation in neonates. Clin Ther 27: 877–899.

Badgett RG, O'Keefe M, Henderson MC. (1997). Using systematic reviews in clinical education. Ann Intern Med 126: 886–891.

Ballantyne M, McNair C, Ung E. (2003). A randomized controlled trial evaluating the efficacy of tetracaine gel for pain relief from peripherally inserted central catheters in infants. Adv Neonatal Care 3: 297–307.

Baños J-E, Ruiz G, Guardiola E. (2001). An analysis of articles on neonatal pain published from 1965 to 1999. Pain Res Manage 6: 45–50.

Bell SG. (1994). The national pain management guideline: implications for neonatal intensive care. Neonatal Netw 13: 9–17.

Bellù R, de Waal KA, Zanini R. (2005). Opioids for neonates receiving mechanical ventilation. The Cochrane Database of Systematic Reviews Issue 3. Online. Available: http://www.nichd.nih.gov/cochrane/Bellu/BELLU.HTM

Bhatt-Mehta V. (1996). Current guidelines for the treatment of acute pain in children. Drugs 61: 760–776.

Blomquist HK, Mjörndal T, Tiger G. (1983). Dicycloverin chloride solution – a remedy for severe infantile colic. Läkartidningen 80: 116–118.

Brady-Fryer B, Wiebe N, Lander JA. (2004/2005). Pain relief for neonatal circumcision. The Cochrane Database of Systematic Reviews Issue 3. Online. Available: http:// www.nichd.nih.gov/cochrane/BradyFryer/BRADYFRYER.HTM

Bucher H-U, Bucher-Schmid A. (1996). Treating pain in the neonate. In: Hansen TN, McIntosh N (eds) Current topics in neonatology, Number 1. W.B. Saunders, London.

Chalmers I (ed.). (2005). The James Lind Library. Online. Available: http://www.jameslindlibrary.org

Chalmers I, Enkin M, Keirse MJNC (eds). (1989). Effective care in pregnancy and childbirth. Oxford University Press, Oxford.

Cochrane AL. (1972). Effectiveness and efficiency: Random reflections on health services. Nuffield Provincial Hospitals Trust, London.

Cochrane AL. (1979). A critical review with particular reference to the medical profession. In: Medicines for the year 2000. Office of Health Economics, London, pp. 1–11.

Cook DJ, Greengold NL, Ellrodt AG, et al. (1997). The relation between systematic reviews and practice guidelines. Ann Intern Med 127: 210–216.

Craven PD, Badawi N, Henderson-Smart DJ, et al. (2003/2005). Regional (spinal, epidural, caudal) versus general anaesthesia in preterm infants undergoing inguinal herniorrhaphy in early infancy. The Cochrane Database of Systematic Reviews Issue 3. Online. Available: http://www.nichd.nih.gov/cochrane/Craven/CRAVEN.HTM

Crombie IK, McQuay HJ. (1998). The systematic review: a good guide rather than a guarantee. Pain 76: 1–2.

Daniel I: 6–16. The Holy Bible.

Darwin C. (1872). The expression of the emotions in man and animals. John Murray, Albemarle Street, London.

Feinstein AR. (1995). Meta-analysis: statistical alchemy for the 21st century. J Clin Epidemiol 48: 71–79.

Fiselier T, Monnens L, Moerman E, et al. (1983). Influence of the stress of venepuncture on basal levels of plasma renin activity in infants and children. Intern J Pediatr Nephrol 4: 181–185.

Gardosi J. (1998). Systematic reviews: insufficient evidence on which to base medicine. Br J Obstet Gynaecol 105: 1–5.

Gradin M, Eriksson M, Holmqvist G, et al. (2002). Pain reduction at venipuncture in newborns: oral glucose compared with local anesthetic cream. Pediatrics 110: 1053–1057.

Greenhalgh T. (1997) How to read a paper. The basics of evidence-based medicine. British Medical Journal Publishing Group, London.

Guyatt GH. (1991). Evidence-based medicine. Ann Intern Med 114 (Suppl 2): A-16.

Guyatt GH. (2004). Foreword. In: Moyer VA, Elliott EJ (eds) Evidence based pediatrics and child health. BMJ Books, London, p xvii–xviii.

Harpin VA, Rutter N. (1983). Making heel pricks less painful. Arch Dis Child 58: 226–228.

Harrison H. (1986). Letter to the editor. Birth 13: 124.

Higgins JP, Thompson SG, Deeks JJ, et al. (2003). Measuring inconsistency in meta-analyses. BMJ 327: 557–560.

Holve RL, Bromberger PJ, Groveman HD, et al. (1983). Regional anesthesia during newborn circumcision. Effect on infant pain response. Clin Pediatr 12: 813–818.

Jadad AR, Cook DJ, Jones A. (1998). Methodology and reports of systematic reviews and meta-analyses: a comparison of Cochrane reviews with articles published in paper-based journals. JAMA 280: 278–280.

Jain A, Rutter N. (2000). Does topical amethocaine gel reduce the pain of venepuncture in newborn infants? A randomized double blind controlled trial. Arch Dis Child Fetal Neonatal Ed 83: F207–F210.

Jordens CF, Hawe P, Irwig LM. (1998). Use of systematic reviews of randomized trials by Australian neonatologists and obstetricians. Med J Aust 168: 267–270.

Kirya C, Werthman MW. (1978). Neonatal circumcision and penile dorsal nerve block – a painless procedure. J Pediatr 92: 998–1000.

Larsson BA, Tannfeldt G, Lagercrantz H, et al. (1998). Alleviation of the pain of venepuncture in neonates. Acta Paediatrica 87: 774–779.

Larsson BA, Gradin M, Lind V, et al. (2002). Swedish guidelines for prevention and treatment of pain in the newborn infant. Läkartidningen 99: 1946–1949.

Lawson JR. (1986). Letter to the editor. Birth 13: 124–125.

Lee SJ, Ralston HJP, Drey EA, et al. (2005). Fetal pain. A systematic multidisciplinary review of the evidence. JAMA 294: 947–954.

Lind J. (1953). A treatise of the scurvey (reprint of the 1753 publication). University Press, Edinburgh.

Lindh V, Wiklund U, Håkansson S. (2000). Assessment of the effect of EMLA® during venipuncture in the newborn by analysis of heart rate variability. Pain 86: 247–254.

Long CP, McCafferty DF, Sittlington NM, et al. (2003). Randomized trial of novel tetracaine patch to provide local anaesthesia in neonates undergoing venepuncture. Br J Anaesth 91: 514–518.

Luke II: 21. The Holy Bible.

Moore J. (2001). No more tears: a randomized controlled double-blind trial of amethocaine gel vs. placebo in the management of procedural pain in neonates. J Adv Nurs 34: 475–482.

Moore J, Stretton J. (2001). Assessment of the benefits of topical anaesthetic application prior to iv cannulation. J Neonatal Nurs 7: 63–67.

MRC Streptomycin in Tuberculosis Trials Committee. (1948). Streptomycin treatment for pulmonary tuberculosis. BMJ ii: 769–782.

Mulrow CD. (1987). The medical review article: state of the science. Ann Intern Med 106: 485–488.

Mulrow CD, Cook DJ, Davidoff F. (1997). Systematic reviews: critical links in the great chain of evidence. Ann Intern Med 126: 389–391.

O'Brien L, Taddio A, Lyszkiewicz DA, et al. (2005). A critical review of the topical local anesthetic amethocaine (Ametop™) for pediatric pain. Pediatr Drugs 7: 41–54.

Ohlsson A. (1994). Systematic reviews – theory and practice. Scand J Clin Lab Invest 54 (suppl 219): 25–32.

Ohlsson A. (1996). Randomized controlled trials and systematic reviews: a foundation for evidence-based perinatal medicine. Acta Paediatrica 85: 647–655.

Ohlsson A, Taddio A, Jadad AR, et al. (2000). In: Anand KJS, Stevens BJ, McGrath PJ (eds) Pain in neonates, 2nd revised and enlarged edition. Pain Research and Clinical Management, Vol 10, pp. 251–268.

Owens ME. (1984). Pain in infancy: Conceptual and methodological issues. Pain 20: 213–230.

Owens ME, Todt EH. (1984). Pain in infancy: Neonatal reaction to heel lance. Pain 20: 77–86.

Oxman AD, Guyatt GH. (1988). Guidelines for reading literature reviews. Can Med Assoc J 138: 697–703.

Palmer LE. (1962). Relief of pain in infant teething; double blind study of a new choline salicylate agent. Ohio Med J 58: 434–435.

Perreault T, Fraser-Askin D, Liston R, et al. (1997). Pain in the neonate. Paediatr Child Health 2: 201–209.

Rawlings DJ, Miller PA, Engel RR. (1980). The effect of circumcision on transcutaneous PO_2 in term infants. Am J Dis Child 134: 676–678.

Rovner S. (1986). Surgery without anesthesia: Can preemies feel pain? The Washington Post Aug 13: HE7–8.

Rushforth JA, Levene MI. (1994). Behavioural response to pain in healthy neonates. Arch Dis Child 70: 174–176.

Sackett DL, Rosenberg WMC, Gray JAM, et al. (1996). Evidence-based medicine: what it is and what it isn't. BMJ 312: 71–72.

Scanlon JW. (1985). Barbarism. Perinatal Press 9: 103–104.

Schwartz G. (1977). Rembrandt. All the etchings reproduced in true size. Utgeverij Gary Schwartz, Maarsen, The Netherlands.

Shah V, Ohlsson A. (1999/2005). Venepuncture versus heel lance for blood sampling in term neonates. The Cochrane Database of Systematic Reviews Issue 3. Online. Available: http://www.nichd.nih.gov/cochrane/ Shah/shah.htm

Shea B, Moher D, Graham I, et al. (2002). A comparison of the quality of Cochrane reviews and systematic reviews published in paper-based journals. Eval Health Prof 1: 116–129.

Simons SH, van Dijk M, Anand KJS, et al. (2003). Do we still hurt newborn babies? A prospective study of procedural pain and analgesia in neonates. Arch Pediatr Adolesc Med 157: 1058–1064.

Sinclair J, Bracken M (eds). (1992). Effective care of the newborn infant. Oxford University Press, Oxford.

Sinclair JC, Haughton DE, Bracken MB, et al. (2003). Cochrane neonatal systematic reviews: a survey of the evidence for neonatal therapies. Clin Perinatol 30: 285–304.

Stevens B, Ohlsson A. (1998). Sucrose in neonates undergoing painful procedures. The Cochrane Library. The Cochrane Collaboration: Issue 2. Update Software, Oxford.

Stevens BJ, Johnston CC, Petryshen P, et al. (1996). Premature Infant Pain Profile: development and initial validation. Clin J Pain 12: 13–22.

Stevens B, Taddio A, Ohlsson A, et al. (1997). The efficacy of sucrose for relieving procedural pain in neonates – a systematic review and meta-analyses. Acta Paediatrica 86: 837–842.

Stevens B, Yamada J, Ohlsson A. (2005). Sucrose in neonates undergoing painful procedures. The Cochrane Library Issue 3. Online. Available: http://www.nichd.nih.gov/cochrane/ Stevens/Stevens.htm

Swenson O (ed.). (1958). Pediatric surgery, second edition. Appleton-Century-Crofts, New York.

Taddio A, Ohlsson A. (2005). Lidocaine-prilocaine cream (EMLA) to reduce pain in male neonates undergoing circumcision. The Cochrane Library Issue 3. Online. Available: http://www.nichd.nih.gov/cochrane/ taddio/taddio1.htm

Taddio A, Ohlsson A, Einarson TR, et al. (1998). A systematic review of lidocaine-prilocaine cream (EMLA) in the treatment of acute pain in neonates. Pediatrics 101: E1. Online. Available: http://www.pediatrics.org/cgi/content/ full/101/2/e1

Taddio A, Ohlsson K, Ohlsson A. (1999). Lidocaine-prilocaine cream for analgesia during circumcision in newborn boys. The Cochrane Library. The Cochrane Collaboration; Issue 3. Update Software, Oxford.

The Cochrane Library, Issue 1 1999. Update Software, Oxford.

The Cochrane Library, Issue 3 2005. John Wiley & Sons, Chichester.

Pain in vulnerable populations and palliative care

Bonnie J Stevens
Linda Johnston
Christine Newman
Maria Rugg

INTRODUCTION

Neonates and infants who are developmentally, neurologically, physically or pharmacologically compromised and those who are receiving end of life supportive or palliative care are the most vulnerable of all infants. They are vulnerable because they cannot act as their own advocates and they are dependent on others for all of their needs including pain relief. Despite their vulnerability, these infants do not need to suffer unrelieved pain. Significant advances in infant pain assessment and management research should extend equally to these infants as to all other infants. However, to date, researchers have generally not included this population in their research studies. Therefore, our knowledge of the validity of existing pain measures and the efficacy and safety of (a) pharmacological (e.g. therapies that involve administration of pharmacologic agents), (b) physical (e.g. therapies that affect sensory systems), (c) behavioural (e.g. therapies that change behaviours), (d) environmental (e.g. strategies that modulate the environment) and (e) supportive (e.g. strategies that empower and support the child and family) therapies, although implemented effectively with healthy infants, are relatively unknown in these infants. Effective pain assessment and management of vulnerable infants, including those receiving end of life care, need to become a major priority of researchers and healthcare providers in settings that accommodate vulnerable infants and their families.

In this chapter, we will define and explore conceptualizations for vulnerability, risk for vulnerability and pain in infants envisioned as those who are most vulnerable or who are receiving palliative or supportive care. In particular, we will consider the applicability of existing pain assessment and management strategies for vulnerable infants and neonates and make recommendations for practice and future research.

CONCEPTUALIZATION OF THE VULNERABLE/AT-RISK NEONATE AND INFANT

Vulnerable, from the Latin *vulnerāre*, means to wound; easily wounded or injured (Taber's Cyclopedic Medical Dictionary 2001). 'At risk' is explained in the epidemiological literature as those persons experiencing a biologic event that can negatively impact on their health. The factors leading to this *risk* can be unalterable such as gender or age; or acquired, such as exposure to a toxin, disease or health-impacting event. 'Vulnerability' to such risk (i.e. the likelihood that a harmful outcome will result) can be defined as a varying state of weakness or strength that can modify risk responses (Leffers et al. 2004).

Flaskerud and Winslow (1998) developed the Vulnerable Populations Model (VPM) to identify the major relationships between resource availability, relative risk and health status. 'Resource availability' refers to the availability of socioeconomic and environmental resources, 'relative risk' is the ratio of risk of poor outcome in groups exposed to risk factors and not receiving resources compared to that of groups who do receive such resources, and 'health status' is measured by disease prevalence, morbidity and mortality rates. This model incorporates research, practice, ethical and policy analysis as having the capacity to impact directly on, as well as modify the relationships between these components.

Purdy (2004) has applied the conceptual framework of vulnerable populations specifically to premature infants where premature birth is the risk factor for many complications such as intraventricular haemorrhage, sepsis, long-term chronic illness and disability. Purdy argues that the VPM is applicable to both the care and follow up of premature infants as it offers an evaluation of relative risk (e.g. perinatal exposure, biophysical risk), resource availability (e.g. perinatal care) and health status (e.g. physical and neurodevelopmental outcomes). Similarly, Leffers et al. (2004) have applied a theoretical construct for risk and vulnerability in two studies of preterm infants where biophysical and developmental risks, for poor health and outcomes, were moderated by the actions of nurse midwives in one study, and by mothers in another study.

The VPM may serve as a framework for considering how pain assessment and management (as healthcare resources) could modify the vulnerability (as a result of exposure to noxious stimuli) of not only premature, but other neonatal and infant subpopulations, and thus impact on their health outcomes. Each of the components in this adaptation of the VPM can be adjusted to reflect the acuity of the healthcare environment in which the neonate or infant is cared for, the potential for altered physical, behavioural responses and/or adverse neurological sequelae as a result of exposure to pain, and the inherent vulnerability of the neonate or infant (see Table 18.1).

Definitions of vulnerable neonates and infants

Vulnerable neonates and infants (i.e. those susceptible to a negative outcome) may be defined according to

Table 18.1 Components and mediating factors of the Vulnerable Populations Model (Flaskerud and Winslow 1998)

Model components	Mediating factors
Resources available	
Pain assessment	
Pain management	Practice
Relative risk	
Prematurity	
Neurological impairment	Ethics
Surgery	
Metabolic disturbance	
Palliative care	Policy
Health status	
Physical outcomes	Research
Behavioural outcomes	
Neurological sequelae	

criteria including gestational age, birth weight, degree of physical or neurological impairment, dependence on medical technologies, presence of conditions associated with extensive tissue damage and those resulting in recurrent or chronic pain, or the social and environmental contexts they inhabit. These groups are not only dependent on caregivers interpreting their needs, but are often limited in the cues they can provide for care providers to make correct interpretation of those needs.

The term 'very low-birth-weight' (VLBW) refers to the baby born weighing less than 1500 g, while babies categorized as 'extremely low-birth-weight' (ELBW) are those born weighing less than 1000 g (Bakewell-Sachs and Blackburn 2001). These neonatal populations have unique management requirements in light of their extremely vulnerable state of development; particularly in terms of their neurodevelopmental and neurobehavioural outcomes. These outcomes may also be impacted by the negative physical environment of the neonatal intensive care unit (NICU) (e.g. noise and lighting) which is not associated with the infant's typical interactions with the environment (Whitfield 2003) and thus, could also affect development. One could describe the VLBW and ELBW infants in the NICU setting as being particularly vulnerable and sensitive, as they are confronted with repeated painful experiences and an environment lacking many of the positive aspects of human contact that are common in the home setting.

Other factors may also contribute to neurological impairment in the neonate and infant and thus enhance their vulnerability. Substance-exposed neonates and infants, such as those of heroin-dependent or moderate to heavy alcohol-drinking mothers are at risk for substantial neurodevelopmental disorders. These may impact not only on their ability to mount a response to a painful stimulus, but also to alter the effectiveness of pharmacological and non-pharmacological pain-reduction strategies (Fike 2003). Periventricular/intraventricular haemorrhage, seen almost exclusively in neonates born less than 32 weeks gestation, can have neurodevelopmental sequelae as can other types of intracranial haemorrhage, seen more often in term infants. Hypoxic-ischaemic encephalopathy (HIE) results from a combination of decreased cerebral perfusion and systemic hypoxia. Depending on the severity of the insult, neurological manifestations can range from seizures and hypotonia to profoundly altered consciousness. The impact of these insults can extend beyond the neonatal period with cerebral palsy (CP) being a common sequelae. Neural tube defects such as spina bifida result in neurologic deficit at the level of and below the defect. Clearly both CP and the associated spasticity and spinal malformations influence a baby's capacity to respond to a painful stimulus and treatment.

Infants requiring surgical management may also be more vulnerable than other groups. Their clinical course in the intensive care environment, with the accompanying exposure to frequent painful insults such as placement of intravenous lines and heel pricks for blood sampling, underlies the stress of the surgical procedure and the postoperative course. These acute (surgery) and sub-acute (postoperative period) events may entail direct involvement of sensory nerves and sensory receptors as well as longer-lasting inflammatory, cytochemical or paracrine responses (McIntosh 1997). Furthermore, prolonged illnesses prior to surgery that are accompanied by inflammatory processes (e.g. necrotizing enterocolitis) may constitute persistent unrelieved periods of pain and may alter an infant's response to both acute and sub-acute painful events. The construct of persistent or chronic pain, although identified as plausible in neonates and infants, requires much attention. Infants receiving muscle relaxants as a part of their clinical management are unable to move spontaneously; thus behavioural responses to painful stimuli are attenuated, making pain assessment tools of little use.

Conceptualization and definition of palliative care for neonates and infants

Current statistics indicate that more children die in the first year of life than in all other age groups of childhood combined and two-thirds of infant deaths occur in the neonatal period (Institute of Medicine report). Despite remarkable strides in neonatal survival, some newborns still die, with many of these deaths resulting from perinatal illnesses (Hoyert et al. 2001). Infants who may require palliative or supportive care include: (a) newborns born at the limit of viability (e.g. ELBW infants), (b) newborns with congenital anomalies or severe neurologic impairments, that are incompatible with prolonged life, (c) newborns and infants with overwhelming illness who are not responding to aggressive life-sustaining medical treatment, and (d) newborns and infants for whom continued medical treatment may prolong suffering (Leuthner 2004). An evolving conceptual framework describes the trajectories of childhood illness and death in children facing life-threatening illness. Figure 18.1 illustrates the varying trajectories of illness and death within this population. Supportive care during this time of palliation must be an integral part of delivering excellent care, including comprehensive pain assessment and management in vulnerable infant populations (Carter and Bhatia 2001, Leuthner et al. 2001, Pierucci et al. 2001, Catlin and Carter 2002).

PAIN ASSESSMENT IN VULNERABLE NEONATES AND INFANTS

Extremely low-birth-weight infants

The gestational age of viability for preterm and ELBW infants continues to decrease. However, concomitant with this improvement in survival is a simultaneous increase in painful procedures associated with diagnostic and newly evolving treatment modalities. This situation and our knowledge of the long-term consequences of pain compel healthcare professionals to identify pain early and manage it safely and effectively (Stevens et al. 2003). Only a few researchers have examined indicators of pain for ELBW infants. Flexing and extending extremities, finger splaying, fisting and mouthing were movements consistent with pain; while startles, twitches, jitters and tremours were not associated with pain (Grunau et al. 2000, Holsti et al. 2004). A few measures have been validated primarily with VLBW infants (and a few ELBW infants) (e.g. Premature Infant Pain Profile (PIPP; Stevens et al. 1996); Pain Assessment Tool (PAT; Hodgkinson et al. 1994, Spence et al. 2003), Douleur Aigue du Nouveau-ne (DAN; Carbajal et al. 1997, 2005, Bellieni et al. 2002)), but generally there has been relatively little research on pain measurement that is applicable to this age group. This general lack of validation of pain indicators and measures with ELBW infants leaves clinicians and researchers with minimal guidance in assessing pain and evaluating treatment strategies.

Common Trajectories of Child Death

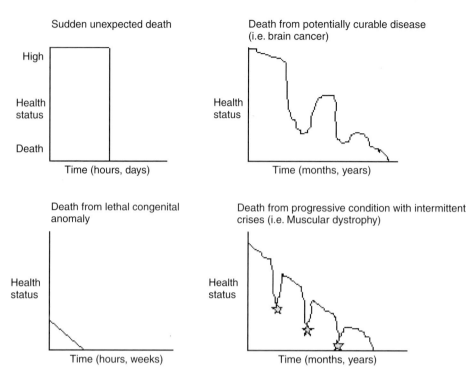

Figure 18.1 Trajectories of childhood illness and death in children facing life-threatening illness (reproduced from Field MJ and Behrman R (2003) with permission from National Academies Press and the Institute of Medicine).

Extrapolation of behaviours from more mature infants negates the physiological and behavioural immaturity of ELBW infants. Inconsistencies with behavioural and physiological pain responses in ELBW infants and their inability to sustain responses over time may simply reflect poor regulation of their CNS development and not the presence or absence of pain. The trajectory exploring how ELBW infants' responses to pain change over time will provide needed information about this vulnerable population for developing pain assessment indicators in this population. Assessment of neonatal pain, available pain measures with their psychometric and clinimetric properties, and descriptions of changes in biobehavioural responses over time are further described in Chapter 6.

Infants with congenital abnormalities or severe neurological impairments

Virtually no pain assessment research has been conducted with newborn infants with severe congenital anomalies. Furthermore, very little is known about pain reactivity in neonates with a significant neurological injury (SNI). While there is an emerging assumption that pain reactivity may be altered in older

children with SNI (Breau et al. 2006), systematic differences in biobehavioural pain reactivity in neonates with SNI have been only minimally addressed. In a study of preterm infants with and without cerebral parenchymal infarction (grade 4 intraventricular haemorrhage) or cystic periventricular leukomalacia, no differences in facial action or measures of cardiac autonomic reactivity were identified following an acute painful event (Oberlander et al. 2002). These authors speculated that although most of the infants with SNI went on to develop cerebral palsy, in the neonatal period, pain responses remained intact. In a prospective observational study of behavioural and physiologic responses to a heel lance of 149 neonates (GA >25–40 weeks) at high (n = 54), moderate (n = 45) and low (n = 50) risk for SNI, Stevens et al. (2001) similarly found that all infants responded to the most painful phase of the heel lance with the greatest change from baseline. However, infants at the highest risk for SNI exhibited the least change in facial expression and physiologic indicators. Infants with the highest severity of illness also demonstrated the highest pitched cries. Infants at all levels of risk for SNI appear to be capable of demonstrating behavioural and physiologic responses to painful procedures, although these responses vary in magnitude based on SNI risk status and severity of illness. Differences in these two studies warrant further investigation to validate indicators for pain assessment in this population.

Pain assessment in critically ill infants

Critical illness has been defined either as severely ill infants in an intensive care environment requiring ventilation or by determining a severity of illness score, such as the Score for Neonatal Acute Physiology (SNAP) or the Clinical Risk Index for Babies (CRIB) (van Dijk et al. 2002). Stevens et al. (1994) demonstrated a significant interaction between severity of illness and behavioural state on physiologic pain response, implying that those who were in quiet sleep and most severely ill were most affected. As management of pain in critically ill adults frequently dictates the administration of sedatives with opioids, pain should be assessed with the level of sedation. One infant pain measure, the Neonatal Pain, Agitation and Sedation Scale (N-PASS; Hummel and Puchalski 2001, Hummel et al. 2003) uniquely combines the measurement of these two constructs; however, minimal establishment of psychometric properties of this measure precludes widespread use in clinical practice.

Behavioural indicators such as tearing and being 'too awake' have also been portrayed as synonymous with pain in critically ill infants (van Dijk et al. 2002). To date, these indicators have not been validated or included in pain measures for these infants. However, instruments such as the Comfort Measure (Ambuel et al. 1992, van Dijk et al. 2000), which included indicators such as calmness-agitation, muscle tone and facial tension in addition to more typical physiologic and behavioural indicators, may be useful to consider.

Foster (2001) suggests that the expert judgement of the nurse is the key factor in assessing pain in critically ill children. However, Foster implies that judgement be articulated by expert nurses, leaving more novice nurses who may be caring for these infants somewhat disadvantaged. Generally, there is a recognized difficulty in making observational differentiations between pain, agitation and sedation; these concepts require further exploration. On rare occasions, these infants receive muscle relaxants that preclude any behavioural responses; in these situations, physiological indicators may be useful in determining pain. As discussed in Chapter 6, other indicators such as biomarkers that may reflect cognitive as well as spinal reflexes in these infants need further exploration.

PAIN MANAGEMENT IN VULNERABLE NEONATES AND INFANTS

Applicability of existing pain interventions

As with all individuals regardless of age, valid measurement of pain is the first step to good management. Once we are aware of 'where we stand' with the infant's current pain status, we are in a much better position to contemplate management strategies. As a general principle, pain management should be multidimensional and considered within the context in which it is experienced. Context, within the conceptualization of vulnerability, refers to the at-risk populations described above, the environments in which their pain is experienced and expressed, the resources available and the quality of existing evidence on pain management strategies. The evidence supporting pharmacologic, environmental, behavioural and physical strategies are described in detail in Chapters 8–12. The following will serve as a few examples of strategies that can generally be applied with most vulnerable infants to promote comfort and pain relief.

Pharmacological strategies

The use of analgesia in vulnerable infants needs to follow similar principles as for administering analgesia in all neonates and infants. Analgesic administration in this population includes opioid analgesics, sedative/hypnotic drugs, non-steroidal anti-inflammatory durgs and acetaminophen, injectable and topical local anaesthetics and sucrose. A group of international experts, the Neonatal Pain Control Group, as part of the Newborn Drug Development Initiative, the US Food and Drug Administration and the National Institute of Child Health and Human Development, have recently reviewed the therapeutic options for pain management for painful procedures, surgery and ventilated infants (Anand et al. 2005). Detailed descriptions of prescribing, administering, titrating and adapting systemic (Chapter 10) and neuraxial and regional analgesia (Chapter 11) are included elsewhere. There are, however, special considerations that require attention when administering pharmacological agents in vulnerable infants; especially those who are most premature and neurologically compromised and/or those who are receiving palliative or supportive care. These considerations relate to the fears, worries and concerns of using opioid analgesics and sedation (either alone or in combination) in infants that are thought to be very fragile; and the relative paucity of research in this population. The meaning attributed to drugs that families may associate with death, addiction and other serious side effects in critically ill infants and those receiving palliative care also need to be taken into account. Issues related to pharmacological interventions in this population are summarized below.

Sucrose, both alone and in combination with pacifiers has received a great deal of attention for procedural pain management; particularly in term and preterm neonates. A series of updated systematic reviews (Stevens et al. 2001) clearly indicates that administration of a 24% sucrose solution either with or without a pacifier approximately 2 minutes prior to a tissue-damaging procedure reduces the pain associated with procedures. However, the consistent implementation of sucrose over multiple repeated painful procedures during the neonatal period has mixed findings of effectiveness (Stevens et al. 2001, Johnston et al. 2002) and reason for caution exists in the most vulnerable ELBW infants (Johnston et al. 2002). As with other pharmacological interventions, many questions on the frequency of administration, dose-related effects, toxicity and repetitive use must be carefully considered to ensure safe and effective use with all vulnerable populations of neonates and infants.

Environmental strategies
The American Academy of Pediatrics released recommendations for paediatric practice and policy with respect to the NICU environment (American Academy of Pediatrics 1987). A number of studies have reported the continuous exposure to noise of babies nursed in an NICU environment without periods of quiet (Bess et al. 1979, Thomas 1989). Zahr and Balian (1995) reported alterations in infants' physical and behavioural responses as a result of exposure to sudden loud noise (80 dB) in an NICU. The implementation of individualized environmental care (IEC) for a population of premature infants resulted in neurological development on a par with their term infant counterparts (Buehler et al. 1995). Cycled lighting in the NICU is the most studied of the light environment interventions although results to date remain inconclusive (Blackburn 1996, Brandon et al. 2002). While researchers have attempted to demonstrate the impact of such lighting on an infant's neurodevelopmental outcome, no attempt has been made to determine the efficacy of this intervention with respect to pain reduction.

The efficacy of music therapy has been examined in a small number of studies of premature infants undergoing routine heel lancing. Music therapy, with or without non-nutritive sucking (NNS), resulted in lower pain scores and reduced physiological measures of heart rate and oxygen saturation (Bo and Callaghan

2000, Butt and Kisilevsky 2000). Some concern exists about the provision of music therapy without consideration for the developmental level of the infant and their inability to regulate the duration or intensity of the input. Music, in the form of lullabies sung by mothers, has also been recently evaluated in terms of procedural pain reduction. In a cross-over study, where the mother's voice was played in the experimental condition and no sound was played in the control condition during routine heel lance, no effect was found on infant pain response, suggesting that auditory stimulation may not be sufficient as an analgesic. While no firm link has been established between environment and pain reduction strategies, the apparent influences on an infant's neurodevelopment suggest consideration should be given by clinicians to promote simple strategies for reducing noise in the nursery and providing cycled lighting.

Behavioural strategies
Developmentally supportive practices implemented as a means of reducing pain in vulnerable populations include swaddling and positioning. These strategies are designed to provide containment and boundaries and enhance feelings of security. The influence of 'tucking' or swaddling on pain responses to heel lance procedures has been studied in populations of medically stable premature infants. Infants, contained in the flexed position prior to, and following, heel lance cried less and spent more time asleep than those infants nursed according to routine practice (Corff et al. 1995). Fearon et al. (1997), in a very small population of infants, suggested positioning reduced behavioural and physiological responses in infants greater than 31 weeks corrected age but had no effect in less-mature infants. Prone positioning and rocking of infants have also been shown to be ineffective strategies for reducing pain associated with heel lance procedures in preterm infants (Campos 1994, Stevens et al. 1999, Grunau et al. 2004).

Physical strategies
Kangaroo care (KC), or more precisely labelled when performed by mothers, kangaroo mother care (KMC), involves placing the term or preterm infant skin-to-skin against a parent's or mother's chest. In a recent cross-over design study of 74 stable preterm neonates using the PIPP tool, Johnston et al. (2003) demonstrated significantly lower scores in infants while they were KMC nursed for 30 minutes prior to and during the procedure when compared to their response when nursed in the control prone position in their isolette. A recent Cochrane review on kangaroo care for lactation success (Anderson et al. 2005) concluded that it was useful in promoting breastfeeding

and decreasing crying; however, pain as an outcome was not addressed. Studies have been conducted with stable term and preterm infant populations. The effectiveness of KMC in reducing procedural and/or chronic pain in unstable or vulnerable infants requiring multiple supportive therapies has not been established.

The analgesic effects of breastfeeding have been studied in healthy term infants. Using both physiological and behavioural measures, infants who were breastfed during a heel lance cried less and had a lesser increase in heart rate in association with the procedure compared with control infants who were swaddled and placed on their side (Gray 2002). Provision of expressed breast milk (EBM) during venepuncture, rather than breastfeeding, reduced crying time and physiological responses when compared to the administration of water to a control group (Upadhyay et al. 2004). Breastfeeding appears to be a simple and cost-effective means of reducing procedural pain in medically stable infants; however, its utility in sick or very preterm infants remains problematic as these infants may not tolerate either holding or oral feeds.

Non-nutritive sucking (NNS) is one of the most common interventions implemented in the neonatal unit to reduce procedural pain. In combination with other developmentally supportive interventions or with non-pharmacological interventions such as sweet-tasting solutions (see Cochrane review by Stevens et al. 2001) NNS has reduced both behavioural and physiological responses to painful procedures in term and preterm neonates when compared to NNS alone (Franck 1987, Blass 1989, Gibbins et al. 2002). Issues of whether vulnerable infants have the capacity to suck or the energy to sustain sucking at a rate to induce serotonin release have not been adequately determined. A more detailed examination of environmental, physical and behavioural interventions to prevent and manage pain and discomfort is provided in Chapter 12.

ASSESSING AND MANAGING PAIN IN NEONATES AND INFANTS RECEIVING PALLIATIVE CARE

Barriers to pain assessment and management

Pain and other symptoms are inadequately assessed and treated in neonates and infants receiving palliative care despite the availability of pain-relieving treatments. Although these infants may be as capable of feeling pain as all other infants, assessment and management of pain brings its own barriers from families as well as healthcare professionals. Some of these barriers have been articulated as: (1) the thought

that infants do not have an adequate integrated cortical function to translate pain experiences. Nurses have also given into this belief by providing higher pain ratings to full-term infants compared to preterm infants (Shapiro 1993); (2) concern that reporting pain may distract physicians from treatment of the underlying disease; (3) alarm that pain means that the disease is worse or that death is imminent; (4) fear of addiction/sedation to complicate existing side effects of disease and treatment; (5) worries about unmanageable adverse effects; (6) avoidance of accepting appropriate pain management due to the negative connotation of 'drugs' and the subclass of opioids (more frequently misknown as 'narcotics') for many cultural groups as well as the public in general; and (7) concern about becoming dependent on or tolerant to pain medications (Jacox et al. 1994, Ersek 1999, McCaffery and Pasero 1999).

Assessment of pain during supportive or palliative care

Assessment of pain at the end of life must be based on an approach that integrates the perspectives of multiple professional and lay care providers. In neonates, it is essential to use scales that incorporate both physiologic and behavioural parameters to assess pain during this time as particular indicators may not be viable in these infants (Walden et al. 2001). It is also crucial to elicit the parents' perspective, as they will contribute valuable information regarding their infant's usual activities and functions and deviations from normal that may indicate persistent underlying pain and discomfort. While no multidimensional pain measures have been specifically established or validated for use in neonates at the end of life, several instruments have been validated in neonates for procedural, postoperative or persistent pain. These could be applicable to this population, given the age and situation of the infant (Duhn and Medves 2004). All neonatal and infant pain measures, their psychometric properties, feasibility and clinical utility are discussed in detail in Chapter 6.

The idea of pain versus suffering at the end of life has been explored in great depth (Sutton et al. 2002). Pain in the terminally ill is complex and includes dimensions of psychological, social and spiritual distress along with the more tangible physical aspects. The principles of family-centred care, which are integral to this vulnerable population, must be considered. The consequences of uncontrolled pain for newborns and infants may include: agitation, depression/anxiety, loss of appetite, sleep disturbance, decreased quality of life and interruption in family life for all family members.

Two primary principles need to be considered when assessing pain in neonates and infants at the end of life and/or receiving palliative care: (a) Involving the family/caregiver when obtaining a pain history. When discrepancies occur between the family/caregiver's report and those of the healthcare professional, these differences need to be explored. For example, the family member may be very distressed about their infant's illness and may be overestimating the child's pain in response to their own suffering. Conversely, the family member may be denying or minimizing their infant's pain, in light of the meaning being attributed to it. (b) Paying careful attention to pain language. Some people may have difficulty using the word 'pain'. 'Discomfort' is the most frequently used alternative. Other terms may include 'hurt' or 'ache'. Some terms suggest emotion, such as 'distressing' or 'horrible'. The meanings of pain words often need to be clarified for the family and their preferences acknowledged. Perception of or verbalization of pain may also be influenced by culture, religion, previous experience and family, institution or societal expectations.

The QUESTT Principle Model (Hockenberry et al. 2003) is appropriate and adaptable for pain in this population and gives a highly organized and comprehensive method of assessment. The acronym can be explained as follows:

- Question the patient; in the case of neonates and infants use family/caregivers;
- Use valid and reliable pain-rating scales;
- Evaluate behaviour/physiologic changes;
- Secure patient/family involvement;
- Take the cause of pain into account; and
- Take action and evaluate results.

Reassessing pain regularly, with changes in activity, treatment or the analgesic regimen is crucial. The frequency of pain assessment is also dependent upon the degree to which the infant's condition or pain state is changing; particularly if it is worsening. More rapidly progressive disease frequently demands more frequent assessment. Families should be coached to report any changes in the pain or the infant's response to pain treatments. Health professionals need to be mindful to assess for presence of pain at each patient contact and to conduct a full reassessment of pain with each new observation of pain, at the appropriate time interval after providing analgesia (15–20 min IV, 45–60 min after PO). Having health professionals and/or parents keep a pain diary (e.g. intensity scores, pain relief, times and doses of breakthrough pain medications given, additional comments about activities or other factors) often assists nurses and parents

in enhanced decision making about customizing pain-relieving strategies.

The meaning of the infant's pain can profoundly affect the family's perception of the pain at end of life. Parents often feel a profound sense of unfounded guilt; reframing of guilt-ridden views may help relieve families of these beliefs, often resulting in improved comfort for all. Cultural and spiritual beliefs regarding the meaning of pain should be examined. In the neonate, the meaning of pain is reflected from the family or caregiver's perspective and by culture. Religious/spiritual beliefs can influence the meaning of pain and consulting appropriate spiritual/religious advisors may help mediate these issues.

Communicating assessment findings cannot be overemphasized enough (McCaffery and Pasero 1999). Clear, objective communication (both verbally and in writing) of the pain assessment findings ultimately improves pain management. Also, descriptions of functional limitations that result from the pain(e.g. the infant cannot tolerate feeds or is so fatigued that they cannot interact with parents) assist with the re-establishment of a 'care plan' for the family and other healthcare providers (i.e. physical therapy, diagnostic imaging, other consulting specialty services). This plan should include pain history, current non-pharmacological and pharmacological therapies, titration of drugs in the event of an acute pain episode, and appropriate contact numbers for easy access to the appropriate primary treatment team.

Pain management in neonates and infants receiving palliative care

The word 'palliate' means to mitigate, alleviate, lessen the severity of (pain or disease) or to give relief. Palliative care was recognized as a medical specialty in 1987 – and was defined as 'the study and management of patients with active, progressive, far-advanced disease for whom the prognosis is limited and the focus of care is the quality of life' (Doyle et al. 1993). The World Health Organization definition focuses on the control of pain, of other symptoms, and of psychological, social and spiritual problems as paramount. The overall goal of palliative care is achievement of the best quality of life for patients and their families (World Health Organization 1990, 1998).

Although the number of neonatal and infant deaths each year may seem small in comparison to our adult counterparts in palliative care, the emotional, social and financial impact is extraordinary. A neonate/infant death is a painful, sorrowful loss for parents, siblings, extended family members, healthcare personnel and others. During the trajectory of diagnosis, illness and death, families suffer from reduced quality of life, loss of family income, inconsistency in the availability and quality of hospice palliative care, and the lack of real choices concerning where their child lives and dies.

Reflecting on what is understood about infants and neonates within the paediatric palliative care population, it is important to understand the basic precepts of paediatric palliative care. The guiding principles surrounding paediatric hospice palliative care (adapted from the Canadian Hospice Palliative Care Association 2006) may be used when considering pain management strategies in life threatening illness:

- All children regardless of age have different skills and different emotional, physical and development issues/needs.
- Religious/cultural beliefs, patterns of coping, disease experience, previous experience with loss/ death, sadness, and other emotions associated with grief, all influence a child's and family's understanding of death (Eiser 1995, McConnell and Frager 2003).
- All children regardless of age are members of many communities, including families, neighbourhoods and schools, and their continuing role in these communities should be incorporated into their dying journey.
- Children experience unique symptoms, such as fatigue, nausea, vomiting and shortness of breath, depression and anxiety, which are not well understood. They experience and express pain differently than adults, and require individualized treatment.

- Children are not as able to advocate for themselves, and often rely on family members to make decisions for them.
- Many life-threatening conditions that affect children are rare and only affect children. Many of the illnesses are familial and may affect more than one child in the family. The diseases are often unpredictable in terms of prognosis, and children and their families may require years of care giving.

Parents bear a heavy responsibility for the care of their child, which may include making decisions in the best interest of the child at a time when they are highly stressed and grieving the loss of their child's health as well as dealing with other losses such as financial stability and the loss of time to spend with other children. Families of children who have life-threatening conditions tend to be younger and have fewer resources. Their quality of life is significantly improved when the ill child's quality of life is enhanced. The grief associated with a child's death has devastating, long-term implications for the entire family. Siblings have unique needs during and after a child's death.

The model shown in Figure 18.2 is adopted from the Canadian Hospice and Palliative Care Association (2004) and shows how infants and their families could be supported through diagnosis, illness, death and bereavement.

Special issues for consideration within palliative care

There are two primary ethical principles in clinical care; beneficence (to do good) and non-maleficence

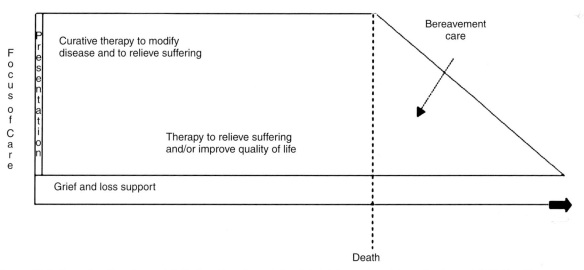

Figure 18.2 Canadian Hospice and Palliative Care Association Model (reproduced from Ferris et al. (2004) with permission from the Canadian Hospice and Palliative Care Association).

(to do no harm). The challenge in all clinical care, but especially efforts directed at palliation, is in seeking a balance between benefits of treatments and the burdens on the infant and family. For example, many assessment and management strategies are based on 'doing good' or relieving pain; however, we need to ensure that the therapies chosen are safe and efficacious so that they minimize harm. These principles are founded on respect for the child and their need to be protected (World Health Organization 1998).

In the case of supportive, end of life or palliative care, doing 'good' and minimizing harm may take on different meanings than in other contexts where pain management is provided as primarily a means to prevent or attenuate pain from single procedures. Health professionals are often faced with re-evaluating what is the meaning of the constructs of good and harm in this particular context. For example, questions such as 'What are the desired effects of this medication? How much is too much or too little? Is physiologic tolerance or psychological dependence an issue?' all are paramount queries with few prescribed answers.

Health professionals may also be confronted with difficult moral and ethical issues. The issue of medical euthanasia in the face of overwhelming suffering of a young child may be raised. By definition, medical euthanasia is the 'intentional, active intervention by a healthcare professional to terminate a life, based on the belief that it is better to end a life of intolerable suffering' (World Health Organization 1998, p. 61). In practical terms, health professionals are often faced with decisions about withdrawal of treatment where burden outweighs the benefit. However, these decisions are clearly not supporting medical euthanasia as is defined above; nor is providing adequate analgesia – even in the unfortunate event that adequate doses to relieve pain may hasten the child's death or lead to the side effect of respiratory depression, to the point where respirations cease. These difficult ethical and moral issues for front-line healthcare providers and parents providing care to these neonates and infants require further exploration with all multiple stakeholders, so that those delivering care can feel comfortable and supported in their deliberations around these issues.

The ability to provide adequate resources to control pain is another difficult issue in palliative care. Unfortunately, adequate supplies of opiates are not universally available; and even when they are, they may not be prioritized for or readily available to all children. In developing countries, children who are dying may not receive adequate analgesia as limited resources are directed towards curative rather than palliative care (World Health Organization 1998, p. 62). These issues, combined with the common misbelief that neonates and infants are incapable of pain perception, leave these infants at particular risk. Collaborative efforts between WHO and humanitarian organizations need to be expanded to promote discussion and concrete action plans between developed and developing countries to ensure effective pain treatment and minimize suffering in all children.

SUMMARY AND FUTURE DIRECTIONS

Pain assessment and management is a universal challenge across neonatal and infant populations due to their developmental, behavioural and communication immaturity. However, particular groups of infants including those who are very preterm at birth, at high risk for various types of impairment, critically ill and compromised physically and pharmacologically, and receiving end of life supportive or palliative care are particularly vulnerable. In this chapter, we have attempted to deconstruct models of risk and vulnerability and apply them to these populations of vulnerable infants. Challenges with pain assessment and management were explored. Key queries about (1) whether existing measures validated in populations of infants who are less vulnerable and (2) the safety and efficacy of pharmacological, environmental, behavioural and physical strategies for pain management in these populations were raised.

Future directions need to focus on the clinical, developmental, moral and ethical issues that face all of us who care for and conduct research with these infants and their families. A research agenda, which includes some of the following questions, may serve to move this relatively unexplored domain forward:

- What is the interplay between the concepts of risk, environment, resources and health status for vulnerable neonates and infants?
- How can existing pain-relieving strategies improve outcomes in this population of vulnerable neonates and infants? What are the most salient outcomes for these infants and their families?
- How can differentiation between pain, agitation and other symptoms benefit these infants? What are the best ways to assess these multiple symptoms?
- What is the professional and non-professional care provider's role in advocating for vulnerable neonates and infants?
- What is the role of local, national, international and professional organizations and agencies in ensuring evidence-based guidelines for pain

prevention and practice and their implementation for vulnerable infants and neonates?

Collaboration of multiple stakeholders to address these and other important questions will provide the basis for a better understanding of how to address pain in this population of neonates and infants. Transfer of knowledge to decision makers at all levels may assist in preventing undue pain and suffering for both these babies and their families.

REFERENCES

Ambuel B, Hamlett KW, Marx CM, et al. (1992). Assessing distress in pediatric intensive care environments: the COMFORT scale. J Pediatr Psychol 17: 95–109.

American Academy of Pediatrics. Committee on Drugs, Section on Anesthesiology and Section on Surgery. (1987). Neonatal anesthesia. Pediatrics 80: 186.

Anand KJS, Johnston C, Oberlander TF, et al. (2005). Analgesia and local anesthesia during invasive procedures in the neonate. Clin Ther 27: 844–876.

Anderson GC, Moore E, Hepworth J, et al. (2005). Early skin-to-skin contact for mothers and their healthy newborn infants. Cochrane Database Syst Rev CD003519.

Bakewell-Sachs S, Blackburn S. (2001). Discharge and follow-up of the high-risk preterm infant. March of Dimes Education Services, White Plains, NY, p. 20.

Bellieni C, Bagnoli F, Perrone S, et al. (2002). Effect of multisensory stimulation on analgesia in term neonates: a randomized controlled trial. Pediatr Res 51: 460–463.

Bess FH, Peek BF, Chapman JJ. (1979). Further observations on noise levels in infant incubators. Pediatrics 63: 100–106.

Bo LK, Callaghan P. (2000). Soothing pain-elicited distress in Chinese neonates. Pediatrics 105: E49.

Blackburn ST. (1996). Research utilization: modifying the NICU light environment. Neonatal Netw 15: 63–66.

Blass EM, Shide DJ, Weller A. (1989). Stress-reducing effects of injesting milk, sugars and fats. A developmental perspective. Ann NY Acad Sci 575: 292–305.

Brandon DH, Holditch-Davis D, Belyea M. (2002). Preterm infants born at less than 31 weeks' gestation have improved growth in cycled light compared with continuous near darkness. J Pediatr 140: 192–199.

Breau L, Stevens BS, Grunau RVE. (2005). Developmental issues in acute and chronic pain in developmental disabilities. In: Symons F, Oberlander T (eds). Pain in individuals with developmental disabilities. Paul H Brookes, Baltimore, pp. 80–108.

Buehler DM, Als H, Duffy FH, et al. (1995). Effectiveness of individualized developmental care for low-risk preterm infants: behavioral and electrophysiologic evidence. Pediatrics 96: 923–932.

Butt ML, Kisilevsky BS. (2000). Music modulates behaviour of premature infants following heel lance. Can J Nurs Res 31: 17–39.

Campos RG. (1994). Rocking and pacifiers: two comforting interventions for heelstick pain. Res Nurs Health 17: 321–331.

Canadian Hospice Palliative Care Association Pediatric hospice palliative care: guiding principles and norms of practice. (March 2006). Online. Available: http://www.chpca.net/ marketplace/pediatric_norms/ pediatric_norms.htm

Carbajal R, Paupe A, Hoenn E, et al. (1997). DAN: une echelle comportementale d'evaluation de la douleur aigue du nouveau-ne. Arch Pediatr 4: 623–628.

Carbajal R, Lenclen R, Jugie M, et al. (2005). Morphine does not provide adequate analgesia for acute procedural pain among preterm neonates. Pediatrics 15: 1494–1500.

Carter BS, Bhatia J. (2001). Comfort/palliative care guidelines for neonatal practice: development and implementation in an academic medical centre. J Perinatol 21: 279–283.

Catlin AJ, Carter BS. (2002). Creation of a neonatal end of life protocol. J Perinatol 22: 184–195.

Corff KE, Seideman R, Venkataraman PS, et al. (1995). Facilitated tucking: a nonpharmacologic comfort measure for pain in preterm neonates. J Obstet Gynecol Neonatal Nurs 24: 143–147.

Doyle D, Hanks GWC, MacDonald N. (1993). Introduction. In: Doyle D, Hanks G, Cherny NI, et al. (eds) Oxford textbook of palliative medicine. Oxford University Press, Oxford, pp. 1–8.

Duhn LJ, Medves JMA. (2004). Systematic integrative review of infant pain assessment tools. Adv Neonatal Care 4: 126–140.

Eiser C. (1995). Children's understanding of the cancer experience. Intern J Pediatr Hematol/ Oncol 2: 357–367.

Ersek M. (1999). Enhancing effective pain management by addressing patient barriers to analgesic use. J Hospice Palliative Nurs 1: 87–96.

Fearon I, Kisilevsky BS, Hains SM, et al. (1997). Swaddling after heel lance: age-specific effects on behavioral recovery in preterm infants. J Dev Behav Pediatr 18: 222–232.

Ferris FD, Balfour HM, Bowen K et al. A model to Guide Hospice Palliative Care: Based on National Principles and Norms of Practice. Canadian Hospice Palliative Care Association (CHPCA), Ottawa, Canada. Online. Available: http://chpca.net/ marketplace/national_norms_of_ practice.htm

Field MJ, Behrman RE. (2003) (eds). Committee on Palliative and End of Life Care for Children and Their Families. When Children Die: Improving Palliative and End-of-Life Care for Children and Their Families. Institute of Medicine of the National Academy of Science, Washington, DC, pp. 1–16.

Fike D. (2003). Assessment and management of the substance-exposed newborn and infant. In: Kenner C, Lott JW (eds) Comprehensive neonatal nursing; a physiologic perspective, 3rd edn, pp. 773–802, WB Saunders, Philadelphia, PA.

Flaskerud JH, Winslow BJ, (1998). Conceptualizing vulnerable populations health-related research. Nursing Res. 47(2): 69–78.

Foster R. (2001). Nursing judgment: the key to pain assessment in critically ill children. J Soc Pediatr Nurs 6: 90–93.

Franck LS. (1987). A national survey of assessment and treatment of pain and agitation in the neonatal intensive care unit. J Obstet Gynecol Neonatal Nurs 16: 387–393.

Gibbins S, Stevens B, Hodnett E, et al. (2002). Efficacy and safety of sucrose for procedural pain relief in preterm and term neonates. Nurs Res 51: 375–382.

Gray L, Miller LW, Philipp BL, et al. (2002). Breastfeeding is analgesic in healthy newborns. Pediatrics 109: 677–686.

Grunau RVE, Holsti L, Whitfield MF, et al. (2000). Are twitches, startles, and body movements pain indicators in extremely low birth weight infants? Clin J Pain 16: 37–45.

Grunau RVE, Weinberg J, Whitfield MF. (2004). Neonatal procedural pain and preterm infant cortisol response to novelty at 8 months. Pediatrics 114: e77–84.

Hockenberry M, Wilson D, Winkelstein M, et al. (2003). Wong's nursing care of infants and children, 7th edn. Mosby, St. Louis, MO.

Hodgkinson K, Bear M, Thorn J, et al. (1994). Measuring pain in neonates: evaluating an instrument and developing a common language. Aust J Adv Nurs 12: 17–22.

Holsti L, Grunau RVE, Oberlander T, et al. (2004). Specific newborn individualized developmental care and assessment program movements are associated with acute pain in preterm infants in the neonatal intensive care unit. Pediatrics 114: 65–72.

Hoyert DL, Freedman MA, Strobino DM, et al. (2001). Annual summary of vital statistics 2000. Pediatrics 108: 1241–1255.

Hummel P, Puchalski M. (2001). Neonatal pain, agitation & sedation scale. Loyola Medical Centre, Maywood, IL. Online. Available: http://www.n-pass.com/research.html

Hummel P, Puchalski M, Creech S, et al. (2003). N-PASS: Neonatal pain, agitation and sedation scale – reliability and validity. Pediatric Academic Societies Annual Meeting, 2003, Seattle Washington (Abstract).

Jacox A, Carr DB, Payne R, et al. (1994). Management of cancer pain. Clinical practice guidance. Agency for Health Care Policy and Research, Clinical Guideline Number 9, Publication No. 94-0592: March 1994. US Govt, Washington DC.

Johnston CC, Filion F, Snider L, et al. (2002). Routine sucrose analgesia during first week of life in neonates less than 31 weeks post-conceptional age. Pediatrics 110: 523–528.

Johnston CC, Stevens BJ, Pinelli, et al. (2003). Kangaroo Care is effective in diminishing procedural pain in neonates. Arch Pediatr Adolesc Med 157: 1084–1088.

Leffers J, Martins D, McGrath M, et al. (2004). Development of a theoretical construct for risk and vulnerability from six empirical studies. Res Theory Nurs Pract 18: 15–34.

Leuthner SR. (2001). Decisions regarding resuscitation of the extremely premature infant and models of best interest. J Perinatol 21: 1–6.

Leuthner SR. (2004). Palliative care of the infant with lethal anomalies. Pediatr Clin North Am 51: 747–759.

McCaffery M, Pasero C. (1999). Pain: Clinical manual, 2nd edn. Mosby, St. Louis, MO.

McConnell Y, Frager G. (2003). (Draft) A Module for the Ian Anderson Continuing Education Program in End-of-Life Care. Dalhousie University, Faculty of Medicine and Pediatric Palliative Care, IWK Health Center, Halifax.

McIntosh N. (1997). Pain in the newborn, a possible new starting point. Eur J Pediatr 156: 173–177.

Oberlander TF, Grunau RVE, Fitzgerald C, et al. (2002). Does parenchymal brain injury affect biobehavioral pain responses in very low birth weight infants at 32 weeks' postconceptional age? Pediatrics 110: 570–576.

Pierucci RL, Kirby RS, Leuthner SR. (2001). End-of-life care for neonates and infants: the experiences and effects of a palliative care consultation service. Pediatrics 108: 653–660.

Purdy IB. (2004). Vulnerable: A concept analysis. Nurs Forum 39: 25–33.

Shapiro CR. (1993). Nurses judgements of pain in term and preterm newborns. J Obstet Gynecol Neonatal Nurs 22: 41–47.

Spence K, Gillies D, Harrison D, et al. (2003). A reliable pain assessment tool for clinical assessment in the neonatal intensive care unit. J Obstet Gynecol Neonatal Nurs 34: 80–86.

Stevens BJ, Johnston CC, Horton L. (1994). Factors that influence the behavioural pain responses of premature infants. Pain 59: 101–109.

Stevens B, Johnston C, Petryshen P, et al. (1996). Premature Infant Pain Profile: development and initial validation. Clin J Pain 12: 13–22.

Stevens B, Johnston C, Franck L, et al. (1999). The efficacy of developmentally sensitive interventions and sucrose for relieving procedural pain in very low birth weight neonates. Nurs Res 48: 35–43.

Stevens B, Yamada J, Ohlsson A. (2001). Sucrose for analgesia in newborn infants undergoing painful procedures. The Cochrane Database of Systematic Reviews, Issue 3. Online. Available: http://www.nichd.nih.gov/cochrane/Stevens/Stevens.htm

Stevens B, McGrath P, Gibbins S, et al. (2003). Procedural pain in newborns at risk for neurologic impairment. Pain 105: 27–35.

Stevens B, Yamada J, Beyene J, et al. (2005). Consistent management of repeated procedural pain with sucrose in preterm neonates: is it effective and safe for repeated use over time? Clin J Pain 21: 543–548.

Sutton LM, Porter LS, Keefe FJ. (2002). Cancer pain at the end of life: A bio-psychosocial perspective. Pain 99: 5–10.

Taber's Cyclopedic Medical Dictionary, 19th edn. (2001). FA Davis, Philadelphia, PA.

Thomas K. (1989). How the NICU environment sounds to a preterm infant. MCN Am J Matern Child Nurs 14: 249–251.

Upadhyay A, Aggarwal R, Narayan S, et al. (2004). Analgesic effect of expressed breast milk in procedural pain in term neonates: a randomized, placebo-controlled, double-blind trial. Acta Paediatr 93: 518–522.

van Dijk M, de Boer JB, Koot HM, et al. (2000). The reliability and validity of the COMFORT scale as a postoperative pain instrument in 0 to 3-year-old infants. Pain 84: 367–377.

van Dijk M, Peters J, Bouwmeester N, et al. (2002). Are postoperative pain instruments useful for specific groups of vulnerable infants? Clin Perinatol 29: 469–491.

Walden M, Penticuff J, Stevens B, et al. (2001). Changes over six weeks in physiologic and behavioral responses of preterm neonates to a painful stimulus. J Natl Assoc Neonatal Nurs 1: 94–106.

Whitfield MF. (2003). Psychosocial effects of intensive care on infants and families after discharge. Semin Neonatol 8: 185–193.

World Health Organization. (1990). Cancer pain relief and palliative care. Report of a WHO Expert Committee, Geneva (WHO Technical Report Series, No. 804).

World Health Organization. (1998). Cancer pain relief and palliative care in children. World Health Organization in collaboration with the International Association for the Study of Pain, Geneva.

Zahr LK, Balian S. (1995). Responses of premature infants to routine nursing interventions and noise in the NICU. Nurs Res 44: 179–185.

Infant pain in developing countries: a South African perspective

Rene Albertyn
Monique van Dijk
Dick Tibboel
Inge de Liefde
Adrian T Bosenberg

Heinz Rode
Jenny Thomas

INTRODUCTION

Infant pain management has attracted ever-increasing attention in the Western world over the last 20 years. As a result, a range of pain assessment instruments have been validated, and randomized controlled trials have tested analgesic efficacy and safety in neonates and infants. Pain assessment and treatment protocols have become part of daily practice in hospitals. Developing countries, however, often lack the resources and infrastructure for pain research and therapy. Therefore, future training and education programs need to direct attention to the specific cultural, economical and disease-related conditions specific for developing countries. From a societal perspective, it is time to employ Western research experience to support the specific clinical questions that have arisen in the developing world. As relevant examples, this chapter will address the challenges associated with the management and assessment of pain in HIV-positive (HIV+) infants as well as in burn-injured infants from a predominantly South African perspective.

PAIN IN HIV-POSITIVE INFANTS

While research on the management and treatment of HIV/AIDS in both adults and older children gets full attention, only a few papers have documented relevant aspects of pain in infants and small children infected with the HIV virus (Hirschfeld et al. 1996, Gaughan et al. 2002, Lolekha et al. 2004). It appears that women and children infected with the HIV virus are at a greater risk for under-treatment of pain and that the clinical course of HIV is more rapid in children than in adults (MacDougall 1998). American literature indicated that, on average, 30–80% of those diagnosed with HIV will experience pain, with 85% of patients estimated to be under-treated for pain (Breitbart et al. 1996). Similar research is lacking in developing countries and, therefore, the incidence of pain and its treatment for these countries is unknown. The fact that infants may contract the HIV virus and subsequently die of HIV-related infections is not widely recognized, as HIV is predominantly perceived as an adult disease. In addition, infant HIV is not recognized as a first-world problem, as it is mostly prevalent in developing countries. Consequently, HIV-related pain in the adult population is well recognized and well investigated, whereas information on pain in the infant group is unrecognized, under-reported and extrapolated from adult patients. While bodies such as the World Health Organization provide basic information on the pharmacological management of pain in HIV-infected individuals 15 years and older, guidelines on the management of pain, discomfort and anxiety in HIV+ infants are non-existent.

Epidemiology of HIV/AIDS

Globally, around 39.4 million people were infected with the HIV virus in 2004 (avert.org 2005a). An estimated 25 million (70%) people infected with the HIV virus are living in sub-Saharan Africa, a region that makes up 10% of the world's population. Around 2.2 million people have died of HIV-related infections in this region with a further 2.1 million new infections reported in 2003. Health surveillance studies have shown a sharp increase in the incidence of HIV infection with 5 million new cases reported in 2004 (avert.org 2005a). Worldwide, approximately 10.5 million children under the age of 5 die each year. Of the 20 countries with the highest incidence of mortality in this age group in the world, 19 are in Africa (World Health Organization 2003a). Since 1981, more than 20 million people have died of HIV-related diseases. Globally, around 2 million children younger than 15 years of age are living with HIV, while an estimated 12 million are orphaned by AIDS.

Reliable information on the morbidity and mortality associated with infant HIV/AIDS in sub-Saharan Africa is scarce. Estimates on HIV infections in South Africa revealed a 28% infection rate in a population of 40 million people. Furthermore, 13% of all the people infected with the HIV virus are living in South Africa. Mother-to-child transmission during pregnancy and birth, and the stigma associated with non-breastfeeding and HIV testing are largely responsible for the high incidence of infant HIV in South Africa. The challenges of HIV are complicated by the South African government's apparent lack of acceptance of the true pathology and disease processes of this illness. In 2001, for instance, the South African government questioned the statistics on HIV infections and AIDS-related mortality. In an ensuing lawsuit the Minister of Health was compelled to implement a mother-to-child transmission program. Only since 2003 has antiretroviral therapy become more available as part of a national program. Despite this turnaround, the Minister of Health continued to advocate a diet of beetroot, olive oil, garlic and African potato for people with HIV (http://www.aids.org.za/hiv.htm and http://www.wsws.org/articles/2004/

feb2004/stha-f16.shtml). There are signs of change, but for the moment, patients are encouraged to improve their diets and ignore the advantages of anti-retroviral agents. A variety of factors such as lack of monitoring facilities and lack of resources are further responsible for the under-reporting of HIV in infants.

Pain management issues

Parental factors

Parents often fear discrimination if their children are identified as being infected with HIV. Infants are, as a rule, not admitted to hospital because they are HIV+, but rather because they are sick. The fact that they are HIV+ is often only determined weeks into the admission phase. South African law dictates that parents must give consent before an infant can be tested for HIV. The high refusal rate is likely to contribute to the under-diagnosing and incorrect treatment of HIV and associated pain in hospitalized infants. These children will be denied the opportunity to receive highly active antiretroviral therapy (HAART) and will die as a result.

Parental illiteracy and poverty are additional factors challenging pain management in children. Around 96% of the patients treated at the Red Cross War Memorial Hospital are extremely poor and from severely disadvantaged communities. Parental illiteracy is a major obstacle in the management of patients after discharge, especially those on palliative care. Few parents can read the instructions on medicine labels; others cannot read the time and as a result are unsure when to administer the next dose of medicine. Correct storage of medicine is further hampered by the unavailability of refrigeration in poorer communities and informal settlements.

Background information: where do the patients come from? A survey was performed in 2004 in a township in Capetown called Brown's Farm with an estimated 1.5 million population. Five inhabitants were trained to do house-to-house surveys and visited in this manner 1364 families. These families live in shacks, small cabins with a corrugated iron roof without indoor electricity or running water. All but two respondents were of South African nationality. Up to 17 people (median of three) may live in a shack under very poor circumstances. Forty percent of these families were unemployed; in the remaining 60% one or two adults were employed, not always regularly. Monthly incomes range from US$0–75 (46.8%) to >US$75–220 (38.9%). Approximately 14% of the respondents earned >220 US$, primarily because both husband and wife were employed. Numbers of children ranged from none (19.4%), one or two

(52.8%), three or four (23.4%) up to 4.4% with five to ten children. Healthcare problems in the 2433 children (0–18 years) of these families were: 121 burns, 77 motor vehicle accidents, 22 head injuries, 21 rapes, seven assaults and three near-drownings. Burns were caused by hot water ($n = 68$), paraffin stove ($n = 15$), open fire ($n = 15$), hot oil ($n = 7$), hot food ($n = 8$) or cloths on fire ($n = 8$).

Of all 2433 children, 283 (11.6%) had been admitted to the Red Cross Children's Hospital; another 30 children elsewhere. Reasons for admissions were, in descending order, respiratory tract problems (mostly asthma) (31%), diarrhoea and/or vomiting (17.3%), accidents and assaults (14.1%), burns (7.3%) and the remaining categories included neurological, heart, gastrointestinal, ear-throat-nose and eye problems.

Healthcare-related factors

The only hospital in sub-Saharan Africa with a paediatric pain team is the 320-bed Red Cross War Memorial Hospital in Cape Town, South Africa. There, two health professionals, comprised of a paediatric anaesthesiologist and a pain specialist (social scientist) are responsible for pain management, covering both inpatients and outpatients.

Pain management in many South African hospitals is, to a large extent, the responsibility of inexperienced health professionals. Being untrained and understaffed, they are often unable to recognize and manage pain and discomfort, especially in young children. For example, South African nurses and doctors receive limited training on issues pertaining to pain management. Pain management is not seen as a priority; rather emphasis is given to the management of the disease process and not to pain. This is illustrated by the often-observed fear of administering opioids such as morphine, which are thought to cause respiratory arrest and death. An evaluation of 121 deceased HIV+ infants under the age of 1 year in the period 2002–2004 in two paediatric wards at the Red Cross Children's Hospital revealed that 84% did not receive any analgesics in the last week of life, despite a variety of painful symptoms related to pneumonia, sepsis, gastroenteritis, meningitis, etc. Six infants received intravenous continuous morphine during their last week of life, thanks to their admission to the intensive care unit, where monitoring is available. Staff shortages and large patient numbers in South African state hospitals additionally contribute to the inadequate management of paediatric pain, as pain management is often not given priority. Prescribed medication is not necessarily given and preprocedural analgesia is often inadequately (wrong timing, incorrect dosing) administered in daily practice.

A number of pain clinics specializing in adult pain are available in South Africa, whereas none are available for children, either in South Africa or on the continent of Africa.

Disease-related factors

HIV develops over time and the World Health Organization has classified HIV/AIDS by four stages (2005).

- Stage I: Associated conditions such as acute retroviral infection, asymptomatic or persistent generalized lymphadenopathy.
- Stage II: Weight loss less than 10% of body weight, minor mucocutaneous manifestations, herpes zoster within the past 5 years, and recurrent upper respiratory tract infections.
- Stage III: Weight loss more than 10% of body weight, unexplained chronic diarrhoea, prolonged fever, oral *Candida*, pulmonary tuberculosis within the past 12 months, severe bacterial infection (e.g. pneumonia).
- Stage IV or 'full-blown AIDS': Unexplained severe wasting or severe malnutrition, recurrent severe bacterial infections, extrapulmonary tuberculosis, HIV encephalopathy.

Disease-related pain conditions can result from both infectious and non-infectious pathological conditions and can be acute or chronic. The diagnosis and presence of the potentially painful symptoms associated with opportunistic infections (i.e. pneumonia, meningitis, gastroenteritis) should be considered in addition to the challenges associated with drug interaction and pre-emptive pain during procedures. Below is a summary of conditions and symptoms indicative of pain and discomfort in HIV+ patients.

- Oral and oesophageal mucositis; aphthous ulcers; *Candida*, herpes and cytomegalovirus. All these symptoms may cause dysphagia, salivary gland infection and ulcerative oesophagitis. Oesophageal and gastrointestinal pain can cause poor oral intake, increased weight loss, malnutrition, failure to thrive and progression to wasting syndrome.
- Wasting syndrome can be associated with chronic diarrhoea (contributing to buttock ulceration and cramping), mouth and throat ulceration, fatigue, fever and weakness (enhancing any pain experience), depression, musculoskeletal pain, abdominal pain and neuropathy secondary to nutritional deficiencies. Pain associated with wasting syndrome is one of the most challenging pain syndromes to treat (Grubman and Oleske 2003).

- Diarrhoea and vomiting are commonly associated with abdominal cramps, oesophagitis and diaper dermatitis.
- Encephalitis and CNS infections may give headache and epileptic seizures as well as variability in consciousness. Neurological and neuromuscular pain is common in children with HIV/AIDS including symptoms and diagnoses such as hypertonicity, spasticity, static and progressive encephalopathy, herpes zoster and myopathy.
- Pneumonia and pulmonary tuberculosis accompanied with severe respiratory distress and coughing may cause both pain and distress.
- Abdominal pain caused by pancreatitis, hepatitis, hepatosplenomegaly, inflammatory and infectious colitis.
- Skin and soft tissue complications such as oral thrush and skin rash are potentially painful and can be associated with both acute and chronic pain.
- The problems of neuropathic pain syndromes, peripheral neuropathy, myelopathy and Karposi's sarcoma do not appear to be a consideration in this age group as they are seldom observed in the age group <1 year.

Side effects of antiretroviral therapy such as skin rash and diarrhoea may induce painful complications such as diaper dermatitis (World Health Organization 2003b). Additionally side effects include fatigue, anorexia, headaches, and neuropathy, some of which are difficult to assess in infants. Furthermore, it is difficult to differentiate between the side effects of HAART and those attributed to the disease process.

LACK OF DRUG RESOURCES

One of the more prominent obstacles in paediatric pain management is the lack of resources. State hospitals in South Africa, normally funded by the South African government, operate on tight budgets. Most patients seen at these hospitals are from disadvantaged communities and cannot pay for medical treatment. In addition, budget constraints only allow for a small selection of analgesic medicines provided by the State Health Department. State hospitals will only stock drugs that are on the essential drug list. This list includes the following analgesic drugs for children; paracetamol, ibuprofen and morphine. Recently the addition of tilidine HCL, codeine and oral clonidine has been requested. Transdermal fentanyl patches, fentanyl lollies and oxycodone are not available. This restriction often necessitates the combining of two medicines for more intense pain relief.

As no clinical trials have as yet been carried out in HIV+ infants, many drugs are used off-label. Neonatal physiology reflects an immature organ function requiring decreased drug doses and longer dosage intervals. Formulations for this group are inappropriate; suppositories are too big, solutions may be problematic (alcohol, tartrazine) and many drugs such as midazolam are only available as tablets for oral administration.

Highly active antiretroviral therapy (HAART)

Antiretroviral therapy is still not freely available for patients who require it. Mother-to-child transmission programs are available throughout South Africa but legislation prevents the HIV testing of a child without parental consent. This lack of consent could lead to under-diagnosing and incorrect treatment of the HIV+ children. Treatment regimens are based on CD4 count levels, and treatment is usually initiated when this level falls below 20%. HAART is complicated by the frequent necessity to administer anti-tuberculosis drugs concurrently. The educational and socio-economic circumstances of families are limiting factors in HAART provision. Parents often have no or a low income, which has an impact on, for example, transport to HIV clinics or hospitals to obtain HAART or follow-up visits. Additionally, those living in informal settlements often do not have access to adequate storage facilities (e.g. refrigerators) for these drugs. In addition, parental illiteracy plays a major role in non-compliance because parents are often not able to follow written instructions for drug administration.

PAIN ASSESSMENT IN HIV+ INFANTS

Background

Pain assessment in HIV+ infants is hampered by several factors. First, pain caused by HIV infection may be chronic, acute or recurrent. It can also originate from different sources, as indicated above. The underlying pathology associated with opportunistic infections can change virtually on a daily basis. Infants diagnosed with HIV or AIDS do not respond to pain/discomfort in the same manner that sick infants in developed countries would. This may be due to a number of factors in addition to the severity of illness. The infants are often from underprivileged circumstances including lack of proper nutrition or hygiene, inadequate housing (e.g. lack of space, no electricity or running water), inadequate or no perinatal care. In addition, infants are often understimulated and developmentally delayed as luxuries such as developmental toys, nurseries, warmth, parental presence (parents are often too sick or have died of HIV-related diseases) are not available for these children.

Second, language barriers and cultural differences limit the use of conventional assessment methods in South African hospitals. South Africa has a multi-cultural and multilanguage society with a total of 11 languages and cultures. Language barriers prevent health caregivers from communicating with the parents and involving them in the assessment process. As a result, the rationale behind the use of a specific pain assessment tool cannot be adequately explained to the parent/caregiver.

More than three dozen pain assessment instruments are now available for neonates and infants (Franck et al. 2000, van Dijk et al. 2004) (see Chapter 6 for a comprehensive review of pain assessment in infants and neonates). Most instruments comprise behavioural assessment including facial expression, crying and often body movements. They have been primarily validated for acute or postoperative pain assessment and have not been tested in the South African HIV+ infant and may not be applicable.

Behavioural indicators

Usually a painful facial expression comprises brow bulge, nasolabial furrow and eye squeeze. However, HIV+ infants often do not show facial expressions of pain. It is not fully clear whether this could be caused by the severity of illness, severe malnutrition, or lack of stimulation earlier in life. Instead of facial grimacing or a 'pain face', they display wide-opened eyes expressing fear or even depression. Only in extremely painful situations, such as diaper change with severe diaper rash, might grimacing and some crying be observed.

Hospitalized infants will normally cry because of separation anxiety, fear of strangers or painful procedures. South African HIV+ infants, however, seem less inclined to express their pain, hunger, discomfort or other sources of distress by crying. One explanation could be attributed to lack of energy caused by opportunistic infections and the management associated with these infections. Hypothetically, one could speculate that HIV+ infants who were born sick cannot discriminate between a state of well-being and a state of being unwell. Consequently, the infant is not given attention or adequate pain treatment.

Severity of illness (for instance meningitis, gastroenteritis and pneumonia) and underdevelopment may result in a limited range of body movements. Even in the awake state, compared to age-related 'normal' ill infants, HIV+ infants will show few, if any, similarities related to the body movements associated with pain. Because of the lack of activity, it is difficult to tell if a child is asleep or awake because of their limited responses. They often seem asleep but are not when observed more closely.

The physical and emotional discomfort in HIV+ infants scale (PEDHIV scale)

In view of the above considerations, we developed a new assessment tool, which focuses on physical and emotional pain and discomfort and takes many potentially painful symptoms into account. The PEDHIV scale assesses the child's behaviour (behavioural state, cry and a numerical rating scale for pain and discomfort). In addition, physical examinations of the mouth (to detect oral lesions or thrush), skin (extent of rash), buttocks (to determine the extent of diaper rash) and breathing (to assess respiratory distress) are recorded. Medical and nursing charts are reviewed for incidences of diarrhoea, vomiting and feeding difficulties. For background information pharmacological treatment details and confirmed diagnoses are noted.

Preliminary results of PEDHIV assessment

During a 7-month period (February to September 2005) the scale was tested in 115 hospitalized infants (58 girls, 57 boys) under the age of 1 year (median age 136 days) diagnosed with HIV stage 2 or 3. A total of 332 assessments were made, with one to 16 assessments per child. One of the two experienced observers (intraclass correlation coefficient 0.89) scored a numeric rating (range 0 to 10) indicating discomfort in almost half of all observations (48.7%) of 4 or higher. Nevertheless, no crying was observed in 73% and only moaning in 20.6% of all observations. Physical examination showed respiratory distress in 37.2% and severe respiratory distress (gasping, nasal flaring, etc.) in 28.4% of observations. Mild to moderate diaper dermatitis was seen in 25.5%, and severe diaper dermatitis (entire diaper area with oozing papules or pustules/erosions) in 20% of observations. Oral lesions or thrush were scored in 20.2% of the observations. The following diagnoses were found to be pain-inducing; 62.6% had pneumonia, 60.9% sepsis, 44.3% gastroenteritis, 38.3% failure-to-thrive and 16.5% meningitis.

PAIN TREATMENT

Pharmacological pain treatment

The World Health Organization (1990) has provided guidelines for the pharmacological approach to pain management. In brief, medication should be prescribed following the WHO 'ladder', medication should be given by the clock (pro re nata prescriptions should be avoided), and oral administration of drugs is recom-mended as opposed to intramuscular or intravenous injections as these cause even more pain.

The WHO analgesic ladder provides a validated simple method for treating children with HIV/AIDS. Mild pain should be treated with a non-opioid plus 1 adjuvant. Pharmacological agents such as acet-aminophen, aspirin, ibuprofen and ketalorac combined with an adjuvant (i.e. tricyclic antidepressants) are proposed for the treatment of minor pain. Moderate pain and persisting pain should be treated with weak opioids (codeine, hydrocodone with acetaminophen) plus 1 non-opioid plus 1 adjuvant (i.e. antidepressants, barbiturates, anxiolytic agents). Morphine, oxycodone, and fentanyl are suggested for the treatment of severe pain, combined with 1 non-opioid plus 1 adjuvant. In addition to the above WHO regimen, provision of anxiolysis is essential. In our experience, midazolam or clonidine have been most useful.

Epidural anaesthesia in neonates and infants

Against the background of the shortage of intensive care unit (ICU) beds and ventilators, methods have to be 'invented' to prevent systemic side effects of opioids such as respiratory depression, yet still providing appropriate analgesia perioperatively. In general, opioids, especially morphine, are used for pain management in children after major surgery (van Dijk et al. 2002). However, morphine has unwanted side effects such as vomiting, reduced gut motility, urinary retention, pruritis, hypotension, bradycardia and respiratory depression. Neonates in particular require a narrower therapeutic window for morphine compared to older children (Bouwmeester et al. 2003a). Therefore, most neonates on morphine need to be mechanically ventilated and closely monitored (Bouwmeester 2002, Bouwmeester et al. 2003b). Apart from these side effects, systemic morphine administration may have still unknown effects on the developing brain (see Chapters 9 and 10 for a review of opioids).

An alternative method of pain management after major surgery is epidural anaesthesia, already well-established in adults (Boos et al. 1996) but not as widely used in some centres for children (see Chapter 11 for a review of neuraxial and regional analgesia and anaesthesia). Children, especially neonates, were thought to be more susceptible to complications such as severe cardiac dysrhythmia with cardiac arrest, respiratory depression and convulsions, due to low levels of protein alpha 1-acid glycoprotein (AAG) and serum albumin (Bosenberg 1998, Mazoit and Dalens 2004). Nevertheless, AAG levels have been found to rise significantly after major surgery, approaching

adult levels within 4 days (Booker et al. 1996, Larsson et al. 1997). This suggests a degree of protection, although AAG has low capacity for binding local anaesthetic drugs. Besides, the epidural space acts as a buffer, preventing a rapid increase in serum concentration. Additionally, neonates are already quite capable of excretion of the analgesic drug (Mazoit and Dalens 2004). Larsson et al. showed that neonates undergoing major abdominal surgery who received a bolus of 1.8 mg/kg of bupivacaine after induction of anaesthesia, followed by continuous bupivacaine infusion of 0.2 mg/kg/h, had relatively unchanged concentrations of bupivacaine between 1–24 hours. Interindividual variation was large, though, and a great many patients showed increasing total plasma concentrations of bupivacaine after 48 hours. No complications were observed, suggesting that technique, dose and medication are safe for these patients (Larsson et al. 1997).

There are several other studies about the efficacy and safety of epidural anaesthesia in children. Jylli et al. (2002) retrospectively evaluated continuous epidural infusion for postoperative pain in patients from 5 days to 20 years old. Postoperative pain relief as measured by clinical judgement was good in 76% of the patients, with only a few minor complications, mostly related to the epidural technique (such as leakage or catheter dislodgement) (Jylli et al. 2002). Moreover, they found that the rate of success was greater in younger children. Bosenberg (1998) studied the effects of epidural anaesthesia in neonates, and found satisfactory postoperative pain relief. The only complications in 240 neonates were one dural puncture, one convulsion and one intravascular migration of catheter. Other studies reported comparable results with rare incidences of complications and satisfactory analgesia (Pietropaoli et al. 1993, Bosenberg 1998, Aram et al. 2001, Jylli et al. 2002, Williams and Howard 2003).

A great additional advantage of epidural anaesthesia in children and neonates is lesser need for muscle relaxants, opioid analgesics and ventilatory support after surgery (Bosenberg 1998). Especially neonates as noted above are very sensitive to the respiratory depressant effects of opioids. In these patients epidural anaesthesia will result in earlier extubation, avoiding ventilator-related complications such as infections and barotrauma, which may result in a shorter duration of stay in the ICU and hospital (McNeely et al. 1997, Bosenberg 1998). These advantages seem ideal especially for developing countries where ventilatory support is often not feasible and ICU care is limited. However, the risk–benefit ratio of epidural analgesia in neonates in developing countries needs to be rationalized. The complication rate is low, but not insignificant. It is recommended that only anaesthesiologists with training and experience in the technique should perform the epidural technique in these small children. In conclusion, in countries with limited resources, epidural anaesthesia can be of great value for pain management in neonates after major surgery due to the low complication rate and good postoperative pain relief.

Non-pharmacological management of pain

The WHO analgesic ladder does not include non-pharmacological pain control, the importance of which should not be underestimated. Massage, reflexology, aromatherapy and heat application are techniques that could supplement the pharmacological regimen. Touch techniques have gained a place in the management of stress and anxiety associated with pain. The beneficial effects of touch in young children are well known, as are the consequences of limited or no tactile stimulation. Unfortunately, evidence from randomized controlled trials is limited and this may be due to the fact that it is difficult to assess the benefits of these non-pharmacological treatments (see Chapter 12 for a review of environmental, physical and behavioural interventions to prevent and manage pain and discomfort). Staff shortages, high patient admission numbers and the absence of parents or caregivers are predominantly responsible for the lack of tactile stimulation often observed in hospitalized children. At the Red Cross Children's Hospital, trained and registered aromatherapists and reflexologists provide these supplementary therapies.

For procedural pain, giving sucrose or applying local anaesthetic cream prior to venepuncture and immunizations are important measures to limit the burden of pain, just as in other countries.

MANAGEMENT OF PAIN IN BURNED INFANTS

Burn injuries in childhood are notorious for the difficulty in management, the pain associated with treatment and the devastating long-term consequences. Occurring in both developed and developing countries, but more greatly associated with poverty, burn injuries are the leading cause of death in children aged 5–14 years. Poor socioeconomic circumstances, financial constraints, lack of resources and unavailability of trained health professionals contribute to the higher morbidity in this age group. The incidence of burn injuries in infancy is not accurately documented in South Africa. In the Red Cross Children's Hospital, 800–1000 children are admitted yearly because of burns. Management requires a proper assessment of pain and anxiety prior to treatment,

then reassessment once treatment has started to check adequacy of the treatment regimen. Treatment options in this group include paracetamol, codeine, tilidene hydrochloride, morphine, ketamine and clonidine. Clonidine has not been used in the neonatal age group. Local anaesthetics should be used whenever possible. Tolerance does occur in this age group and it is important to give enough drugs for analgesia in addition to provide a safe environment for the baby. The principles of management should include knowing and using a few drugs well. Table 19.1 shows the pharmacological protocol for the change of burn dressings used in the Red Cross Children's Hospital. However, as previously indicated, availability of analgesics and sedatives is limited.

Other limitations of current pain management have emerged from a small study performed from March until July 2005 on the burn unit of the Red Cross Children's Hospital. In 49 burn patients with a median age of 4 years (interquartile range 2 to 8 years), we performed a total of 131 assessments around daily change of dressings (COD). In the Table 19.1 protocol, premedication should be given

Table 19.1 Red Cross Children's Hospital protocol for change of dressing

Change of dressing medications	
To be given 30 minutes prior to dressing change:	
Midazolam: 0.5 mg/kg/dose (anxiolysis only)	
Paracetamol + codeine:	1 ml/kg/dose
Each ml contains paracetamol	20 mg/ml
+ codeine	1 mg/ml
Paracetamol: (singly) 20 mg/kg/dose	
Ibuprofen: 6 mg/kg/dose (as long as there are no contraindications)	
Valoron: 1 mg/kg/dose 1 drop = 2.5 mg	
Number of drops = Body weight divided by 2.5	
Ketamine: 2 mg/kg/dose per os	
Options: Midazolam + paracetamol + codeine + ibuprofen Midazolam + paracetamol + ibuprofen + valoron Midazolam + paracetamol + valoron Midazolam + paracetamol + valoron + ketamine per os Midazolam + paracetamol + ketamine per os	

Note: the intravenous formulations of ketamine and midazolam can be used orally, mixed with syrup to taste.

30 minutes prior to COD. In practice, however, the median time was 2 and 2.25 hours for tilidine HCL and midazolam, respectively. Shortage of nurses and lack of education on the relevance of timely administration of these drugs contribute to less than optimal pain management. Medications that are only prescribed in developing countries, for instance Valoron® drops consisting of tilidine HCL, although satisfactory in daily practice should be further investigated in these paediatric burn patients. Treatment efficacy should be determined by assessing both pain and anxiety in the burn patient during COD, in rest and during activities. For this reason a combined pain/anxiety tool is currently being tested for children older than 2 years. For the neonate and infant under the age of 2 years, an age-specific tool needs to be developed. This tool should incorporate the fact that sick and traumatized infants will respond to pain and discomfort differently than what is described in the available literature.

CULTURAL DILEMMAS

Working in South Africa with any health issue including HIV/AIDS requires some acknowledgement of cultural aspects. One such aspect is the influential role of the estimated 200 000 traditional healers or 'sangomas' in South Africa as compared to 23 000 trained doctors (Watson 2005). In rural areas an estimated 85% of the population first consult a traditional healer for illnesses against 70% in other areas. In September 2004, a bill passed by the South African government allowed the licensed traditional healer to prescribe sick leave and offer cures for some diseases, excluding AIDS. Traditional healers will nevertheless prescribe herbs such as *Hypoxis* (African potato) and *Sutherlandia* for the cure of AIDS (Mills et al. 2005a). It is feared that these herbs may inhibit drug metabolism of antiretroviral drugs and may cause unknown side effects (Mills et al. 2005b).

CONCLUSION

Very little literature currently exists on the specific management of pain in neonates, infants and older children in developing countries. Children are still seen as mini-adults, their drug doses are extrapolated from adult doses and health caregivers often base their ideas of paediatric pain assessment on how adults would respond in the same situation. Right now, children are suffering because of the existing and perhaps growing ignorance of those destined to care for them. Lack of knowledge around and acknowledgement of the existence of paediatric pain are key contributors to this situation.

Although analgesics may be prescribed they are often not given at all or not given at the correct times. Nursing is understaffed and the level of training of nurses varies enormously. Specific training and specialization should be offered to health professionals such as nurses, (para) medical students and intern doctors. Parental education is a creative challenge in finding ways to communicate with parents. Furthermore, pharmacokinetic and pharmacodynamic studies are needed to determine how analgesic drugs are metabolized in the severely ill, undernourished infant with multiple organ failure. With the increased administration of HAART, drug–drug interactions between HAART and analgesics, opioids and sedatives need to be studied.

Cultural differences in parental and child perception and coping with pain should be examined.

Appropriate pain and discomfort assessment tools should be validated for HIV+ infants and burn patients. These instruments should also be tested outside South Africa to establish optimal external validity. The ultimate goal is to implement these in daily practice.

There is an urgent need for collaboration with developed world partners to combine knowledge and resources from one side and the practical experiences and questions from the other side. Western experience (research) should be applied to support specific paediatric pain-related problems in the developing world. Very little in the world of pain assessment can be directly extrapolated from first-world information. Indigenous research is necessary to answer specific questions – but the ability to do professional and scientific research is lacking in developing countries. A recently initiated collaboration between the Red Cross Children's Hospital in Capetown, South Africa and the Erasmus MC-Sophia Children's Hospital in Rotterdam, The Netherlands is a first step in this direction.

REFERENCES

Aram L, Krane EJ, Kosloski LJ, et al. (2001). Tunneled epidural catheters for prolonged analgesia in pediatric patients. Anesth Analg 92: 1432–1438.

avert.org (2005a). World HIV & AIDS statistics. Online. Available: http://www.avert.org/worldstats.htm

avert.org (2005b). The different stages of HIV infection. Online. Available: http://www.avert.org

Booker PD, Taylor C, Saba G. (1996). Perioperative changes in alpha 1-acid glycoprotein concentrations in infants undergoing major surgery. Br J Anaesth 76: 365–368.

Boos K, Beushausen T, Ohrdorf W. (1996). [Peridural catheter for postoperative long-term analgesia in children]. Anasthesiol Intensivmed Notfallmed Schmerzther 31: 362–367.

Bosenberg AT. (1998). Epidural analgesia for major neonatal surgery. Paediatr Anaesth 8: 479–483.

Bouwmeester J. (2002). Evaluation of pain management in neonates after oesophageal atresia. Paediatric pain management: from personal-biased to evidence-based. Rotterdam, thesis.

Bouwmeester NJ, Hop WC, van Dijk M, et al. (2003a). Postoperative pain in the neonate: age-related differences in morphine requirements and metabolism. Intensive Care Med 29: 2009–2015.

Bouwmeester NJ, Van Den Anker JN, Hop WC, et al. (2003b). Age- and therapy-related effects on morphine requirements and plasma concentrations of morphine and its metabolites in postoperative infants. Br J Anaesth 90: 642–652.

Breitbart W, Passik S, McDonald MV, et al. (1996). Pain in AIDS: A call for action. Clinical Updates. Vol IV, Issue 1.

Franck LS, Greenberg CS, Stevens B. (2000). Pain assessment in infants and children. Pediatr Clin North Am 47: 487–512.

Gaughan DM, Hughes MD, Seage 3rd GR, et al. (2002). The prevalence of pain in pediatric human immunodeficiency virus/acquired immunodeficiency syndrome as reported by participants in the Pediatric Late Outcomes Study (PACTG 219). Pediatrics 109: 1144–1152.

Grubman S, Oleske JM. (2003). Palliative care for children infected with HIV. In: Shearer W, Hanson I (eds). Medical management of AIDS in children. WB Saunders, Philadelphia, pp. 349–360.

Hirschfeld S, Moss H, Dragisic K, et al. (1996). Pain in pediatric human immunodeficiency virus infection: incidence and characteristics in a single-institution pilot study. Pediatrics 98: 449–452.

Jylli L, Lundeberg S, Olsson GL. (2002). Retrospective evaluation of continuous epidural infusion for postoperative pain in children. Acta Anaesthesiol Scand 46: 654–659.

Larsson BA, Lonnqvist PA, Olsson GL. (1997). Plasma concentrations of bupivacaine in neonates after continuous epidural infusion. Anesth Analg 84: 501–505.

Lolekha R, Chanthavanich P, Limkittikul K, et al. (2004). Pain: a common symptom in human immunodeficiency virus-infected Thai children. Acta Paediatr 93: 891–898.

MacDougall DS. (1998). Pediatric HIV: evaluation, management, and rehabilitation. J Int Assoc Physicians AIDS Care 4: 16–25.

Mazoit JX, Dalens BJ. (2004). Pharmacokinetics of local anaesthetics in infants and children. Clin Pharmacokinet 43: 17–32.

McNeely JK, Farber NE, Rusy LM, et al. (1997). Epidural analgesia improves outcome following pediatric fundoplication. A retrospective analysis. Reg Anesth 22: 16–23.

Mills E, Cooper C, Seely D, et al. (2005a). African herbal medicines in the treatment of HIV: Hypoxis and Sutherlandia. An overview of evidence and pharmacology. Nutr J 4: 19.

Mills E, Foster BC, van Heeswijk R, et al. (2005b). Impact of African herbal medicines on antiretroviral metabolism. Aids 19: 95–97.

Pietropaoli JA, Jr, Keller MS, Smail DF, et al. (1993). Regional anesthesia in pediatric surgery: complications and postoperative comfort level in 174 children. J Pediatr Surg 28: 560–564.

van Dijk M, Bouwmeester J, Duivenvoorden HJ, et al. (2002). Efficacy of continuous versus intermittent morphine administration after major surgery in 0 to 3-year old infants: a double-blind randomised controlled trial. Pain 98: 298–306.

van Dijk M, Simons S, Bouwmeester NJ, et al. (2004). Pain assessment in neonates. Paediatric and Perinatal Drug Therapy 6: 97–103.

Watson J. (2005). Traditional healers fight for recognition in South Africa's AIDS crisis. Nat Med 11: 6.

Williams DG, Howard RF. (2003). Epidural analgesia in children. A survey of current opinions and practices amongst UK paediatric anaesthetists. Paediatr Anaesth 13: 769–776.

World Health Organization. (1990). Cancer pain relief and palliative care. Report of a WHO expert committee [World Health Organization Technical Report Series, 804] Geneva, Switzerland, pp. 1–75.

World Health Organization. (2003a). Global Health: today's challenges. Geneva, Switzerland, pp. 7–12.

World Health Organization (2003b). Managing antiretroviral side effects. HIV/AIDS antiretroviral newsletter. Geneva, Switzerland, pp. 1–8.

World Health Organization (2005). Interim WHO clinical staging of HIV/AIDS and HIV/AIDS case definitions for surveillance. Online: Available: http://www.who.who.int/hiv/pub/guidelines/casedefinitions/en/index.htm

Health policy and health economics related to neonatal pain

Shoo K Lee

INTRODUCTION

Pain and suffering of babies were frequently overlooked in the past, and some even argued that since babies have no subsequent recollection of events during infancy, pain and suffering during that time are irrelevant (Levy 1960, D'Apolito 1984, Shearer 1986). Today, this idea would seem preposterous, and in the modern neonatal intensive care unit (NICU), much attention is given to minimizing pain and suffering (Anand et al. 1987, Hatch 1987, Yaster 1987). Critically ill babies requiring assisted ventilation and multiple procedures are routinely sedated and treated with analgesics, handling is minimized and cuddling and bodily contact are encouraged to provide warmth and comfort, and to foster bonding and development (Als et al. 1986). However, everything in health care comes at a cost, financial or otherwise. Consequently, any therapy must be evaluated both by its benefits and its costs, and caregivers must constantly ask themselves whether their treatment is appropriate, how much is too much, under what conditions is it appropriate to provide sedation and analgesia, and at what cost. Unfortunately, measuring and managing pain in babies is challenging, and applying a valuation to pain is even more so. These are difficult issues that raise dilemmas with respect to policy development, and particularly for babies who cannot speak for themselves. In this chapter, we will consider issues that deal with health policy and economics related to neonatal pain.

CHALLENGES OF NEONATAL ANALGESIA IN HEALTH POLICY

Pain is a common problem across all ages. Moulin et al. (2002) reported that 29% of adult Canadians reported suffering from chronic non-cancer pain. Blyth et al. (2001) similarly reported a prevalence of 17% and 20% among Australian men and women respectively. A hospital-wide survey of children indicated that 49% reported moderate to severe pain in the previous 24 hours and 21% had clinically significant ongoing pain (Cummings et al. 1996). There are few studies of the prevalence of pain in babies, but data on the number of painful procedures that infants undergo while in the NICU suggest that at least in that context, the prevalence is high. In the Canadian Neonatal Network, Lisonkova et al. (2003) reported that in 2003, 52% of babies receiving assisted ventilation in the NICU were treated with sedation or analgesia for pain or discomfort during their stay. This percentage is probably an underestimate of the real prevalence, since there are few guidelines concerning use of analgesia for babies and there is considerable interhospital variation in the use of analgesics among NICUs (Lisonkova et al. 2003, Anand et al. 2004). Among Canadian NICUs, the incidence of analgesic and sedative use varied from 22% to 79% (Lisonkova et al. 2003).

Neonatal pain poses some unique health policy challenges. First, the recognition that pain is an important issue and needs to be treated in babies, is a relatively recent phenomenon. Consequently, although it has a high prevalence rate, it is seldom reported as part of public health or hospital statistics, and receives low priority and attention from policy makers and healthcare professionals alike (Glasziou 2002). The lack of emphasis and information about its prevalence, treatment and outcomes compound the lack of general awareness about neonatal pain. It is therefore imperative to have better data and to raise awareness about neonatal pain among both the public and health professional constituencies in order to make more timely progress on many policy issues.

Second, it is difficult to reach consensus about how best to evaluate and measure neonatal pain, when to treat, what therapies to use, and how best to manage pain over time. Unlike adults, who can verbalize or otherwise indicate discomfort and degrees of pain, babies communicate their feelings only through cry, facial and body expressions, and physiological change (Izard et al. 1980, Levine and Gordon 1982, Grunau and Craig 1987). Recently, there have been great strides in the development of reliable and valid pain measures and currently over three dozen measures exist (Duhn and Medves 2004) (see Chapter 6 for a complete review of pain assessment in infants). However, interpretation of pain scores is difficult under the best circumstances. Much of the knowledge about treatment of neonatal pain was derived from pain in adults and therefore is not always appropriate to extrapolate for infants. Efficacy and safety data specific to babies are not readily available for many pharmacological agents and treatments. Special consideration needs to be given to the fact that major organ and neurological systems are still in the process of development in babies and are more susceptible to any potentially adverse effects of pharmacological agents (Prechtl 1984, Flower 1985). Without good data, fashioning consensus for practice guidelines is difficult, and health professionals will continue to manage pain in varied ways.

After much consultation, the American Academy of Pediatrics and Canadian Paediatric Society (2000) and the National Institutes of Health/National Institute of Child Health and Human Development (NIH/NICHD) (Anand et al. 2005a) recently published consensus statements on the management of pain in infants. These valuable resources offer practical advice to practitioners on various aspects of pain assessment and management, including procedure-related pain, operative pain and trauma-related pain. They also emphasize the need for the practitioner to anticipate and recognize pain, the ethical mandate to treat pain and suffering, and that the treatment approach should be multimodal and meet the individual child's needs.

Third, better methods are needed to tailor treatments for individual babies because of differences in co-morbidities, drug metabolism and drug interactions (Glasziou 2002). The majority of medications used in children are 'off-label' (i.e. not tested for safety and efficacy in children as required by the US Food and Drug Administration (FDA) regulations), because of difficulties associated with ethical evaluation of drugs in the paediatric population (Anand et al. 2005b). Yet, babies are inherently different from adults in that their bodies and major organ systems are still developing and their physiology constantly changing. Consequently, drugs that are considered efficacious and safe for adults may have different effects in babies (see reviews on pharmacologic agents in Chapters 8–11). In particular, the long-term effects of pain or prolonged treatment with various pharmacological agents are still not well understood (see Chapters 4 and 5). Thus, it is important to properly test drugs for all treatments before using them in babies on a routine basis, and even more important to individualize drug therapy in babies than in adults to ensure safety and efficacy.

Fourth, there are unique organizational, financial and legal barriers to developing and implementing the most appropriate treatments. For instance, the small size of the market for neonatal therapeutic agents is a deterrent to conducting expensive clinical trials and leads to the phenomenon of 'orphan drugs', for which there is a need but not a sufficiently large market to entice development by pharmaceutical industries (Peabody et al. 1995). To address these barriers, healthcare organizations and governments must take proactive roles to establish specific social policies to ensure adequate research, development and supply of neonatal therapeutic agents (Arno et al. 1995).

To address this issue, the FDA issued a Pediatric Rule in 1994 that allowed the labelling of drugs for paediatric use based on extrapolation of efficacy in adults and additional pharmacokinetics, pharmacodynamics and safety studies in paediatric patients, if the course of the disease and the response to the drug are similar in children as in adults. Unfortunately, few well-conducted studies resulted from this Rule. Subsequent legislation was passed in 1997 that provided an additional 6-month exclusivity period for marketing to pharmaceutical companies for paediatric drug testing. Then, in 2002, Congress passed the Best Pharmaceuticals for Children (BPCA) Act (http://www. nichd.nih.gov/oppb/bpca/#bpca-act) to provide for the funding of paediatric drug studies through a collaborative process between industry and NIH/FDA.

Fifth, current knowledge translation processes for healthcare professionals to update their procedures and therapies remain largely ineffective and slow. The development of tools for accessing medical resources (e.g. Medline and Pubmed systems for searching the published literature, Cochrane Library of Systematic Reviews – see Chapter 17) has significantly improved access to information for health professionals (http://www.ncbi.nlm.nih.gov/entrez/query. fcgi?db=pubmed; Guyatt et al. 2000). However, the cadre of published information is large, and health professionals may not have the resources, time or expertise to sort through the volumes of material and find the information they need (Del Mar et al. 2001). Furthermore, the evidence suggests that even when information is readily available, it is often difficult to persuade healthcare professionals to change their practice accordingly (Lee et al. 2001). More recently, interactive and participatory methods using concepts like continuous quality improvement have shown promise for improving our ability to translate knowledge into practice and policy (Horbar et al. 2001).

Finally, there are potential ethical and medico-legal considerations relevant to health policy. Since babies are not able to give informed consent, parents are the usual accepted surrogates. Difficulties arise, however, when parents refuse consent for therapies that caregivers feel are in the best interests of the child. In these cases, the courts usually rule in the infant's favour and mandate the treatment. Although this has not been legally tested for pain management, it is commonly assumed that the legal precedent set for other treatments may apply. Furthermore, pain is now becoming a consideration in personal injury damage litigation for infants and children. Since babies are incompetent to give informed consent for clinical trials, the President's Commission for the Study of Ethical Problems in Medicine and Biomedical and Behavioral Research (1983) recommended that decisions made on such patients' behalf must protect the best interest of the patient and, therefore, limits may be placed on the range of acceptable decisions that surrogates may make. Institutional ethics committees adopt

much stricter ethical guidelines for clinical trials and research in babies than in adults, and studies that deal with neonatal pain may incur an even higher level of scrutiny. Infants who need chronic care are another important group who need particular attention because it would be inconsistent for society to undertake tremendous initiatives through neonatal intensive care to save their lives but not provide adequate resources to care for them and to relieve their pain and suffering.

COSTS OF NEONATAL PAIN

Costs are both financial and emotional, and affect the individual, family, caregivers and society at large. Consequently, any consideration of the costs of treating neonatal pain must take into account a whole range of perspectives and factors.

Financial costs

Neonatal intensive care for sick babies is very expensive and often prolonged. Lee and Anderson (2004) recently reported that in 2002, the average in-hospital cost (excluding physician fees and surgical patients) of neonatal intensive care in British Columbia, Canada was Can$1702 per day for very sick babies requiring tertiary level (Level 3) intensive care and Can$1315 per day for less sick babies requiring intermediate level (Level 2) neonatal care. Nursing care costs accounted for over 50% of the total NICU cost, whereas pharmacy and drug costs (excluding parenteral nutrition) accounted for less than 3% of the total NICU costs. Since drugs for sedation and pain control comprised only a fraction of total drug costs, the pharmacotherapy costs for pain management are relatively low compared with the overall costs of neonatal intensive care, even after accounting for the nursing cost of pain assessment and drug administration. In addition to hospital costs, the babies' families often incur out-of-pocket costs arising from loss of work, hospital visits, transportation and child care costs for siblings. However, for the most part, these costs are incurred irrespective of pain management and therefore cannot be strictly considered a cost of treating neonatal pain.

Costs are also incurred after initial discharge from hospital. For preterm babies less than 1000 g birth weight, about half are subsequently hospitalized during the first 3 years of life for various illnesses, and they require substantially more ambulatory care than term babies. Shankaran et al. (1988) estimated that direct medical costs incurred by these babies average between US$60 and US$1200 monthly, compared with US$22 to US$26 for healthy term babies. Given that these results were published in 1988, it is likely that these costs have increased substantially. In some instances, pain management remains an issue during re-hospitalization, and costs are incurred as a result, particularly if sedation and pain management are needed during assisted ventilation or procedures. However, these costs are within the range of costs incurred during initial hospitalization and are therefore modest. Costs are also incurred by parents, in paying for early intervention programmes and special education programmes. Raphael et al. (1985) estimated that special needs students incur annual expenses of US$7026, about twice that for regular students.

The extent to which analgesia is used at home during the early infant period for pain relief is also not well documented and may be an underestimated problem. The use of alternative therapies for pain relief, such as acupuncture, acupressure, herbal remedies and others are also paid for personally by parents and have not been articulated. These therapies are reviewed in Chapter 21. The costs of these therapies, as well as those of environmental, behavioural and physical therapies, have not been well documented for babies, but nevertheless represent direct costs to parents.

Walker et al. (1984) examined the cost–benefit of NICU care and estimated that costs ranged from $362 992 per survivor for infants weighing between 600 g and 699 g birth weight to $40 647 per survivor for those weighing between 900 g and 999 g birth weight. In contrast, the net present value of expected lifetime earnings ranged from zero earnings for infants weighing between 600 g and 699 g birth weight to $77 084 for those weighing between 900 g and 999 g birth weight. It should be noted that the costs described above do not consider quality of life. Boyle et al. (1983) used the concept of QALY (quality adjusted life years) to estimate that for babies less than 1000 g at birth, neonatal intensive care cost C$102 500 per additional survivor, C$9300 per life year gained and C$22 400 per quality adjusted life year gained. In this kind of analysis, the dimension of pain is captured, not separately but as part of the overall individual ratings of quality of life. We did not find studies that examined quality of life adjustment strictly as a function of pain. Thus, it is not possible to separate out the effect of pain singly on the quality of life. This area remains fertile for future investigations.

Non-financial costs

Non-financial costs are more difficult to measure, but nonetheless, they impose real burdens on the babies, families and society. These include pain and suffering of the baby, emotional costs to the parents and families, and financial burden placed on society. These costs have not been explored and require attention

in the future to truly understand the impact of pain and pain management on all of these individuals.

Pain and suffering of the baby

Pain and suffering of the baby are difficult to quantify or attach a value to, but they should not be overlooked as costs. Most adults are willing to pay for pain relief and indeed they do. A conservative estimate of the annual cost of chronic pain in the US was reported in excess of US$40 billion (Sheehan et al. 1996). In Canada, pain is the most common, debilitating and perplexing symptom reported by Canadians and in one province alone (Ontario), pain-related illness costs are estimated at approximately 5 billion dollars per year (Moulin et al. 2002). It could be argued that if babies were able to express themselves, they would be willing to pay for pain relief to relieve their suffering. Similarly, it is reasonable to assume that most parents would be willing to pay for pain relief for their babies, although the extent to which they would valuate this option has not been properly studied.

Emotional costs to parents

Parents suffer deep emotional distress when they have a sick baby (Lee et al. 1991). This is made worse if they perceive their baby to be suffering acute or persistent pain (Gale et al. 2004). In addition to anxiety and concern for their baby, parents may also feel overwhelmed by feelings of helplessness, guilt and even anger towards the caregivers for causing them such emotional distress. Some parents suffer interruptions in their jobs and lives, and the stress can lead to personal and marital breakdowns. The stress does not necessarily abate after the baby is discharged from hospital, particularly if the baby suffers from physical or mental disabilities, or continues to have pain. Tilford et al. (2005) reported that parents' divorce rates doubled if ex-preterm or handicapped children have chronic pain versus those who do not have chronic pain. Finally, the special needs of these infants and the stress imposed on the family may result in unrealized opportunities and unfulfilled aspirations, further imposing financial and non-financial costs on the family.

Burden on society

Although pain and its attributable costs primarily affect the individual who is suffering, it should not be forgotten that we live in an interlinked world in which societies must balance the needs of many groups of people. Costs expended on health care for babies must be balanced against the health, welfare and educational needs of others including the ageing population where pain and dementia are also noted to be major problems. The costs of caring for babies with long-term disabilities place a significant burden on the resources of many countries, developed and developing alike. When pain and suffering of babies cause job dislocation and absence from work for their parents, it impacts on their workplace and affects economic productivity. Thus, there is a ripple effect that is not always obvious to the observer at a cursory glance.

THE FUTURE

The challenges that lie ahead are complex and multifaceted, and include technological, economic, ethical and social dimensions. Advancing technological and medical capabilities promise to open new possibilities for neonatal treatments, including gene therapy, new assisted ventilation modalities and fetal surgery among others. Some, if not all, will require preventative and ongoing pain assessment and management. Improved methods for assessing and monitoring pain prevalence, treatments and outcomes are needed, including assessment of the long-term effects of pain and its treatment on the neonate. Although pain guidelines exist, it is still challenging to ensure that they are implemented in practice. Pain management should be a routine part of treatment of babies and efforts should be made to increase awareness of neonatal pain and its treatment among both the public and health professional sectors. This will require public discussion of ethical and social issues related to neonatal pain. In the final analysis, the problems and issues related to pain are really all human in nature, and their solutions should be handled with understanding and compassion.

REFERENCES

Als H, Lawhon G, Brown E, et al. (1986). Individualized behavioral and environmental care for the very low birth weight preterm infant at high risk for bronchopulmonary dysplasia: neonatal intensive care unit and developmental outcome. Pediatrics 78: 1123–1132.

American Academy of Pediatrics/Canadian Paediatric Society. (2000). Prevention and management of pain and stress in the neonates. Pediatrics 105: 454–461 and Paediatric Child Health 5: 31–38.

Anand KJS, Sippell WG, Aynsley-Green A. (1987). Pain, anesthesia and babies. Lancet 2: 543–545.

Anand KJS, Hall RW, Desai N, et al. (2004). Effects of morphine analgesia in ventilated preterm neonates: Primary outcomes from the NEOPAIN randomized trial. Lancet 363: 1673–1682.

Anand KJS, Johnston CC, Oberlander T, et al. (2005a). Analgesia and local anesthesia during invasive procedures in the neonate. Clin Ther 27: 844–876.

Anand KJS, Aranda J, Johnston CC, et al. (2005b). Analgesia for neonates: Study design and ethical issues. Clin Ther 27: 813–843.

Arno PS, Bonuck K, Davis M. (1995). Rare diseases, drug development, and AIDS: the impact of the Orphan Drug Act. Milbank Q 73: 231–252.

Blyth FM, March LM, Bunabie AJM, et al. (2001). Chronic pain in Australia: a prevalence study. Pain 89: 127–134.

Boyle MH, Torrance GW, Sinclair JG, et al. (1983). Economic evaluation of neonatal intensive care of very low birth weight infants. New Engl J Med 308: 1330–1337.

Cummings EA, Reid GJ, Finley GA, et al. (1996). Prevalence and source of pain in pediatric inpatients. Pain 68: 25–31.

D'Apolito K. (1984). The neonate's response to pain. Am J Matern Child Nurs 9: 256–258.

Del Mar CB, Silagy CA, Glasziou PP, et al. (2001). Feasibility of an evidence-based literature search service for general practitioners. Med J Aust 175: 134–137.

Duhn L, Medves J. (2004). A systematic integrative review of infant pain assessment tools. Adv Neonatal Care 4: 126–140.

Flower MJ. (1985). Neuromaturation of the human fetus. J Med Philos 10: 237–251.

Gale G, Franck LS, Kool S, et al. (2004). Parents' perceptions of their infant's pain experience in the NICU. Intern J Nurs Stud 41: 51–58.

Glasziou PR. (2002). Analgesia and public health: what are the challenges? Am J Ther 9: 207–213.

Grunau RVE, Craig KD. (1987). Pain expression in neonates: facial action and cry. Pain 28: 395–410.

Guyatt GH, Haynes RB, Jaeschke RZ, et al. (2000). Users' guides to the medical literature: XXV Evidence-based medicine: principles for applying the users' guides to patient care. JAMA 284: 1290–1296.

Hatch DJ. (1987). Analgesia in the neonate. Br Med J 294: 920.

Horbar JD, Rogowski J, Plsek PE, et al. (2001). Collaborative quality improvement for neonatal intensive care. Pediatrics 107: 14–22.

Izard CE, Huebner RR, Risser D, et al. (1980). The young infant's ability to produce discrete emotional expressions. Dev Psychol 16: 132–140.

Lee SK, Anderson L. (2004). BC perinatal services costing project: Report on costs in the neonatal intensive care unit. Centre for Healthcare Innovation and Improvement, January 2004, Vancouver, BC, Canada.

Lee SK, Penner PL, Cox M. (1991). The impact of very low birth weight infants on the family and its relationship to parental attitudes. Pediatrics 88: 105–109.

Lee SK, Normand C, McMillan DD, et al. (2001). Evidence for changing guidelines for routine screening for retinopathy of prematurity. Arch Pediatr Adolesc Med 155: 387–395.

Levine JD, Gordon NC. (1982). Pain in prelingual children and its evaluation by pain-induced vocalization. Pain 14: 85–93.

Levy DM. (1960). The infant's earliest memory of inoculation: a contribution to public health procedures. J Gen Psychol 96: 3–46.

Lisonkova S, Lee SK, Bavinton HB, et al. (2003). Canadian Neonatal Network™ 2003 Annual Report Volume 3. Canadian Neonatal Network™, Vancouver, BC, Canada.

Moulin DE, Clark AJ, Speechley M, et al. (2002). Chronic pain in Canada – prevalence, treatment, impact and the role of opioid analgesia. Pain Res Manage 7: 179–184.

Peabody JW, Ruby A, Cannon P. (1995).
The economics of orphan drug policy
in the US. Can the legislation be
improved? Pharmacoeconomics
8: 374–384.

Prechtl HFR (ed). (1984). Continuity of
neural functions from prenatal to
postnatal life. Blackwell, Oxford.

President's Commission for the Study
of Ethical Problems in Medicine and
Biomedical and Behavioral Research.
(1983). Deciding to forgo life-
sustaining treatment. US Government
Printing Office, Washington DC.

Raphael ES, Singer JD, Walker DK.

(1985). Per pupil expenditures on
special education in three
metropolitan school districts. J Educ
Finance 11: 69–88.

Shankaran S, Cohen SN, Linver S, et al.
(1988). Medical care costs of high risk
infants after neonatal intensive care: a
controlled study. Pediatrics
81: 372–378.

Shearer MH. (1986). Surgery on the
paralysed, unanesthesized newborn.
Birth 13: 79.

Sheehan J, McKay J, Ryan M, et al.
(1996). What cost chronic pain? Ir
Med J 89: 218–219.

Tilford JM, Grosse SD, Robbins JM,
et al. (2005). Health state preference
scores of children with spina bifida
and their caregivers. Qual Life Res
14: 1087–1098.

Walker DJ, Feldman A, Vohr BR, et al.
(1984). Cost–benefit analysis of
neonatal intensive care for infants
weighing less than 1,000g at birth.
Pediatrics 74: 20–25.

Yaster M. (1987). Analgesia and
anesthesia in neonates. J Pediatr
111: 394–396.

Complementary and alternative approaches to pain in infancy

Jennie CI Tsao
Marcia L Meldrum
Lonnie K Zeltzer

INTRODUCTION

Complementary and alternative medicine (CAM) has been defined as those interventions not generally provided by US hospitals and clinics, nor widely taught in medical schools (Eisenberg et al. 1993). The Cochrane collaboration defines CAM as 'a broad domain of healing resources that encompasses all health systems, modalities and practices and their accompanying theories and beliefs, other than those intrinsic to the politically dominant health systems of a particular society or culture in a given historical period' (Zollman and Vickers 1999). According to the National Center for Complementary and Alternative Medicine (NCCAM; http://nccam.nih.gov/health/whatiscam/), CAM may be grouped into five domains: mind–body interventions (e.g. relaxation), biologically-based therapies (e.g. herbal medicine), manipulative/body-based methods (e.g. massage), alternative medical systems (e.g., acupuncture) and energy therapies (e.g. energy healing). It is evident from these disparate definitions that one of the difficulties in the study of CAM is lack of consensus regarding what practices are considered CAM at any specific point in time.

Researchers have not specifically investigated the prevalence of CAM use in infants and neonates; rather, the few existing studies have included children of all ages. One recent study (Bellas et al. 2005) reported on paediatric insurance claims data for CAM practitioners in Washington state, which requires such services to be covered by private health insurance. It was estimated that the rate of CAM use was 3.2% for infants (aged 0–1 year), a percentage similar to the rate for children aged 2–5 years (3.0%) but lower than that for older children (6–12 years – 5%; 13–17 years – 9.8%). Among infants, 1.8% received chiropractic care, 1.4% received naturopathic medicine, 0.1% received acupuncture and 0% received massage. Reasons for CAM use were not examined separately by age; however, CAM use was elevated in children with back pain and cancer. In other studies that have not clearly distinguished between infants and older children, estimates of CAM use have varied from as low as 2% (Davis and Darden 2003) to as high as 20–30% (Simpson et al. 1998, Ottolini et al. 2001). Rates of CAM use among paediatric patients with chronic conditions such as cancer, rheumatoid arthritis and cystic fibrosis range from 30% to 73% (Stern et al. 1992, Grootenhuis et al.

1998, Neuhouser et al. 2001). In many of these conditions, pain may be a significant problem.

Increased awareness of the number of painful medical procedures that infants, especially preterm neonates in the neonatal intensive care unit (NICU), must undergo (Simons et al. 2003), as well as concerns regarding potential adverse effects of pharmacological agents, has led to a growing interest in alternative, non-pharmacological interventions for acute, procedural pain in infants and neonates. There are no published estimates regarding the prevalence of CAM use for procedural pain in hospitals and NICUs and it is likely that rates vary widely. Existing research has focused on procedural pain in infants; no published work was located that examined the effects of CAM for other pain problems. This chapter reviews the existing literature regarding the efficacy of CAM approaches for painful medical procedures in these particularly vulnerable populations.

CAM INTERVENTIONS FOR PROCEDURAL PAIN

Sucrose and non-nutritive sucking (NNS)

Minor procedures (heel lance/venipuncture)

The most frequently studied non-pharmacological approach for procedural pain in infants is the oral administration of sucrose with or without non-nutritive sucking (NNS) (e.g. pacifiers). It is believed that the effects of sucrose and NNS are mediated by both endogenous opioid and non-opioid systems (Gunnar et al. 1988), although the underlying mechanisms may differ. A recent Cochrane review examined 21 studies (1616 infants) using sucrose with and without NNS for procedural pain (mostly heel lance) (Stevens et al. 2004). Studies were only included if they met established standards for methodological quality of randomized controlled trials. The review found that, in general, sucrose led to decreased physiological (heart rate) and behavioural (cry behaviours, facial action) pain indicators and composite pain scores. When the results of three studies (Johnston et al. 1999, Stevens et al. 1999, Gibbins et al. 2002) using the Premature Infant Pain Profile (PIPP) scale (Stevens et al. 1996) were pooled, sucrose was found to significantly reduce pain scores compared to control conditions following heel lancing. The authors concluded that sucrose is a safe and effective intervention for reducing infants' procedural pain, with the greatest analgesic effect realized when sucrose is administered approximately 2 minutes before the pain stimulus – an interval thought to coincide with endogenous opioid release (Stevens et al. 2004).

Despite these recommendations, the authors of the review (Stevens et al. 2004) also pointed out important caveats. First, they noted that there was general lack of adequate information regarding assurance of the blinding of the randomization process. In fact, 13 of the 21 studies reviewed were not double-blinded since additional interventions (e.g. pacifiers) precluded double-blinding. Second, it was noted that sample sizes were generally small. Third, it was pointed out that few studies provided details regarding the painful procedure and thus it was not possible to determine if procedures were comparable in intensity, frequency or duration. Fourth, most studies did not define pain nor did they provide a conceptual framework for how pain was related to the measured outcomes. The authors also indicated that only six studies evaluated adverse effects, although these effects were minor and no medical interventions were required. The reviewers recommended further research on procedures other than heel lancing as well as studies on repeated administrations of sucrose. Finally, they called for additional work to examine the use of sucrose with other behavioural and pharmacological interventions for more invasive procedures, as well as the use of sucrose in very low-birth-weight (VLBW), unstable/ventilated neonates.

The review also noted that use of a pacifier for sucrose delivery may promote NNS, which may have helped reduce pain-related distress (Campos 1994) and enhance calming effects (Blass 1994). Nevertheless, the authors indicated that the calming effects of NNS have not been sustained following cessation of contact whereas the administration of sucrose has been found to persist beyond the cessation of contact for several minutes (Stevens et al. 2004). A number of studies have examined NNS without sucrose for reduction of procedural pain. One meta-analysis of the effects of NNS (Shiao et al. 1997) reviewed three studies examining needle insertions or heel sticks (Field and Goldson 1984, Campos 1989, Miller and Anderson 1993). When the results of these studies were combined, the total weighted effect size (i.e. adjusted for number of subjects) of NNS on heart rate during painful stimulation was 1.05, indicating a large effect. The authors concluded that NNS appears to have a positive effect on heart rate in infants during painful procedures. They speculate that the underlying mechanism for these effects may be the influence of NNS on cardiac vagal tone (Shiao et al. 1997). However, it should be noted that only two of three studies used random assignment (Field and Goldson 1984, Miller and Anderson 1993). Non-random assignment increases the possibility that observed differences may have been due to factors other than the intervention.

A more recent review (Pinelli et al. 2002) concluded that the overall effects of NNS were generally
positive leading to reduced cry behaviour (Miller and
Anderson 1993, Corbo et al. 2000), lower scores on
the PIPP (Stevens et al. 1996), and reduced heart rate
(Miller and Anderson 1993, Corbo et al. 2000). However, the review authors also noted several methodological problems. For example, cry behaviours were
evaluated using a subjective, non-validated scale in
one study (Miller and Anderson 1993). One novel
study tested the impact of NNS, music therapy, combined NNS and music therapy, and no intervention
control on term and preterm neonates undergoing
heel lance (Bo and Callaghan 2000). All three interventions resulted in improved outcomes but the NNS
and music therapy condition had the greatest effect
on pain behaviour; music alone had the strongest
effect on heart rate. However, as pointed out in the
review, it was unclear whether the neonates were
randomly assigned to conditions and the assessors
of pain behaviours were not blinded to group assignment which may have biased their ratings of pain
response.

Major procedures (circumcision)

The above reviews did not include studies examining
pain in relation to circumcision. An early study
randomly assigned 18 healthy newborns to receive
either pacifier or no pacifier during circumcision
(Gunnar et al. 1984). Behavioural state was assessed
by two observers and inter-rater reliability was high,
although it was probably not feasible for raters to be
blinded to condition. Results indicated that newborns
given the pacifier cried significantly less and engaged
in less motor activity than controls. This well-
conducted though small study supports the use of
NNS for circumcision pain. A number of studies by
Blass and colleagues have also shown beneficial effects
of sucrose and pacifier for circumcision pain. Thus,
Blass and Hoffmeyer (1991) found that infants who
were given sucrose on a pacifier before and during
circumcision cried 31% of the time compared to
no-intervention controls who cried 67% of the time.
Pacifier alone reduced crying time to 49%. Cry duration (audiotaped) was evaluated by a single coder
who was unaware of group assignment. A more recent
study in 119 term neonates randomly assigned to
receive dorsal penile nerve block (DPNB), sucrose
or standard care prior to circumcision (Herschel et al.
1998) found that sucrose appeared to be as beneficial
as DPNB in reducing elevations in heart rate and
excessive movement, compared to standard care. The
authors recommended use of sucrose when physicians/
parents are uncomfortable with DPNB. Unfortunately,

this study did not include any behavioural measures
for the assessment of pain response.

Another group of studies reported that sucrose
in combination with other interventions resulted
in lowered circumcision pain (Stang et al. 1997,
Kaufman et al. 2002, Razmus et al. 2004). One study
on 80 term newborns found that pacifier with sucrose
and DPNB led to reduced behavioural distress compared to DPNB and pacifier with water (Stang et al.
1997). Although a well-validated scale was used to
assess behavioural distress (i.e. Brazelton Neonatal
Behavioral Assessment Scale (Brazelton 1973)), only
one rater was used; use of multiple raters together
with evidence of good inter-rater reliability would
have strengthened the findings. In a recent study
(Kaufman et al. 2002) comparing two commonly used
circumcision procedures (i.e. Mogen; Gomco), all
infants were given a eutectic mixture of local anaesthetic (EMLA) cream and either pacifier with sucrose
or pacifier with water. Results indicated that sucrose
was more effective than water in reducing crying and
facial grimacing although the findings mainly held
for the longer procedure (Gomco). The authors concluded that: (1) the shorter (Mogen) procedure should
be used unless contraindicated; (2) sucrose on a pacifier
is more effective than water on pacifier (although
pacifier alone is more effective than no intervention);
(3) combined interventions, in this case EMLA, sucrose
and shorter procedure, lead to enhanced analgesia.
This was a well-conducted study – raters were unaware
of experimental condition and inter-coder reliability
was reported at 95% agreement. On the other hand,
behavioural ratings were conducted using a relatively
new software program with unknown psychometric
properties.

Existing work suggests that sucrose/NNS with and
without other pharmacological interventions appears
to reduce pain related to circumcision. Further research
using well-validated behavioural pain measures are
warranted.

Music therapy

It is recognized that music has been used since anti-
quity to enhance well-being as well as to alleviate
pain and suffering (Kemper and Danhauer 2005). As
noted in recent reviews (Standley 2002, Kemper and
Danhauer 2005), music can be distinguished from
noise in that the latter exists without controls for
volume, duration or cause/effect relations. Exposure
to excessive noise has resulted in documented adverse
health effects such as increased heart rate and sleep
disturbance in infants hospitalized in the NICU
(Kellman 2002). Music, on the other hand, can be
defined as an intentional auditory activity with

organized elements (e.g. melody, rhythm). The clinical application of music may involve music therapy delivered in live performances by trained music therapists, or as recorded music administered through headphones or free-standing speakers. Several studies have supported the use of music to improve health outcomes in neonates, although the methodological quality of such work varies widely and relatively few have focused on pain response.

In one study (Marchette et al. 1991), the effects of music were studied in 121 full-term neonates undergoing unanaesthetized circumcision. Participants were randomly assigned to one of six conditions: classical music (tape-recorded), intrauterine sounds (tape-recorded), pacifier, music and pacifier, intrauterine sounds and pacifier, or control (no intervention). Pain outcome variables were heart rate, dysrhythmias, blood pressure, transcutaneous oxygen level and behavioural state. The latter was measured using the Brazelton scale (Brazelton 1973) and assessed by two raters whose inter-rater reliability was 0.97. Results indicated that the interventions did not have a significant beneficial effect on the variables assessed. The authors noted that baseline measures were not available and the inclusion of such measures may have offered evidence of more positive findings.

In a more recent study (Joyce et al. 2001), the effects of recorded music and EMLA were examined in 23 healthy term neonates undergoing circumcision. Pain response was assessed using the Riley Infant Pain Scale (RIPS), which has shown adequate reliability and validity (Joyce et al. 1994, Schade et al. 1996). All procedures were videotaped and independent raters who were unaware of group assignment conducted the ratings. Unfortunately, the design of this study was such that it is difficult to interpret the results. It appears that half of the neonates were assigned to receive EMLA ($n = 11$) and the other half to receive the placebo cream ($n = 12$). Similarly, half of the infants were assigned to receive music ($n = 11$) or no music ($n = 12$). However, it is unclear which infants received which combination of interventions. Thus, even though the results indicate that infants who received music had lower pain ratings, it is not known what proportion of these infants received EMLA vs. placebo. Future research would ideally compare these interventions in a more complete design, which would test each intervention individually as well as in combination.

Another study (Malone 1996) investigated the effects of live music therapy for pain related to intravenous starts, venipunctures, injections and heel sticks in 20 paediatric patients aged 0–7 years and 20 controls who did not receive the intervention, matched on age and type of procedure. This study was unusual in that the music intervention was delivered by a trained music therapist. Results indicated that the music group showed less behavioural distress than controls during pre- and post-needle stages, although there were no differences during needle insertion. However, this study had several limitations including lack of information regarding who conducted the behavioural ratings, whether the rater was aware of group assignment, and the psychometric properties of the rating scale used. Another limitation concerns possible differences in number of parents who were present across conditions. The presence of parents may have impacted on the behaviour of the child as well as the staff. Finally, nurses and IV therapists were instructed to 'maintain their normal modes of consolation or distraction' in the control condition and it is not known if these varied across participants.

Butt and Kisilevsky (2000) examined the impact of music on procedural pain in 14 preterm infants in the NICU who received heel lances. In a crossover design, neonates were tested twice, receiving music (recorded lullabies) or no music at each occasion. Pain response was assessed by The Neonatal Facial Coding System (NFCS) (Grunau and Craig 1987), which has demonstrated reliability (Craig et al. 1993) and validity (Grunau and Craig 1987, Craig et al. 1993, Johnston et al. 1993). Inter-rater reliability (0.77; $P < 0.01$) was assessed using a randomly selected and independently coded subset of tapes. Results indicated that older infants (post-conceptual age greater than 31 weeks) demonstrated a more rapid recovery in heart rate, behavioural state and facial expressions of pain in the music compared to the no-music condition. Unfortunately, it is not known who was the primary rater and whether raters were aware of group assignment. Another important limitation is that order effects for the music and no-music conditions were not tested (i.e. whether the order in which the conditions were administered was related to outcome). Possible order effects should have been examined as sensitization or habituation may have occurred on the second heel lance.

The studies reviewed above suggest that music may assist in reducing pain response in infants undergoing painful medical procedures, although methodological limitations preclude any definitive statements of therapeutic effects. As pointed out by Kemper and Danhauer (2005), music is a cost-effective strategy with few associated risks, as long as common sense volume controls are instituted (see also Standley (2002) for NICU guidelines). It is unknown, however, whether live or recorded music produces superior effects or whether these modalities can be differentiated in terms of possible therapeutic mechanism(s). It appears that music may function primarily as a form of distraction that indirectly influences pain response. Distraction may facilitate habituation to painful stimuli (Arntz et al. 1991), possibly because engaging in an alternate, attentionally demanding task limits the capacity to process pain (Farthing et al. 1984). Currently, it is not known whether music exerts any additional effects on pain above and beyond distraction, or whether music functions as a superior distractor compared to other stimuli.

Kangaroo care

Kangaroo care (KC) is defined as holding the newborn skin-to-skin against the mother's body, at an upright 40° to 60° angle, and with its body covered by the mother's blouse or shirt, with or without additional covering for warmth. Ludington-Hoe et al. (2003) monitored temperature and vital signs and determined that this intervention was safe for preterm infants. KC is advocated as a natural, non-invasive, method of providing analgesia during heel sticks and other painful procedures. Evaluation of this method in a well-controlled study is complex, both because it may be difficult to blind observers to the condition and because mothers may introduce an unknown factor of bias by additional touch or verbal interactions, unless otherwise instructed.

Gray et al. (2000) randomized 30 healthy, full-term newborns to skin-to-skin or no-contact groups prior to heel stick. Mothers in the treatment group received the infants in bed and were instructed to hold the baby securely, and not to rub its head. They were allowed to speak or make comforting sounds. The control group rested quietly in the crib. Outcome measures were cry behaviours (audiotaped), facial grimacing and heart rate. Assessors of cry behaviours were blinded as to study condition, but those assessing facial grimaces were aware of group assignment from viewing the videotape. Results indicated that skin-to-skin contact significantly reduced crying by 85% and grimacing by 65% over the control group. Heart rates of the babies held by their mothers did not increase significantly over baseline whereas heart rates of the control infants increased significantly during and after the procedure. Skin-to-skin contact thus appeared to provide an analgesic effect in this study. Limitations of the trial included the failure to blind the observers assessing facial grimacing and the unknown factor introduced by differential levels of verbal or touch comforting offered by mothers.

Johnston et al. (2003) evaluated KC in 74 preterm neonates using a single-blind crossover design, with each neonate undergoing heel stick under both KC

and swaddled crib positions in randomized order. The KC condition involved being held upright by the mother with maximal skin-to-skin contact; mothers were asked not to vocalize or to touch the child's head with their faces during the procedure. The control group lay prone swaddled in a blanket with the heel left accessible. The PIPP (Stevens et al. 1999) was used to assess pain response. Facial actions were recorded using a camera focused on the infant's face only and placed so that the mother could not be seen and the condition could not be identified. Thus, this is one of the few studies reviewed in this chapter where attempts were made to blind raters to condition. Post-hoc assessment of the effectiveness of the blinding however was not reported. In addition, this study, unlike most of those discussed, explicitly stated that raters were unaware of study hypotheses. Inter-rater reliability, however, was not reported and the number of raters was not specified. Nevertheless, results indicated PIPP scores were significantly lower in the KC condition compared to control following heel stick; there were no effects of order or illness severity.

Thus, existing evidence supports KC as a safe alternative analgesic for both preterm and term infants. KC may exert its effects via state regulation (de Leeuw et al. 1991, Ludington-Hoe et al. 2000); maternal touch has been implicated in the development of humans and animals (Fleming et al. 1999). However, as noted by Johnston et al. (2003), their study had a 40% refusal rate indicating that those mothers who were not as comfortable with the procedures may not have been as effective in providing KC to their infants. Further research on the generalizability of KC and maternal attitudes toward it are warranted.

Olfactory stimuli

Olfactory comfort through providing a familiar smell is a simple intervention, which can be done without moving the baby or risking a change in temperature. In one controlled trial (Goubet et al. 2003), 51 stable preterm infants were randomized to receive venipuncture or heel stick. Within each procedure, infants were divided into three subgroups: familiar odour (FAM), unfamiliar odour (NFAM), and no odour (CONT). The FAM group had a vanillin-scented scarf placed in their incubators overnight and then removed. The following morning, the FAM and NFAM groups were given the scented scarf, while the CONT group received a scarf with no odour. The observers scoring pain responses were unaware of group assignment, but were not blinded to type of procedure. Results indicated no group differences in infants given heel sticks. However, in those given venipuncture, the FAM group showed no increase in crying over baseline levels whereas both the NFAM and CONT groups increased crying significantly during the procedure. These findings support the use of familiar odours in infants undergoing venipuncture. Although high inter-rater reliability was reported in this study, it is unclear whether infants were randomly assigned to condition subgroups. Moreover, there was no effect of the familiar odour when infants were subjected to heel sticks. These findings replicate other studies that have failed to find reductions in crying following heel sticks among infants exposed to olfactory stimulation (Kawakami et al. 1997).

Swaddling

A number of studies have evaluated the effectiveness of swaddling, or 'facilitated tucking' (side-lying or supine position with flexed limbs close to the trunk) to relieve procedural pain. Fearon et al. (1997) studied responses to heel sticks in 15 preterm infants assigned to swaddling and standard care; all infants received both conditions and thus served as their own controls. They found that facial activity (scored using the NFCS; (Grunau and Craig 1987)) and heart rate decreased more rapidly in swaddled infants aged ≥31 weeks; younger infants, however, returned spontaneously to baseline regardless of condition. Limitations include the use of pacifiers and other sensory stimulations for some of the infants were provided with pacifiers and other sensory stimulation. In addition, potential order effects were not tested. Corff et al. (1995) used a similar design in 30 preterm neonates given facilitated tucking or no intervention across two separate heel sticks. Results indicated faster return to baseline heart rate and reduced cry behaviours when infants were given tucking during and after heel stick. However, order effects were not specifically examined. Prasopkittikun and Tilokskulchai (2003) conducted a meta-analysis of four cross-over studies (108 neonates) of swaddling during routine heel sticks. Although mean effect sizes ranged from moderate (0.53) to large (0.79) suggesting that swaddling effectively attenuated pain scores relative to control conditions, all of the studies reviewed were unpublished masters' theses making it impossible to evaluate the quality of the research. Ward-Larson et al. (2004), in a prospective randomized crossover design, examined facilitated tucking in 40 VLBW infants compared to standard NICU care for pain related to endotracheal suctioning using the PIPP. Results indicated that PIPP scores were significantly lower in the tucking vs. standard care condition. Although order effects were examined and none found, the lead investigator was the only rater, allowing possible bias in the findings.

Taken together, these studies provide preliminary support for the use of swaddling to reduce pain related to heel sticks. It is thought that by supplying motoric boundaries, swaddling may facilitate self-regulation and decreased physiological responsivity to painful stimulation (Corff et al. 1995). A limitation of all these studies is that the observer scoring facial expression could not be blinded, and was in some cases doing the swaddling or tucking herself. In addition, most of the studies to date have used cross-over designs and yet order effects were not consistently examined. The suggested conclusion is that swaddling, tucking or some kind of tactile support may assist the infant in recovering from procedural pain but additional, more rigorous research is needed, particularly on procedures other than heel sticks.

Sensorial saturation

A novel approach developed by Bellieni and colleagues (2001, 2002) incorporates several CAM modalities in a method termed 'sensorial saturation'. Sensorial saturation consists of simultaneously lying the infant on its side with limbs flexed but free to move; looking the infant in the face closely to attract attention; massaging the infant's face and back; speaking to the infant gently; allowing the infant to smell pleasant fragrance on the therapist's hands; instilling glucose with a syringe to stimulate sucking. In 17 preterm neonates in the NICU undergoing heel prick (Bellieni et al. 2001), sensorial saturation led to reduced pain response, as measured by the PIPP (Stevens et al. 1996) compared to glucose administered to induce sucking, glucose administered without sucking, water administered orally without sucking, control (no intervention). Each neonate received all the conditions in random order across five different heel pricks. Pain response was assessed by two independent raters who were unaware of condition assignment, with one exception – it was not possible to mask the sensorial saturation condition since the therapist was visible in the videotapes of the procedure. Thus, it is possible that bias was introduced in the ratings. Furthermore, this study used univariate tests (paired t-tests) to compare each condition with the other; multivariate analyses comparing all conditions simultaneously as well as testing for possible order effects would have been more appropriate.

Bellieni and colleagues (2002) conducted a second, larger scale study with 120 term neonates undergoing heel lance. Neonates were randomly assigned to one of six groups: glucose with sucking; glucose without sucking; water with sucking; sensorial saturation; sensorial saturation without glucose; control (no intervention). Pain response was measured using the Douleur Aiguë du Nouveau-né (DAN) scale (Carbajal et al. 1997). Results indicated that sensorial saturation (with glucose) was more effective than the other conditions in reducing pain response, although water with sucking and glucose with sucking also reduced pain scores relative to control. Mean duration of crying decreased from 25 seconds in the control group to 7 seconds in the glucose plus sucking condition and 2.8 seconds for sensorial saturation. These findings replicate the earlier study on preterm neonates in a larger sample. However, as in the earlier study, it was not possible for sensorial saturation conditions to be masked. Moreover, the authors did not state how many behavioural raters were used and whether any reliability checks were conducted across raters.

Despite these limitations, the work by Bellieni and associates supports the analgesic effects of multi-sensory stimulation in newborns undergoing heel sticks. Non-painful stimulation, by engaging a number of channels (i.e. auditory, tactile, visual, olfactory, vestibular and gustatory), is thought to compete with painful stimulation (Bellieni et al. 2001, 2002). Notably, the second study by Bellieni's group indicated that sensorial saturation *without* glucose did not have an analgesic effect; but rather increased awareness of the painful stimulus and irritated the neonate (Bellieni et al. 2002). Thus, the authors maintain that the inclusion of glucose leads to maximal analgesia, which is superior to that of glucose alone. The authors conclude that in order for sensorial saturation to function properly, it requires a 'favorable background situation' (Bellieni et al. 2002, p. 462) such as an infant already engaged in sucking a sweet liquid. Interestingly, however, prior work did not reveal an incremental analgesic effect of simulated rocking with sucrose (Johnston et al. 1997). Thus, further research is necessary to determine the optimal therapeutic ingredients within the sensorial saturation approach (in addition to glucose) that produce its analgesic effects.

CONCLUSION

The studies reviewed above suggest that several CAM approaches show promise in alleviating pain related to medical procedures in term and preterm infants. The most rigorous research has examined the effects of sucrose with and without pacifier to promote NNS.

Additional research is warranted for other potentially useful CAM interventions. For example, massage therapy appears not to have been tested as an analgesic intervention in newborns, except as part of Bellieni et al.'s 'saturation' approach. Many NICU physicians and nurses continue to maintain a 'minimal touch' policy, based on the well-known finding by Long et al. (1980) that excessive handling, as in diaper changes or examinations, was associated with major risk of oxygen desaturation. A number of researchers (Field 2002), however, have championed standardized massage of medically stable preterm infants as contributing to growth and weight gain. Dieter et al. (2003) found, in a randomized study of 32 premature newborns, that the massaged babies averaged 53% greater daily weight gain than their controls, after just 5 days. As massage often contributes to the comfort and relief of adult pain patients, therefore, a controlled evaluation of its efficacy in low-risk neonates would appear to be strongly indicated.

Further work is also needed to more fully test the effects of combined CAM and pharmacological approaches, particularly for more invasive procedures such as circumcision. As noted above, the quality of existing research varies greatly and the field would benefit from greater attention to crucial methodological issues including proper randomization, blinding of behavioural raters when feasible, use of appropriate statistics and reporting of effect sizes, use of validated instruments for assessment of pain and adequate sample sizes. Currently, it is unknown which CAM approaches are best suited for which painful procedures. It is hoped that future studies will help guide clinicians in applying the optimal combination of CAM and conventional interventions that will produce the greatest analgesic effect, tailored for each type of painful medical procedure that infants must undergo. Further research on CAM for non-procedure acute or persistent pain in neonates, such as that associated with surgery, mechanical ventilation and necrotizing enterocolits, is warranted.

ACKNOWLEDGEMENTS

Research by the authors is supported in part by R01 DE12754-01A1 awarded by the National Institute of Dental and Craniofacial Research (PI: Zeltzer) and R01 MH063779 awarded by the National Institutes of Mental Health (PI: Jacob).

REFERENCES

Arntz A, Dreessen L, Merckelbach H. (1991). Attention, not anxiety, influences pain. Behav Res Ther 29: 41–50.

Bellas A, Lafferty WE, Lind B, et al. (2005). Frequency, predictors, and expenditures for pediatric insurance claims for complementary and alternative medical professionals in Washington State. Arch Pediatr Adolesc Med 159: 367–372.

Bellieni CV, Buonocore G, Nenci A, et al. (2001). Sensorial saturation: an effective analgesic tool for heel-prick in preterm infants: a prospective randomized trial. Biol Neonate 80: 15–18.

Bellieni CV, Bagnoli F, Perrone S, et al. (2002). Effect of multisensory stimulation on analgesia in term neonates: a randomized controlled trial. Pediatr Res 51: 460–463.

Blass EM. (1994). Behavioral and physiological consequences of suckling in rat and human newborns. Acta Paediatr Suppl 397: 71–76.

Blass EM, Hoffmeyer LB. (1991). Sucrose as an analgesic for newborn infants. Pediatrics 87: 215–218.

Bo LK, Callaghan P. (2000). Soothing pain-elicited distress in Chinese neonates. Pediatrics 105: E49.

Brazelton TB. (1973). Neonatal behavioral assessment scale. Lippincott, Philadelphia.

Butt ML, Kisilevsky BS. (2000). Music modulates behaviour of premature infants following heel lance. Can J Nurs Res 31: 17–39.

Campos RG. (1989). Soothing pain-elicited distress in infants with swaddling and pacifiers. Child Dev 60: 781–792.

Campos RG. (1994). Rocking and pacifiers: two comforting interventions for heelstick pain. Res Nurs Health 17: 321–331.

Carbajal R, Paupe A, Hoenn E, et al. (1997). APN: evaluation behavioral scale of acute pain in newborn infants. Arch Pediatr 4: 623–628.

Corbo MG, Mansi G, Stagni A, et al. (2000). Nonnutritive sucking during heelstick procedures decreases behavioral distress in the newborn infant. Biol Neonate 77: 162–167.

Corff KE, Seideman R, Venkataraman PS, et al. (1995). Facilitated tucking: a nonpharmacologic comfort measure for pain in preterm neonates. J Obstet Gynecol Neonatal Nurs 24: 143–147.

Craig KD, Whitfield MF, Grunau RV, et al. (1993). Pain in the preterm neonate: behavioural and physiological indices. Pain 52: 287–299.

Davis MP, Darden PM. (2003). Use of complementary and alternative medicine by children in the United States. Arch Pediatr Adolesc Med 157: 393–396.

De Leeuw R, Colin EM, Dunnebier EA, et al. (1991). Physiological effects of kangaroo care in very small preterm infants. Biol Neonate 59: 149–155.

Dieter JN, Field T, Hernandez-Reif M, et al. (2003). Stable preterm infants gain more weight and sleep less after five days of massage therapy. J Pediatr Psychol 28: 403–411.

Eisenberg DM, Kessler RC, Foster C, et al. (1993). Unconventional medicine in the United States: prevalence, costs, and patterns of use. N Eng J Med 328: 246–252.

Farthing GW, Venturino M, Brown SW. (1984). Suggestion and distraction in the control of pain: test of two hypotheses. J Abnorm Psychol 93: 266–276.

Fearon I, Kisilevsky BS, Hains SM, et al. (1997). Swaddling after heel lance: age-specific effects on behavioral recovery in preterm infants. J Dev Behav Pediatr 18: 222–232.

Field T. (2002). Preterm infant massage therapy studies: an American approach. Semin Neonatol 7: 487–494.

Field T, Goldson E. (1984). Pacifying effects of nonnutritive sucking on term and preterm neonates during heelstick procedures. Pediatrics 74: 1012–1015.

Fleming AS, O'day DH, Kraemer GW. (1999). Neurobiology of mother–infant interactions: experience and central nervous system plasticity across development and generations. Neurosci Biobehav Rev 23: 673–685.

Gibbins S, Stevens B, Hodnett E, et al. (2002). Efficacy and safety of sucrose for procedural pain relief in preterm and term neonates. Nurs Res 51: 375–382.

Goubet N, Rattaz C, Pierrat V, et al. (2003). Olfactory experience mediates response to pain in preterm newborns. Dev Psychobiol 42: 171–180.

Gray L, Watt L, Blass EM. (2000). Skin-to-skin contact is analgesic in healthy newborns. Pediatrics 105: e14.

Grootenhuis MA, Last BF, De Graaf-Nijkerk JH, et al. (1998). Use of alternative treatment in pediatric oncology. Cancer Nurs 21: 282–288.

Grunau RV, Craig KD. (1987). Pain expression in neonates: facial action and cry. Pain 28: 395–410.

Gunnar MR, Fisch RO, Malone S. (1984). The effects of a pacifying stimulus on behavioral and adrenocortical responses to circumcision in the newborn. J Am Acad Child Psychiatry 23: 34–38.

Gunnar MR, Connors J, Isensee J, et al. (1988). Adrenocortical activity and behavioral distress in human newborns. Dev Psychobiol 21: 297–310.

Herschel M, Khoshnood B, Ellman C, et al. (1998). Neonatal circumcision. Randomized trial of a sucrose pacifier for pain control. Arch Pediatr Adolesc Med 152: 279–284.

Johnston CC, Stevens B, Craig KD, et al. (1993). Developmental changes in pain expression in premature, full-term, two- and four-month-old infants. Pain 52: 201–208.

Johnston CC, Stremler RL, Stevens BJ, et al. (1997). Effectiveness of oral sucrose and simulated rocking on pain response in preterm neonates. Pain 72: 193–199.

Johnston CC, Stremler R, Horton L, et al. (1999). Effect of repeated doses of sucrose during heel stick procedure in preterm neonates. Biol Neonate 75: 160–166.

Johnston CC, Stevens B, Pinelli J, et al. (2003). Kangaroo care is effective in diminishing pain response in preterm neonates. Arch Pediatr Adolesc Med 157: 1084–1088.

Joyce BA, Schade JG, Keck JF, et al. (1994). Reliability and validity of preverbal pain assessment tools. Issues Compr Pediatr Nurs 17: 121–135.

Joyce BA, Keck JF, Gerkensmeyer J. (2001). Evaluation of pain management interventions for neonatal circumcision pain. J Pediatr Health Care 15: 105–114.

Kaufman GE, Cimo S, Miller LW, et al. (2002). An evaluation of the effects of sucrose on neonatal pain with 2 commonly used circumcision methods. Am J Obstet Gynecol 186: 564–568.

Kawakami K, Takai-Kawakami K, Okazaki Y, et al. (1997). The effects of odors on human newborn infants under stress. Infant Behav Develop 20: 531–535.

Kellman N. (2002). Noise in the intensive care nursery. Neonatal Netw 21: 35–41.

Kemper KJ, Danhauer SC. (2005). Music as therapy. South Med J 98: 282–288.

Long JG, Alastair GS, Philip MB, et al. (1980). Excessive handling as a cause of hypoxemia. Pediatrics 65: 203–207.

Ludington-Hoe SM, Nguyen N, Swinth JY, et al. (2000). Kangaroo care compared to incubators in maintaining body warmth in preterm infants. Biol Res Nurs 2: 60–73.

Ludington-Hoe SM, Ferreira C, Swinth J, et al. (2003). Safe criteria and procedure for kangaroo care with intubated preterm infants. J Obstet Gynecol Neonatal Nurs 32: 579–588.

Malone AB. (1996). The effects of live music on the distress of pediatric patients receiving intravenous starts, venipunctures, injections, and heel sticks. J Music Ther 33: 19–33.

Marchette L, Main R, Redick E, et al. (1991). Pain reduction interventions during neonatal circumcision. Nurs Res 40: 241–244.

Miller HD, Anderson GC. (1993). Nonnutritive sucking: effects on crying and heart rate in intubated infants requiring assisted mechanical ventilation. Nurs Res 42: 305–307.

Neuhouser ML, Patterson RE, Schwartz SM, et al. (2001). Use of alternative medicine by children with cancer in Washington state. Prev Med 33: 347–354.

Ottolini MC, Hamburger EK, Loprieato JO, et al. (2001). Complementary and alternative medicine use among children in the Washington, DC area. Ambul Pediatr 1: 122–125.

Pinelli J, Symington A, Ciliska D. (2002). Nonnutritive sucking in high-risk infants: benign intervention or legitimate therapy? J Obstet Gynecol Neonatal Nurs 31: 582–591.

Prasopkittikun T, Tilokskulchai F. (2003). Management of pain from heel stick in neonates: an analysis of research conducted in Thailand. J Perinat Neonatal Nurs 17: 304–312.

Razmus IS, Dalton ME, Wilson D. (2004). Pain management for newborn circumcision. Pediatr Nurs 30: 414–417, 427.

Schade JG, Joyce BA, Gerkensmeyer J, et al. (1996). Comparison of three preverbal scales for postoperative pain assessment in a diverse pediatric sample. J Pain Symptom Manage 12: 348–359.

Shiao SY, Chang YJ, Lannon H, et al. (1997). Meta-analysis of the effects of nonnutritive sucking on heart rate and peripheral oxygenation: research from the past 30 years. Issues Compr Pediatr Nurs 20: 11–24.

Simons SH, Van Dijk M, Anand KS, et al. (2003). Do we still hurt newborn babies? A prospective study of procedural pain and analgesia in neonates. Arch Pediatr Adolesc Med 157: 1058–1064.

Simpson N, Pearce A, Finlay F, et al. (1998). The use of complementary medicine in paediatric outpatient clinics. Ambulatory Child Health 3: 351–356.

Standley JM. (2002). A meta-analysis of the efficacy of music therapy for premature infants. J Pediatr Nurs 17: 107–113.

Stang HJ, Snellman LW, Condon LM, et al. (1997). Beyond dorsal penile nerve block: a more humane circumcision. Pediatrics 100: E3.

Stern RC, Canda ER, Doershuk CF. (1992). Use of nonmedical treatment by cystic fibrosis patients. J Adolesc Health 13: 612–615.

Stevens B, Johnston C, Petryshen P, et al. (1996). Premature Infant Pain Profile: development and initial validation. Clin J Pain 12: 13–22.

Stevens B, Johnston C, Franck L, et al. (1999). The efficacy of developmentally sensitive interventions and sucrose for relieving procedural pain in very low birth weight neonates. Nurs Res 48: 35–43.

Stevens B, Yamada J, Ohlsson A. (2004). Sucrose for analgesia in newborn infants undergoing painful procedures. Cochrane Database Syst Rev, CD001069.

Ward-Larson C, Horn RA, Gosnell F. (2004). The efficacy of facilitated tucking for relieving procedural pain of endotracheal suctioning in very low birthweight infants. MCN Am J Matern Child Nurs 29: 151–156; quiz 157–158.

Zollman C, Vickers A. (1999). What is complementary medicine? BMJ 319: 693–696.

Parenting and pain during infancy

Rebecca R Pillai Riddell
Christine T Chambers

AN INFANT'S PAIN BEHAVIOUR: AN INSTINCTIVE TRIGGER FOR PARENTAL CAREGIVING BEHAVIOUR

For years, infants have suffered needlessly due to failures to recognize pain and the resultant lack of pain management (Anand and Craig 1996, Craig 1997, American Academy of Pediatrics and American Pain Society 2001). Parents, nurses and physicians all play important and distinct roles in assessing and managing infant pain. In the absence of an absolute index of pain severity and the lack of verbal self-report, both parents' and health professionals' reactions to infant pain can be seen as informed guesses regarding the infant's pain experience. Given their personal investment and lack of technical knowledge about infant pain, parents seem to confront a more emotionally distressing, ambiguous and challenging task than that faced by health professionals. However, in some cases, parents may be in the unique position to advocate for appropriate pain care for their infants. For example, the surge of research on infant pain that began in the 1980s can be credited in large part to parental advocacy that was initiated when it was discovered that seriously ill premature infants had undergone major surgeries without anaesthesia due to prevailing myths that infants did not feel pain (American Pain Society 2005).

Despite their important and potentially vulnerable role, it is surprising to discover that there has been relatively little research examining parental assessment and management of infant pain. While the context of infant pain is a topic that has received discussion in previous editions of this book, this is the first edition in which a chapter explicitly dedicated to parents and their role in caring for an infant in pain is included. In addition to providing a review of the sparse research that has been conducted on this topic to date with both full-term and preterm infants, this chapter provides an overview of theoretical perspectives on parent–infant relationships that can be used to guide future research on this important topic.

Over the past four decades, exploration of how infants and parents (particularly mothers) interact in distress contexts has exploded with the ongoing refinement of an overarching attachment theory of this dyadic relationship (Bowlby 1982) and the development of well-validated measures of related constructs. For example, the Strange Situation Paradigm

(Ainsworth et al. 1978), which measures the quality of an infant's attachment to their mother, and the Adult Attachment Interview, which measures the coherence of an adult's account of their own childhood attachment experiences (George and Soloman 1996).

Bowlby's theory of instinctive behaviour (Bowlby 1982) is wholly relevant to the study of parenting the infant in pain, because it gives central importance to the role of the infant in distress and specifically addresses painful situations. Bowlby's theory, developed in great detail over three volumes and 13 years, borrowed heavily from the fields of psychoanalysis, experimental psychology, ethology and neurophysiology, although Bowlby later distanced himself from traditional psychoanalysis due to concerns regarding the inability to test the scientific rigour of psychoanalytic models. According to Bowlby, behavioural observation, not historical recollection, was the key to empirical model testing. By shunning extreme behaviourism and the condemnation of cognitions to the nebulous 'black box', Bowlby integrated cognitive mechanisms into his theory of understanding instinctive behaviour. In essence, he took a cognitive-behavioural approach to understanding the caregiver–infant relationship even before the cognitive-behavioural orientation became an established psychological tradition in its own right.

Bowlby understood instinctive behaviours (which he defined as a pattern of behaviours, with obvious survival value, that follow a similar pattern across members of a species and will manifest in some form even if all opportunities for learning the pattern are absent; Bowlby 1982, p. 38) as orchestrated by behavioural control systems. Behavioural control systems select movements in a non-random manner in order to bring an organism progressively nearer to an end goal that, in some way, increases survival probability. Behavioural control systems can be activated or deactivated by either internal (e.g. organism's perceptions) or external cues (e.g. environmental stimuli). Moreover, in higher-level species, such as humans, control systems will incorporate feedback from the current course of action and correct behaviour if it is deemed necessary to achieve the goal. Two specific behavioural control systems are of direct relevance to this chapter: the attachment system and the caregiving system.

The overall goal of the attachment behavioural system is to attain and maintain close proximity to a caregiver figure when security is an issue (Marvin and Britner 1999). Thus in a strict Bowlbyian use of the term attachment, only behaviours that serve to increase proximity to a caregiver in order to regulate

safety should be seen as a part of the attachment behavioural system. When describing activating triggers for the attachment system he stated 'a child's attachment behaviour is activated especially by pain, fatigue and anything frightening, and also by the mother being or appearing to be inaccessible' (Bowlby 1988, p. 3). In the case of the infant in pain, behaviours such as facial expressions, vocal activity and body movements can all be seen as instinctive behaviours enacted to bring a caregiver close during a time of perceived danger. One's attachment representations or internal working model of attachment (cognitive filters based on representations of oneself and others which are based on caregiving experiences during childhood but are continually revised throughout life; Thompson 1999, p. 267) are beginning to be linked to how pain is experienced throughout the lifespan. For example, a child's cognitive schema of separation from a caregiver was found to be related to their cognitive schema for painful situations (Walsh et al. 2004). How an adult copes with chronic pain has also been theorized to be related to early attachment experiences (Kolb 1982, Anderson and Hines 1994).

Thus, the goal of the attachment system in infancy is to enact behaviours when the infant is distressed that will elicit a distress-reducing response from a caregiver. However, it is theorized that the caregiver's responses to the infant's attachment behaviours are controlled by a reciprocal behavioural control system, referred to as the caregiving system. While Bowlby proposed the concept of the caregiving behavioural system, and felt strongly about it being the product of biopsychosocial influences (Bowlby 1988), research on this system has only recently become the subject of methodical inquiry. The caregiving system is more multifaceted than the attachment system because the parent has access to a greater breadth and depth of information than the infant when enacting attachment behaviours. Based on this exponentially higher level of complexity, it is important to recognize that while an infant's cues should activate the caregiving system, what the parent chooses to do in response to those cues appears to have more to do with the internal organization of the parent's caregiving system than the infant's actual behaviour (George and Solomon 1999, Pillai Riddell et al. 2004, Nader 2005).

The caregiving system is not one that lies dormant until adulthood. Immature forms of caregiving behaviour are seen throughout the lifespan (Marvin and Britner 1999). In normative circumstances, once an individual is in a position of responsibility for a child, the caregiving system is ultimately triggered by the caregiver's perceptions of danger to the child. The goal of the caregiving system is to increase the proximity between parent and child to serve the end goal of protection, in a manner that complements the child's attachment system's end goal of safety. While the infant's attachment system and the parent's caregiving system have complementary goals, it is important to recognize that both infant and caregiver must implicitly agree on whether a stimulus, such as pain, is a threat to the infant's security. Given the developing cognitive ability of the infant, this places greater onus on the caregiver to be able to discern what the infant considers a threat to security.

Bowlby's theory regarding the reciprocal systems of attachment and caregiving directs attention to the importance of understanding the infant in pain from both the child and parent perspective. Expanding this perspective in greater depth for the infant in pain, the Sociocommunication Model (Craig et al. 1996) approaches the infant in pain with attention to the caregiver, the infant and the dynamic interplay between the two.

UNDERSTANDING INFANT PAIN IN A DYADIC CONTEXT

The Sociocommunication Model of Infant Pain

Attempting to understand the infant in pain necessitates an understanding of the dyadic relationship between the infant and caregiver (Craig et al. 2002). For almost a decade, Craig and colleagues (Prkachin and Craig 1995, Craig et al. 1996, 2002, Craig and Pillai Riddell 2003) have worked to develop a comprehensive model to conceptualize infant pain assessment and management. The Sociocommunication Model of Infant Pain (Fig. 22.1) purports an understanding of infant pain as a sequence of nonlinear stages within the child, within the caregiver, and between the child and caregiver. This model emphasizes interdependence of stages by depicting feedback loops (i.e. arrows in both directions) among stages. The model also suggests that larger spheres of influence (e.g. family, community, culture) separately influence the infant and the caregiver.

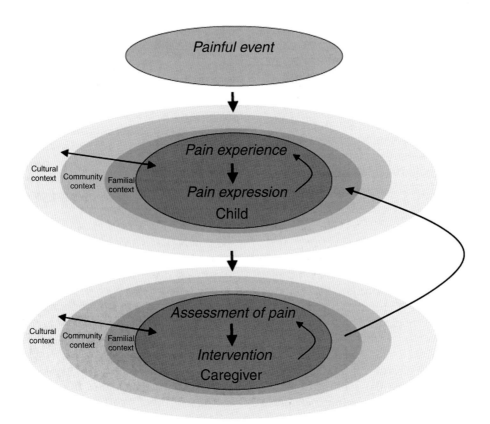

Figure 22.1 Social influences on the Sociocommunication Model of Pain (reproduced from Craig and Pillai Riddell 2003 with permission from the International Association for the Study of Pain).

Pain experience

It is theorized that the biological composition of the infant (e.g. nervous system thresholds), the infant's past experiences with pain, and the different social contexts (e.g. in the hospital alone, at home with a parent) in which the infant experiences the painful stimuli would all factor into the infant's internal experience of pain. Pain is a subjective experience and, regardless of one's ability to verbally communicate, a caregiver can never obtain a definitive understanding of the child's internal pain experience. However, representative indicators can give caregivers a working understanding of the infant pain experience.

Pain expression

Healthy infants almost invariably react to tissue stress and damage with vigorous vocal and non-vocal activity, thereby providing a means for inferring their subjective state. In light of the infant's dependency on caregivers for survival, motor programmes such as cry, body movements and facial activity tend to clearly depict that the infant is distressed. Once again it is hypothesized that aspects of the social context (such as the presence of mother versus father) in which an infant undergoes a pain stimulus will impact the infant's pain expression.

Assessment of pain

During the next step, infant caregivers become aware of and interpret the infant's expression of pain. The caregiver may or may not initiate an information-gathering process that will result in clarification of whether the distress relates to pain or not. This attribution of pain is hypothesized to be impacted by factors such as the sensitivities of the caregiver, their knowledge level (of the specific child, of possible alternatives to distress, of children in general, of common pain cues or indicators, etc.), their attitudes and the context of the surrounding environment.

Action dispositions

Once the caregiver has processed the information gathered and made decisions as to whether the infant is in pain, the stage is set for action dispositions to alleviate the infant's pain. Depending on the caregiver's assessment of the level of pain, different pain-relieving behaviours may be enacted (e.g. cuddling, administering medication, withdrawal of an aversive stimuli) to aid the infant. Initial action dispositions should not be seen as simply the last step in the process because the caregiver's first intervention may not alter the infant's pain experience and/or expression appropriately thus requiring further pain assessment and a new management strategy.

Bowlby's theory, regarding an infant's instinct to secure safety from their parent and for a parent's instinct to protect their infant, provides a broader theoretical context and specific mechanisms in which to understand how the infant in distress is impacted by their caregiver and vice versa. Focusing in on the specific example of the infant in pain, Craig has postulated how each step between the infant's internal experience of pain to the caregiver's pain management is influenced by the dynamic relationship between caregiver and child. What follows are a series of case examples that illustrate these various potential influences.

A PARENT'S CAREGIVING BEHAVIOUR: THE IMPACT ON AN INFANT'S PAIN

Extrapolating from previous discussions, one can speculate that the infant's experience and expression of pain will be subsequently impacted by the caregiver's ability to detect an infant's pain signals and discern an appropriate course of action. Furthermore, it has also been suggested that the influence of parenting behaviour on infant pain expression may become greater as the infant and parent build a relationship over time (Sweet et al. 1999). Given the minimal amount of literature regarding how the infant's pain is impacted by the dyadic relationship between parent and child, the following scenarios integrate templates of well-validated infant and parental categories of attachment in distress contexts (Ainsworth et al. 1978, George and Solomon 1996) and suggest possible outcomes within the context of pain (Craig et al. 1996). Based on the attachment intervention literature, it is important to point out that the outcomes that follow could be modified with parent and/or infant intervention (Bakersmans-Kranenburg et al. 2003).

An optimal situation would have a caregiver sensitively assess the infant's pain signals and take appropriate action to soothe both the physical and emotional dimensions of the infant's pain. Should that course of action not result in a reduction in the infant's pain behaviours, an optimal caregiver would be aware of this and attempt another strategy for pain reduction. Over time, the infant becomes secure in knowing the caregiver will respond to the infant's pain and, as a result, the emotional and behavioural dysregulation that results from unheeded pain is moderated.

A caregiver with low sensitivity (i.e. the tendency to dismiss infant pain behaviours and require intense infant pain expression before taking action) or inconsistent sensitivity (i.e. sometimes requiring intense infant pain behaviours vs. sometimes not requiring intense infant pain behaviours to take action) would be less effective at managing the infant's pain. Principles of operant conditioning would generally suggest a few possible scenarios developing over time: (a) the infant's most intense pain behaviours would be positively reinforced by parental attention and less intense reactions would be extinguished because they were not reinforced or, (b) the infant with the less-sensitive/less-consistent parent may cause the child to mount less-vigorous signalling to a caregiver (e.g. Sweet et al. 1999) because the child has either learned to modulate their pain experience by themselves or has learned that his/her energy is wasted on trying to elicit help from a caregiver.

In another more disruptive scenario, if a parent consistently attempted to comfort the child's pain in frightening or paradoxical ways (e.g. completely over-reacting to the infant's pain signal in a way that exacerbates the infant's distress), this would be confusing to the infant as the potential source of safety has now become a potential source of distress/danger. Thus, in response to the parent's paradoxical behaviour, over time the infant's responses could become disorganized (Benoit 2000), resulting in odd behaviours in the pain context such as a high level of inconsolability to an objectively mild pain stimulus or low/no level of reactivity ('spacing out') to a highly painful stimulus.

Aside from the generally consistent and sensitive caregiver, any of the above infant pain caregiving scenarios (i.e. low/inconsistent sensitivity and paradoxical sensitivity) could contribute to a more stressful experience for the infant, thus exacerbating the infant's perceived intensity of the pain. Research has suggested a positive relationship between inappropriate parental behaviours and physiological stress responses (Field 1994, Luecken and Lemery 2004). Moreover, while not attributable to parenting but rather health professional caregiving within a hospital environment, longitudinal analyses of infants who were subjected to painful medical procedures without benefit of appropriate pain assessment and/or management express pain differently than infants who have not experienced lapses in the caregiving relationship (Grunau et al. 1994, Taddio et al. 1997).

Theoretical underpinnings are an important basis from which to understand the literature in the area of parenting the infant in pain. The focus of this chapter will now turn to a review of empirical research conducted to date that addresses the parenting context of both full-term and preterm infants in pain.

RESEARCH ON PARENTING A FULL-TERM INFANT IN PAIN

While the role of parents in the pain experience of older children has received considerable attention (Chambers 2003), the role they play with infants who are wholly or more dependent on their parents for pain assessment and management has been sparsely and only recently researched.

Assessment

Three studies (Craig et al. 1988, Pillai Riddell et al. 2004, Nader 2005) have examined parental judgements of neonatal pain associated with routine procedures such as heel lance and immunizations. When presented with infants in pain, parents in all three studies consistently acknowledged significant levels of pain. Akin to findings with medical professionals, behavioural indicators such as facial activity, cry and body movements were reported to be most important in parents' decision-making process regarding the infants in pain. However, despite the consistent finding that behavioural indicators are reported by parents to be most important to their pain judgements, Nader (2005) found that behavioural reactivity only predicted a relatively small percentage of the variability in parents' pain judgements, and that 85% of the variance could not be accounted for by the various other behavioural and contextual cues (e.g. infant age) included in his model. Moreover, Pillai Riddell (2004) found, despite controlling for behavioural reactivity (all infants judged had similar levels of facial movements, body movements and cry), a trend in parental pain judgements that suggested intra-individual factors of the parents were also very influential. These studies suggest that while parents consistently attribute significant levels of pain to the infant they may lack awareness of how much their personal biases influence these pain judgements.

Other studies that explore parental pain judgements of infants have taken a comparative slant and examined differences between how medical professionals and parents attribute pain (Xavier Balda et al. 2000, McClellan et al. 2003, Pillai Riddell 2004). Xavier Balda et al. (2000) found that health professionals (i.e. nurses, doctors, residents and nurses' aids) were less able to correctly discriminate between pain and non-pain infant faces than parents when utilizing a photographic discrimination task. Similarly, despite using completely different methodologies (in vivo judgements vs. a video judgement task), both McClellan et al. and Pillai Riddell found that parents attributed significantly more pain to infants than health professionals did. Follow-up analyses by Pillai Riddell suggest that these differences are in part due to parents (and, to a similar extent, nurses) relying on a different pain judgement process that included a broader range of cues than physicians. Other factors speculated to play into this difference could relate to an 'institutional insensitivity' due to repeated exposure to infants in distress that desensitizes health professionals (Xavier Balda et al. 2000) or, although the parents were not judging their own children, one could conceive that parents would be more emotionally available to their own child thus having lower thresholds for detecting pain in children (Emde et al. 1985). These findings with regard to infant pain are similar to those reported among older children, in that parents tend to show better agreement with children's self-reports of pain as compared to nurses and physicians, who frequently underestimate children's pain (Manne et al. 1992). Despite the consistent finding that parents appear to attribute greater pain to the infant as compared to health professionals, it is impossible to conclude that they are more accurate. Accuracy in infant pain judgements is not possible to determine due to the infant's inability to self-report on their subjective experience. Regardless, what has not been established in these studies is whether parents and other caregivers manage infant pain differently based on their pain judgements.

Management

While parents are frequently involved in the management of their older children's pain, only recently has the role of parents in the management of their infant's pain been explored. Among older children, there are a number of parental behaviours that have been consistently linked to increases in child distress and pain during medical procedures, such as immunizations and intravenous insertions (Blount et al. 1989, 1997). For example, through detailed coding of parent–child interactions using the Child Adult Medical Procedure Interaction Scale (CAMPIS; Blount 1989, 1997), it has been established that parental use of criticism, reassurance, empathy, apologies and giving control have been found to frequently precede children's behavioural displays of distress and pain. While the mechanism behind how these various primarily well-intentioned parental behaviours may be linked with child distress is not well understood, it has been suggested that these behaviours may serve as a signal to the child that the parent is anxious or concerned, and may also serve to reinforce the display of child distress once it has been initiated (Chambers et al. 2002). Similar studies have extended this research to parents and their infants (Sweet and

McGrath 1998, Sweet et al. 1999), showing that parents who use reassurance with their infants have children who subsequently show increases in pain and distress during painful procedures.

It is acknowledged that parental approaches to reassurance are likely to be qualitatively different when used with infants as opposed to older children (e.g. reliance on more non-verbal vs. verbal behaviours intended to reassure). As a result, Cohen and colleagues recently developed the Measure of Adult and Infant Soothing and Distress (MAISD; Cohen et al. 2005). In their study, they describe a number of parent and/or nurse behaviours that are intended to soothe infants during painful medical procedures, including distraction, offering food or a toy, rocking, verbal reassurance, physical comfort, pacifying and rubbing. Results of this study mirrored those reported with older children, in that adult use of distraction promoted successful diversion of infant attention from the painful procedure, whereas use of reassurance was linked with increases in child distress.

Other work on parental soothing attempts during painful procedures has yielded mixed results. While some studies have found no evidence for the effectiveness of maternal soothing in reducing infant distress during painful medical procedures (e.g. Alfven 1986, Lewis and Ramsay 1999, Ipp et al. 2004), these null findings are likely attributable to the manner in which maternal soothing was coded (e.g. a gross score for maternal soothing attempts such as maternal presence versus absence or coarse categories of soothing amount rather than examining specific soothing behaviours). Studies in which more detailed analyses of maternal soothing behaviours are conducted generally find that certain maternal behaviours are indeed related to reductions in child distress. For example, among newborns receiving heel sticks, Campos (1994) found that use of pacifiers and rocking were both effective in reducing distress responses. In another study, maternal holding in combination with sweet taste had combined effects that acted on different behavioural and physiological systems during heel stick (Gormally et al. 2001). Crying, grimacing and heart rate were significantly reduced when infants were held and breastfed by their mothers as compared to infants in a control group who received the procedure swaddled in their bassinets as per standard care (Gray et al. 2002).

Maternal use of different soothing strategies likely changes and evolves as infants grow older. For example, one study found that mothers' use of affection and touching decreased from 2 to 6 months of age during inoculation, whereas maternal holding/rocking and vocalization increased over time (Jahromi et al. 2004). At both ages, holding/rocking and vocalization were associated with decreases in infant reactivity. The change in maternal use of soothing strategies over time may reflect increased insight on the part of the parent in regards to which soothing behaviours are most effective in reducing their infants' distress. Moreover, based on an infant's social development, the ability of who (e.g. mother versus other caregiver) will be able to soothe the infant in distress will narrow as the infant builds bonds with specific caregivers (Marvin and Britner 1999).

Furthering the idea that parent–infant interactions influence how an infant experiences and expresses pain, there is evidence that the effects of maternal soothing behaviours during painful procedures may extend far beyond the immediate procedure period. For example, Axia and Bonichini (2005) found that maternal soothing during vaccination at 3 months was associated with faster infant quieting during a subsequent vaccination at 5 months. Interestingly, the effects of maternal soothing were evident only when infant distress was not too high. The finding of ineffective maternal soothing during high levels of infant distress was also reported by Jahromi et al. (2004) and could reflect that high levels of distress disrupt an infant's ability to be regulated by otherwise helpful soothing behaviours on the part of the mother.

In addition to the physical and emotional soothing strategies employed by mothers in the above studies, distraction as an intervention for infant pain is an area that shows promise. There is good evidence that distraction is effective in reducing the pain and distress experienced by preschoolers and older children during medical procedures (Uman et al. 2005). Recent research has extended these findings to infants. For example, Cohen (2002) found that nurse-directed distraction (e.g. with an age-appropriate toy and video) was effective in reducing infant behavioural distress. In this study, nurses were used as the primary means of delivering the distraction intervention; however there is evidence that parents can be equally effective in providing evidence-based non-pharmacological pain care to their infants with relatively minimal instruction. For example, Felt and colleagues (2000) randomly assigned parents to either a standard care or intervention group. Parents in the intervention group received basic information about techniques (e.g. distraction) that could be used to help their infants during immunization. Infants of parents in the intervention group were more likely to use behavioural strategies than parents in the control group, and the infants in the intervention group showed reductions in both behavioural and biochemical indicators of distress during and following the immunization.

In summary, the study of parental behaviour in the context of infant pain provides insight into the potentially powerful role of parents as agents of pain relief for their infants. Moreover, the strategies that have been found to be helpful in these studies are relatively simple and cost-effective, and can be used by parents who, as described below, are highly motivated to learn how they can be involved in delivering pain care to their children.

RESEARCH ON PARENTING A PRETERM INFANT IN PAIN

Special consideration of parent and infant perspectives in the neonatal intensive care unit (NICU)

In high-risk pregnancies and deliveries, medical and technological advances come physically and emotionally between the mother and her newly born child. Mothers are most often physically distanced from their pained infant by an incubator and may wait weeks or even months before being able to comfortably soothe her child in her arms. Recalling the tenet that infants are biologically predisposed to need proximity to a caregiver during times of distress and that caregivers are also predisposed with complementary needs to provide protection, it is disturbing to note that during this most sensitive period of attachment development preterm infants and their parents are necessarily separated (Marvin and Britner 1999). Not only do preterm infants face repetitive stressful events (e.g. invasive painful procedures, painful disease processes) without direct proximity to their mother, at one of the most physically and psychologically malleable stages of their lives, they are also extremely limited in their ability to communicate distress to any caregiver.

Although research in the area is relatively new, it has been shown that preterm infants engage with their mothers less, provide fewer positive behaviours with their mothers, show less interest in their mothers and have mothers who report less satisfying mother–infant interactions (Edwards et al. 2003). While the impact of maternal depression on sensitivity to infant cues has been found to be of significant concern even with full-term infants (e.g. Crockenberg and Leerkes 2003), Poehlman and Fiese (2001) found an additive effect in that depressed mothers with preterm infants were more likely to be insecurely attached to their mothers than preterm infants without depressed mothers. Despite findings that many mothers can experience long-term psychological disturbances after giving birth to a preterm infant (e.g. Kaplan and Mason 1960, Eriksson and Pehrsson 2002), which could significantly influence the mother–child attachment relationship of infants who are already physically and psychologically vulnerable, it is still not common practice in hospitals to provide psychological support to parents of preterm infants (Brisch et al. 2003). Accordingly, it is important to consider the direct effect of prematurity on parents when understanding the preterm infant in pain. Months after their child had left the NICU, many parents reflect back to their time in the NICU as the 'worst major life event they have experienced' (Whitfield 2003).

A series of recent papers by Franck and colleagues (Franck et al. 2004, 2005, Gale et al. 2004) have explored parental perceptions regarding pain in the NICU in greater detail. The series of studies included data from a multiple-choice and long-answer survey with 257 parents from nine neonatal units across two countries (England and United States). In a complementary study (Gale et al. 2004), an in-depth qualitative analysis of focus group and interview data, with both parents of children currently in the NICU and parents who have had children in the NICU in the last 2 years, was conducted. The issue of unrelieved pain in their child and feelings of parental helplessness were consistent across the different samples and methodologies employed in these studies. Parental concerns about infant pain were strongly related to levels of parental stress. Moreover, important implications for clinical practice were highlighted in that most parents wanted more information about infant pain assessment and management and wanted to be consulted regarding how they wished to be involved in their infant's care.

Literature in the area of infant pain within an intensive care setting advocates that clinicians and researchers take a developmentally sensitive approach in understanding the compromised needs on both the side of the infant and the parent. While it is important to recognize the primary importance of the parent–child relationship, it is also necessary to proceed with interventions that are accompanied by a sensitive understanding of the idiosyncratic needs of both child (e.g. level of medical compromise) and parent (e.g. cultural norms; personality; comfort level in medical settings).

Current research on parenting a preterm infant in pain

Most research regarding pain with preterm populations is conducted within the context of tertiary care hospital nurseries. Because of their complicated medical conditions, front-line decisions regarding the assessment and management of pain are often left in the hands of medical professionals. Franck et al.'s

(2001) survey demonstrated that approximately 50% of parents reported not being given any instruction regarding how to assess or manage their infant's pain. However, developmentally sensitive care that acknowledges the symbiotic relationship of parent and infant is taking hold in more nurseries as modern medical science turns to more traditional methods of child care to soothe the premature infant.

An exemplar in this direction is the renaissance of the parent as a direct regulator of an infant's physiological and psychological response. Skin-to-skin contact, or kangaroo care, has been explored in the neonatal nursery as an intervention with infants to help both the parent and infant to overcome the separation trauma associated with a NICU stay and to physiologically stabilize the preterm infant (Tessier et al. 1998). The introduction of kangaroo care in hospital nurseries has been associated with remarkable outcomes such as reductions in the apnoeic attacks of very small preterm infants, increasing parental bonds to the infant, and even improving spousal behaviours towards each other when in proximity of the infant (Feldman et al. 2003), all without causing any iatrogenic physiological stress (de Leeuw et al. 1991). However, the kangaroo care literature is rife with published studies that utilize different time requirements for skin-to-skin contact that range from 1 hour a day to 24 hours a day with infants of differing degrees of medical severity, thus clear conclusions are not possible. While kangaroo care appears to be a promising parental intervention specifically in the area of acute pain with both preterm and full-term infants (Gray et al. 2000, Johnston et al. 2003), more work specifically exploring variables such as illness severity (e.g. how stable does the infant have to be before starting), effectiveness of kangaroo care in relation to time spent (i.e. dose–response relationship), and its contraindications needs to be done.

CONCLUSION

Infancy is characterized as a time when the child is wholly dependent on his/her caregivers yet is equipped with innate predispositions to elicit protection from caregivers. Moreover, similarly reciprocal predispositions in the caregiver also help guarantee the survival of the infant. Given that the template for pain experience and expression is significantly malleable through infancy, it is crucial that both clinicians and scientists continue to explore how to best alleviate infant pain within the context of the infant–caregiver relationship.

To further this relatively new line of inquiry in infant pain, the considerable theoretical and empirical contributions in the area of developmental psychology should be consulted. In particular, as should be clear from this chapter, there is much to be gained from referring to studies in which parent–infant relationships in the context of negative infant emotional states are examined. While frequently framed as examining infant 'distress', many of these studies actually employ painful stimuli (e.g. immunization) as the source of distress. The relationship between well-established attachment security categories and pain will likely lead to fruitful work regarding environmentally influenced individual differences in how pain experience and expression develop across the lifespan. Use of well-validated measures of dimensions of the parent–

infant relationship within the context of infant pain will be important. Our review suggests that the most useful research to date has focused on attitudes and behaviours relating to specific caregiving behaviours rather than more general cognitive constructs or behaviours.

As one of the clearest causes of danger to an infant during a time of extreme developmental plasticity, the study of infant pain provides a unique opportunity in which clinicians and scientists can make a difference across the lifespan. However, the primary importance of the parent–child relationship during infancy suggests that making this difference is also the privilege and responsibility of the parent.

REFERENCES

Ainsworth MD, Blehar MC, Waters E, et al. (1978). Patterns of attachment: a psychological study of the strange situation. Erlbaum, Hillsdale, NJ.

Alfven G. (1986). Pain and the mother–child interaction. Lancet 8517: 1222.

American Academy of Pediatrics and American Pain Society. (2001). The assessment and management of acute pain in infants, children and adolescents. Pediatrics 108: 793–797.

American Pain Society. (2005). Jeffery Lawson award for advocacy in children's pain relief. Online. Available: http://www.ampainsoc.org/awards/lawson.htm

Anand KJS, Craig KD. (1996). Editorial – new perspectives on the definition of pain. Pain 67: 3–6.

Anderson DJ, Hines RH. (1994). Attachment and pain. In: Grzesiak RC, Ciccone DS (eds) Psychological vulnerability to chronic pain. Springer, New York, pp. 137–152.

Axia G, Bonichini S. (2005). Are babies sensitive to the context of acute pain episodes? Infant distress and maternal soothing during immunization routines at 3 and 5 months of age. Infant Child Develop 14: 51–62.

Bakermans-Kranenburg MJ, Van Ijzendoorn MH, Juffer F. (2003). Less is more: meta-analyses of sensitivity and attachment interventions in early childhood. Psychol Bull 129:195–215.

Benoit D. (2000). Attachment and parent–infant relationships: a review of attachment theory and research. Ontario Assoc Child Aid Soc J 44: 13–23.

Blount RL, Corbin S, Sturges JW, et al. (1989). The relationship between adult's behavior and child coping and distress during BMA LP procedures: A

sequential analysis. Behav Ther 20: 585–601.

Blount RL, Cohen LL, Frank NC, et al. (1997). The Child–Adult Medical Procedure Interaction Scale-Revised: An assessment of validity. J Pediatr Psychol 22: 73–88.

Bowlby J. (1982). Attachment, 2nd edn. Tavistock Institute of Human Relations, USA.

Bowlby J. (1988). A secure base: parent child attachment and healthy human development. Basic Books, New York, p. 3.

Brisch KH, Bechinger D, Betzler S, et al. (2003). Early preventive attachment-oriented psychotherapeutic intervention program with parents of a very low birth weight premature infant: results of attachment and neurological development. Attach Human Develop 5: 120–135.

Campos RG. (1994). Rocking and pacifiers: two comforting interventions for heelstick pain. Res Nurs Health 17: 321–331.

Chambers CT. (2003). The role of family factors in pediatric pain. In: McGrath PJ, Finley GA (eds) Pediatric pain: biological and social context. IASP, Seattle, pp. 99–130.

Chambers CT, Craig KD, Bennett SM. (2002). The impact of maternal behavior on children's pain experiences: An experimental analysis. J Pediatr Psychol 27: 293–301.

Cohen LL. (2002). Reducing infant immunization distress through distraction. Health Psychol 21: 207–211.

Cohen LL, Bernard RS, McClellan CB, et al. (2005). Assessing medical room behavior during infants' painful procedures: The Measure of Adult and

Infant Soothing and Distress (MAISD). Child Health Care 34: 81–94.

Craig KD. (1997). Implications of concepts of consciousness for understanding pain behaviour and the definition of pain. Pain Res Manage 2: 111–116.

Craig KD, Pillai Riddell R. (2003). Social influences, culture and ethnicity. In: Finley GA, McGrath PJ (eds) Pediatric pain: biological and social context. IASP Press, Seattle, pp. 159–182.

Craig KD, Grunau R, Aquan-Assee J. (1988). Judgements of pain in newborns: facial activity and cry as determinants. Can J Behav Sci 20: 442–449.

Craig KD, Lilley CM, Gilbert CA. (1996). Social barriers to optimal pain management in infants and children. Clin J Pain 12: 232–242.

Craig KD, Korol CT, Pillai RR. (2002). Challenges of judging pain in vulnerable infants. Clin Perinatol 29: 445–458.

Crockenberg S, Leerkes E. (2003). Parental acceptance, postpartum depression, and maternal sensitivity: mediating and moderating processes. J Fam Psychol 17: 80.

de Leeuw R, Colin EM, Dunnebier EA, et al. (1991). Physiological effects of kangaroo care in very small preterm infants. Biol Neonate 59: 149–155.

Edwards H, Davis L, Mohay H. (2003). Mother–infant interaction in premature infants at three months after nursery discharge. Intern J Nurs Pract 9: 374–381.

Emde RN, Izard CE, Huebner RR, et al. (1985). Adult judgements of infant emotions: replication studies within and across laboratories. Infant Behav Develop 8: 79–88.

Eriksson B, Pehrsson G. (2002). Evaluation of psycho-social support to parents with an infant born preterm. J Child Health Care 6: 19–33.

Feldman R, Weller A, Sirota L, et al. (2003). Testing a family intervention hypothesis: the contribution of mother: infant skin-to-skin contact (kangaroo care) to family interaction, proximity, and touch. J Fam Psychol 17: 94–107.

Felt BT, Mollen E, Diaz S, et al. (2000). Behavioral interventions reduce infant distress at immunization. Arch Pediatr Adolesc Med 154: 719–724.

Field T. (1994). The effects of mother's physical and emotional unavailability on emotion regulation. Monogr Soc Res Child Develop 59: 208–227.

Franck LS, Scurr K, Couture S. (2001). Parent views of infant pain and pain management in neonatal intensive care units. Newborn Infant Nurs Rev 1: 106–113.

Franck LS, Cox S, Allen A, et al. (2004). Parental concern and distress about infant pain. Arch Dis Child Fetal Neonatal Ed 89: F71–75.

Franck LS, Alison A, Cox S, et al. (2005). Parents' views about infant pain in neonatal intensive care. Clin J Pain 21: 133–139.

Gale G, Frank LS, Kools S, et al. (2004). Parents' perceptions of their infant's pain experience in the NICU. Intern J Nurs Stud 41: 51–58.

George C, Solomon J. (1996). Attachment and caregiving: the caregiving behavioral system. In: Cassidy J, Shaver PR (eds) Handbook of attachment: theory, research, and clinical applications. The Guilford Press, New York, pp. 649–670.

George C, Solomon J. (1999). Measurement of attachment security in infancy and childhood. In: Cassidy J, Shaver PR (eds) Handbook of attachment: theory, research, and clinical applications. The Guildford Press, New York, pp. 287–316.

Gormally S, Barr RG, Wertheim L, et al. (2001). Contact and nutrient caregiving effects on newborn infant pain response. Develop Med Child Neurol 43: 28–38.

Gray L, Watt L, Blass EM. (2000). Skin-to-skin contact is analgesic in healthy newborns. Pediatrics 105: e14.

Gray L, Miller LW, Philipp BL, et al. (2002). Breastfeeding is analgesic in healthy newborns. Pediatrics 109: 590–593.

Grunau R, Whitfield M, Petrie JH, et al. (1994). Early pain experience, child and family factors, as precursors of somatization: a prospective study of extremely premature and fullterm children. Pain 56: 353–359.

Ipp M, Taddio A, Goldbach M, et al. (2004). Effects of age, gender and holding on pain response during infant immunization. Can J Clin Pharmacol 11: e2–e7.

Jahromi LB, Putnam SP, Stifter CA. (2004). Maternal regulation of infant reactivity from 2 to 6 months. Develop Psychol 4: 477–487.

Johnston CC, Stevens B, Pinelli J, et al. (2003). Kangaroo care is effective in diminishing pain response in preterm neonates. Arch Pediatr Adolesc Med 157: 1084–1088.

Kaplan D, Mason EA. (1960). Maternal reactions to premature birth viewed as an acute emotional disorder. Am J Orthopsychiatry 30: 539–552.

Kolb L. (1982). Attachment and pain complaints. Psychosomatics 23: 413–425.

Lewis M, Ramsay DS. (1999). Effect of maternal soothing on infant stress response. Child Develop 70: 11–20.

Luecken LJ, Lemery KS. (2004). Early caregiving and physiological stress responses. Clin Psychol Rev 24: 171–191.

Manne SL, Jacobsen PB, Redd WH. (1992). Assessment of acute pediatric pain: Do child self-report, parent ratings, and nurse ratings measure the same phenomenon? Pain 48: 45–52.

Marvin R, Britner P. (1999). Normative development: the ontogeny of attachment. In: Cassidy J, Shaver PR (eds) Handbook of attachment: theory, research, and clinical applications. The Guildford Press, New York, pp. 44–67.

McClellan CB, Cohen LL, Joseph KE. (2003). Infant distress during immunization: a multimethod assessment. J Clin Psychol Med Settings 10: 231–238.

Nader R. (2005). Age related differences in infant pain expression and parental judgements of pain throughout the first year of life. Doctoral dissertation, University of British Columbia.

Pillai Riddell RR. (2004) Attributions of pain to infants: a comparative analysis of parents, nurses and paediatricians. Doctoral dissertation, University of British Columbia.

Pillai Riddell R, Badali MA, Craig KD. (2004). Parental judgements of infant pain: importance of perceived cognitive abilities, behavioural cues and contextual cues. Pain Res Manage 9: 73–80.

Poehlmann J, Fiese BH. (2001). The interaction of maternal and infant vulnerabilities on developing attachment relationships. Develop Psychopathol 13: 1–11.

Prkachin KM, Craig KD. (1995). Expressing pain: the communication and interpretation of facial pain signals. J Nonverbal Behav 19: 191–203.

Sweet SD, McGrath PJ. (1998). Relative importance of mothers' versus medical staffs' behavior in the prediction of infant immunization pain behavior. J Pediatr Psychol 23: 249–256.

Sweet SD, McGrath PJ, Symons D. (1999). The roles of child reactivity and parenting context in infant pain response. Pain 80: 655–661.

Taddio A, Katz J, Ilersich AL, et al. (1997). Effect of neonatal circumcision on pain response during subsequent routine vaccination. Lancet 349: 599–603.

Tessier R, Cristo M, Velez S, et al. (1998). Kangaroo mother care and the bonding hypothesis. Pediatrics 102: 17–24.

Thompson RA. (1999). Early attachment and later development. In: Cassidy J, Shaver PR (eds) Handbook of attachment: theory, research, and clinical applications. The Guildford Press, New York, pp. 265–286.

Uman LS, Chambers CT, McGrath PJ, et al. (2005). Psychological interventions for needle-related procedural pain and distress in children and adolescents (Protocol). Cochrane Database Syst Rev CD005179.

Walsh TM, Symons DK, McGrath PJ. (2004). Relations between young children's responses to the depiction of separation and pain experiences. Attach Human Develop 6: 53–71.

Whitfield MF. (2003). Psychosocial effects of intensive care on infants and families after discharge. Semin Neonatol 8: 185–193.

Xavier Balda R, Guinsburg R, de Almeida MF, et al. The recognition of facial expression of pain in full-term newborns by parents and health professionals: Arch Pediatr Adolesc Med 154: 1009–1016.

CHAPTER

23

Future directions for clinical research in infancy

KJS Anand
Bonnie J Stevens
Patrick J McGrath

Recent attention to pain in neonates and young infants has resulted in a better understanding of the underlying anatomy and physiology of pain transmission in this population, validated measures and methods for the assessment of acute or postoperative pain in pre-verbal patients, as well as the determination of safety and efficacy of various interventions for the treatment of pain in neonates and older infants. For such a rapidly developing field, particularly within the context of prolific scientific, technological and intellectual advances resulting from the instantaneous sharing of ideas and inventions in an Internet-based culture, it may be impossible to predict or even outline the future directions that pain research will take. It has been said, however, that 'leaders lay the train tracks, managers make trains run on time'. To provide leadership and direction in the field of neonatal and paediatric pain, therefore, we believe that future research should be directed at:

- clarifying the developmental neurobiology and physiology of pain;
- reaching beyond acute pain, to describe the epidemiology, biology and clinical features of persistent/chronic pain, visceral pain, or neuropathic pain in early life;
- developing measures and methods for assessment for persistent, recurring or chronic pain in infants and further validating measures for acute pain;
- designing drugs based on the unique expression of neurotransmitters and receptor populations in early life;
- defining pharmacogenetics and pharmacogenomics of the developing pain system;
- developing novel techniques for the neuroimaging of pain;
- articulating processes for knowledge transfer to enhance the translation of scientific knowledge into clinical practice;
- exploring infant pain management in the home and community to reach those not treated at hospitals or tertiary medical centres;
- expanding the focus on the globalization of pain research and pain therapies to enhance access and availability beyond developed countries.

In general, future trends for research may be broadly classified into the biology, assessment, management and the societal context for pain in the neonate and young infant. Because this volume is mainly directed towards clinicians and clinical scientists, the sections below will be focused primarily on the assessment and management of pain in early life.

PAIN ASSESSMENT TECHNIQUES

That 'diagnosis precedes treatment' is perhaps the foremost axiom in clinical practice. Consequently, first and foremost, we need valid and reliable methods or measures for assessing pain, the effects of pain, or the efficacy of analgesic interventions in neonates or infants. Given there is no biologic measure identified as the gold standard for assessing pain in infants (Warnock and Lander 2004), physiological, bio-behavioural and behavioural indicators are frequently used as surrogate markers of self-report to infer the existence of pain in non-communicating or vulnerable populations. Although there were few measures to assess pain in infants only a decade ago, a recent systematic integrative review of infant pain assessment measures by Duhn and Medves (2004) indicates that there are now approximately three dozen univariate, multivariate and composite measures for assessing pain in infants. However, the behavioural and physio-logical indicators comprising these measures are notoriously difficult to quantify and validate based on the currently available subjective methodology. Therefore, only a few have well-established validity, reliability, clinical utility and feasibility for assessing acute procedural and postoperative pain and none have been validated for infants that are either extremely premature, mechanically ventilated or chemically paralyzed.

Measures of pain

We have carefully focused pain assessment on the behavioural (e.g. facial expression, body movements, flexion reflex and cry) and physiological (i.e. heart rate, respiratory rate, blood pressure, oxygen saturation, vagal tone, palmar sweating) indicators in response to acute painful procedures (i.e. most frequently heel lance). Biomarkers have also been employed; however, while multiple biomarkers are available to determine neonatal pain reactivity, no single biomarker can characterize all aspects of neonatal pain. Furthermore, the response patterns of biomarkers vary differently under different contextual and illness conditions. To date, there has been minimal consideration of con-textual factors that influence these responses (e.g. sleep/wake states, stage of development, severity of illness, risk for impairment). Measures to quantify the reactivity (magnitude, latency, duration of responses) and regulation (rate, duration, pattern of recovery) of biomarkers, and how to use biomarkers as outcome measures or developmental probes need to be addressed when studying pain-related outcomes. Even when differences in biomarkers are statistically different from a baseline to pain condition, such differences may not be clinically meaningful.

Other clinically relevant outcome measures (both short term and long term) need to be developed for sick newborns or young infants receiving brief or prolonged analgesia. Outcomes specifically related to pain must be discovered, as differentiated from the effects of underlying illness or developmental immaturity. For example, recent data suggest that mechanical ventilation itself may be associated with abnormal neurologic outcomes, including cerebral palsy and cognitive delay (Laptook et al. 2005). Whether concomitant exposure to analgesia or seda-tion attenuates or enhances these outcomes remains currently unclear (Simons et al. 2003, Anand et al. 2004).

Specific types of pain

Clearly, our attention has been focused on acute pain, occurring from tissue injury. Prolonged pain states are also distinguishable because a defined stimulus (e.g. surgical procedure, skin or mucosal burns, meningitis, or multiple heel sticks) and a definable endpoint are readily discernible. The assessment of prolonged pain, however, challenges healthcare professionals because the psychophysiological activation responses (overt pain behaviours and signs of sympathetic nervous system arousal) are often absent (Anand 1997). Accordingly, assessing prolonged pain in infants currently depends on observing disruptions in behavioural or functional activity over a period of hours rather than minutes (Debillon et al. 2001, Hummel et al. 2003). Even more problematic is the pain with no discernible endpoint. Chronic pain has been defined in adults as a pathological pain state without apparent organic cause that has persisted beyond the normal period for tissue healing (usually 3 months) (Bonica 1953, Jovey et al. 2003). Both persistent and chronic pain are entities that have been little explored in the infant population. The assessment of other types of pain, such as visceral or neuropathic pain, also remains un-explored in this population. It is possible that the lack of clinical methods to diagnose these types of pain in infancy may contribute to the relatively low incidence among infants and neonates.

We have made major advances in pain assessment over the past few years. However, critical reviews of the multiplicity of pain measures suggest that we need to validate existing measures and concentrate on determining the clinical utility and feasibility of valid and reliable measures for practice, expand the search for novel indicators or combinations of indicators of pain, turning our efforts away from finding recombinations of established indicators (such as facial activity, body movements and heart rates). We also need to focus on special populations of infants who have received less than adequate pain assessment and management as well as on the unresolved measurement issues across ages, populations and situations as outlined in Chapter 6. Then, and only then, would we have scientifically valid tools to investigate the efficacy and clinical applicability of various pain management approaches for infant and neonatal patients as discussed below.

PAIN MANAGEMENT APPROACHES

Although considerable progress has been made in studying the safety, efficacy, dose response, and clinical outcomes related to a few pharmacological, behavioural and environmental methods for pain relief in neonates and infants, major gaps in our knowledge continue to hinder optimal clinical practice. Multicentre clinical trials with adequate sample sizes are needed to assess the occurrence of uncommon adverse effects or safety concerns. These study designs and sample sizes should allow validated evaluation of therapeutic efficacy and dose–response relationships, while avoiding exposure to pain in neonates and infants. Ethical constraints also apply to placebo or no-treatment control groups among neonates or infants, particularly when sufficient data exist to provide standard treatment to control groups. Population-based pharmacokinetic approaches seem appropriate for this patient group, while avoiding the detrimental effects of repeated blood sampling in the same patient. Future studies should examine if multimodal analgesia, as in adults, can improve clinical outcomes in neonates and infants.

Future studies should also include assessments of drug efficacy and safety following repeated doses of analgesic, sedative or other drugs because pain occurs repeatedly and, in most cases, analgesia needs to be used repeatedly. In this regard, dose-ranging studies must identify the minimum effective dose so that cumulative drug exposures can be minimized. Future study designs should also consider the evaluation of specific analgesics in combination with other pharmacologic agents, or with behavioural, physical and psychological interventions, in order to improve analgesic efficacy and minimize the side effects.

Pharmacological considerations

Pharmacogenetics and pharmacogenomics

The promise of pharmacogenetics and pharmacogenomics, particularly with the potential to 'individualize' analgesic therapy, has spurred a great deal of research in industry and academia. This research hinges on the premise that the genetic variability caused by single nucleotide polymorphisms (SNPs) may explain some of the large interindividual differences in analgesic requirements (Evans and Relling 1999, Evans and McLeod, 2003, Weinshilboum 2003). For example, in the β-opioid receptor (MOR) gene, a nucleotide substitution at position 118 (A118G), predicts an amino acid change at codon 40, from asparagine (*asn*) to aspartate (*asp*), with threefold increases in β-endorphin binding affinity (Bond et al. 1998) and reduced potency of M6G in humans (Hollt 2002, Lotsch et al. 2002). Another abundant SNP of the cathechol-O-methyltransferase (COMT) gene encodes the substitution of valine (*val*) by methionine (*met*) at codon 158, reducing COMT enzyme activity by three- to fourfold, with diminished activation of the endogenous μ-opioid system in response to pain ($met^{158}met < val^{158}met < val^{158}val$) and higher sensory/affective ratings of pain (Zubieta et al. 2003). Pilot data suggest that both these SNPs may reduce the need for postoperative morphine analgesia in infants, but only effects of the COMT mutation were significant (P = 0.034), because fewer patients were homozygous for the $asp^{40}asp$ MOR (Simons et al. 2004). Other similar examples and their relevance to infant pain are described in Chapter 8.

Ongoing and future research will design additional creative approaches to investigate the pharmacogenetics and pharmacogenomics of analgesia and sedation, with a particular focus on the early developmental expression of genes encoding opioid and other receptors, molecules mediating their signal-transduction mechanisms, and enzymes involved in the degradation of analgesic/sedative drugs.

Pharmacokinetics and pharmacodynamics

Despite recent progress, there are still large gaps in our understanding of the pharmacokinetics and pharmacodynamics of analgesic and sedative drugs in the neonate. As noted in Chapters 9 and 10, currently available data are limited, even for commonly used drugs such as morphine, fentanyl, ibuprofen, acetaminophen or other agents, particularly among preterm neonates and infants beyond the neonatal period. Novel approaches such as the use of nonlinear modelling techniques or population pharmacokinetics require the measurement of plasma drug levels in large numbers of neonates. Because the neonatal and infant populations are highly heterogeneous, the methods for population pharmacokinetics may offer a greater ability to address the effects of clinical covariates and to estimate interindividual variability in pharmacokinetics and dosing

(Hunt et al. 1999, Swart et al. 2004). These types of analyses are noted in Chapter 9, but need to be extended to analgesics and sedatives used in infancy, both currently used and novel drugs.

Future research must address several questions that remain unanswered at present. Taking opioid drugs as an example, have the pharmacokinetics of morphine, fentanyl, hydromorphone, methadone, remifentanil, oxycodone, codeine and dexmedetomidine been described completely in neonates and infants? How does metabolism change with postconceptional age, postnatal age, medical and surgical conditions (including abdominal surgery), genetic polymorphisms, gender, or drug–drug interactions? What pharmacokinetic/pharmacodynamic models for opioid effects are best suited for neonates and infants? Can we use pharmacokinetic parameters to explain the analgesic dose response? Do metabolites of morphine or other opioids contribute to analgesia in infants? Is immaturity of the blood–brain barrier an important factor in age-related differences in opioid dose-response, both for analgesia and for respiratory depression? Similar questions can be generated for other analgesic drug classes that are used for neonates or infants.

Research considerations for opioids

Ideally designed opioid drugs would have proven efficacy against different types of pain, a rapid onset and well-defined duration of action, effective via enteral, parenteral or neuraxial routes, minimal side effects or tolerance and withdrawal, and negligible effects on the developing brain, spinal or peripheral mechanisms. Long-acting drugs such as morphine and methadone may be favourable for prolonged or persistent pain, whereas short-acting drugs like fentanyl, alfentanil or remifentanil may be indicated for procedural pain (Anand et al. 2005b). Very little is known about the pharmacology of these drugs at different gestational ages, among neonates or infants with different diagnoses, or varying degrees of critical illness. In addition, the need for studies investigating repeated administration must be emphasized, to evaluate their safety and efficacy over short periods (24–48 hours) as well as cumulative exposure over the entire hospital stay.

Neonates and infants are exposed to many invasive procedures that do not cause severe enough pain (e.g. heel sticks, peripheral venous cannulation) to warrant the use of powerful opioid agents, particularly if repetitive dosing is required and if the infant is not ventilated. Individual patients may have more than tenfold differences in the doses required to produce opioid analgesia. Individual differences in drug

responsiveness are accentuated because the currently available methods for assessment of pain intensity involve observation of behavioural and physiological indicators, either singly or in combination, the response characteristics of which are not highly correlated (Anand et al. 2005a). Genetic differences caused by single nucleotide polymorphisms (SNPs) may also explain some interindividual differences in analgesic requirements among infants (Evans and McLeod 2003, Weinshilboum 2003). Further research on opioid analgesia in infants must include an assessment of these genetic, metabolic, developmental and other variables.

Unanswered questions related to opioids

Future research must address the numerous unanswered questions concerning the use of opioid agents in neonates and infants. What clinical paradigms can be used to study efficacy or dose responses to opioid analgesia? Can opioids be dosed effectively in neonates or infants using formal criteria that combine scoring of valid pain indicators, assessment of vital signs, sedation scoring and contextual factors? Are these criteria reproducible and reliable when used for dosing opioids in individual patients? Can adverse effects be decreased by using opioid antagonists with opioid agonists? What doses of opioids suppress hormonal/metabolic stress responses or immune responses to injury or inflammation? Are there useful surrogate measures of the opioid effect in neonates or infants, including processed electroencephalography (EEG), respiratory response curves, changes in pupillary diameter, or suppression of nerve stimulation at frequencies specific for C-fibres, A-δ fibres, or A-β fibres?

What duration of opioid administration results in tolerance in neonates and infants? Is this risk decreased by using specific opioid drugs or drug combinations? What factors are critical to the development of tolerance? Is the time course of development of tolerance different for different opioids? Are the opioid side effects or tolerance altered in the presence or absence of ongoing pain? How can opioid withdrawal be assessed, prevented and treated in infants? Does dexmedetomidine have advantages over enteral opioid conversion and weaning (in terms of time, safety, or risk of withdrawal)? Is codeine ineffective because it is a prodrug requiring hepatic metabolism, which is immature in infants?

With respect to clinical safety, are there better ways of predicting, monitoring and preventing ventilatory depression in neonates and infants receiving opioids? At equianalgesic doses, do the commonly used opiates differ in their side-effect profiles? When and how do opioids cause seizures in infants? Can strategies be developed to prevent or minimize paralytic ileus or biliary spasm in infants receiving opioids? What is the incidence of urinary retention after receipt of opioids in infants?

Unanswered questions related to opioid antagonists

There are numerous questions concerning the use of opioid antagonists in neonates and infants. Can low- or ultra-low dose infusions of naloxone reduce opioid adverse effects in neonates or infants? Are there any adverse effects of low- or ultra-low dose administration of opioid antagonists in neonates or infants? Are doses of the longer-acting antagonist nalmefene as effective as intermittent doses or infusions of the shorter-acting naloxone? In addition to decreasing adverse effects (urinary retention, ileus, pruritus), does the combination of opioid antagonists and opioid analgesics delay or decrease the onset of tolerance? If there is an effect, would dose escalation be retarded and/or weaning be more rapid? What are the effects of gender, postnatal or gestational age on the pharmacokinetic parameters of opioid antagonists?

Opioid antagonists methylnaltrexone (Yuan et al. 1997, 2000, 2002, Yuan and Foss 2000, Foss 2001) and alvimopan (ADL 8-2698) (Liu et al. 2001, Schmidt 2001, Taguchi et al. 2001) are active at gastrointestinal opioid receptors, are poorly absorbed and do not cause systemic adverse effects, but can reduce opioid-induced ileus in adults. Can these drugs be used for preventing paralytic ileus and feeding intolerance in neonates or infants receiving prolonged opioid therapy?

Research considerations for sedatives/hypnotics

The role of sedatives/hypnotics for pain management in neonates or infants may include: (a) their effects as adjuvant drugs for invasive procedures associated with tissue injury, (b) their role as primary analgesic agents for clinical conditions not associated with tissue injury. Sedatives like ketamine, for example, have potent analgesic effects and can be used as primary agents for most neonates and infants. Future investigations should be designed to examine the role of these drugs in combination with opioids or other agents and as primary agents. The pharmacology of these drugs remains unclear, together with unknown effects of the variations in gestational age, postnatal age or severity of illness. The potential neurotoxic effects of sedatives, general anaesthetics and antiepileptic drugs in preterm neonates and older infants need to be investigated in models that closely approximate the doses, duration and clinical contexts for use in human infants (Anand and Soriano 2004,

Soriano et al. 2005). Genetic and developmental differences that focus on the GABA/benzodiazepine receptor may explain some of the variability in drug effects noted from the use of these drugs. The effects of these drugs in infants who are neurologically compromised and other considerations listed for the use of systemic opioids should also apply to this class of drugs.

Unanswered questions related to sedatives and hypnotics

There are numerous questions concerning the efficacy of sedative–hypnotics in neonates and infants. Are there valid sedation scales for use in infancy? Are these scales specific to sedation as opposed to pain or other conditions? Are surrogate markers, including processed EEG measures, useful as markers of depth of sedation in infants? How are these measures affected by developmental maturity? Are clonidine and dexmedetomidine effective as analgesics in neonates and young infants? Do these drugs have safety/efficacy advantages compared with standard opioids when used for postoperative analgesia or other indications?

Concerning safety in clinical use, can neonates or older infants with congenital heart disease, sepsis, or other conditions tolerate sedative–hypnotics along with opioids for sedation/analgesia during mechanical ventilation or following major surgery? What are the respiratory, haemodynamic, neuro-endocrine, immunologic or long-term effects of sedative–hypnotics in neonates and infants? How do sedative–hypnotics influence respiratory control in preterm and full-term neonates? Are the studies of neurodegeneration in neonatal rats administered NMDA antagonists pertinent to human neonates and infants? Can sedative–hypnotics be neuroprotective in some infants? How do general anaesthetics and sedatives affect brain metabolism in infancy? How rapidly does tolerance develop to benzodiazepines and how can withdrawal symptoms from benzodiazepines be assessed and treated in infancy?

With respect to uptake, distribution and metabolism, how do hepatic and renal maturation affect metabolism and excretion of benzodiazepines and other sedatives? Does abdominal surgery, with or without increased intra-abdominal pressure, impair metabolism of sedative–hypnotics in infants? Which vehicles, solvents and additives are toxic for neonates or infants? Should neonates and infants only receive preservative-free formulations?

Research considerations for NSAIDs

Sparse information is available on the pharmacology, safety or efficacy of NSAIDs used as analgesic agents in neonates and older infants (Litalien and Jacqz-Aigrain 2001, Kokki 2003). Drugs such as indometacin, ibuprofen, sulindac or mefenamic acid have been used for closure of patent ductus arteriosus in preterm neonates, but information on their analgesic efficacy and safety is not available (Ng et al. 1996, 1997). NSAIDs may be associated with serious adverse effects in various organ systems as well as toxic drug interactions, therefore, without proof of efficacy their routine use for neonatal analgesia cannot be recommended (Camu et al. 2001, Kokki 2003, Morris et al. 2003). In children, acetaminophen and other NSAIDs have opioid-sparing properties when used for postoperative pain (Kokki 2003) and it is likely that they may have similar benefits in neonates and infants. Repeated procedures usually lead to inflammation (e.g. repeated heel lances, chest tube insertions), which may provide suitable indications for the use of these drugs in infancy. Future research should compare the efficacy of acetaminophen and other NSAIDs, as well as the combined effects of acetaminophen and other NSAIDs for analgesia in infants, as has been done for their antipyretic effects in these age groups (Litalien and Jacqz-Aigrain 2001).

Unanswered questions related to NSAIDs

Concerning efficacy, do NSAIDs, COX-2 selective inhibitors, acetaminophen or propacetamol provide clinically important analgesia in early life? Are there age-related differences in the analgesic responses to these agents? Do these agents provide clinically important opioid-sparing effects after surgery? Studies should measure efficacy not only in terms of reduction in pain scores, but also in terms of reduced opioid requirements, side effects, and reduced duration or frequency of postoperative ventilatory support.

Pharmacokinetic data are available on single-dose administration of acetaminophen in preterm and term neonates (Howard et al. 1994, Shah et al. 1998, van Lingen et al. 1999a, 1999b), but there is little information on older infants (Hopkins et al. 1990, Bremerich et al. 2001) or the effects of repeated dosing on pharmacokinetic/pharmacodynamic parameters. No information is available concerning the pharmacokinetic/pharmacodynamic parameters of other NSAIDs in neonates or infants. How does metabolism change with postconceptional age, postnatal age, medical and surgical conditions, pharmacogenetics and drug interactions? What are the best methods for pharmacokinetic/pharmacodynamic modelling of the actions of NSAIDs, COX-2-selective inhibitors, and acetaminophen in neonates and infants?

Concerning safety, these drugs have major adverse effects in adults involving the hepatic (acetaminophen/ propacetamol), renal, coagulation, cardiovascular (including cerebral blood flow) and gastrointestinal systems. Do all NSAIDs or the COX-2 selective inhibitors increase the risks for necrotizing enterocolitis (NEC), gastritis, intracranial haemorrhage, pulmonary hypertension and nephropathy in critically ill neonates or infants? Are there significant differences in the risk–benefit ratios for these agents? How is the dosing of acetaminophen or propacetamol influenced by gestation or postnatal age, critical illness or different disease states?

Research considerations for local anaesthetics

Increasing use of topical and injectable local anaesthetics in neonates and infants has been supported by various research studies over the past 10 years. Given these recent advances, it remains unclear what are the acceptable extrapolations of local anaesthetic efficacy from children and what needs to be investigated in infancy. For example, studies in children demonstrate that EMLA decreases pain from venipuncture, venous cannulation, lumbar puncture, intramuscular injections and other acutely painful procedures (Dutta 1999). With this information readily available, is it necessary to test each condition in neonates and infants as well? Or is it reasonable to suggest that local anaesthesia can be used for similar procedures in neonates/infants without proof of benefit? Similarly, the burning pain caused by lidocaine infiltration may be counteracted with co-administration of topical anaesthetics or systemic analgesia; however, these measures have not been proven in neonates or infants. Similar examples of procedures where evidence is lacking in neonates and older infants are lumbar puncture, venous cut-down, intramuscular or subcutaneous injections.

Important outcomes may include longer-term measures of regular analgesic use, such as the potential to decrease the long-term hypersensitivity to pain. This notion is supported by a previous study demonstrating that regular treatment of heel lancing pain with EMLA reduced the development of primary hyperalgesia (Fitzgerald et al. 1989). Studies investigating combination therapy with other analgesics or environmental interventions for various procedures are also lacking (Taddio et al. 2000, Geyer et al. 2002). With respect to topical local anaesthetics, newer formulations such as LMX.4 appear to offer the best risk–benefit profile in infants and future investigations should focus on these preparations.

Recent research shows that the developmental expression of sodium channels in early life is distinct from that of adults or older children (Yiangou et al. 2000). Local anaesthetic drugs like 2-chloroprocaine may offer specific advantages for use in neonates and infants, with a favourable risk–benefit profile. Based on clinical observations and pharmacokinetic/pharmacodynamic considerations, no local anaesthetic except 2-chloroprocaine can be given safely at infusion rates high enough to be effective as a sole analgesic in infants (Berde 2004). Future research should also develop protocols to investigate these drugs for local, topical or neuraxial use in infancy.

Unanswered questions related to local anaesthetics

What measures should be used to assess the efficacy of local anaesthetics in infants or preterm/term neonates? Can surrogate measures be developed that correlate with the dermatomal level of blockade (e.g. thermography, laser-Doppler measurement of skin blood flow) that can be correlated with pain scores and outcomes of different local anaesthetic procedures? Does the use of local anaesthetics decrease opioid requirements following surgery or intensive care? What are the pharmacokinetic/pharmacodynamic profiles for each of these drugs? How does the metabolism and elimination of local anaesthetics change with postconceptional age, postnatal age, medical and surgical conditions, pharmacogenetics or concomitant drug therapy? What are the methods for pharmacokinetic/pharmacodynamic modelling of the actions of local anaesthetics (at nerve sites, or local injection sites) in neonates and infants?

Lidocaine is considered safer than other amide local anaesthetics because blood levels can be monitored. Questions concerning safety include the development of surrogate measures to define blood concentrations associated with the risks of seizures or arrhythmias. What are the infant disease states or drug characteristics that modify these risks? Specifically, are ropivacaine, chloroprocaine or levobupivacaine significantly safer than bupivacaine in infancy (Spencer et al. 1992, Tobias et al. 1997)? What are the physiological effects of high-spinal or epidural blockade on blood pressure? How common are infections from epidural catheters in neonates or infants? What are the risks associated with bleeding in the epidural space during catheter placement? How can these risks be reduced? Is the local neurotoxicity of local anaesthetics a concern in neonates or infants? How can these risks be assessed in animal models or human epidemiologic studies? Future research must address these questions as well as compare the relative efficacy and safety of different local anaesthetics in neonates and infants.

Research considerations for non-pharmacological approaches

As discussed in Chapter 12, several investigators have evaluated the efficacy of non-pharmacological, environmental and behavioural comfort measures in relieving procedural pain. For example, sucrose exhibits an analgesic effect in neonates and infants (Blass and Shah 1995, Bucher et al. 1995) and this analgesic effect is obtained with 2 ml of sucrose (12% or higher) if given 2 minutes before acute pain (Stevens et al. 2004). Non-nutritive sucking on a pacifier also produces neonatal analgesia if the rate of sucking is >30 per minute (Blass 1997, Blass and Watt 1999). Future research may help to define how the integration of these two modalities occurs at different gestational or postnatal ages. Other characteristics of sucrose analgesia need to be investigated, such as duration of analgesic effect, efficacy of repeated doses, side effects (hyperglycaemia, diuresis, metabolic acidosis), and other physiological effects (e.g. hormonal changes, cardiovascular responses) during the newborn and infant period. Other sugars such as lactose and fructose may also have similar or more potent effects on pain responses in infancy.

Environmental measures, behavioural interventions and developmental care may improve the infant's ability to cope with and recover from painful procedures, such as nesting, positioning, reduction in light or noise levels and physical handling. However, the impact of these measures needs to be explored further. An individualized package of developmental nursing care includes many of these components (NIDCAP; Neonatal Individualized Developmental Care Assessment Program), and was noted to improve the clinical and long-term developmental outcomes of preterm infants (Als et al. 1994). Future studies must replicate these results in larger randomized trials and study the mechanisms leading to the improved long-term outcomes.

Unanswered question related to sucrose analgesia

Despite recent systematic reviews and meta-analyses on the efficacy and safety of sucrose (Stevens et al. 2004) and studies investigating the effects and mechanisms of analgesia produced by other sweet-tasting substances (dextrose, breast milk, others) in neonates and infants, many questions remain unanswered. These are particularly related to the dosing, drug interactions, and long-term effects of sucrose (or other substances used similarly). How much sucrose should be given during a single procedure? Is there is a dose–response curve or a threshold effect? Do the more intensely painful procedures require higher doses than less painful procedures? How much sucrose can be given each day without negative long-term effects? Which are the neonatal populations most at risk for developing adverse long-term neurobehavioural effects? What are the dose–response relationships with adverse metabolic effects, such as hyperglycaemia or metabolic acidosis? Is opioid responsiveness altered in children who were exposed to sucrose in the neonatal period? What is the upper limit of age or development at which sucrose analgesia remains effective? Are the dose–response relationships altered for different age groups?

Does sucrose have an interactive effect with other analgesic agents? What are optimal outcome measures where sucrose is used as analgesic (e.g. behavioural responses may show significant differences while cardiac/physiologic measures may not)? What are the interactions of sucrose therapy with additional non-pharmacological measures, such as non-nutritive sucking, rocking, kangaroo care and others? What do we know about sucrose metabolism and efficacy at the extremes of illness and prematurity? What are the long-term consequences of sucrose in relation to clinical, behavioural and neurodevelopmental outcomes of neonates and infants?

Research considerations related to analgesic drug delivery

Drug formulations

The rapid developmental changes occurring in preterm and term neonates and older infants significantly alter the gut sensitivity, fragility, bioavailability, disposition, metabolism and elimination of analgesic drugs. There are limited data on the effects of development on these processes during infancy. Analgesics are available in a variety of dosage forms (including enteral, parenteral, transcutaneous, transmucosal and intrapulmonary formulations). There is a need to identify and develop age-appropriate analgesic formulations and safe additives (American Academy of Pediatrics 1985, 1997):

- Oral formulations: There are few studies in infants regarding the rate and extent to which absorption is affected by high intragastric pH (>4) and developmental changes in intraluminal pH. Data are required on the influence of immature biliary function on the solubility of lipophilic agents, and effects of low CYP1A1 activity on drug metabolism (Suchy et al. 1981, Stahlberg et al. 1988). Oral formulations must be tested for stability, allow accurate dosing without requiring multiple dilutions or compounding procedures, and give due consideration to the restrictions of fluid volume in preterm neonates.

- Topical formulations: Immature development of the epidermis in preterm neonates is associated with high skin permeability to lipophilic drugs such as diamorphine (Barrett et al. 1993), but low permeability to other less lipophilic drugs (e.g. lidocaine (Barker and Rutter 1995)). Skin permeability does not appear to alter the clinical toxicity of EMLA cream (Gourrier et al. 1995, Stevens et al. 1999). The full potential for the use of topical formulations has not been exploited in infants, preterm and term neonates (Fitzgerald et al. 1989, Barrett and Rutter 1994, Southam 1995, Larsson et al. 1996, Barr 1999, Paut et al. 2000).

- Intravenous formulations: Immature drug metabolism (delayed glucuronidation or oxidation via the cytochrome P450 pathway) and decreased renal function (low glomelular filtration rate) may lead to cumulative increases in plasma concentrations, poor drug elimination, and increased drug toxicity in infancy (Barrett et al. 1996, Alcorn and McNamara 2002a, 2002b). The effects and stability of additive agents (e.g. propylene glycol, alcohol, sodium benzoate) in the vehicle for intravenous drugs also need to be considered. Drug concentration in the formulations used for neonates and infants must allow individualized dosing, since the dilution of higher-strength formulations may result in loss of stability, dosage errors, fluid volume overload and increased pharmacy costs.

- Intramuscular and subcutaneous formulations: Use of these routes for drug dosing causes acute pain and is limited by the decreased muscle mass and the delicate skin of neonates and infants. The intramuscular and subcutaneous routes of administration should be avoided except in extreme circumstances.

- Rectal formulations: A decreased and variable absorption of rectal acetaminophen in neonates (term, preterm, older infants) was noted in multiple studies (Hopkins et al. 1990, Birmingham et al. 1997, Lin et al. 1997, van Lingen et al. 1999a, 1999b, Bremerich et al. 2001). Rectal formulations of lipophobic drugs are unlikely to provide therapeutic drug levels for analgesia in infants; however, limited information is available for lipophilic drugs.

Local/topical drug delivery

Pain receptors are located in the dermis, therefore, topical analgesia requires absorption or infiltration across the epidermis. The main barrier to transdermal absorption of drugs is the stratum corneum, which is traversed by lowering the melting point of drugs (e.g.

EMLA) or binding to a lipophilic vehicle (e.g. LMX.4). Future techniques for non-invasive drug delivery in neonates and infants may include:

- Laser drug delivery: Ablation of the stratum corneum with a pulsed Er:Yag laser (2.94 mm) (Flock et al. 1997) allows the rapid penetration of local anaesthetics such as lidocaine or EMLA to areas of treated skin, providing topical analgesia (in <1 minute). Diffusion studies showed a dramatic increase in skin permeation rates of lidocaine and were effective in reducing the pain from lancet pinprick in adult volunteers (Koh et al. 1998). A similar laser has been shown to be a suitable and safer replacement for conventional lancets for drawing capillary blood for use in microanalysis (Marchitto et al. 1998).
- Iontophoretic drug delivery: Iontophoresis has been used for 30 years, using an electrical current to transfer charged local anaesthetics through the epidermis to the dermal nociceptors. Local anaesthetics mixed with a vasoconstrictor are applied to the active negative electrode and the positive electrode is placed on another part of the body (Zempsky et al. 1998).
- Injection devices: Initial studies showed that the use of a spring-loaded lance reduced the duration of neonatal distress resulting from heel pricks (McIntosh et al. 1994). Other devices were found to be superior with fewer repeat procedures than heel puncture for blood sampling (Barker et al. 1994). Novel injection devices utilizing compressed gases or spring-loaded pistons can deliver local anaesthetics at high velocity through a narrow orifice (Dermal Powderject (PowderJect Technologies, Inc., Fremont, CA), Biojector 2000® (Bioject, Inc., Portland, OR), Medi-Ject system (Medi-Ject Corporation, Minneapolis, MN)), providing drug delivery localized to a small area of skin.
- Biodegradable polymer microspheres: Current formulations of local anaesthetic drugs cause sodium channel blockade for short periods of time. Encapsulating local anaesthetics into biodegradable polymer microspheres or matrices may prolong analgesia and diminish systemic toxicity (Malinovsky et al. 1995). By increasing the molecular weight of a lidocaine-containing co-polymer paste, it was possible to obtain local anaesthetic action that lasts for 12, 24, 48, 72 or 120 hours (Sato et al. 1995). Newer formulations can develop techniques for prolonged blockade of peripheral nerves or sympathetic ganglia, which may be utilized for the management of

postoperative pain, sympathetically maintained pain or other types of chronic pain. Incorporating drugs such as fentanyl or morphine into these polymers may allow us to achieve prolonged epidural or regional anaesthesia without motor blockade.

Systemic drug delivery

Systemic analgesia can be achieved using various routes of administration in neonates and infants, most of which are invasive or aversive. Alternate methods using non-invasive means to deliver systemic analgesia or sedation may include:

- Iontophoresis system: Iontophoretic delivery of 25 or 40 µg of fentanyl (Southam 1995) has been developed into a self-contained adhesive patch that is easy to use, activated by pushing a button on the patch. The device delivers fentanyl analgesia non-invasively through the skin over a period of 10 minutes, and was safe and effective for adults undergoing surgery (Brown et al. 1998, Moodie et al. 1998). Further innovations may broaden the use of this device for providing fentanyl analgesia to neonates or infants undergoing surgical or other invasive procedures.
- Intratracheal delivery: A non-invasive method of drug delivery for ventilated neonates and infants with limited venous access includes intratracheal administration of fentanyl or other analgesics. Rabbits randomized to receive intratracheal or intravenous fentanyl showed no differences in pharmacokinetic parameters, indicating good absorption through the pulmonary parenchyma (Irazuzta et al. 1996, Cohen and Dawson 2002). Given these encouraging results, future studies should investigate similar approaches to drug delivery in preterm or term neonates or older infants.
- Injection devices: As described above, various injection devices use compressed gases to propel high-velocity medication in the dermis, subcutaneous tissue or muscle. These devices can be used to deliver preoperative medications or systemic analgesics to neonates and infants in a variety of settings, resulting in a faster onset of analgesic or sedative effects (Schmitz et al. 1998).
- Microdialysis: Preliminary animal studies have shown that microdialysis perfusion is a powerful technique for transdermal drug delivery (Ault et al. 1992). Future studies may allow us to administer analgesia into the epidural space or directly to the brain using strategically placed microdialysis probes (Quan and Blatteis 1989). Several factors determine the uptake of these drugs, including the

rate of perfusion, surface area of the semipermeable membrane, the molecular size, protein binding and physicochemical properties of the drug, and enzymatic degradation at the site of delivery.

Comparative studies

Previous analgesic trials including neonates or infants have commonly compared one analgesic agent against a placebo control and very few comparative studies have been published (e.g. comparing morphine with fentanyl (Ionides et al. 1994, Lejus et al. 1994, Franck et al. 1998, Saarenmaa et al. 1999), or morphine with diamorphine (Wood et al. 1998), or various interventions for circumcision or heelsticks). Future comparative studies should evaluate:

- Methods for local/topical analgesia: Comparison of topical preparations for procedural pain are required in preterm neonates, term neonates and older infants (e.g. comparing EMLA vs. amethocaine, LMX.4 vs. amethocaine, EMLA vs. lidocaine, or other drugs).
- Regional analgesic techniques: Although used infrequently for neonates or older infants these techniques can relieve the pain caused by various invasive procedures. Future studies should compare the efficacy and safety of different drugs (lidocaine, bupivacaine, ropivacaine) or drug combinations with clonidine (Constant et al. 1998, Luz et al. 1999), ketorolac, fentanyl (Porter et al. 1998), morphine or naloxone in neonates and infants.
- Systemic analgesia approaches: Studies comparing the efficacy and safety of fentanyl vs. alfentanil, morphine vs. fentanyl, ketamine vs. morphine or fentanyl, remifentanil vs. alfentanil, and other drug combinations. Optimal dosing regimens for long-acting and short-acting systemic analgesics, or combinations of analgesic and sedative drugs need to be developed, specifically for preterm neonates, term neonates and older infants.

Starting from a nascent field 20 years ago, remarkable strides have been made in the development of analgesic approaches for neonates and infants. While much of this knowledge has been applied to improve the clinical care of infants, there remains a significant gap between current knowledge and medical practice. This gap is partly related to inadequate evidence that can be derived from methodologically sound randomized controlled trials, but is also related to professional attitudes that discount the importance of pain and maintain a resolute adherence to traditional ways of providing care to infants and newborns. More research on pain management approaches would be essential, but not sufficient for bringing about the required changes in clinical practice. In this regard, the roles of social, economic and professional factors cannot be over-emphasized for changing practice, as discussed in the section below.

THE SOCIAL CONTEXT

Major research issues that derive from the social context of infant and neonatal pain are of critical importance in expanding our understanding of pain in the infant and neonate. Much of this research will require recruitment of a broader range of scientists than are currently involved in pain research on infants and neonates. Sociologists, marketers, anthropologists, economists, social psychologists and health systems researchers will be needed to contribute appropriate skills to the mix of researchers that currently consists primarily of nurses, physicians and psychologists.

Social factors

A more detailed examination of the social factors that permit the continuation of inadequate pain management in infants and neonates while they are being medically cared for is needed. This research will require sophisticated techniques that examine practices at the local, regional and national levels. Both individual decision making and group practices such as the adoption of national, disciplinary or local practice guidelines should be investigated.

The wide variation in care and patient outcomes in pain provides an important resource for research on infant and neonatal pain measurement, management and prevention in clinical settings. How do centres with better outcomes differ from those with less than optimum outcomes? Are there other variation parameters such as time of day, patient load and staffing levels that influence outcomes?

Finally, we need research on the processes leading to infant and neonatal research. What prompts budding researchers to enter this area? Why have some environments fostered this area of research? Is there a need for national and international networks in neonatal and infant pain? What can sustain such collaborative research networks?

Leadership and marketing

Detailed examination of the development of empathy and desensitization to infant pain in adult caregivers might help explain individual differences in caregiving. Similarly, leadership in advancing better pain management in clinical settings deserves closer scrutiny to determine the characteristics of effective leadership in this area.

Marketing has driven many aspects of our society but has not been used in advancing the agenda of better pain management in infants and neonates. Investigation of the use of pain management in infants and neonates as a marketing strategy in locations where health centres compete for patients is warranted. In addition, research on parental consumer preferences using techniques such as discrete choice modelling (Train 2003) could be used to inform the development of more consumer-oriented, pain-sensitive programmes. Similar studies could be undertaken with professionals to determine what types of approaches would be acceptable and effective for professionals. Other marketing research might help in determining the most effective way to change attitudes and behaviour in infant and neonatal pain.

Knowledge transfer

The methods of knowledge transfer in infant and neonatal pain management by nurses, physicians and other health professionals, especially the sustainability of knowledge transfer, must be better understood. What factors determine if very promising methods such as audit and feedback are introduced and sustained? Can the electronic health record be used in prompting analgesic methods with each painful procedure? How does the culture of a unit change from permitting painful procedures without analgesia to seeing painful procedures without analgesia as unacceptable? How do legitimate scientific disagreements affect clinical knowledge transfer? Research has a major role in determining ways of constantly changing practice to reflect current scientific knowledge.

The development of ways to reduce pain during immunization has become more important with the increasing number of immunizations given to infants and young children. It has included many different strategies including topical analgesics (Halperin et al. 2002), distraction (Cohen 2002), sucrose, parental holding and oral stimulation. Parents consider the reduction of pain to be very important in infant and child immunization and report they would pay to reduce pain (Meyerhoff et al. 2001) but most infants receive no pain protection when they are immunized. Why is this so and what can be done to change it?

Role of the family

Research that investigates the important role of parents in advocating for pain management in neonates and infants is needed. What prompts a parent to advocate for better pain management for their infant? What prevents parents from advocating? What sustains advocacy over time? What is the role of professionals and professional associations in helping parents advocate for better pain management? Are there differences between advocacy efforts that succeed and those that fail?

The role of the family in pain management has just begun to be examined (Chapter 22) and differences among families in their views and behaviours about pain need to be delineated. Ethnic and socioeconomic factors have not been widely examined and may yield better understanding of infant and neonatal pain. The role of intergenerational teaching and learning and factors such as maternal depression in comfort strategies are needed.

Health economics

Economic research that determines the short-term and long-term costs of poorly managed infant and neonatal pain is needed. In addition, studies are required that compare different regimens for managing pain. As new drugs emerge and are approved by regulatory agencies, health centres will need to decide if the costs of these new drugs make them superior to the old standbys. How will we develop economic indices for reductions in pain and suffering in babies and in anxiety in parents? Can sophisticated but expensive drugs for pain be justified to the payers of the health system? How will drug companies be attracted to examining pain drugs for infants and neonates? How will we know if the influence of drug companies is appropriate in the prescribing of new drugs for pain?

The initiation of pain research on infants and neonates in developing countries (see Chapter 19) has opened up opportunities to examine social, economic and cultural factors in pain. Are the methods used in the developed world helpful in the developing world? What can we in the developed world learn from methods in the developing world?

Social research in infant and neonatal pain has been lacking in the past. The social processes underlying infant and neonatal pain are often ignored because it is difficult to see social differences from within a given society. However, well-designed research on the social context of pain will yield benefits to infants and neonates worldwide.

REFERENCES

Alcorn J, McNamara PJ. (2002a). Ontogeny of hepatic and renal systemic clearance pathways in infants: part I. Clin Pharmacokinet 41: 959–998.

Alcorn J, McNamara PJ. (2002b). Ontogeny of hepatic and renal systemic clearance pathways in infants: part II. Clin Pharmacokinet 41: 1077–1094.

Als H, Lawhon G, Duffy FH, et al. (1994). Individualized developmental care for the very low-birth-weight preterm infant. Medical and neurofunctional effects. JAMA 272: 853–858.

American Academy of Pediatrics Committee on Drugs. (1985). "Inactive" ingredients in pharmaceutical products. Pediatrics 76: 635–643.

American Academy of Pediatrics Committee on Drugs. (1997). "Inactive" ingredients in pharmaceutical products: Update. Pediatrics 99: 268–278.

Anand KJS. (1997). Long-term effects of pain in neonates and infants. In: Jensen TS, Wiesenfeld-Hallin Z (eds) Proceedings of the 8th World Congress on Pain, Vol. 8. IASP Press, Seattle, pp. 881–892.

Anand KJS, Soriano SG. (2004). Anesthetic agents and the immature brain: are these toxic or therapeutic agents? Anesthesiology 101: 527–530.

Anand KJS, Hall RW, Desai NS, et al. (2004). Effects of pre-emptive morphine analgesia in ventilated preterm neonates: Primary outcomes from the NEOPAIN trial. Lancet 363: 1673–1682.

Anand KJS, Aranda JV, Berde CB, et al. (2005a). Analgesia for neonates: Study design and ethical issues. Clin Ther 27: 814–843.

Anand KJS, Johnston CC, Oberlander T, et al. (2005b). Analgesia and local anesthesia during invasive procedures in the neonate. Clin Ther 27: 844–876.

Ault JM, Lunte CE, Meltzer NM, et al. (1992). Microdialysis sampling for the investigation of dermal drug transport. Pharm Res 9: 1256–1261.

Barker DP, Rutter N. (1995). Lignocaine ointment and local anaesthesia in preterm infants. Arch Dis Child Fetal Neonatal Ed 72: F203–204.

Barker DP, Latty BW, Rutter N. (1994). Heel blood sampling in preterm infants: which technique? Arch Dis Child Fetal Neonatal Ed 71: F206–F208.

Barr GA. (1999). Antinociceptive effects of locally administered morphine in infant rats. Pain 81: 155–161.

Barrett DA, Rutter N. (1994). Transdermal delivery and the premature neonate. Crit Rev Ther Drug Carrier Sys 11: 1–30.

Barrett DA, Rutter N, Davis SS. (1993). An in vitro study of diamorphine permeation through premature human neonatal skin. Pharm Res 10: 583–587.

Barrett DA, Barker DP, Rutter N, et al. (1996). Morphine, morphine-6-glucuronide and morphine-3-glucuronide pharmacokinetics in newborn infants receiving diamorphine infusions. Br J Clin Pharmacol 41: 531–537.

Berde C. (2004). Local anesthetics in infants and children: an update. Paediatr Anaesth 14: 387–393.

Birmingham PK, Tobin MJ, Henthorn TK, et al. (1997). Twenty-four-hour pharmacokinetics of rectal acetaminophen in children: an old drug with new recommendations. Anesthesiology 87: 244–252.

Blass EM. (1997). Interactions between contact and chemosensory mechanisms in pain modulation in 10-day-old rats. Behav Neurosci 111: 147–154.

Blass EM, Shah A. (1995). Pain-reducing properties of sucrose in human new-borns. Chem Senses 20: 29–35.

Blass EM, Watt LB. (1999). Suckling- and sucrose-induced analgesia in human newborns. Pain 83: 611–623.

Bond C, LaForge KS, Tian M, et al. (1998). Single-nucleotide polymorphism in the human mu opioid receptor gene alters beta-endorphin binding and activity: possible implications for opiate addiction. Proc Natl Acad Sci USA 95: 9608–9613.

Bonica JJ. (1953). The management of pain of cancer. J Mich State Med Soc 52: 284–290.

Bremerich DH, Neidhart G, Heimann K, et al. (2001). Prophylactically administered rectal acetaminophen does not reduce postoperative opioid requirements in infants and small children undergoing elective cleft palate repair. Anesth Analg 93: 1626–1627.

Brown CR, Moodie JE, Bisley EJ. (1998). Safety and efficacy of Transfenta in the treatment of postoperative pain: A double blind, single center, placebo-controlled trial. Proceedings of the 17th Annual Scientific Meeting, American Pain Society, San Diego, Nov. 5–8.

Bucher HU, Moser T, von Siebenthal K, et al. (1995). Sucrose reduces pain reaction to heel lancing in preterm infants: a placebo-controlled, randomized and masked study. Pediatr Res 38: 332–335.

Camu F, Van de Velde A, Vanlersberghe C. (2001). Nonsteroidal anti-inflammatory drugs and paracetamol in children, Acta Anaesthesiol Belg 52: 13–20.

Cohen LL. (2002). Reducing infant immunization distress through distraction. Health Psychol 21: 207–211.

Cohen SP, Dawson TC. (2002). Nebulized morphine as a treatment for dyspnea in a child with cystic fibrosis. Pediatrics 10: e38.

Constant I, Gall O, Gouyet L, et al. (1998). Addition of clonidine or fentanyl to local anaesthetics prolongs the duration of surgical analgesia after single shot caudal block in children. Br J Anaesth 80: 294–298.

Debillon T, Zupan V, Ravault N, et al. (2001). Development and initial validation of the EDIN scale, a new tool for assessing prolonged pain in preterm infants Arch Dis Child 85: F36–F40.

Dutta S. (1999). Use of eutectic mixture of local anesthetics in children. Indian J Pediatr 66: 707–715.

Duhn L, Medves J (2004). A systematic integrative review of infant pain assessment tools. Adv Neonatal Care 4: 126–140.

Evans WE, McLeod HL. (2003). Pharmacogenomics – drug disposition, drug targets, and side effects. New Engl J Med 348: 538–549.

Evans WE, Relling MV. (1999). Pharmacogenomics: translating functional genomics into rational therapeutics. Science 286: 487–491.

Fitzgerald M, Millard C, McIntosh N. (1989). Cutaneous hypersensitivity following peripheral tissue damage in newborn infants and its reversal with topical anaesthesia. Pain 39: 31–36.

Flock ST, Lehman P, Franz T, et al. (1997). Transdermal drug delivery with a Transmedica Er:YAG laser device. TRANSMEDICA Inc, Little Rock, AR. Online. Available: http://www.transmedicainc.com

Foss JF. (2001). A review of the potential role of methylnaltrexone in opioid bowel dysfunction. Am J Surg 182: 19S–26S.

Franck LS, Vilardi J, Durand D, et al. (1998). Opioid withdrawal in neonates after continuous infusions of morphine or fentanyl during extracorporeal membrane oxygenation. Am J Crit Care 7: 364–369.

Geyer J, Ellsbury D, Kleiber C, et al. (2002). An evidence-based multidisciplinary protocol for neonatal circumcision pain management, J Obstet Gynecol Neonatal Nurs 31: 403–410.

Gourrier E, Karoubi P, el Hanache A, et al. (1995). Utilisation de la creme EMLA chez le nouveau-ne a terme et premature. Etude d'efficacite et de tolerance. Arch Pediatr 2: 1041–1046.

Halperin BA, Halperin SA, McGrath P, et al. (2002). Use of lidocaine-prilocaine patch to decrease intramuscular injection pain does not adversely affect the antibody response to diphtheria-tetanus acellular pertussis-inactivated poliovirus-*Haemophilus influenzae* type b conjugate and hepatitis B vaccines in infants from birth to six months of age. Pediatr Infect Dis J 21: 399–405.

Hollt V. (2002). A polymorphism (A118G) in the mu-opioid receptor gene affects the response to morphine-6-glucuronide in humans. Pharmacogenetics 12: 1–2.

Hopkins CS, Underhill S, Booker PD. (1990). Pharmacokinetics of paracetamol after cardiac surgery. Arch Dis Child 65: 971–976.

Howard CR, Howard FM, Weitzman ML. (1994). Acetaminophen analgesia in neonatal circumcision: the effect on pain. Pediatrics 93: 641–646.

Hummel P, Puchalski M, Creech S, et al. (2003). N-PASS: Neonatal pain, agitation and sedation scale – reliability and validity. Pediatric Academic Societies Annual Meeting, Seattle, Washington (Abstract).

Hunt A, Joel S, Dick G, et al. (1999). Population pharmacokinetics of oral morphine and its glucuronides in children receiving morphine as immediate-release liquid or sustained-release tablets for cancer pain. J Pediatr 135: 47–55.

Ionides SP, Weiss MG, Angelopoulos M, et al. (1994). Plasma beta-endorphin concentrations and analgesia-muscle relaxation in the newborn infant supported by mechanical ventilation. J Pediatr 125: 113–116.

Irazuzta JE, Ahmed U, Gancayco A, et al. (1996). Intratracheal administration of fentanyl: Pharmacokinetics and local

effects. Intensive Care Med 22: 129–133.

Jovey RD, Ennis J, Gardner-Nix J, et al. (2003). Use of opioid analgesics for the treatment of chronic non-cancer pain: a consensus statement and guidelines from the Canadian Pain Society, 2002. Pain Res Manag 8(Suppl A): 3–28.

Koh JL, Harrison D, Flock ST, et al. (1998). Local anesthesia by topical application of lidocaine after stratum corneum ablation with 2.94 micrometer Er:Yag laser radiant energy. Proceedings of the 17th Annual Scientific Meeting, American Pain Society, San Diego, Nov. 5–8.

Kokki H. (2003). Nonsteroidal anti-inflammatory drugs for postoperative pain: a focus on children. Paediatr Drugs 5: 103–123.

Laptook AR, O'Shea TM, Shankaran S, et al, for the NICHD Neonatal Network. (2005). Adverse neuro-developmental outcomes among extremely low birth weight infants with a normal head ultrasound: Prevalence and antecedents. Pediatrics 115: 673–680.

Larsson BA, Norman M, Bjerring P, et al. (1996). Regional variations in skin perfusion and skin thickness may contribute to varying efficacy of topical, local anaesthetics in neonates. Paediatr Anaesth 6: 107–110.

Lejus C, Roussiere G, Testa S, et al. (1994). Postoperative extradural analgesia in children: comparison of morphine with fentanyl. Br J Anaesth 72: 156–159.

Lin YC, Sussman HH, Benitz WE. (1997). Plasma concentrations after rectal administration of acetaminophen in preterm neonates. Paediatr Anaesth 7: 457–459.

Litalien C, Jacqz-Aigrain E. (2001). Risks and benefits of nonsteroidal anti-inflammatory drugs in children: a comparison with paracetamol. Paediatr Drugs 3: 817–858.

Liu SS, Hodgson PS, Carpenter RL, et al. (2001). ADL 8-2698, a trans-3,4-dimethyl-4-(3-hydroxyphenyl) piperidine, prevents gastrointestinal effects of intravenous morphine without affecting analgesia. Clin Pharmacol Ther 69: 66–71.

Lotsch J, Skarke C, Grosch S, et al. (2002). The polymorphism A118G of the human mu-opioid receptor gene decreases the pupil constrictory effect of morphine-6-glucuronide but not that of morphine. Pharmacogenetics 12: 3–9.

Luz G, Innerhofer P, Oswald E, et al. (1999). Comparison of clonidine 1 microgram kg^{-1} with morphine 30 micrograms kg^{-1} for post-operative caudal analgesia in children. Eur J Anaesthesiol 16: 42–46.

Malinovsky JM, Bernard JM, Le Corre P, et al. (1995). Motor and blood pressure effects of epidural sustained-release bupivacaine from polymer microspheres: a dose-response study in rabbits. Anesth Analg 81: 519–524.

Marchitto KS, Perkins LA, Martin R, et al. (1998). Laser lancet and capillary blood microanalysis. TRANSMEDICA Inc, Little Rock, AR. Online. Available: http://www.transmedicainc.com

McIntosh N, van Veen L, Brameyer H. (1994). Alleviation of the pain of heel prick in preterm infants. Arch Dis Child Fetal Neonatal Ed 70: F177–F181.

Meyerhoff AS, Weniger BG, Jacobs RJ. (2001). Economic value to parents of reducing the pain and emotional distress of childhood vaccine injections. Pediatr Infect Dis J 20(11 Suppl): S57–62.

Moodie JE, Brown CR, Bisley EJ, et al. (1998). Efficacy and safety of Transfenta in the management of postoperative pain on days 1, 2, and 3 after surgery. Proceedings of the 17th Annual Scientific Meeting, American Pain Society, San Diego, Nov. 5–8.

Morris JL, Rosen DA, Rosen KR. (2003). Nonsteroidal anti-inflammatory agents in neonates. Paediatr Drugs 5: 385–405.

Ng PC, So KW, Fok TF, et al. (1996). Fatal haemorrhagic gastritis associated with oral sulindac treatment for patent ductus arteriosus. Acta Paediatr 85: 884–886.

Ng PC, So KW, Fok TF, et al. (1997). Comparing sulindac with indomethacin for closure of ductus arteriosus in preterm infants. J Paediatr Child Health 33: 324–328.

Paut O, Camboulives J, Viard L, et al. (2000). Pharmacokinetics of transdermal fentanyl in the peri-operative period in young children. Anesthesia 55: 1202–1207.

Porter J, Bonello E, Reynolds F. (1998). Effect of epidural fentanyl on neonatal respiration. Anesthesiology 89: 79–85.

Quan N, Blatteis CM. (1989). Microdialysis: a system for localized drug delivery into the brain. Brain Res Bull 22: 621–625.

Saarenmaa E, Huttunen P, Leppaluoto J, et al. (1999). Advantages of fentanyl over morphine in analgesia for ventilated newborn infants after birth: a randomized trial. J Pediatr 134: 144–150.

Sato S, Baba Y, Tajima K, et al. (1995). Prolongation of epidural anesthesia in the rabbit with the use of a biodegradable copolymer paste containing lidocaine. Anesth Analg 80: 97–101.

Schmidt WK. (2001). Alvimopan* (ADL 8-2698) is a novel peripheral opioid antagonist. Am J Surg 182: 27S–38S.

Schmitz ML, Fanurik D, Harrison RD, et al. (1998). A comparison of midazolam premedication of pediatric patients by the oral route or subcutaneous needleless injection. Proceedings of the Annual Spring Meeting, Society for Pediatric Anesthesia, Phoenix, AZ, February 1998.

Shah V, Taddio A, Ohlsson A. (1998). Randomised controlled trial of paracetamol for heel prick pain in neonates. Arch Dis Child Fetal Neonatal Ed 79: F209–211.

Simons SHP, van Dijk M, van Lingen RA, et al. (2003). Routine morphine infusion in preterm newborns who received ventilatory support: A randomized controlled trial. JAMA 290: 2419–2427.

Simons SHP, van der Werf M, van der Marel CD, et al. (2004). Pharmacogenetics of morphine in neonates and infants: analyses of 2 single nucleotide polymorphisms. Pediatr Res 55: A1566.

Soriano SG, Anand KJS, Rovnaghi CR, et al. (2005). Of mice and men: Should we extrapolate rodent experimental data to the care of human neonates? Anesthesiology 102: 866–869.

Southam MA. (1995). Transdermal fentanyl therapy: system design, pharmacokinetics and efficacy. Anticancer Drugs 6: 29–34.

Spencer DM, Miller KA, O'Quin M, et al. (1992). Dorsal penile nerve block in neonatal circumcision: chloroprocaine versus lidocaine. Am J Perinatol 9: 214–218.

Stahlberg MR, Hietanen E, Maki M. (1988). Mucosal biotransformation rates in the small intestine of children. Gut 29: 1058–1063.

Stevens B, Johnston C, Taddio A, et al. (1999). Management of pain from heel lance with lidocaine-prilocaine (EMLA) cream: is it safe and efficacious in preterm infants? J Develop Behav Pediatr 20: 216–221.

Stevens B, Yamada J, Ohlsson A. (2004). Sucrose for analgesia in newborn infants undergoing painful procedures, The Cochrane Database Syst Rev Issue 3 CD001069.

Suchy FJ, Balistreri WF, Heubi JE, et al. (1981). Physiologic cholestasis: elevation of the primary serum bile acid concentrations in normal infants. Gastroenterology 80: 1037–1041.

Swart E, Zuideveld K, de Jongh J, et al. (2004). Comparative population pharmacokinetics of lorazepam and midazolam during long-term continuous infusion in critically ill patients. Br J Clin Pharmacol 57: 135–145.

Taddio A, Pollock N, Gilbert-MacLeod C, et al. (2000). Combined analgesia and local anesthesia to minimize pain during circumcision, Arch Pediatr Adolesc Med 154: 620–623.

Taguchi A, Sharma N, Saleem RM, et al. (2001). Selective postoperative inhibition of gastrointestinal opioid receptors. New Engl J Med 345: 935–940.

Tobias JD, Mateo C, Ferrer MJ, et al. (1997). Intrathecal morphine for postoperative analgesia following repair of frontal encephaloceles in children: comparison with intermittent, on-demand dosing of nalbuphine. J Clin Anesth 9: 280–284.

Train K. (2003). Discrete choice methods with simulation. Cambridge University Press, Cambridge, UK.

van Lingen RA, Deinum HT, Quak CM, et al. (1999a). Multiple-dose pharmacokinetics of rectally administered acetaminophen in term infants. Clin Pharmacol Ther 66: 509–515.

van Lingen RA, Deinum JT, Quak JM,

et al. (1999b). Pharmacokinetics and metabolism of rectally administered paracetamol in preterm neonates. Arch Dis Child Fetal Neonatal Ed 80: F59–63.

Warnock R, Lander J. (2004). Foundations of knowledge about neonatal pain. J Pain Symptom Manage 27: 170–179.

Weinshilboum R. (2003). Inheritance and drug response. New Engl J Med 348: 529–537.

Wood CM, Rushforth JA, Hartley R, et al. (1998). Randomised double blind trial of morphine versus diamorphine for sedation of preterm neonates. Arch Dis Child Fetal Neonatal Ed 79: F34–39.

Yiangou Y, Birch R, Sangameswaran L, et al. (2000). SNS/PN3 and SNS2/NaN sodium channel-like immunoreactivity in human adult and neonate injured sensory nerves. FEBS Lett 467: 249–252.

Yuan CS, Foss JF. (2000). Oral methylnaltrexone for opioid-induced constipation. JAMA 284: 1383–1384.

Yuan CS, Foss JF, Osinski J, et al. (1997). The safety and efficacy of oral methylnaltrexone in preventing morphine-induced delay in oral-cecal transit time. Clin Pharmacol Ther 61: 467–475.

Yuan CS, Foss JF, O'Connor M, et al. (2000). Methylnaltrexone for reversal of constipation due to chronic methadone use: a randomized controlled trial. JAMA 283: 367–372.

Yuan CS, Wei G, Foss JF, et al. (2002). Effects of subcutaneous methylnaltrexone on morphine-induced peripherally mediated side effects: a double-blind randomized placebo-controlled trial. J Pharmacol Exp Ther 300: 118–123.

Zempsky WT, Anand KJS, Sullivan KM, et al. (1998). Lidocaine iontophoresis for topical anesthesia before intravenous line placement in children. J Pediatr 132: 1061–1063.

Zubieta JK, Heitzeg MM, Smith YR, et al. (2003). COMT val158met genotype affects mu-opioid neurotransmitter responses to a pain stressor. Science 299: 1240–1243.

Index

Rostral ventromedial medulla (RVM),
    pain processing and, 27, 58
'Rule of ones', protein intolerance
    enteritis/colitis, 206
'Rule of threes', infant colic
    diagnosis/definition, 93

S

Sacral plexus, 169
Scale for Use in Newborns (SUN), 73t
Score for Neonatal Acute Physiology
    (SNAP-II), 84, 255
Score for Neonatal Acute Physiology
    Perinatal Extension (SNAPE-II),
    84
Sedation/sedatives
    assisted ventilation, 273–4
    ethical issues, 215
    opioids, 143, 148
    research, 303
    see also specific drugs
Seizures
    intravascular injection of local
        anaesthetics, 157
    opioid-induced, 149
Self-report pain measures, 69
Sensorial saturation, pain management,
    284–5
Sensory effects of neonatal pain *see*
    Hyperexcitability/sensitization
Sensory neurons
    central innervation, 13–14
    embryonic specification, 12
    opioid receptor expression, 17–18
    visceral afferents, 27
Sensory receptors
    fetal development, 192
    postnatal development, 13
    see also Nociceptors; *specific types*
Sensory transduction
    enteric nervous system, 203
    polymodal nociceptors, 13
Sex differences, analgesia and
    nociception, 50–1
Siblings
    attachment issues, 181
    neonates' contact with, pain response
        effects, 181–2
Signal transduction pathways
    enteric nervous system, 203
    pharmacogenetics/pharmacogenomics,
        106–9
    polymodal nociceptors, 13
Significant neurological injury (SNI),
    pain assessment, 84, 254–5
Simethicone, infant colic management,
    98
Single nucleotide polymorphisms
    (SNPs), 301, 302
Size models (pharmacological), 120–3
    allometric 3/4 model, 121–2, 121f,
        123, 123f
    body surface area and, 121
    comparison between models, 122–3,
        123f

linear, 120
linear per kilogram model, 122–3, 123f
surface area model, 122, 123f
weight and dose, 120
Skin injury and hypersensitivity, 3
    hyperinnervation and, 18–19, 60
Skin-to-skin care *see* Kangaroo care (KC)
Sleeping, co-bedding, 181–2
Social context, 5, 178–82, 219–34
    definition, 219
    health knowledge democratization,
        220–1
    NICU as, 220
    pain management influences, 223–30
        health professionals, 227–30
        pharmaceutical industry and, 222–3
    research issues, 308–9
    significant others, 178–82
        fathers, 180–1
        mothers, 178–9
        siblings, 181–2
    see also Cultural issues
Social costs (of neonatal pain), 276–7
Socially approved pain, 221–2
Sociocommunication Model of Infant
    Pain, 68, 291–2, 291f
Socioeconomic status (SES), maternal
    stress and, 51
Somatic afferents, medullary nuclei, 27,
    28
Somatic pain, long-term consequences,
    3, 48
Somatization, preterm *vs.* full-term
    infants, 20, 48
Somatosensory cortex
    development, 18, 35
    pain processing, 35–6
    primary (S1), 35
    secondary (S2), 35
Somatotopic maps
    cortical, development, 35
    dorsal horn development, 13
    'fractured', cerebellum, 37
    nerve injury effects, 19
Sound
    environmental context, 182–3
    fetal response to, 195
South Africa, 6–7
    burns management, 6, 269–70, 269t
    drug resource problems, 266
    HIV infection/AIDS, 6, 264–7
        cultural issues, 270
        see also HIV infection/AIDS
Spared nerve injury (SNI) model, 19
Spina bifida, vulnerable neonates, 253
Spinal afferents, enteric nervous system
    (ENS), 202–3
Spinal anaesthesia/analgesia
    adjuvant drugs, ketamine, 156
    risks, 157
Spinal cord
    development, 13–14
        dorsal horn *see* Dorsal horn
            development
        embryonic, 192

neurotransmitter receptor
    expression, 14, 16–17
    see also Pain pathway development
opioid receptors, 58
pain pathways *see* Spinal pain
    pathways
visceral afferents, 203
see also Dorsal horn
Spinal pain pathways
    brainstem neurons and, 27, 28
    development *see* Pain pathway
        development
    visceral organs, 203–4
Spinothalamic tract (STT), 32
    enteric nervous system, 203–4
Splanchnic innervation, visceral organs,
    202
Standards of care, 212
    changes associated, 225–7, 230–2
Stereoisomers
    ketamine, 131
    keterolac, 127
Strange Situation Paradigm, 289–90
Stress
    childbirth, 196–7
    mild neonatal, beneficial effects, 61
    neonatal intensive care unit, 45
        cortisol responses and, 48
        light-associated, 5, 182–3
        long-term consequences, 46
        noise-associated, 5, 182–3, 229
    parental, 229
    preterm infants, 51
    prenatal
        programming and, 197
        see also Fetal pain
    preterm infants, 48, 49, 50
        parental stress, 51
        *see also neonatal intensive care unit
            (above)*
    responses to *see* Stress response
Stress-induced analgesia (SIA), 28, 29,
    63, 63f
'Stress-inoculation', 61
Stress response
    acute, 61
    adult, 194
    analgesia due to, 28, 29, 63, 63f
    fetal, 194–5
    hypoalgesia and, 20
    learning and, 50
    long-term changes following neonatal
        pain, 48–9, 50, 61–4, 168, 208
        adult stress behaviours and, 62–3
        animal models, 61–4, 197
        hyperactive stress response, 61
        maternal factors, 51–2, 63–4
        opiate system changes, 62
        visceral pain, 62
    long-term changes following non-
        noxious stressors, 61–2
    neural substrates, 61
        endogenous opiates/receptors, 62
        HPA axis, 33, 48–9, 51, 61
        nucleus tractus solitarius and, 28